Medical Intelligence Unit

New Bacterial Vaccines

Ronald W. Ellis, Ph.D.
Shire Biologics Inc.
Northborough, Massachusetts, U.S.A.

Bernard R. Brodeur, Ph.D.
Unité de Recherche en Vaccinologie
Centre Hospitalier Universitaire de Québec
Québec, Canada

Landes Bioscience / Eurekah.com
Georgetown, Texas
U.S.A.

Kluwer Academic / Plenum Publishers
New York, New York
U.S.A.

New Bacterial Vaccines

Medical Intelligence Unit

Eurekah.com / Landes Bioscience
Kluwer Academic / Plenum Publishers

Printed in the U.S.A.

Kluwer Academic / Plenum Publishers, 233 Spring Street, New York, New York, U.S.A. 10013
http://www.wkap.nl/

Please address all inquiries to the Publishers:
Eurekah.com / Landes Bioscience, 810 South Church Street
Georgetown, Texas, U.S.A. 78626
Phone: 512/ 863 7762; FAX: 512/ 863 0081
www.Eurekah.com
www.landesbioscience.com

ISBN 0-306-47832-3

New Bacterial Vaccines edited by Ronald W. Ellis and Bernard R. Brodeur, Landes / Kluwer dual imprint / Landes series: Medical Intelligence Unit

Library of Congress Cataloging-in-Publication Data

New bacterial vaccines / [edited by] Ronald W. Ellis, Bernard R. Brodeur.
p. ; cm. -- (Medical intelligence unit)
Includes bibliographical references and index.
ISBN 0-306-47832-3
1. Bacterial vaccines.
[DNLM: 1. Bacterial Vaccines. 2. Drug Design. 3. Technology, Pharmaceutical. WC 200 B1318 2003] I. Ellis, Ronald W. II. Brodeur, Bernard R. III. Series.
QR189.5.B33B342 2003
615'.372--dc21

2003012218

To all the individuals over the last century who have devoted themselves to the field of vaccinology and, in so doing, have saved lives and enhanced the quality of life for innumerable people worldwide.

CONTENTS

Preface xv

1. **Genomics and Proteomics in Vaccine Design** 1
John L. Telford, Mariagrazia Pizza, Guido Grandi and Rino Rappuoli
A Brief History of Bacterial Vaccines 1
Genome Technologies in Vaccine Design 2
From Genome to Vaccine Design 4
Proteomics in Vaccine Design 7
Identification of Antigens Important for Infection 8
Future Prospects 9

2. **Universal Proteins As an Alternative Bacterial Vaccine Strategy** 12
Bernard R. Brodeur, Denis Martin, Stéphane Rioux, Nathalie Charland and Josée Hamel
Introduction 12
Meningococcal NspA Protein 15
Group B Streptococcal Sip Protein 19
Pneumococcal BVH Proteins 26
Conclusions 28

3. **DNA Vaccines** 30
John J. Donnelly
Summary 30
Elements of the Technology 30
Bacterial Vaccines 31
Results of Initial Clinical Studies 33
Adjuvants and Delivery Vehicles for DNA Vaccines 34
Conclusions 37

4. **Live, Attenuated *Salmonella* Vaccine Vectors** 45
Sims K. Kochi and Kevin P. Killeen
Introduction 45
Live, Attenuated *Salmonella* Vaccines and Vectors 46
Summary 57

5. **Mucosal Immunity** 63
Michael W. Russell
Introduction 63
Distinct Features of the Mucosal Immune System 65
Strategies and Routes of Mucosal Immunization 68
Selected Approaches to Mucosal Immunization 69
Selected Applications of Mucosal Immunization 73
The Future for Mucosal Immunization 74

6. **New Technologies for Bacterial Vaccines** **80**
Ronald W. Ellis
Introduction 80
Live Vaccines 83
Subunit/Inactivated Vaccines 84
DNA 88
Formulation of Antigens 88
Conclusion 90

7. ***Chlamydia trachomatis* and *Chlamydia pneumoniae* Vaccines** **93**
Svend Birkelund and Gunna Christiansen
Summary 93
Chlamydia Biology and Diseases 93
Diagnosis, Treatment and Prevention 94
Chlamydia Surface-Exposed Components 96
Humoral Immune Response to *C. trachomatis* 98
Mapping of Neutralizing Epitopes on MOMP with Mouse MAbs 99
Humoral Immune Response to *C. pneumoniae* 99
Cellular Immunity to *C. trachomatis*, T-Helper Cell Response 103
Cytotoxic T-Cell Response 103
Vaccines 103
Animal Vaccines and Vaccine Studies 104
Vaccine Development 104
Conclusion and Perspectives 105

8. ***Escherichia coli* Vaccines** **110**
Myron M. Levine and Michael S. Donnenberg
Summary 110
Introduction 110
Clinical Syndromes and Causative Agents 111
Vaccine Development Strategies and Experience with Vaccine Candidates 115

9. **A Vaccine for Gonorrhea** **128**
P. Frederick Sparling, Christopher E. Thomas and Weiyan Zhu
Summary 128
Introduction: Gonorrhea Is a Persistent Clinical Problem 128
Natural History of Infection 129
Surface Structures: Variability in Expression and Antigenicity 129
Key Surface Antigens and Their Roles in Pathogenesis 129
Stress Proteins 136
Lessons Learned about Expression of Gonococcal Antigens from Studies of Infection in Patients and Human Volunteers 137
Summary: Pathogenic Strategies Employed by Gonococci during Infection 139

21. **Typhoid Vaccines** **326**
Deborah House and Gordon Dougan
Introduction 326
Epidemiology 326
Licensed Typhoid Vaccines 327
New Typhoid Vaccines 331
The Future 333

22. **Vaccines against *Vibrio cholerae*** **339**
James D. Campbell and James B. Kaper
Overview 339
Immunobiology 340
Strategies for a Cholera Vaccine Based on Epidemiology and Immunobiology 341
Efforts to Date 342
The Future 345

Index **351**

17. **Vaccines for *Pseudomonas aeruginosa*** **260**
Gregory P. Priebe and Gerald B. Pier
Secreted Products: Exotoxin A, Alkaline Protease, Elastase 260
LPS 262
Mucoid Exopolysaccharide (MEP) 265
Outer Membrane Proteins (OMPs) 266
Flagella 267
Pili 268
Components of the Type III Secretion System 268
Other Aspects of Immunity to *P. aeruginosa* 269
Vaccine Approaches to Elicit Antibody-Mediated and Cell-Mediated Immunity 272
Considerations and Conclusions 273

18. ***Staphylococcus aureus* Vaccine** **283**
Jean C. Lee
Summary 283
Introduction 283
Capsular Polysaccharide (CP) 284
Poly-N-Acetyl Glucosamine (Polysaccharide Intercellular Adhesin) ... 288
Protein Vaccines 288
Toxoids 290
Conclusion 291

19. ***Streptococcus pneumoniae* Vaccines** **294**
James C. Paton and David E. Briles
Abstract 294
Introduction 294
Polysaccharide Vaccines 295
Polysaccharide-Protein Conjugate Vaccines 297
Purified Protein Vaccines 300
Combination Protein Vaccines 303
Mucosal Vaccination Strategies 304
DNA Vaccines 305
Concluding Remarks 305

20. **New Generation Tuberculosis Vaccines for Targeted Populations** **311**
Uli Fruth and Michael J. Brennan
Mycobacterial Pathogenesis 311
Host Response to Infection with *Mycobacterium tuberculosis* 312
The Problem of Persistent Infection with *M. tuberculosis* 313
Lessons Learned from BCG Vaccine 314
Improving the BCG Vaccine 315
Novel Vaccine Approaches 316
Preclinical Testing of New TB Vaccines 319
TB Vaccines for Targeted Populations 320
Progress Towards the Clinical Investigation of Novel TB Vaccines ... 320
Summary 321

13. **Lyme Disease Vaccine** 202
Janine Evans and Erol Fikrig
Epidemiology and Ecology 202
Bacteriology 203
Animal Models 205
Pathogenesis 205
Immunologic Response to the Spirochete 206
Immunization 207
Mode of Action 208
Human Trials 208
Additional Considerations 210
Future Vaccines 211
Note 212

14. ***Moraxella catarrhalis*** 217
Timothy F. Murphy
Introduction 217
Infections Caused by *Moraxella catarrhalis* 217
Epidemiology and Respiratory Tract Colonization 219
Immune Response to Infection 219
Animal Models 220
Vaccine Development 221
Future Directions 224

15. ***Neisseria meningitidis* Vaccines** 229
Carl E. Frasch and Margaret C. Bash
Summary 229
Introduction 229
Immunobiology of Meningococcal Infection 230
Strategies for New Vaccines 232
Meningococcal Conjugate Vaccines 232
Vaccines for Group B 236
Genomics As a Vaccine Approach 238
Prospects for the Next Five Years 239

16. **A Vaccine for Nontypable *Haemophilus influenzae*** 244
Allan W. Cripps and Jennelle M. Kyd
Summary 244
NTHI Infections and Disease 244
Vaccination Strategies for Nontypeable *Haemophilus influenzae* 248
Potential Vaccine Candidates 249
Conclusions and Future Directions 252

The Immune Response 140
Animal Models for Studying Vaccines 142
Possible Vaccine Candidates 142
Questions 143
Conclusions 145

10. Group A Streptococcus Vaccine Research: Historical Synopsis and New Insights 155
Sean D. Reid, Kimmo Virtaneva and James M. Musser
Group A *Streptococcus* Distribution, Disease Complexity, Resurgence and Impact 155
Disease in the United States and Other Western Countries 155
Resurgence of Invasive Disease 156
Replacement of GAS M Protein Serotype in Host Populations 157
GAS Disease in Developing Countries 157
Historical Account of Early GAS Vaccine Efforts 158
Protective Immunity by Type-Specific IgG 158
Nontype-Specific Protection and Mucosal Immunity 159
Additional GAS Vaccine Candidates 160
GAS Mediated Autoimmunity in Human Infection 163
Newly Described Extracellular Proteins and Antigens of GAS 163
Post Genomic Strategies to Study Host-Pathogen Interactions 165
Final Comments 167

11. Academic Pursuits of Vaccines against Group B *Streptococcus* 174
Lawrence C. Paoletti
Introduction 174
Ecological Niches of GBS 174
Epidemiology of GBS Disease 174
GBS Targets of Protective Immunity 176
Clinical Trials with GBS Vaccines 178
Target Populations to Receive GBS Vaccines 184
Future of GBS Vaccine Research and Implementation 185
Summary 186

12. Helicobacter pylori Vaccines 192
Gabriela Garcia and Jacques Pappo
Summary 192
Host Immune Program and Disease Pathogenesis 192
Raison D'être for Vaccination 193
Surrogate Models of Human Vaccine Efficacy 193
Vaccine Effector Pathways and Post-Immunization Gastritis 195
H. pylori Vaccine Targeting and Antigen Discovery 196
Clinical Trials 197

EDITORS

Ronald W. Ellis, Ph.D.
Shire Biologics Inc.
Northborough, Massachusetts, U.S.A.
rellis@ca.shire.com
Chapter 6

Bernard R. Brodeur, Ph.D.
Unité de Recherche en Vaccinologie
Centre Hospitalier Universitaire de Québec
Québec, Canada
Bernard.Brodeur@crchul.ulaval.ca
Chapter 2

CONTRIBUTORS

Margaret C. Bash
Laboratory of Bacterial Polysaccharides
Center for Biologics Evaluation and Research
Food and Drug Administration
Bethesda, Maryland, U.S.A.
Chapter 15

Svend Birkelund
Department of Medical Microbiology and Immunology
University of Aarhus
Denmark
Chapter 7

Michael J. Brennan
Senior Investigator
Laboratory of Mycobacterial Diseases
Center for Biologics Evaluation and Research
Food and Drug Administration
Bethesda, Maryland, U.S.A.
Brennan@CBER.FDA.GOV
Chapter 20

David E. Briles
Department of Microbiology
The University of Alabama at Birmingham
Birmingham, Alabama, U.S.A.
dbriles@uab.edu
Chapter 19

James D. Campbell
Center for Vaccine Development
Department of Pediatrics
University of Maryland School of Medicine
Baltimore, Maryland, U.S.A.
Chapter 22

Nathalie Charland
Unité de Recherche en Vaccinologie
Centre Hospitalier Universitaire de Québec
Québec, Canada
Chapter 2

Gunna Christiansen
Department of Medical Microbiology and Immunology
University of Aarhus
Denmark
Chapter 7

Allan W. Cripps
University of Canberra
Canberra, Australia
allan.cripps@canberra.edu.au
Chapter 16

John J. Donnelly
Immunology and Infectious Diseases
Chiron Research and Development
Chiron Corporation
Emeryville, California, U.S.A.
john_donnelly@chiron.com
Chapter 3

Michael S. Donnenberg
Division of Infectious Diseases
Department of Medicine
University of Maryland
School of Medicine
Baltimore, Maryland, U.S.A.
Chapter 8

Gordon Dougan
Centre for Molecular Microbiology
and Infection
Department of Biological Sciences
Imperial College of Science, Technology
and Medicine
London, England
Chapter 21

Janine Evans
Yale University
Section of Rheumatology
Department of Internal Medicine
New Haven, Connecticut, U.S.A.
Chapter 13

Erol Fikrig
Yale University
Epidemiology and Public Health
Section of Rheumatology
Department of Internal Medicine
New Haven, Connecticut, U.S.A.
erol.fikrig@yale.edu
Chapter 13

Carl E. Frasch
Laboratory of Bacterial Polysaccharides
Center for Biologics Evaluation
and Research
FDA
Bethesda, Maryland, U.S.A.
Chapter 15

Uli Fruth
Vaccines and Biologicals
World Health Organization
Geneva Switzerland
furthu@who.int
Chapter 20

Gabriela Garcia
AstraZeneca R&D Boston
Waltham, Massachusetts, U.S.A.
Chapter 12

Guido Grandi
Istituto Ricerche Immunobiologiche
Siena
Chiron S.r.l.
Siena, Italy
Chapter 1

Josée Hamel
Unité de Recherche en Vaccinologie
Centre Hospitalier
Universitaire de Québec
Québec, Canada
Chapter 2

Deborah House
Centre for Molecular Microbiology
and Infection
Department of Biological Sciences
Imperial College of Science, Technology
and Medicine
London, England
Chapter 21

James B. Kaper
Center for Vaccine Development
Department of Microbiology
and Immunology
University of Maryland School
of Medicine
Baltimore, Maryland, U.S.A.
Chapter 22

Kevin P. Killeen
AVANT Immunotherapeutics. Inc.
Needham, Massachusetts, U.S.A.
Chapter 4

Sims K. Kochi
AVANT Immunotherapeutics. Inc.
Needham, Massachusetts, U.S.A.
Chapter 4

Jennelle M. Kyd
University of Canberra
Canberra, Australia
jennelle.kyd@canberra.edu.au
Chapter 16

Jean C. Lee
Channing Laboratory
Department of Medicine
Brigham and Women's Hospital
and Harvard Medical School
Boston, Massachusetts, U.S.A.
jean.lee@channing.harvard.edu
Chapter 18

Myron M. Levine
Center for Vaccine Development
University of Maryland
School of Medicine
Baltimore, Maryland, U.S.A.
Chapter 8

Denis Martin
Unité de Recherche en Vaccinologie
Centre Hospitalier
Universitaire de Québec
Québec, Canada
Chapter 2

Timothy F. Murphy
Department of Medicine
and Microbiology
University of Buffalo, SUNY
Buffalo, New York, U.S.A.
murphyt@acsu.buffalo.edu
Chapter 14

James M. Musser
Laboratory of Human Bacterial
Pathogenesis
Rocky Mountain Laboratories
National Institute of Allergy
and Infectious Diseases
National Institutes of Health
Hamilton, Montana, U.S.A.
and Department of Pathology
Baylor College of Medicine
Houston, Texas, U.S.A.
Chapter 10

Lawrence C. Paoletti
Channing Laboratory
Department of Medicine
Brigham and Women's Hospital
Harvard Medical School
Boston, Massachusetts, U.S.A.
lpaoletti@channing.harvard.edu
Chapter 11

Jacques Pappo
AstraZeneca R&D Boston
Waltham, Massachusetts, U.S.A.
Chapter 12

James C. Paton
Department of Molecular Biosciences
Adelaide University
Adelaide, S.A.
Australia
james.paton@adelaide.edu.au
Chapter 19

Gerald B. Pier
Channing Laboratory
Department of Medicine
Brigham and Women's Hospital
Microbiology and Molecular Genetics
Harvard Medical School
Boston, Massachusetts, U.S.A.
gpier@channing.harvard.edu
Chapter 17

Mariagrazia Pizza
Istituto Ricerche Immunobiologiche
Siena
Chiron S.r.l.
Siena, Italy
Chapter 1

Gregory P. Priebe
Departments of Anesthesia (Medical/Surgical Intensive Care Unit) and Medicine (Division of Infectious Diseases), Children's Hospital Boston
and Channing Laboratory
Department of Medicine
Brigham and Women's Hospital
Harvard Medical School
Boston, Massachusetts, U.S.A.
gpriebe@rics.bwh.harvard.edu
Chapter 17

Rino Rappuoli
Istituto Ricerche Immunobiologiche
Siena
Chiron S.r.l.
Siena, Italy
rino_rappuoli@chiron.it
Chapter 1

Sean D. Reid
Department of Microbiology and Immunology
School of Medicine
Wake Forest University
Winston-Salem, North Carolina, U.S.A.
Chapter 10

Stéphane Rioux
Unité de Recherche en Vaccinologie
Centre Hospitalier
Universitaire de Québec
Québec, Canada
Chapter 2

Michael W. Russell
Departments of Microbiology & Immunology and of Oral Biology
Witebsky Center for Microbial Pathogenesis and Immunology
University at Buffalo
Buffalo, New York, U.S.A.
russellm@buffalo.edu
Chapter 5

P. Frederick Sparling
University of North Carolina
School of Medicine
Division of Infectious Disease
Chapel Hill, North Carolina, U.S.A.
Chapter 9

John L. Telford
Istituto Ricerche Immunobiologiche
Siena
Chiron S.r.l.
Siena, Italy
Chapter 1

Christopher E. Thomas
University of North Carolina
School of Medicine
Division of Infectious Disease
Chapel Hill, North Carolina, U.S.A.
Chapter 9

Kimmo Virtaneva
Laboratory of Human Bacterial Pathogenesis
Rocky Mountain Laboratories
National Institute of Allergy and Infectious Diseases
National Institutes of Health
Hamilton, Montana, U.S.A.
Chapter 10

Weiyan Zhu
University of North Carolina
School of Medicine
Division of Infectious Disease
Chapel Hill, North Carolina, U.S.A.
Chapter 9

PREFACE

Vaccines are one of the most highly cost-effective modalities in healthcare. It has been estimated that vaccination was responsible for over 10 years of the total increase in the average human lifespan worldwide during the 20th century, an increase second in impact only to that of clean water. There are over 10 million deaths annually worldwide as well as considerable morbidity, mostly among young children, that are attributable to infectious diseases. A very large number of these deaths could be prevented by increased use of existing vaccines, while the great majority of these deaths would be preventable by the future wide-scale use of effective new vaccines now being developed. The development of new vaccine technologies as well as the emergence of new mechanisms for the funding of vaccine development, purchase and distribution worldwide offer hope that the fruits of these technologies will reach an ever-increasing number of people.

There is an increasingly broad array of new technologies that are being applied to developing vaccines. Such technologies are based on breakthrough discoveries in the fields of immunology, biochemistry, molecular biology and related areas. The broad applications of such discoveries should result in the creation of many new vaccines that have not been feasible to date. Alternatively it should be possible to improve existing vaccines in terms of their safety and efficacy. There are ca. 40 new vaccines (not including competing versions of the same product) that were developed and introduced during the 20th century. It is noteworthy that about half of these new vaccines were introduced during the 1980s and 1990s, with many of these based on new technologies such as recombinant proteins and conjugates. Therefore, the development of new vaccine technologies offers yet further potential for considerably reducing mortality and morbidity from infectious diseases worldwide.

Almost all vaccines that have been approved for general use are directed toward the prevention of bacterial or viral diseases. There are many experimental vaccines for immunotherapeutic purposes and applications outside the field of infectious diseases, e.g., autoimmunity and cancer.

This book is focused upon unmet needs for bacterial vaccines. The increase in drug resistance among many bacterial species has increased the need for new bacterial vaccines. Moreover, an increased understanding of the immunobiology and molecular mechanisms of pathogenesis have helped to elucidate the type of immunity needed for protection as well as the most appropriate vaccine strategy for achieving such immunity.

The field of vaccine discovery has been rejuvenated by the application of new molecular technologies. In particular, genomics and proteomics have been applied to several bacterial genomes for discovering new vaccine antigens (Chapter 1). Classical antigen discovery has relied upon the physical or immunological identification of the most abundant bacterial surface proteins, and vaccines such as acellular pertussis and Lyme disease (Chapter 13) have employed such vaccine antigens and been developed successfully. However, the inherent nature of such discovery technologies has limited the number of available vaccine antigens. It has become straightforward to sequence complete bacterial genomes and annotate these sequences into genes for predicting the structure and potential surface-exposure of the encoded vaccine antigens. Other techniques enable the highly sensitive analysis of the expression of the complete genomic complement of proteins, either at the level of protein or mRNA. Through these technologies, novel antigens have been discovered for several bacteria, with the most extensive definition of new candidates being for *Neisseria meningitidis* vaccine antigens (Chapter 15). Indeed, the genomes of almost all pathogens described in the chapters of this book have been sequenced and annotated, thus providing for the definition of a plethora of new vaccine antigens. This new information will provide many opportunities for vaccinologists to investigate new antigens.

Proteins have been successfully developed as antigens for many vaccines. The protein antigens most versatile for vaccine development are those that are broadly conserved and expressed in all strains of a given species of bacteria (Chapter 2). Several technologies, including genomics and proteomics, have been applied to discovering such vaccine antigens. While the physical purification of the most abundant surface proteins has been a very commonly used and facile technique, the detection of novel proteins by immune sera offers a proven biological basis for antigen discovery. These and related techniques have resulted in the discovery of promising candidate vaccine antigens for diverse bacteria such as *Streptococcus agalactiae* (Chapter 11), *Neisseria meningitidis* (Chapter 15), and *Streptococcus pneumoniae* (Chapter 19).

The newest design for vaccines is DNA vaccines (Chapter 3). The technical basis for this approach is that the gene for a vaccine antigen is cloned in an expression vector that, upon injection into the host, is taken up by cells, transcribed and translated into the vaccine antigen. This form of immunological presentation elicits specific antibodies and also stimulates cell-mediated immune responses, e.g., cytotoxic T lymphocytes, better than do most subunit vaccines such as proteins or polysaccharide conjugate vaccines. However, DNA vaccines have not yet shown consistent success at stimulating levels of antibodies as high as do subunit vaccines. DNA vaccines have been applied most extensively to viral vaccines but also are being developed for bacterial vaccines. Enhancements of DNA vaccine potency, such as DNA-specific formulations and use of nonreplicating viral vectors, offer the opportunity for further augmentation of immune responses.

Live vaccines are attenuated bacterial strains that are able to replicate in the host, thereby triggering a potentially broader immune response than that stimulated by a subunit or DNA vaccine. Live bacteria have been developed into vectors that express "foreign" vaccine antigens of other bacteria. The most extensively developed live vectors are *Salmonella* vectors (Chapter 4). Such vaccines offer the advantage of presenting antigens in a way similar to how they are presented during an actual bacterial infection. However, such vaccines have been technically challenging to develop in terms of achieving an appropriate level of attenuation; the vector can be overattenuated and not be sufficiently immunogenic, or the vector can be underattenuated and induce adverse effects in subjects. An appropriately attenuated vector with a foreign antigen expressed in immunogenic fashion would hold promise for the development of new types of vaccines.

Most bacterial species, and indeed almost all of the bacterial species described in this book, enter the body via a mucosal route. The immune system has adapted to these microbial threats by having the highest levels of lymphocytes and antibodies, in particular secretory IgA, at mucosal sites. Thus, the establishment of effective mucosal immunity through vaccination could impede the establishment of bacterial infections (Chapter 5). Some of the approaches that have achieved preclinical successes in achieving effective mucosal immunization include the use of detoxified enterotoxins as mucosal adjuvants, enterotoxin B subunits as carriers, mucosal delivery systems such as microparticles, and live bacterial vectors. While these strategies have proven effective in achieving mucosal immunization and protection in diverse animal models, none of these strategies has yet achieved a clear clinical proof of principle. These and other strategies, which are becoming defined and elucidated through further studies of immunological mechanisms, remain an area of intensive focus throughout all of vaccinology, not just for bacterial vaccines.

Numerous technologies have contributed to the design and formulation of novel vaccines (Chapter 6). Vaccines can be divided into three general categories: live, subunit/inactivated, and DNA. There are several subcategories of specific designs within each of these three general groups. One or more of these specific designs may be applicable for developing a vaccine for a particular bacterial disease. Each design has different potential advantages and disadvantages in terms of immunobiology, potential safety and efficacy, production, and ability to be analytically and biologically characterized. All of these factors need to be weighed when selecting a design early in a development program. Given the long timeframe and large expense for development, such decisions assume significant weight. Among these technologies, polysaccharide (Ps) conjugates and protein subunit vaccines have been licensed recently, while live vectors and DNA vaccines also are being actively developed.

Chlamydia species are structurally quite similar. *C. trachomatis* is a major cause of blindness and genital infections, while *C. pneumoniae* causes pneumonia and also is suspected in the development of arteriosclerosis (Chapter 7). These species have a unique biphasic development cycle alternating between elementary bodies (EB) and reticulate bodies. Inactivated whole-cell EB vaccines were shown to induce relatively short-lived clinical protection. Much attention has focused upon the major outer membrane protein (MOMP), which constitutes the majority of OMPs but which shows some sequence variability. However, there has not been sufficient attention to *Chlamydia* species as targets for vaccine programs to enable many other alternative approaches to go forward yet.

Escherichia coli have been implicated in a range of diseases of the gastrointestinal (GI) tract and of the urinary tract as well as meningitis and sepsis. It has been noted that there are many subspecies of *E. coli*, which have divergent surface structures that appear to direct the pathogenicity of the bacteria to different extents in the GI tract and elsewhere. This has complicated the development of *E. coli* vaccines in that each subspecies has required its own vaccine strategy (Chapter 8). Different vaccine antigens have been defined for the diverse subspecies of *E. coli*, including inactivated whole cells, adhesins, fimbriae, lipopolysaccharide (LPS) O antigen, and enterotoxins. There is a licensed vaccine for enterotoxigenic *E. coli* consisting of inactivated whole cells combined with the recombinant B subunit of cholera toxin (CT). There also have been fimbriae adhesin, O antigen conjugate and live recombinant vaccines in clinical evaluations, and other live oral enteric vaccine vectors have been used to express recombinant *E. coli* antigens.

Gonorrhea has been a major sexually-transmitted disease of mankind for centuries. Although on the wane, this disease has proven refractile to control. Thus, vaccines against *Neisseria gonorrheae* remain an important objective (Chapter 9). Given that there is minimal evidence for naturally-acquired immunity to reinfection, a candidate vaccine needs to be potent enough to induce a much stronger immune response than that stimulated by natural *N. gonorrheae* infection. Some of the gonococcal antigens that have been investigated as candidate vaccine antigens include lipo-oligosaccharide, porin proteins, pili, stress proteins and other OMPs, some of which have been evaluated in clinical studies but without successes reported to date. While a purified pilus vaccine induced only type-specific protection against challenge, this vaccine did provide a clinical proof-of-principle that an injected vaccine could stimulate the production of antibodies that block mucosal gonococcal infection.

Streptococcus pyogenes (Group A Streptococcus) causes diseases ranging from rheumatic fever to pharnygitis to the dreaded necrotizing fascitis and is responsible for a high toll of morbidity as well as healthcare costs. The dominant GAS surface antigen is M protein, which is both protective as well as highly type-specific in its antigenic profile. Aspects of the biology of this protein as well as new technologies have resulted in the definition of new vaccine antigens based on both M protein and other proteins (Chapter 10). There has been only one candidate GAS vaccine in clinical studies to date. However, the impact of GAS diseases suggests that we can expect an increasing number of candidate GAS vaccines in future studies.

Streptococcus agalactiae (Group B Streptococcus) is the most common cause of neonatal meningitis. Although antibiotic therapy in late-stage pregnancy has reduced the incidence of early-onset neonatal GBS meningitis, GBS vaccines (Chapter 11) would be highly desirable for preventing late-stage neonatal meningitis and GBS diseases in the elderly and for obviating the use of antibiotics and resultant prospects for antibiotic resistance. A vaccination program for GBS would involve immunizing women who are pregnant or of child-bearing age, a public-health challenge distinct from vaccination programs of other bacterial pathogens.

Helicobacter pylori has proven to be a very challenging vaccine target (Chapter 12). This bacterium is etiologically linked to stomach ulcers, and persistent *H. pylori* infections are a major risk factor for the development of gastric carcinoma as well as other serious diseases of the gastrointestinal tract. Since *H. pylori* chronically infects mucosal surfaces, vaccination strategies have been targeted toward inducing mucosal immunity following oral delivery. There are many promising *H. pylori* antigens that have been defined as vaccine candidates. However, the formulation and vaccine design that can best deliver these antigens for the stimulation of effective mucosal immunity in the GI tract remains to be defined.

Lyme disease has become recognized only during the last two decades. This disease is caused by *Borrelia burgdorferi* that is transmitted by *Ixodes ricinus* ticks. An effective first-generation vaccine was developed against *B. burgdorferi* and licensed (Chapter 13). However, this vaccine was not widely utilized and subsequently was withdrawn from commercial distribution. Other *B. burgdorferi* vaccine antigens have been defined, in particular outer surface proteins, and these may offer the opportunity for a second-generation vaccine that might enjoy increased utilization relative to that the initial vaccine.

Acute otitis media (AOM) is caused mostly by three bacterial pathogens. Among these, *Moraxella catarrhalis* (Chapter 14) is the third-leading cause of AOM in young children and also causes lower respiratory tract infections and pneumonia in the elderly. *M. catarrhalis* is a common colonizer of the nasopharynx and upper respiratory tract. Since *M. catarrhalis* lacks a capsular Ps, a range of protein and saccharide antigens have been investigated as candidate vaccine antigens. These have included lipo-oligosaccharide, iron-binding proteins, and several OMPs. However, none of these have advanced to date to clinical evaluations. It might be that having a combination vaccine including pneumococcal, non-typable *H. influenzae* and *M. catarrhalis* antigens to broadly cover pediatric AOM diseases would be the biggest spur to *M. catarrhalis* vaccine development.

Neisseria meningitidis causes meningitis and invasive diseases and, among bacteria, is responsible for the second highest burden of such diseases in young children and highest in young adults. The available Ps vaccine is targeted to four meningococcal serogroups, but it does not target serogroup B and is not immunogenic in young children. The serogroup C Ps conjugate vaccine has been shown to be effective at preventing disease in infants, children and young adults. This suggests that conjugate vaccines for other major serogroups also would be effective. However, given that the serogroup B Ps is a self-antigen, a conjugate vaccine approach is risky. Thus, there have been considerable efforts toward defining protein-based vaccines that would be effective for serogroup B or for all meningococcal serogroups (Chapter 15). There are several vaccines based on OMPs that are effective at preventing disease caused by sub-serogroup B strains, but to date none of these has been shown to be effective for all serogroup B strains. However, the application of genomics, proteomics, and serological screening has led to the definition of several new protein antigens that are promising vaccine candidates.

Highly effective Ps conjugate vaccines are available for *Haemophilus influenzae* type *b* (Hib), which was the leading cause of pediatric meningitis before the Hib conjugate vaccine era. Nontypable *H. influenzae* (NTHI), which lacks a capsular Ps, is the second leading cause of AOM in children and also causes pulmonary diseases, especially in the elderly and infirm. Like *M. catarrhalis*, NTHI is a common colonizer of the nasopharynx and upper respiratory tract. Unlike Hib, NTHI has remained refractile to success vaccine development (Chapter 16). Early investigations into NTHI vaccines employed killed whole cells and extracts as vaccine antigens, with some indications of transient reductions of the rate of NTHI diseases. There is a group of 7-8 OMPs that have been evaluated as candidate antigens in experimental NTHI challenge models, in particular the chinchilla. However, only some of these have been effective group-common vaccine antigens, and only few of these have advanced to the stage of clinical evaluations. As noted above, a combination with pneumococcal and *M. catarrhalis* vaccine antigens likely would prompt further development.

Nosocomial infections have been increasing in frequency as a result of an increased number of hospital stays and the development of life-saving technologies that have spared life while resulting in more and prolonged stays in intensive-care units. *Pseudomonas aeruginosa* and *Staphylococcus aureus*, which are not pathogenic for healthy individuals, can cause life-threatening infections in infirm or immunologically compromised subjects. Therefore, effective *P. aeruginosa* and *S. aureus* vaccines would be very important for control of these nosocomial infections. The acute nature of these infections in hospitalized subjects means that it is very important to raise antibody levels rapidly in order to provide for protection. Monoclonal antibodies that can bind to bacteria and mediate their inactivation and that can be administered upon entry to acute care also are being developed. Many *P. aeruginosa* antigens have been investigated as vaccine antigens (Chapter 17), including secreted proteins, mucoid exopolysaccharide, flagella, pili, LPS, and OMPs. Vaccines composed of conjugated LPS and OMPs have been evaluated in advanced clinical trials. While many *S. aureus* vaccine antigens also have been evaluated (Chapter 18), most attention has focused on capsular Ps conjugate vaccines. A bivalent Ps conjugate vaccine showed promising efficacy in a recent clinical efficacy study in end-stage renal dialysis patients undergoing hemodialysis.

Pneumococcal diseases arguably account for more morbidity, mortality and health-care costs than any other bacterial diseases. *Streptococcus pneumoniae* vaccines have been going through different generations of development (Chapter 19). There are >90 serotypes of pneumococcal bacteria based on capsular Ps serotype. The first-generation vaccine consists of Ps from 23 pneumococcal serotypes; while effective in preventing invasive diseases in adults, it is nonimmunogenic in young children and is relatively ineffective at preventing pneumonia in the elderly, hence is not widely used. The second-generation vaccine is a Ps conjugate vaccine, consisting of a mixture of seven conjugates of the major disease-causing serotypes in infants. This vaccine is highly effective in preventing invasive pneumococcal diseases in infants and also is effective in preventing pneumococcal AOM. Further 9- or 11-valent conjugate vaccines are in development. These vaccines will prevent most but not all pediatric disease. In addition, serotype substitution has been observed in clinical studies and in the field, whereby non-vaccine serotypes have been observed in increased frequency in groups immunized with the conjugate vaccine. Furthermore, these conjugate mixtures are complicated and costly to produce. Therefore, increased attention has turned to vaccines based on proteins that are conserved and expressed across all serotypes and that induce protection in experimental animal models. Such vaccines have been evaluated in earlier clinical studies and offer the opportunity for effective third-generation vaccines.

Tuberculosis has been a scourge of mankind throughout recorded history. *Mycobacterium tuberculosis* (Chapter 20) is responsible for causing more disease than almost any other pathogen. A live vaccine has been available for decades for the prevention of TB infections, but very widely divergent rates of efficacy have been reported in clinical trials for this vaccine. There have been numerous attempts to improve this vaccine as well as to define alternative TB vaccines. However, the ability to evaluate new TB vaccines has been hampered by funding and by a relative lack of sites at which to conduct clinical efficacy trials. Hopefully the public-health need for a more effective TB vaccine will result in advances toward full clinical development of new TB vaccines.

There are many bacteria that cause enteric diseases. Foremost among these are *Salmonella typhi*, the cause of typhoid fever, and *Vibrio cholerae*, the cause of cholera. There are several available vaccines for preventing typhoid fever (Chapter 21), which has a worldwide distribution. These vaccines include an inactivated whole-cell vaccine, a capsular Ps (Vi) vaccine, and a live attenuated vaccine (Ty21a), the first two of which are injected and the third oral. Some new typhoid vaccines under development include a Vi conjugate vaccine, a genetically attenuated live oral vaccine with increased immunogenicity, and *S. typhi* strains as live vectors. *V. cholerae* causes endemic disease and widespread epidemics as well as pandemics. The most commonly used cholera vaccines are oral (Chapter 22), based on the stimulation of mucosal immunity in the intestine. The first available vaccine has been an oral inactivated whole-cell vaccine combined with recombinant B subunit of CT, while the second vaccine is a oral live recombinant vaccine in which the gene for the A subunit of CT has been deleted. Investigations in future cholera vaccines include broadening serotype coverage and improving vaccine formulation to enable wider-scale use. In addition, *V. cholerae* strains are being developed into live vectors for expressing vaccine antigens of other enteric pathogens.

While recent technologies have expanded the horizons for new and improved vaccines, considerable staff and financial resources must be available to support vaccine development. From the time that an initial lead has been identified, it takes an average of ~10 years and well over $100 million to develop a new vaccine. Furthermore, the success rate from the time of entry to development to availability on the market is only about 10-20%. Therefore, given this long timeframe, large cost and high risk, it is very important to design and implement a Product Development Plan early during this time-period in order to map out all the technologies and resources (money, people, facilities) necessary for optimizing the likelihood of success of the program.

We hope that *New Bacterial Vaccines* will serve as a comprehensive reference on the major aspects of developing new bacterial vaccines. Since vaccination remains the most cost-effective and one of the most practical ways for preventing infectious diseases (and potentially for treating some diseases), the development and widespread applications of new technologies should spawn new bacterial vaccines that have not been approachable technically, with consequent impact on reducing mortality and morbidity worldwide. This book should prove useful for scientists, developers of vaccines and biotechnology products, clinicians, regulators, and health-care practitioners.

Ronald Ellis is very grateful for the many collaborations in vaccines that he has had over the last 20 years with numerous colleagues in Shire Biologics, BioChem Pharma, Astra, Merck and collaborating companies and academic investigators. The loving support and encouragement of his wife Danielle and children Yaakov and Miriam have been indispensable throughout his career and the course of preparation of this book. He is indebted to the Almighty for the strength to collaborate in preparing this book.

Bernard Brodeur thanks his colleagues Nathalie Charland, Josée Hamel, Denis Martin and Stephane Rioux, who assisted him in preparing this book.

Finally, Ron and Bernard thank all the authors for their outstanding contributions to the field of bacterial vaccines and for their chapters, which should make this book a definitive reference for the field of new bacterial vaccines.

Ronald W. Ellis
Bernard R. Brodeur

Chapter 1

Genomics and Proteomics in Vaccine Design

John L. Telford, Mariagrazia Pizza, Guido Grandi and Rino Rappuoli

A Brief History of Bacterial Vaccines

In 1881, Louis Pasteur, the father of bacterial vaccines and immunology, demonstrated publicly the first vaccine against a bacterial infection. His vaccine, against anthrax in sheep, consisted of *Bacillus anthracis* attenuated by high-temperature growth in his laboratory. At Pouilly-Le-Fort, a small village close to Paris, he vaccinated 25 sheep then challenged these plus 25 controls with a virulent strain of *B. anthracis*. All 25 control sheep died, and all 25 immunized sheep survived. This remarkably successful experiment silenced even his most vocal detractors and paved the way for the development of antibacterial vaccines for use in man. Remarkably, the anthrax vaccine produced today and used to immunize American soldiers is produced in a similar fashion except that a stable partially attenuated strain is used. The second bacterial vaccine was produced by Ramon in 1924 and was essentially a formaldehyde-inactivated supernatant from cultures of *Corynebacterium diphtheriae*. Again, current vaccines against diphtheria are produced in the same way except that the inactivated toxin that confers protection is partially purified from the culture supernatant. The story continues with the inactivated whole-cell vaccine against *Bordetella pertussis* (whooping cough) first produced in the late 1940s and still used today in developing countries. It is unlikely that these vaccines would gain FDA approval today. They are still accepted because several decades of use has demonstrated that they are reasonably safe and very effective. It should not be forgotten that these vaccines, together with the smallpox and polio vaccines, essentially eliminated the major causes of childhood mortality in the industrialized world.

With the development of modern molecular biology and microbiology came a more directed approach to the development of new vaccines. In this approach, the bacterium is studied in order to understand which factors are important in pathogenesis, then the selected subunit antigens are produced in pure form either directly from the bacterium or through recombinant DNA technology. An excellent example of this approach is the genetically-detoxified pertussis toxin[1] that is the major component in a modern acellular vaccine against whooping cough.[2] In addition, highly purified or synthetic polysaccharides have been used in a number of vaccines against encapsulated bacteria. These vaccines are currently becoming considerably more effective by conjugating the polysaccharide with a protein carrier.[3] This development is a consequence of our better understanding of the immune response and the role of T cells in development of both high-affinity antibodies and immunological memory. Nevertheless, in the last 25 years, these approaches have led to the development of only a handful of new bacterial vaccines, at least in part due to the mistaken conclusion that antibiotics had conquered bacterial infection and the perception that vaccines were not commercially important.

More recently, vaccine research and development has gained new impetus for a number of reasons. First, it has become clear that our fight against bacterial infection is not over and, second, it has been realized that vaccines represent the most cost effective of all medical interventions. Most importantly, however, has been the extremely rapid development of genomic

New Bacterial Vaccines, edited by Ronald W. Ellis and Bernard R. Brodeur.

technologies in the last six years since the first complete sequence of a bacterial genome was determined. It is now possible to determine the complete genome sequence of a bacterial pathogen in a very few months at very low cost. To date the genomes of over one hundred bacteria have already been determined.[4] Add to this the genome-related technologies of proteomics and complete genome microarray hybridization, and the stage is set for a new paradigm in the invention of novel vaccines.

Genome Technologies in Vaccine Design

Genome Sequencing and Data Mining

DNA sequencing has become a completely automated, high-throughput procedure. Essentially, random overlapping libraries representing the complete genome in small fragments are prepared in plasmid vectors, and the insert of each plasmid is sequenced in both directions from primers complementary to plasmid sequences flanking the insert. Random sequence is determined to a calculated 8- to 10-fold coverage of the genome. Sophisticated bioinformatics tools then compare the sequences and generate long sequence overlaps known as contigs (from contiguous sequence). After this procedure, the genome is usually found in a relatively small number of large contigs. Closure means filling in the gaps and involves libraries of larger fragments in lambda vectors and cloning of specific PCR products using primer sequences at the extremities of the contigs. The result is the complete genome in one continuous sequence.

A number of bioinformatics tools are then used to annotate the genome. This procedure involves programs that identify open reading frames (ORFs), signal peptides and membrane-spanning regions. In addition, the complete sequence is compared with all other known sequences in the databases to identify genes with similarity to any other known gene. In this way, all possible genes and potential protein products encoded by the genome are identified.

Proteomics

While the availability of the complete genome sequence permits the identification of all potential protein products, this information is not sufficient to permit the identification of the subset of proteins (the proteome) that are actually expressed at any stage of the life of the bacteria. It is well known that bacterial pathogens express subsets of the genomic complement under different conditions of growth and during different stages of infection. To address this problem, highly reproducible methods of separating the proteins from extracts of the bacteria have been developed. These involve 2D-gel electrophoresis and high-resolution chromatography. The novel applications of these techniques depend on the availability of the genome sequence. Very small quantities of highly purified protein, e.g., extracted from a single spot on a 2D gel, can be subjected to specific enzyme degradation and analyzed by mass spectroscopy. The experimental result then is compared with theoretical results expected for the same specific degradation of all predicted proteins from the genome sequence. In this way, the protein can be identified unambiguously as the product of a specific gene. This procedure has been used to identify protein spots in 2D gels of extracts of membrane preparations, thus identifying potential surface exposed antigens.

2D-gel electrophoresis is limited and time-consuming, particularly for analyzing membrane protein fractions due to the physico-chemical nature of these proteins. There are several reasons for this, including the fact that the pI of membrane proteins is frequently in the alkaline range and hence cannot be detected in standard gels. Furthermore, many membrane proteins are poorly soluble or insoluble in the aqueous solution required for the electrophoresis. In order to circumvent these problems, novel approaches are being investigated for high-throughput identification of proteins in complex mixtures. One promising approach involves specific protease digestion of a protein extract followed by loading onto a capillary column packed with a strong cation-exchange resin and reverse-phase matrix material. The bound peptides are then eluted

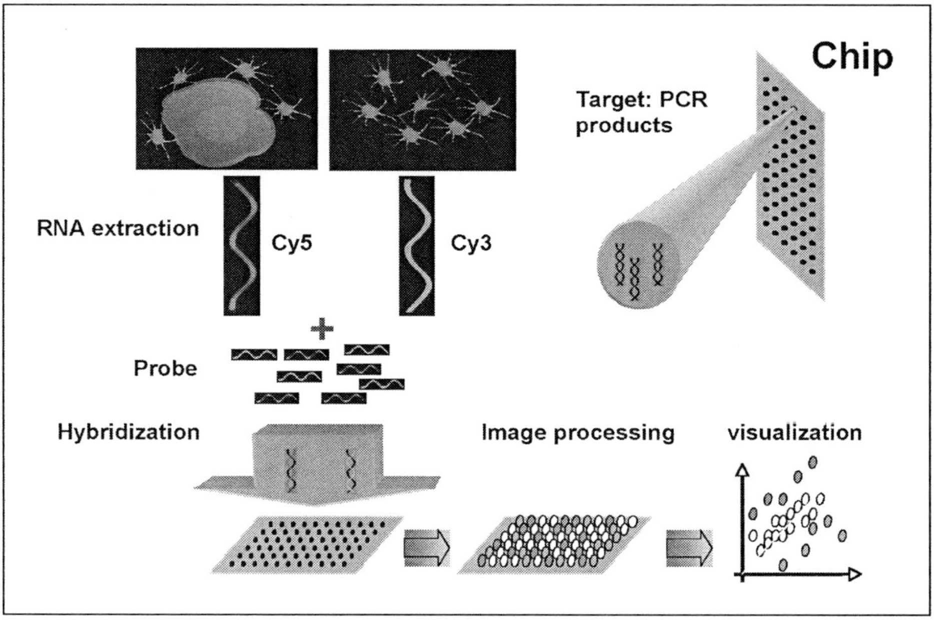

Figure 1. DNA microarray hybridization. Schematic diagram of the use of whole genome DNA chips to assess differences in gene expression under different conditions of bacterial growth. RNA is extracted from control bacteria grown in vitro or under experimental conditions (e.g., in contact with host cells). From each of these RNA preparations, a cDNA probe, labeled with either a red or a yellow fluorescent dye, is prepared. The probes are mixed and used to hybridize to PCR products of every open reading frame in the bacterial genome spotted onto a solid support in orderly arrays. After hybridization, the chips are analyzed automatically to measure the level of red and yellow fluorescence of each spot. The ratio of the intensities is a direct measure of the ratio of expression of each gene under the two conditions. Thus, genes that are differentially regulated between the two growth conditions can be identified.

from the column and applied directly to mass spectroscopy. Very advanced computer algorithms have been written which are capable of taking the mass data and matching the proteins in the mixture to predicted proteins in the genome database. This approach has enormous potential for automation and the design of high-throughput analysis of complex protein mixtures.

DNA Microarrays

DNA microarrays are produced by applying small quantities of specific DNA in spots in ordered high-density arrays on a solid substrate, usually glass slides. Currently up to 10000 DNA spots can be arrayed in a single cm^2 of the chip surface. This process is completely automated. This means that every predicted gene in the genome of a bacterial pathogen, usually prepared by PCR, can be applied to a single chip. These chips are then hybridized with a mixture of two different probes labeled with two different colored fluorescent markers. By comparing the intensity of the two fluorescent markers, the relative hybridization to the probes to each gene can be determined very precisely. The process is shown schematically in Figure 1. This procedure can be used to compare hybridization of genomic DNA from two different strains of bacteria (complete genome hybridization or CGH) to identify genes present or absent in the two genomes. Alternatively they can be hybridized with cDNA prepared from mRNA isolated from bacteria grown under different growth conditions (for example in vivo versus in vitro growth) to identify genes regulated during infection and thus possible virulence factors.

Signature-Tagged Mutagenesis

Another recent technology of use in vaccine design, which does not strictly depend on but is facilitated by genome sequencing, is signature-tagged mutagenesis (STM).[5] In this procedure, a bacterial pathogen is subjected to random transposon-mediated mutagenesis in such a way that each mutant is "tagged" with a specific short DNA sequence tag. Comparison, by hybridization, of the tags found in arrays representing all mutants capable of growing in vitro with mutants that survive passage through an animal host identifies genes essential for the infectious process.

From Genome to Vaccine Design

The development of the above technologies has revolutionized approaches to the study of bacterial pathogenesis and to vaccine design. The availability of complete genome sequences and recent advances in cloning and expression technology now mean that every single antigen in the gene repertoire of a pathogen can be tested for its capacity to induce a protective immune response. In addition, microarray technology and proteomics give additional information on potential antigens and their expression (see Fig. 2). We will illustrate the use of these technologies by describing the recent identification of novel candidate antigens for a vaccine against serogroup B meningococcal disease.[6]

Meningococcus, A Major Cause of Bacterial Meningitis

Neisseria meningitidis is an encapsulated Gram negative diplococcus that colonizes the mucosal membrane of the nasopharynx. It is an exclusively human pathogen colonizing ~30% of the human population where, in most cases, it lives essentially as a commensal causing no serious harm. In a significant number of cases, the bacterium traverses the mucosa to invade the bloodstream, where it can cause fulminant septicemia. It also has the capability to cross the blood-brain barrier and to infect the meninges causing meningitis. Death is a frequent outcome of infection, and up 25% of survivors suffer long-term serious neurological sequelae such as deafness or retardation (reviewed in ref. 7).

There are five major serogroups of the *N. meningitidis* polysaccharide capsule (A, B, C, Y, W135). The capsular polysaccharide (Ps) can induce a protective humoral immune response, but the protection is highly specific for the serogroup and does not confer cross-protection to the other serogroups. Ps vaccines are available for serogroups A, C, Y and W135. When conjugated to a protein carrier, the Ps antigens are considerably more immunogenic and are capable of inducing an immune response even in children under two years of age.[8] However, there is no currently available vaccine against serogroup B, mainly because the serogroup B Ps is identical to an epitope found on human Ps. Hence, it is not immunogenic in humans, and attempts to break tolerance to the antigen are likely to cause problems of autoimmunity.[9] Attempts to design protein-based vaccines have failed conspicuously. In fact, other than a single protein (NspA),[10] all surface-exposed antigens studied to date are so highly variable among different serogroup B strains that they confer only homologous protection and fail to protect against isolates from different geographic locations.[11]

Reverse Vaccinology

Four decades of study using classical approaches to vaccine design failed to produce an effective vaccine against even a majority of disease causing serogroup B meningococcus. It was clearly time to try a different approach. The approach taken has been called reverse vaccinology because, instead of starting with the bacteria and trying identify then clone and sequence protective antigens, the complete genome sequence was first determined then predicted proteins were cloned, expressed and tested in an assay of immunogenicity (shown schematically in Fig. 2).

The complete genome of strain M58 of serotype B consists of 2,272,351 base pairs with an average G+C content of 53%.[12] The genome is predicted to encode 2158 proteins, of which 1158 have been assigned putative function based on homology with known proteins in the

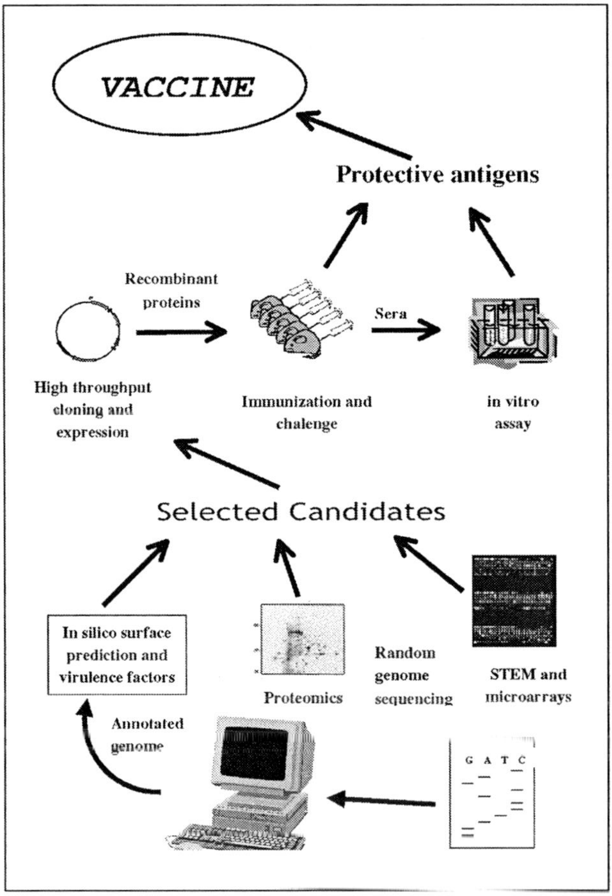

Figure 2. Reverse vaccinology. Schematic diagram of the process of identifying novel vaccine candidates beginning from the complete genome sequence of a pathogen. After assembly of the annotated genome, each predicted open reading frame is analyzed for the presence of sequences capable of encoding signal peptides, membrane-spanning regions, or the motifs associated with surface location such as the LPXTG motif of cell-wall-anchored proteins in Gram positive bacteria. In addition, use of similarity searches identifies homologs of known surface-exposed proteins or virulence factors from other bacterial species. To these candidates are added proteins that have been identified as interesting from proteomic or microarray studies. Recombinant forms of these candidates then are expressed in *E. coli* and tested for their capacity to induce protective immunity in in vitro or in vivo models.

bacteria. An initial selection of potential antigens was made based on predictions of exposure of the antigen on the bacterial surface. A series of computer programs were used to identify potential signal peptides (PSORT, SignalP), membrane-spanning regions (TMPRED), lipoproteins (Motifs) and homology to known surface proteins in other bacteria (FastA). In addition, predicted proteins homologous to known virulence factors or protective antigens from other pathogens were selected. This resulted in an initial selection of 575 potential vaccine candidates.[6]

Each of the 575 candidate genes was cloned by PCR into vectors for expression in *E. coli*. The genes were cloned in two vectors designed to express the antigen either with a tag of six histidine residues or as a fusion protein with glutathione-S-transferase to permit single-step purification by affinity chromatography. The two different vectors were used to increase the

Table 1. Selection of protective antigens of meningococcus B

Selection Step	# of Proteins
Total ORFs	2158
Surface predicted	575
Successfully cloned and expressed	350
Surface expression (FACS positive)	91
Serum bactericidal activity	28

possibility of producing a soluble recombinant protein. 350 of the putative proteins were successfully cloned and purified in this way (Table 1). Each recombinant protein then was used to immunize groups of four CD1 mice. This strain of mice was used, as it is outbred and thus reduces the possibility of poor response due to MHC restriction. Each of the sera was tested in immunoblot of bacterial extracts and in flow cytometry with whole killed bacteria. From these experiments, 91 novel surface-exposed proteins were identified for serogroup B meningococcus. The complexity of the proteins on the surface of this bacterium had previously not been appreciated.

A key requirement for the reverse vaccinology approach is the availability of a relatively rapid test of the capacity to induce a protective immune response. Fortunately, this is available for meningococcal disease. Protection is tightly correlated with the capacity to induce a high titer, complement (C')-dependent bactericidal response in the sera. In fact, this is the accepted surrogate for protection against disease for most regulatory authorities and has been used as the basis of registration of meningococcal vaccines. The assay is relatively rapid and sensitive. The mouse sera raised against the recombinant antigens were each tested in this assay. 28 novel antigens capable of inducing a protective bactericidal titer were identified, a notable result considering that only a handful of antigens have been identified in the last four decades.

Seven of the candidate antigens were selected on the basis of their bactericidal titers and flow cytometry profile for further analysis. The major question remaining was whether these antigens would be conserved among different strains of *N. meningitidis* or if (like most antigens to date) they would be highly variable and thus not cross-protective. To address this question, a panel of 22 serotype B meningococcus strains representing all the major lineages involved in disease[13] was collected. PCR analysis and blot hybridization showed that the genes for each of these antigens were present in all 22 strains. Interestingly, most were also present in strains of serotypes A,C,Y and W135 indicating that they may induce protective immunity across serotypes (Table 2). Furthermore, sequence analysis of the PCR products revealed that the predicted amino acid sequence of five of the seven antigens did not vary more than ~2% among different serotype B isolates.

Finally, these antigens were shown to induce bactericidal antibodies against two other strains of serogroup B meningococcus for which suitable human C' was available. Thus in a relatively short time span of just over two years from the start of the sequencing project, at least five new vaccine candidates with enormous potential for inclusion in a serogroup B meningococcal vaccine have been identified. We await with anticipation the development and clinical evaluation of these antigens.

Reverse Vaccinology for Pneumococcus

More recently the reverse vaccinology approach has been validated by the identification of novel candidate protein antigens for a vaccine against *Streptococcus pneumoniae.*[14] Capsular Ps vaccines are available against this pathogen. However, there are many different capsular serotypes and there is little or no cross-protection among them.[15] An almost identical approach to

***Table 2. Conservation of genes encoding protective antigens in isolates of* neisseria**

Gene	Serogroup B (22 isolates)	ACYXZW (9 isolates)	*N. gonorrhoeae* (3 isolates)	*N.lactamica* (1 isolate)	*N. cinerea* (1 isolate)
gna33	+	+	+	+	+
gna992	+	+	-	+/-	+/-
gna1162	+	+	+	+	+
gna1220	+	+	+	+/-	+/-
gna1946	+	+	+	+	+/-
gna2001	+	+	+	+	+/-
gna2132	+	+	+	+	-

that taken for serogroup B meningococcus was taken to tackle *S. pneumoniae*. However, these authors used more stringent criteria in their *in silico* screening for potentially secreted proteins. This led to the selection of 110 ORFs (out of 2687 ORFs in the genome) for expression in *E. coli*. Ninety-seven of these ORFs were successfully expressed and purified. A second difference in the approach to *S. pneumoniae* candidates was due to the lack of an in vitro assay of protective capability. Hence an animal challenge model was used. This involved immunizing adult mice with the recombinant proteins, then challenging them with a lethal dose of *S. pneumoniae*. The screen of the 97 antigens revealed 6 antigens capable of inducing protective immunity. Analysis of the gene sequences of these antigens in different pneumococcal strains indicated that they were generally very well conserved. Cross-protection of some of the antigens against heterologous strains also was demonstrated.

Thus, in two independent studies, the reverse vaccinology approach has permitted the identification of novel conserved protective antigens against two different bacteria, one a Gram negative diplococcus and the other a Gram positive coccus. The remarkable conservation of the antigens identified in both cases deserves note. Previously reported surface antigens in both of these pathogens have been shown to be highly variable in primary amino acid sequence; hence it was surprising that the reverse vaccinology approach had identified conserved antigens. Previously identified antigens, however, are generally abundant surface proteins that are likely to be under severe immunological pressure. Antigens selected by reverse vaccinology are selected based on their capacity to induce protection and the only bias in their selection is the constraint that they would be predicted to be on the surface of the bacterium. Thus antigens that are expressed at relatively low levels or antigens whose expression is regulated during infection may be identified that may not have been identified by classical methods and that are not under such strong selection pressure by the immune system.

Proteomics in Vaccine Design

Physical analysis of the proteome has the advantage over gene prediction that it permits the identification of proteins actually expressed in a particular compartment (e.g., the membrane) or under different conditions of growth. In addition, it permits the relatively rapid comparison of proteins expressed by different strains of the same bacteria. Both these approaches are being taken to the design of novel bacterial vaccines.

Analysis of the proteome of the membrane compartment is a more direct way to identify potentially surface-exposed proteins and hence vaccine candidates. Reliance on *in silico* predictions of signal peptides and transmembrane spanning regions is of necessity limiting, as it is clear that protein secretion from bacteria is still only partially understood. This is illustrated by a recent analysis of the extracellular subproteome of *Bacillus subtilis*, in which it was shown that the *in silico* predictions dramatically underestimated the number of proteins actually secreted into the medium.[16] Although this approach is still relatively underused, its importance is becoming increasingly clear. For example, an analysis of the membrane compartment of *H. pylori*[17] has identified a number of potential vaccine candidates currently awaiting testing in animal models and further uses of this approach are expected in the near future.

G. Grandi and colleagues have recently combined reverse vaccinology and proteome technologies to identify surface-exposed antigens of *Chlamydia pneumonia*.[18] Little is known of the molecular genetics of this obligate intracellular pathogen, as it is difficult to manipulate and is not amenable to genetic analysis. The bacterium has two distinct developmental phases, a spore-like infectious form, the elementary bodies (EBs), and an intracellular replicative form, the reticulate bodies.[19] The objective of the study was to identify surface exposed antigens expressed in the EBs, as these are likely to be good candidates for a vaccine designed to induce a humoral immune response capable of preventing infection of the target cells. The authors identified 157 putative surface-exposed proteins by *in silico* analysis of the *C. pneumoniae* genome (of a total of 1073 ORFs in the genome). They then employed recombinant forms of these proteins expressed in *E. coli* to raise antisera that were used to assess surface location on the EBs by flow cytometry. Finally, 2D-gel electrophoresis and mass spectroscopy were used to confirm the expression of the antigens in the EB phase of development. In this way 53 novel FACS$^+$ antigens were identified, 41 of which were confirmed by immunoblot or 2D-gel identification.

Proteome comparisons are likely to become increasingly important for the study of bacterial pathogenesis. Comparison of virulent strains of a pathogen with nonvirulent or commensal strains of the same bacteria should permit the identification of proteins involved in virulence. Recently, a comparative study of the proteomes of *Mycobacterium tuberculosis* and *M. bovis* BCG has been undertaken.[20] The proteomes of these two bacteria were found to be highly similar. In fact, this analysis identified only 13 proteins that were specific to virulent strains of *M. tuberculosis* and not expressed in *M. bovis* BCG. These proteins are nevertheless likely to be potential targets for vaccine development and drug discovery. This approach also has been taken to analyze the proteome of BCG grown in vitro compared to that of BCG after infection of macrophages.[21] Several proteins were identified whose expression is upregulated in macrophages and thus may be important for the infectious process.

In contrast, comparison of the proteomes of three isolates of *Helicobacter pylori* revealed very few proteins in common to all three strains, indicating that there is sufficient variation in the protein sequences of these strains to substantially alter their migration profiles.[22] In this case, it is likely that the proteins found in common will be the best candidates for vaccine design or drug discovery. The more rapid strategies for proteome analysis currently being developed will result in a dramatic increase in the use of this approach to study bacterial pathogenesis (reviewed in ref. 23).

Identification of Antigens Important for Infection

Signature-Tagged Mutagenesis

STM is an extremely powerful technique to identify genes in a pathogen of importance for the infectious process.[5] There are two advantages of this approach for the design of novel vaccines. On the one hand, the technique potentially allows the identification of attenuated mutants that fail to cause productive infection and hence may be used as live vaccines. On the other, proteins identified as being essential for infection or disease are likely to be good candidates for inclusion in subunit vaccines. Both these strategies in fact have been used. To date STM analysis has been performed on over a dozen pathogens (reviewed in ref. 24) leading to the identification of a number of vaccine candidates. An interesting and perhaps unexpected outcome of these studies has been the assignment of biological function to a number of gene products of ORFs identified by genome sequences and of otherwise unknown function. The availability of complete genome sequence information can enhance the power of STM studies.

Lau et al[25] have combined an STM approach with complete genome information on *S. pneumoniae* to identify genes flanking mutational inserts, often in the same operon, which also may be involved in pathogenesis.

DNA Microarrays

Whole genome DNA microarrays are a powerful addition to the post-genomic technologies for vaccine design.[23] Hybridization of chips containing DNA spots representing every gene in the genome with RNA extracted from the bacteria allows the complete transcriptome (every expressed RNA in the cell) to be determined in a rapid and precise fashion. Comparison of the transcriptome of bacteria grown in vitro with that of bacteria isolated from infected animal models can rapidly identify all genes regulated during different stages of infection and in vivo growth. Although gene microarrays have been used to study changes in host gene expression upon infection,[26,27] to date little has been published on changes in bacterial transcriptomes during infection. This may be due in part to difficulties in obtaining sufficient high quality RNA from in-vivo-grown bacteria, but such problems are likely to be overcome in the near future. Array technology has been used to study differences in the transcriptome of serogroup B meningococcus between normal bacterial culture and after adhesion to epithelial cells. This study identified >300 genes whose expression was either up- or down-regulated on adhesion. Of particular interest is that several of the most up-regulated genes during the adhesion process were shown to encode proteins capable of inducing bactericidal antibodies on immunization of mice.[28]

Another use of whole genome DNA microarrays is to compare the genomes of related bacteria. DNA chips containing the genome of one strain of bacteria for which the genome sequence is known can be hybridized with total genomic DNA from different strains or related bacteria for which genome sequence data do not exist, thus permitting the identification of genes present in one strain and absent in another.[29,30] Recently, we have used this technique to compare the genomes of 22 strains of *Streptococcus agalactiae* (Group B streptococcus) comprising examples of all nine known serotypes with the genome of a serotype V isolate of which we had determined the complete genome sequence.[31] The analysis revealed a number of regions of the genome that are highly variable and, more importantly, those genes common to all strains. This latter group contains the best candidates for a vaccine capable of cross-serotype protection.[32]

Future Prospects

Genomics has introduced a new paradigm in approaches to bacterial pathogenesis. Instead of starting at the end, i.e., by trying to understand virulence and identify the factors involved, the new approach is to start at the beginning with the complete information of the genome and the gene products and then to identify among these the important factors in virulence. In this respect, comparative genomics will surely become a major endeavor in the future. To date, the complete genome sequence of >100 bacteria has been determined,[4] and valuable information has been derived from their comparisons. As genome sequencing becomes even easier and cheaper, the ability to compare related bacteria, pathogens versus commensals of the same or related species and even bacteria with different or similar pathogenic profiles will produce new concepts of bacterial pathogenesis. An essential part of the development of genomics will be the development of new bioinformatics tools to handle the increasing quantity of raw data. Algorithms capable of comparing whole-genome sequences from large numbers of organisms will be necessary, as will expert systems capable of extracting useful and relevant information in a rational form that can be understood by scientists interested in bacterial pathogenesis (reviewed ref. 32).

It also will be necessary to integrate the large amount of data that will be generated from proteomics and microarray technologies. It is conceivable that, in the very near future, we will have complete information on which genes are expressed and which proteins are made at every stage of the life cycle of a number of bacterial pathogens. Add to this the comparisons of gene expression between pathogenic and nonpathogenic bacteria. STM strategies will be enhanced enormously by the use of microarrays to identify what effect an attenuating mutation has on the transcriptosome and proteosome expressed in the mutant. Hence, there is a real risk that our capacity to analyze data will fall behind our capacity to generate it.

In this new scenario, we would expect that the number of candidate antigens for new vaccines would increase dramatically, promising ever more ways of combating bacterial infections. The major limit in new vaccine development is more likely to be the availability of suitable in vitro or in vivo models of infection and disease in which to test the new molecules. This is less amenable to high-throughput technologies and will require suitable investment both in time and money in order to take full advantage of the genomic revolution in vaccine design. Secondly, although immunology has made striking advances in recent years, we still understand too little about the immune response in most bacterial infections. We need to understand better the role of the innate response and how this influences the adaptive response in order to design better vaccines. In particular, we need to understand the role of adjuvants better. Major breakthroughs in our understanding of the role of Toll-like receptors (TLR) in the function of novel adjuvants such as oligonucleotides peptides containing the CpG motifs may lead to new concepts in adjuvant design. One might envisage a genomic high-throughput approach to the identification of novel TLR ligands. Finally, mucosal adjuvants that would permit the design of subunit vaccines for oral or intranasal delivery would radically alter the current philosophy of vaccine design. In this respect, the potential of nontoxic mutants of *E. coli* heat-labile toxins as mucosal adjuvants is particularly promising.[33]

In conclusion, it is clear that genomics-based technologies are revolutionizing approaches to vaccine development. The ability to address the whole microorganism at the level of every single gene and protein through the use of high-throughput technologies is having a profound effect on the study of bacterial pathogenesis at every level. Not only are new vaccines being developed but also genomics technologies also are being used to identify novel targets for small-molecule therapeutics. We believe that the developments both in new vaccines and new antibiotics will allow us to gain once again the upper hand in our fight against bacterial infectious disease, at least for a while.

References

1. Pizza M, Covacci A, Bartoloni A et al. Mutants of pertussis toxin suitable for vaccine development. Science 1989; 246(4929):497-500.
2. Podda A, De Luca EC, Titone L et al. Acellular pertussis vaccine composed of genetically inactivated pertussis toxin: Safety and immunogenicity in 12- to 24- and 2- to 4-month-old children. J Pediatr 1992; 120(5):680-5.
3. Lesinski GB, Westerink MA. Novel vaccine strategies to t-independent antigens. J Microbiol Methods 2001; 47(2):135-49.
4. Fraser CM, Eisen JA, Salzberg SL. Microbial genome sequencing. Nature 2000; 406(6797):799-803.
5. Chiang SL, Mekalanos JJ, Holden DW. In vivo genetic analysis of bacterial virulence. Annu Rev Microbiol 1999; 53:129-54.
6. Pizza M, Scarlato V, Masignani V et al. Identification of vaccine candidates against serogroup b meningococcus by whole-genome sequencing. Science 2000; 287(5459):1816-20.
7. van Deuren M, Brandtzaeg P, van der Meer JW. Update on meningococcal disease with emphasis on pathogenesis and clinical management. Clin Microbiol Rev 2000; 13(1):144-66.
8. Zollinger WD. New and improved vaccines against meningococcal disease. In: Levine MM, Woodrow GC, Cobon GS, eds. New generation vaccines. New York: Decker, 1997:468-488.
9. Hayrinen J, Jennings H, Raff HV et al. Antibodies to polysialic acid and its n-propyl derivative: Binding properties and interaction with human embryonal brain glycopeptides. J Infect Dis 1995; 171(6):1481-90.
10. Martin D, Cadieux N, Hamel J et al. Highly conserved neisseria meningitidis surface protein confers protection against experimental infection. J Exp Med 1997; 185(7):1173-83.
11. Rosenstein NE, Fischer M, Tappero JW. Meningococcal vaccines. Infect Dis Clin North Am 2001; 15(1):155-69.

12. Tettelin H, Saunders NJ, Heidelberg J et al. Complete genome sequence of neisseria meningitidis serogroup b strain mc58. Science 2000; 287(5459):1809-15.
13. Maiden MC, Bygraves JA, Feil E et al. Multilocus sequence typing: A portable approach to the identification of clones within populations of pathogenic microorganisms. Proc Natl Acad Sci USA 1998; 95(6):3140-5.
14. Wizemann TM, Heinrichs JH, Adamou JE et al. Use of a whole genome approach to identify vaccine molecules affording protection against streptococcus pneumoniae infection. Infect Immun 2001; 69(3):1593-8.
15. Pelton SI. Acute otitis media in the era of effective pneumococcal conjugate vaccine: Will new pathogens emerge? Vaccine 2000; 19(Suppl 1):S96-9.
16. Antelmann H, Tjalsma H, Voigt B et al. A proteomic view on genome-based signal peptide predictions. Genome Res 2001; 11(9):1484-502.
17. Chakravarti DN, Fiske MJ, Fletcher LD et al. Application of genomics and proteomics for identification of bacterial gene products as potential vaccine candidates. Vaccine 2000; 19(6):601-12.
18. Montigiani S, Falugi F, Scarselli M et al. Genomic approach for analysis of surface proteins in chlamydia pneumoniae. Infect Immun 2002; 70(1):368-79.
19. Chlamydia: Intracellular biology, pathogenesis and immunity. In: Stephens RS, ed. Americam Society for Microbiology. Washington DC: 1999.
20. Jungblut PR, Schaible UE, Mollenkopf HJ et al. Comparative proteome analysis of mycobacterium tuberculosis and mycobacterium bovis bcg strains: Towards functional genomics of microbial pathogens. Mol Microbiol 1999; 33(6):1103-17.
21. Monahan IM, Betts J, Banerjee DK et al. Differential expression of mycobacterial proteins following phagocytosis by macrophages. Microbiology 2001; 147(Pt 2):459-71.
22. Jungblut PR, Bumann D, Haas G et al. Comparative proteome analysis of helicobacter pylori. Mol Microbiol 2000; 36(3):710-25.
23. Grandi G. Antibacterial vaccine design using genomics and proteomics. Trends Biotechnol 2001; 19(5):181-8.
24. Mecsas J. Use of signature-tagged mutagenesis in pathogenesis studies. Curr Opin Microbiol 2002; 5(1):33-7.
25. Lau GW, Haataja S, Lonetto M et al. A functional genomic analysis of type 3 streptococcus pneumoniae virulence. Mol Microbiol 2001; 40(3):555-71.
26. Maeda S, Otsuka M, Hirata Y et al. Cdna microarray analysis of helicobacter pylori-mediated alteration of gene expression in gastric cancer cells. Biochem Biophys Res Commun 2001; 284(2):443-9.
27. Yoshimura T, Tomita T, Dixon MF et al. Adams (a disintegrin and metalloproteinase) messenger rna expression in helicobacter pylori-infected, normal, and neoplastic gastric mucosa. J Infect Dis 2002; 185(3):332-40.
28. Tettelin H, Masignani V et al. Complete genome sequence and compatitive genomic analysis of an emerging human pathogen, serotype V Streptococcus agalactiae. Proc Natl Acad Sci USA 2002; 99:12391-96.
29. Bjorkholm B, Lundin A, Sillen A et al. Comparison of genetic divergence and fitness between two subclones of helicobacter pylori. Infect Immun 2001; 69(12):7832-8.
30. Dorrell N, Mangan JA, Laing KG et al. Whole genome comparison of campylobacter jejuni human isolates using a low-cost microarray reveals extensive genetic diversity. Genome Res 2001; 11(10):1706-15.
31. Grifantini R, Bantolini E et al. Previously unrecognized raccine candidates against group B meningococcus by DNA micro arrays. Nat Biotech 2002: 90:914-921.
32. Claverie JM, Abergel C, Audic S et al. Recent advances in computational genomics. Pharmaco genomics 2001; 2(4):361-72.
33. Pizza M, Giuliani MM, Fontana MR et al. Mucosal vaccines: Non toxic derivatives of LT and CT as mucosal adjuvants. Vaccine 2001; 19(17-19):2534-41.

Chapter 2

Universal Proteins As an Alternative Bacterial Vaccine Strategy

Bernard R. Brodeur, Denis Martin, Stéphane Rioux, Nathalie Charland and Josée Hamel

Introduction

In the last two decades, discoveries in biological sciences have allowed vaccine research to expand rapidly. Progress in the understanding of the regulatory mechanisms of the immune response to infection, molecular biology, genomics, proteomics and bioinformatics have revolutionized the way vaccines are designed. Vaccinology has established its own credibility, and it is no longer only a subject in microbiology and immunology classes but a true complex discipline. Vaccines are no longer just crude and complex preparations of killed or attenuated microorganisms but can be defined as proteins, polysaccharides (Ps), or nucleic acids that are delivered to the immune system as single entities, as part of complex particles, or by live attenuated agents or vectors, thereby inducing specific responses that inactivate, destroy, or suppress pathogens.[1]

Despite the recent advances in vaccinology, new strategies for vaccine development are still needed. The traditional approaches have failed to provide effective vaccines for many infectious diseases (Table 1). Furthermore, new vaccines must meet high standards of safety and characterization. It is foreseeable that the future trend will be toward subunit vaccines. Today, there are many effective human vaccines directed to prevent disease caused by various infectious agents.[2] Among existing bacterial vaccines, the *Haemophilus influenzae* type b conjugated vaccine is a good example of recent vaccine success. This formulation proved the clinical effectiveness of Ps conjugates in preventing bacterial disease. Not only was the vaccine effective in preventing meningitis, it also reduced carriage of the bacteria in the upper respiratory tract. With other gram negative encapsulated bacteria, however, variations in serotypes that can cause disease create a different paradigm. In the case of Group B *Streptococcus* (GBS), *Neisseria meningitidis* and *Streptococcus pneumoniae* there are at least 9, 12 and 90 different capsular Ps serotypes, respectively. In addition, the *N. meningitidis* group B capsular Ps is poorly immunogenic and is identical to polysialic acid found on normal human tissues. Generating antibodies to this antigen could potentially be harmful.[3,4] Finally, preliminary data suggest that vaccination with multivalent conjugated Ps may result in substitution of colonizing serotypes not included in the vaccine. For all these reasons, conjugate vaccines are only one strategy for developing successful vaccines. Alternative strategies, such as protein-based vaccines, may offer solutions in other cases.

Ideally, a vaccine should be:

1. Safe and efficacious in the target population
2. Capable of inducing a long-term protective immunity
3. Administered as a single dose and in combination with other vaccines
4. Stable in various conditions

New Bacterial Vaccines, edited by Ronald W. Ellis and Bernard R. Brodeur.

5. Able to eliminate asymptomatic carriers when indicated, and finally
6. Manufacturable in a cost-effective way

In order to meet all these requirements, we are focusing our efforts on protein-based vaccines. Already, the major active component of a few bacterial vaccines, such as diphtheria and tetanus toxoids, acellular pertussis and Lyme disease vaccines are proteins. There are several advantages in using proteins as immunogens. Bacterial proteins can be highly conserved and surface-exposed or secreted by all strains of a defined pathogen regardless of serotype. They can be highly immunogenic and can induce a cross-protective serotype-independent immune response. Proteins elicit T-cell-dependent immune responses generating memory cells for long-term immunity. Furthermore, proteins can be engineered genetically to improve immunogenicity and mixed efficiently to create new combination vaccines. Recombinant proteins can be produced in large quantities in fermentors.

Modern vaccinologists are faced with a dual hypothesis when searching for new vaccines: the top-down approach versus the bottom-up approach. The former consists of using bioinformatics to mine bacterial genomes. After analysis of databases for motifs, identification of homologs, structure-function determination, identification of pathogenicity islands and/or performing subtractive hybridization using the genome of pathogenic bacteria versus commensal bacteria, it is possible to select several virtual vaccine candidates. Following recombinant protein expression, the antigens are evaluated and characterized using numerous in vitro and in vivo pre-clinical tests. The bottleneck of this approach is in testing of large numbers of gene candidates. The bottom-up approach to vaccine development consists of studying naturally acquired immunity, comparing human acute versus convalescent antibody specificity and understanding mechanisms of protective immunity in animal models of infection. The next step is to identify those antigens implicated in the protective immune response. These antigens should be expressed and accessible at the surface of the pathogens during the course of infection. The protective epitope should show minimal molecular and antigenic variation. Finally,

Table 1. Partial list of bacterial human pathogens for which vaccines are not available or need further development.

Bacterial Species
Burkholderia cepacia
Campylobacter jejuni
Chlamydia spp
Enterotoxigenic *Escherichia coli*
Escherichia coli and *Proteus spp* (urinary tract infections)
Helicobacter pylori
Klebsiella spp
Moraxella catarrhalis
Mycobacterium leprae
Neisseria gonorrhoeae
Non typable *Haemophilus influenzae*
Pseudomonas aeruginosa
Serogroup B *Neisseria meningitidis*
Shigella spp
Staphylococcus aureus
Streptococcus agalactiae (group B)
Streptococcus mutans
Streptococcus pneumoniae
Streptococcus pyogenes (group A)

the recombinant protein should be able to confer protection against a lethal challenge in an animal model that mimics as closely as possible the human infection of the particular pathogen.

In our laboratory, we have combined both methods of investigation to circumvent pitfalls that could be encountered by using solely the genomic or the immunological strategy for the discovery of vaccine antigens (Fig. 1). Our preferred strategy to rapidly identify new protective immunogens is to screen genomic libraries with:

1. Human sera
2. Sera obtained from animals immunized with an antigenic protein fraction conferring protection
3. Protective monoclonal antibodies (MAbs)

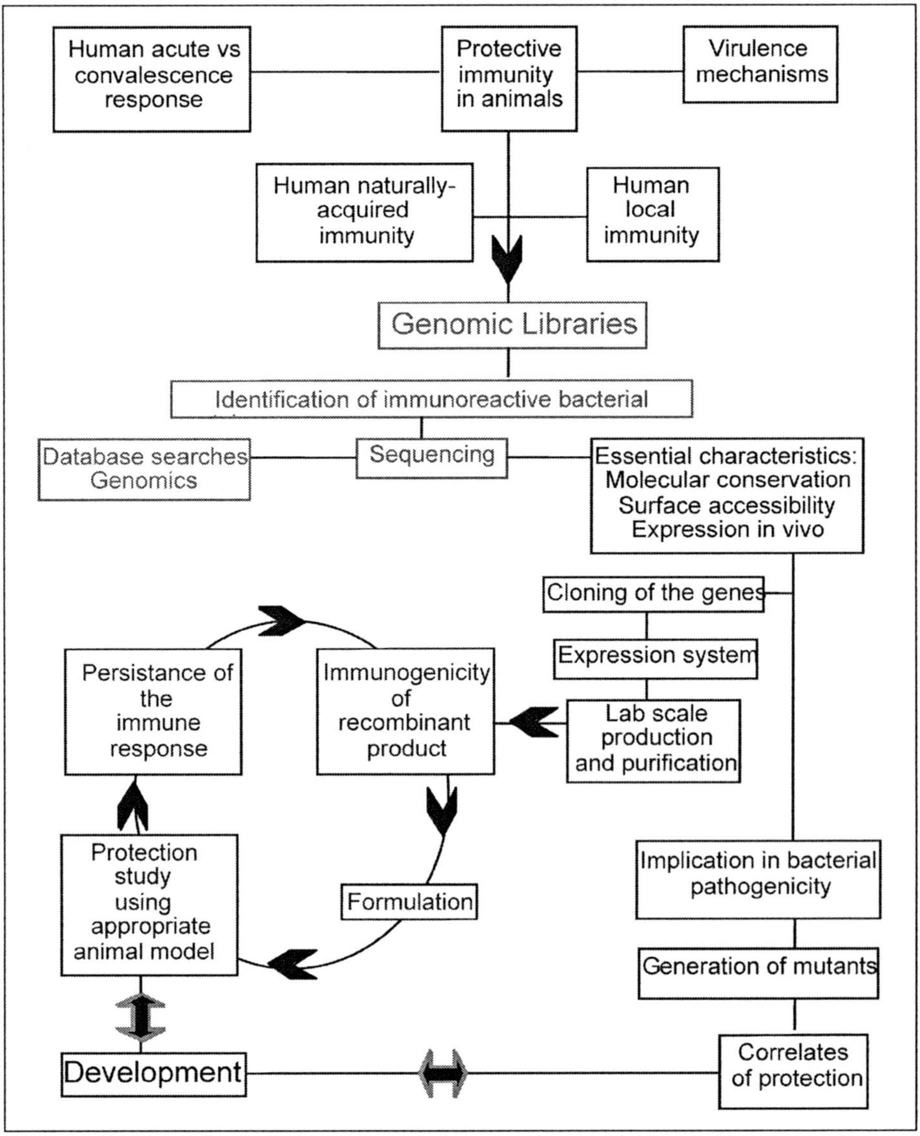

Figure 1. Schematic representation of the dual strategy to identify novel vaccine candidates.

At the same time, immunoreactive antigens are rapidly identified using proteomics and genomics analysis. The corresponding DNA is cloned, expressed and the proteins are tested for immunogenicity and protection in the corresponding animal model of infection. This chapter has been organized to discuss at length the essential parameters to consider for developing a protein-based vaccine. Preclinical evidence supporting protein-based vaccines for *N. meningitidis* serogroup B, GBS and *S. pneumoniae* is presented. The *N. meningitidis* serogroup B NspA vaccine has been tested in humans and was shown to be safe and immunogenic.

Meningococcal NspA Protein

As presented in the *N. meningitidis* vaccine chapter, non-capsular surface antigens, which mainly consist of outer membrane proteins (OMPs) and lipopolysaccharides, are considered as prospective *N. meningitidis* vaccine candidates. However, one of the main problems with most of the already described meningococcal OMPs is their antigenic heterogeneity. Indeed, the interstrain variability of the major OMPs restricts their protective efficacy to a limited number of antigenically related meningococcal strains. Several strategies based on either outer membrane vesicles, which contain most of the major surface proteins, or purified OMPs are being explored in order to broaden the protective potential of protein-based meningococcal vaccines. The identification of universal or, at least, widely distributed proteins with antigenically conserved surface-exposed regions would offer a solution to the great heterogeneity of the major meningococcal OMPs. Described in the following paragraphs are the different steps which led to the discovery and partial characterization of such an antigen, named NspA for Neisserial surface protein A.

MAbs were used to identify the NspA protein.[5] To generate cross-reactive MAbs that are directed against conserved antigens, mice were immunized with different combinations of outer membrane preparations extracted from serologically distinct meningococcal strains. To select broadly reactive Mabs, a panel of meningococcal strains, which represented the major disease-causing groups of strains including serogroups A, B, and C strains, was used during the initial screening. Only MAbs which recognized the majority of these strains were then selected for further characterization. Some of these MAbs were found to react with >99% of the meningococcal strains tested.[5,6] Since MAbs are specific for one particular epitope, it clearly indicated that highly conserved antigenic regions were indeed present on meningococcal cells. These MAbs were found to be directed against a low molecular weight heat-modifiable protein, which was later called NspA.[7]

One of these MAbs was then used to screen a λGEM-11 chromosomal library constructed from a serotype B meningococcal strain in order to identify the gene coding for the NspA protein.[5] Sequence analysis of the meningococcal inserts present on reactive clones revealed a 525-nucleotides open reading frame, which encodes a 174-amino-acid-residue polypeptide. Comparison of this sequence with the sequences compiled in the available databases indicated that the *nspA* gene shared homologies with members of the Neisserial opacity protein family (Opa), which are found in the meningococcal outer membrane. DNA hybridization clearly established that the *nspA* gene is present in the genome of all meningococcal strains tested, but it also indicated that highly conserved homologs were present in the closely related species *N. gonorrhoeae*, *N. lactamica* and *N. polysaccharea*. Characterization of the gonococcal NspA protein was presented by Plante et al. [8] Conclusive proof of the high level of molecular conservation (>96% identity) of this protein was obtained following cloning and sequencing by our group[5,6] and by Moe et al[9] of additional *nspA* genes from divergent serogroups A, B and C meningococcal strains. It was recently reported that the organization of NspA protein in the meningococcal outer membrane closely resembled the structure of other known meningococcal proteins, such as the meningococcal OpA proteins.[9] Structure predictions indicated that the NspA protein contains eight transmembrane β-strands with four surface-exposed loops (Fig. 2).

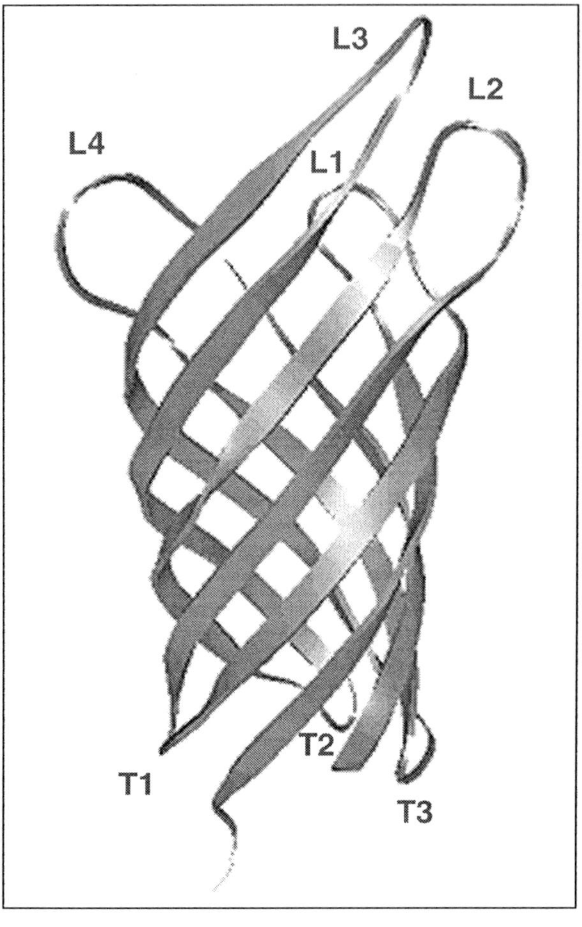

Figure 2. 3-D model of the meningococcal NspA protein. This model was developed from the crystal structure of the refolded *E. coli* OmpA (PDB ID: 1QJP)[30] using Swiss-Pdb Viewer[31]. The eight transmembrane β-strands are connected with three tight turns (T1, T2, T3) on the periplasmic side and four surface-exposed loops (L1, L2, L3, L4) on the outer surface. This figure was prepared using 3D-Mol Viewer from Vector NTI suite 7.0 (InforMax, Inc.).

The *nspA* gene was cloned into the expression vector pWKS30 in order to obtain sufficient amounts of purified protein to evaluate its protective potential in a mouse model of infection.[5] BALB/c mice were immunized three times with 20 μg of immunoaffinity-purified recombinant NspA protein and the mice were then challenged with a lethal dose of a serogroup B strain. Eighty % of the NspA-immunized mice survived the bacterial challenge, compared to less than 20% in the control groups.[5] Analysis of the sera collected from the mice that survived the lethal meningococcal challenge revealed the presence of cross-reactive antibodies that attached to and killed the four serogroup B strains tested. In addition, passive immunization of mice with NspA-specific MAbs confirmed the protective potential of the protein. Indeed, administration of an NspA-specific MAb 18 h before challenge reduced by >75% the levels of bacteremia recorded for mice challenged with 10 out of 11 meningococcal strains tested.[6] These results indicated that this highly conserved protein could induce protective immunity against meningococcal infection.

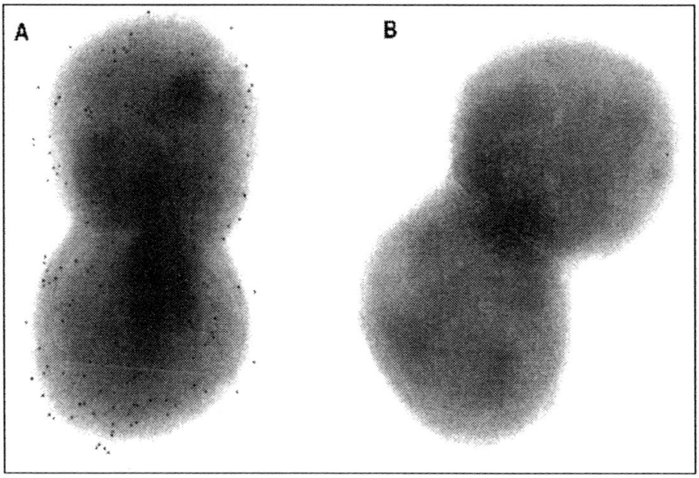

Figure 3. Electron micrographs of whole cells of meningococcal strain 608B probed with the MAb Me-7 (A) or an *H. influenzae* porin-specific MAb P2-4 (B) and followed by gold-labeled goat anti-mouse immunoglobulin G (Reprinted from: Cadieux N, Plante M, Rioux CR et al. 1999. Infection and Immunity: 67: 4955-4959).

NspA-specific MAbs proved to be valuable tools to study the NspA protein on the surface of intact meningococcal cells. The photograph presented in Figure 3A clearly demonstrated that MAb Me-7 recognized the NspA protein on intact meningococci and that this protein is evenly distributed at the surface of the cells. Exposure of NspA at the surface of intact meningococcal cells was further studied using cytofluorometric assays. Figure 4 presents the attachment of 9 representative NspA-specific MAbs to the surface of two serogroup B (608B[5] and CU385[10]), one serogroup A (F8238)[11] and one serogroup C (C11)[11] meningococcal strains. For each MAb, the concentration was adjusted to 1 µg/mL and early exponential-phase meningococcal cells were used to perform the cytofluorometry assay. None of these MAbs reacted with the 608BΔ*nspA* mutant strain in which the *nspA* gene was inactivated by the insertion of a transposon (data not shown). This result indicated that none of these MAbs attached nonspecifically at the surface of live meningococcal cells.

According to the level of attachment to intact meningococcal cells, the NspA-specific MAbs were classified in three groups (Fig. 4). In the first group, MAbs such as Me-7, Me-9, Me-11, Me-13 and Me-15 attached efficiently at the cell surface of the four strains tested, indicating that their epitopes are located on surface-exposed regions of the protein. The binding of MAbs, such as Me-10, Me-12 and Me-14, which were classified in the second group, was more variable since they recognized their corresponding epitopes at the surface of one or two strains out of the four tested. Finally, MAbs such as Me-16, which did not bind to any intact meningococcal cells were classified in the third group. Immunoblots clearly indicated that the MAbs in the latter group reacted well with purified NspA when it was not inserted into the meningococcal outer membrane (data not shown).

Globally these binding data suggested that some epitopes present on the NspA protein are exposed and accessible to specific antibodies at the cell surface of serologically distinct meningococcal cells, while other epitopes are accessible to antibodies on a limited number of strains. Since the NspA protein is highly conserved and is produced by all strains tested to date, the lack of binding of the group II MAbs to certain meningococcal strains is most probably not related to amino acid variation or lack of protein expression. One might postulate that other antigens present at the meningococcal cell surface might mask the epitopes recognized by the

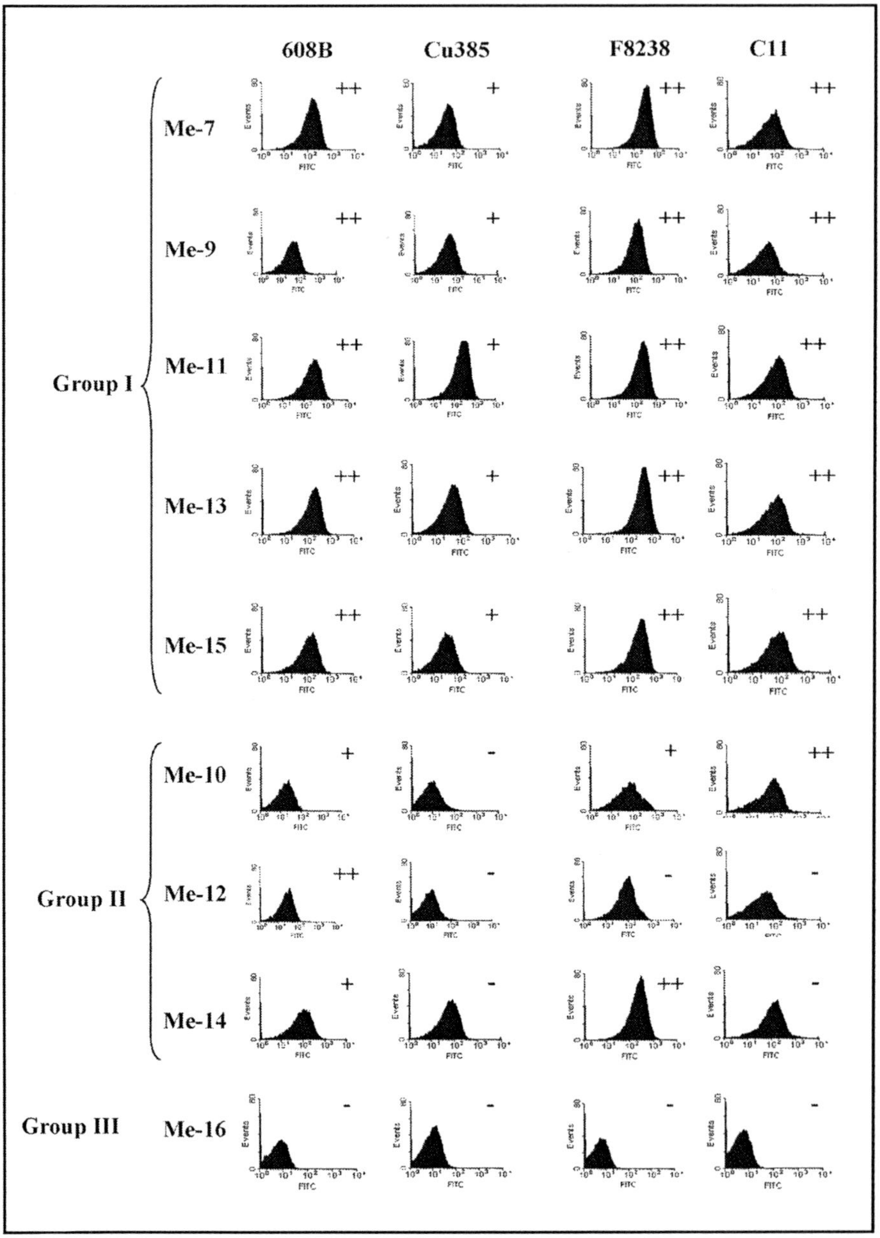

Figure 4. Evaluation by flow cytometry of NspA-specific MAbs accessibility at the surface of two serogroup B meningococcal strain 608B (B:2a:P1.2:L3), CU385 (B:4:P1.15:L3,7,9), one serogroup A strain F8238 (A:4,21) and one serogroup C strain C11 (NT:P1.1:L3,7,9). Exponentially growing meningococcal cells were sequentially incubated with NspA-specific or control MAbs, followed by fluorescein isothiocyanate (FITC)-conjugated anti-mouse immunoglobulin secondary antibody. The bactericidal activity of each MAb is presented as the concentration of antibody resulting in a 50% decrease of CFU/mL after 60 min of incubation compared to control CFU: ++, 0.5-49 µg of antibody/mL; +, 50-99 µg of antibody/mL; - no bactericidal activity at >100 µg of antibody/mL.

MAbs in the second group or that the tertiary structure of the protein might be slightly different in these strains, thus preventing the binding of antibodies to certain epitopes. It was reported that the Ps capsule could shield NspA epitopes and prevent binding of antibodies to meningococcal strains that produce large amounts of Ps.[9] However, the relationship between Ps production, lack of binding and bactericidal activity of NspA-specific antibodies was not clearly established. Indeed, anti-NspA antibodies could bind to the surface and kill a meningococcal strain which was determined to be a high Ps producer, while a low-producer strain was negative for surface binding and resistant to bactericidal activity. Considering this latter observation, one might postulate that other mechanisms, such as conformational changes, may also explain the lack of binding and bactericidal activity observed for certain MAbs.

MAbs classified in group I, which recognize their specific epitopes at the surface of all four strains, were found to be bactericidal against the four meningococcal strains tested (Fig. 4). For group I MAbs, the data suggest a correlation between surface binding and bactericidal activity. However, it is difficult to establish any relation for the MAbs classified in group II. As an example, the meningococcal strain C11 was resistant to the bactericidal activity of MAbs Me-12 and Me-14 even though it was positive for surface binding. Moe et al.[10] also reported similar findings using different NspA-specific MAbs. Interestingly, one of the two strains, the serogroup B Cu385 strain, for which their MAbs were positive for surface binding but resistant to complement-mediated bacteriolysis, was sensitive in our experimental conditions to the bactericidal activity of group I MAbs.

The epitopes recognized by group III MAbs were easily located using overlapping 15- to 20-amino-acid-residue synthetic peptides covering the full length of the NspA protein. As an example, MAb Me-16 was found by ELISA to react with two separate peptides located between residues 41-55 (GSAKGFSPRISAGYR) and 141-150 (VDLDAGYRYNYIGKV). Closer analysis revealed that these two peptides shared the AGYR residues, which are underlined in the peptide sequences. According to the NspA model (Fig. 2), these two regions are embedded inside the meningococcal outer membrane, and antibodies directed against these regions do not attach to intact meningococcal cells. Interestingly, MAbs that were classified in groups I and II did not react with any of these peptides. This result is important since it suggested that these MAbs recognized conformational epitopes. These epitopes can be easily modified or lost during the production, purification and formulation of meningococcal OMPs, as observed with PorA[12-14] and Opc proteins.[15] Antibodies raised against these incorrectly folded proteins are of limited use since they often are less biologically active. To localize these conformational epitopes, a series of truncated NspA proteins were constructed where different combinations of potential surface-exposed loops were deleted. To maintain the conformation of these modified NspA proteins, they were expressed in *E. coli* membranes or inserted into liposomes. Preliminary results indicated that the epitopes recognized by the MAbs in groups I and II are located on the surface-exposed loops 2 (amino acid residues 51-62) and/or 3 (amino acid residues 91-106) (Fig. 2).

In conclusion, the NspA protein induces cross-bactericidal antibodies that can protect against meningococcal infections. We have shown that the surface-exposed loops of the NspA are the targets for these important cross-bactericidal antibodies.

Group B Streptococcal Sip Protein

As presented in the GBS vaccine chapter, GBS protective immunity can be induced by capsular Ps antigens and surface proteins. However, it was observed that protection conferred by capsular Ps is type-specific.[16] Based on current information about serotype distribution, a Ps conjugate vaccine would have to contain types Ia, Ib, II, III and V to prevent the majority of diseases in North America, but would also have to be modified to be effective in other parts of the world such as in Japan where other serotypes are more prevalent.[17] An alternative strategy for protecting neonates and infants would be to develop a GBS vaccine based on an ubiquitous protein. The following paragraphs describe the discovery of a universal surface protein named Sip, for Surface immunogenic protein.

The Sip protein was identified by the immunoscreening of a genomic library prepared from the GBS serotype Ia/c strain C388/90 in λZAPII with a pool of human normal sera collected from volunteers with no known history of GBS disease. The reactive clones were further tested with mouse polyvalent sera collected after immunization with whole-cell preparations from the GBS serotype I a/c strain C388/90.[18] One phage clone, which was recognized by all these sera, was selected for characterization. Immunoblots using phage lysate from this clone revealed that the antibodies present in these sera reacted with a protein band with an approximate molecular mass of 53 kiloDaltons (kDa).[18] Sequence analysis of the GBS chromosomal insert indicated that the polypeptide, which was reactive with human and mouse sera, was encoded by a 1305-bp open reading frame (ORF), later identified as the *sip* gene. Comparison of the nucleotide sequence with sequences compiled in the available databases indicated that, besides GBS, coding regions with homology (62% identity) to the *sip* gene were also present in two streptococcal species, *S. pneumoniae* and *S. pyogenes.*[18] Analysis of functional domains on the Sip protein suggested the presence of a LysM peptidoglycan-binding domain. Such domains were initially identified in many enzymes involved in cell wall degradation but were also found in a number of other proteins, many of which are known to be associated with bacterial cell wall.[19] This analysis suggests that the Sip protein could be involved in cell wall degradation. However, further studies will be required in order to confirm this hypothesis and to determine the role of the Sip protein in the pathogenesis of GBS disease.

To evaluate the level of molecular conservation, *sip* genes were cloned and sequenced from six serologically distinct GBS strains. The nucleotide and deduced amino acid sequences of these six *sip* genes were found to be highly conserved. Indeed, at the amino acid level, these predicted proteins differ in only 8 out of the 434 residues, making them ~98% identical.[18] In addition, these differences were not clustered in any particular region of the Sip protein. More importantly, immunoblots clearly demonstrated that the Sip protein was produced by every GBS strain tested, which included representative isolates of all serotypes (Fig. 5).

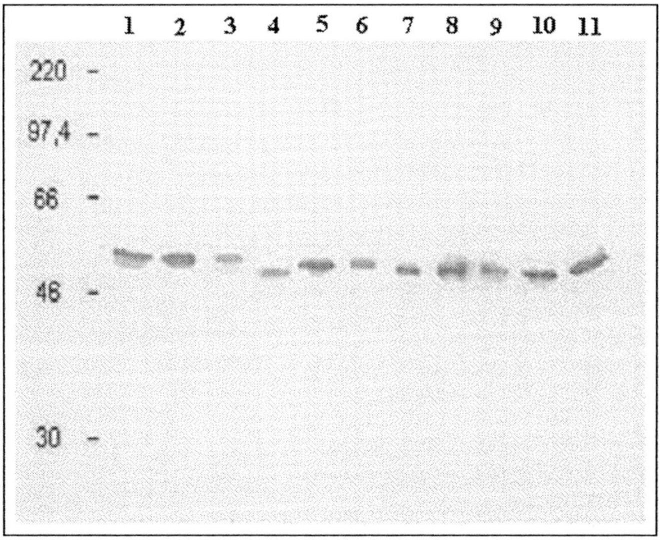

Figure 5. Immunoblots showing the reactivity of the Sip-specific MAb 5A12 with the following GBS whole-cell preparations obtained from strains: lane 1, C388/90 (Ia/c); lane 2, ATCC 12401 (Ib); lane 3, NCS 246 (IIR); lane 4, COH1 (III); lane 5, NCS 97R331 (IV); lane 6, NCS 535 (V); lane 7, NCS 9842 (VI); lane 8, NCS 7271 (VII); lane 9, NCS 970886 (VIII); lane 10, ATCC 27956 (bovine isolate); and lane 11, 1 μg of purified rSip protein. Size standards are marked on the left (in kDa) (Reprinted from: Brodeur BR, Boyer M, Charlebois I et al. 2000. Infection and Immunity: 68: 5610-5618).

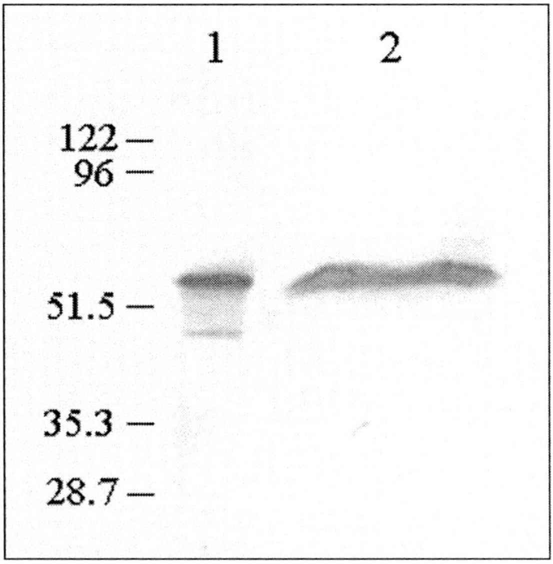

Figure 6. Immunoblots probed with the Sip-specific Mab 5A12 showing the reactivity with the GBS culture pellet (lane 1) and supernatant (lane 2) obtained after overnight incubation at 37°C in the presence of 8% CO_2 in Todd-Hewitt broth.

It was also essential to clearly establish that the Sip protein was not only highly conserved but that it was accessible at the surface of intact GBS cells. Sequence analysis did not reveal the presence of a cell wall anchoring motif (LPXTG), which is often present at the C-terminal region of Gram positive surface proteins, but a 25-amino-acid signal peptide was identified at the N-terminal portion of the Sip protein. The presence of this signal sequence, which is cleaved in the mature protein, was confirmed by N-terminal amino acids sequencing. The presence of a cleavable signal sequence is a strong indication that this protein could be exported outside the cell where it could be associated to the bacterial cell wall.[18] Analysis of GBS culture supernatant confirmed that a portion of the Sip protein is indeed secreted (Fig. 6). The importance of this finding in relation to GBS pathogenesis still has to be determined.

Proteins present at the GBS cell surface were labeled with a water-soluble biotin analog, the sulfo-NHS-biotin reagent, which reacts with the primary amines of a protein and whose negative charge keeps biotinylation localized at the cell surface, so that the reagent does not pass through the cell membrane. Immunoblot analysis of the GBS biotin-labeled surface proteins indicated that a major protein band with an approximate molecular mass of 53 kDa was labeled with biotin (Fig. 7, lane 1). This protein band was shown, using the Sip-specific MAb 5A12, to correspond to the Sip protein (Fig. 7, lane 2). These results suggested that the Sip protein was exposed at the surface of GBS cells and was one of the major biotin-labeled surface proteins of GBS. Flow cytometry analysis confirmed that the Sip protein is not only present at the surface of intact GBS cells, but that portions of the protein are accessible to specific antibodies. Indeed, the antibodies present in the sera collected from mice and rabbits immunized with recombinant Sip (rSip) protein efficiently attached to the cell surface of all GBS strains tested, which included strains representing the 9 capsular serotypes and a bovine isolate (Fig. 8). In addition, examination of GBS cells by immuno-gold electron microscopy revealed that the Sip-specific antibodies attached preferentially at the GBS surface on the septal region (Fig. 9A) or polar sites (Fig. 9B). These results clearly demonstrated that the Sip protein is exposed at the surface of intact cells, an important characteristic for a vaccine candidate.

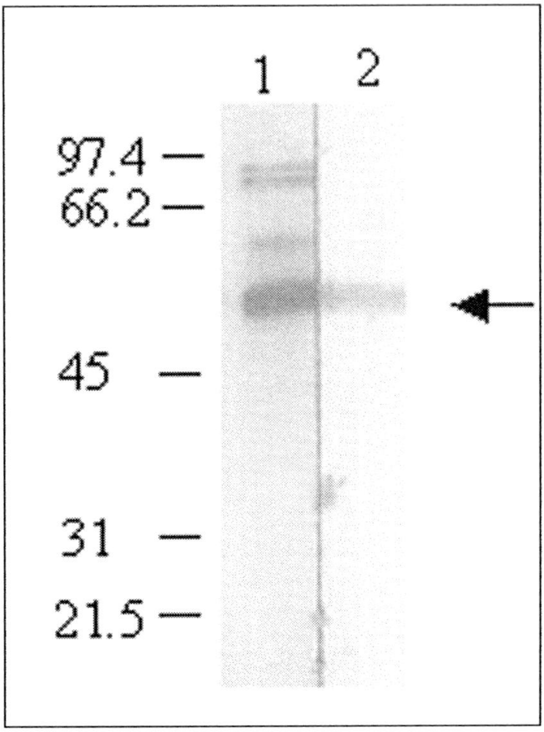

Figure 7. Immunoblots of the biotinalyted surface-exposed proteins of GBS strain C388/90 serotype Ia/c reacted with streptavidin-conjugated alkaline phosphatase (lane 1) or with the Sip-specific MAb 5A12 (lane 2). Arrow indicates the location of the Sip protein. Size standards are marked on the left (in kDa).

Once established that the Sip protein is accessible to specific antibodies at the GBS cell surface, it was important to determine the protective potential of the Sip protein. Groups of CD-1 adult mice were immunized three times with 20 μg of purified rSip protein. Three weeks after the third immunization, mice were challenged with different GBS strains. Eighty percent of mice immunized with purified rSip protein were protected against challenge with the homologous strain C388/90 (Ia/c) (Table 2). More importantly, the response induced after immunization with purified rSip protein efficiently protected adult mice against experimental infection with heterologous GBS strains representing serotypes Ib, II/R, III, V and VI (Table 2). When pooled together, the protection data indicate that 91% of mice immunized with purified rSip protein survived the lethal challenge compared to only 20% for the mice which received the adjuvant alone (Table 2). Analysis of the sera collected from these mice indicated that the purified rSip protein induced a strong humoral immune response with antibodies reactive against the rSip protein as well as the native Sip protein produced by representative strains of every GBS serotype.[18] These results clearly indicated that the Sip protein is an antigen able to confer cross-protective immunity against all GBS serotypes. This is an advantage compared to other GBS surface proteins, such as the alpha and beta C proteins and the Rib protein.[20,21] Indeed, these proteins were not found to be present in all clinical isolates[21,22] and protection was shown to be restricted to strains that produce the specific protein.[23]

Although these results suggested that these Sip-specific antibodies could play a role in the prevention of GBS infection, it was essential to clearly establish a direct link between the presence of Sip-specific antibodies and protection of neonates. Indeed, Baker and Kasper[24]

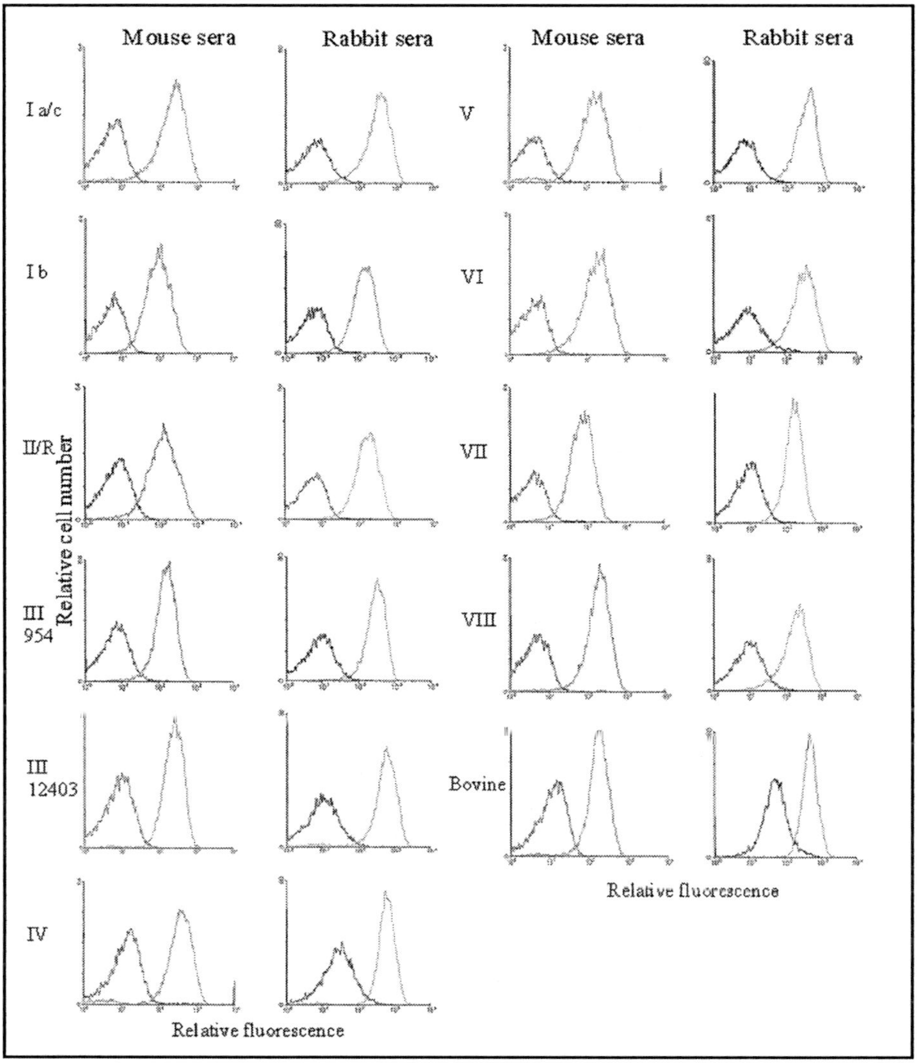

Figure 8. Evaluation by flow cytometry of the accessibility of antibodies to the Sip protein at the surface of 11 distinct GBS strains, which included representative isolates of all serotypes. GBS cells were successively incubated with either mouse anti-Sip or control sera diluted 1/100 (left panel) or rabbit anti-Sip or control sera diluted 1/150 (right panel) followed by the corresponding FITC-conjugated secondary antibody. In each graph, the left peak represents the binding of control serum, while the right peak represents the binding of Sip-specific serum to intact GBS cells.

demonstrated the existence of a correlation between maternal antibody deficiency at delivery and susceptibility to neonatal infection. These findings suggested that vaccination of pregnant women could become a very efficient prophylactic strategy to prevent GBS infection in neonates. Indeed, this approach could stimulate transplacental transfer of GBS-specific antibodies from the mother to the fetus, thus considerably increasing the level of protective antibodies present at the time of delivery.[25]

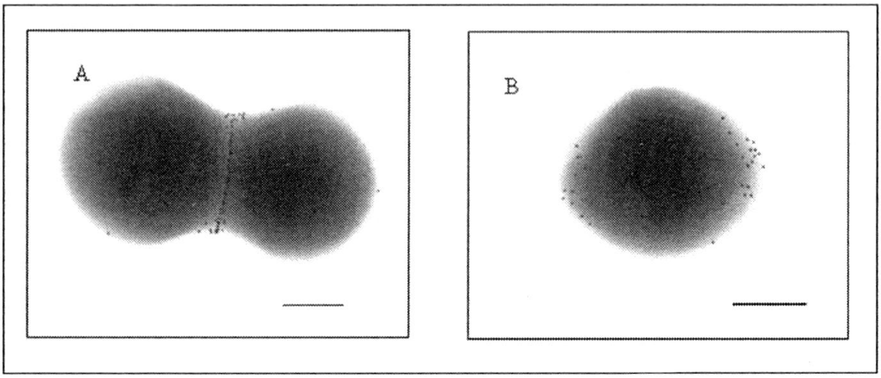

Figure 9. Transmission electron micrographs of whole cells of a GBS serotype III strain NCS 954 probed with mouse anti-Sip and gold-conjugated secondary antibody. The Sip-specific antibodies attached preferentially on the septal region (A) or polar sites (B). Bars, 200 nm. (Reprinted from: Rioux S, Martin D, Ackermann H-W et al. 2001. Infection and Immunity: 69: 5162-5165).

Table 2. Survival of CD-1 mice immunized with purified recombinant Sip protein

Strains Used for Challenge (serotype)	Groups	Number of Mice Surviving the GBS Challenge/ Total (%)[1]	P^2
C388/90 (I a/c)	rSip	8/10 (80)	0.0007
	Control	0/10 (0)	
ATCC 12401 (Ib)	rSip	10/10 (100)	0.0031
	Control	3/10 (30)	
NCS 246 (II)	rSip	10/10 (100)	0.0031
	Control	3/10 (30)	
NCS 954 (III)	rSip	7/10 (70)	0.019
	Control	1/10 (10)	
NCS 535 (V)	rSip	10/10 (100)	0.01
	Control	5/10 (50)	
NCS 9842 (VI)	rSip	10/10 (100)	< 0.0001
	Control	0/10 (0)	

[1]Number of survivors was evaluated for 14 days after challenge. The mice were immunized subcutaneously three times with 20 μg of purified rSip protein or adjuvant only. After immunization, the mice were challenged intraperitoneally with an LD_{90} dose of a GBS strain. [2]Fisher's exact test was determined against control group.

To study this possibility, we selected the mouse neonatal model since it is very well suited to test in offspring the efficacy of antibodies acquired transplacentally from actively vaccinated dams.[26] Indeed, in the absence of a mature immune system, protection in newborn pups can only be achieved via the acquisition of protective maternal antibodies. The potential of Sip-specific antibodies to protect neonates against infection was first evaluated by passive administration of semi-purified rabbit antibodies. Pregnant mice on day 16 of gestation were injected intravenously with partially purified rabbit antibodies directed against the Sip protein. The pups were challenged between 24 h to 48 h after birth with a lethal dose of the serotype Ia/c

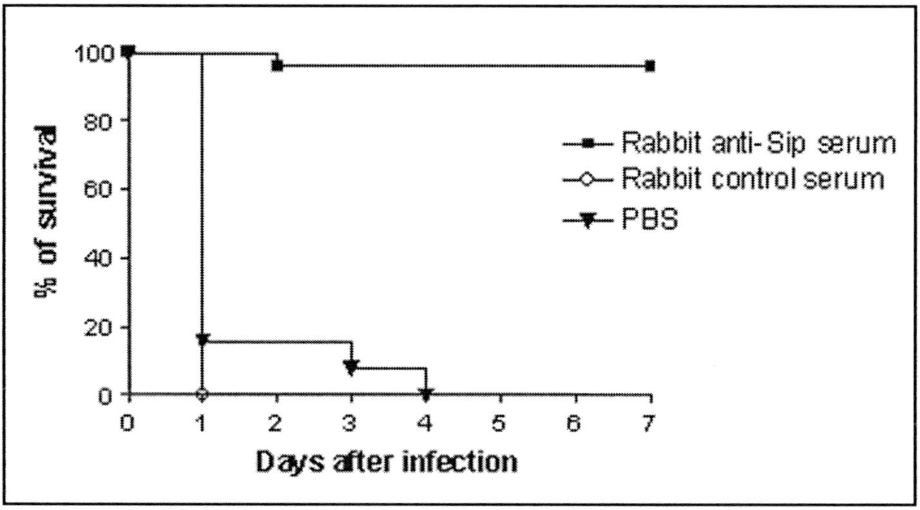

Figure 10. Passive protection of neonatal mice against challenge with serotype Ia/c GBS strain C388/90. CD-1 pregnant mice were injected intravenously two days before delivery with either 500 μL of partially purified rabbit anti-Sip hyperimmune serum or rabbit pre-immune serum. One-day-old pups were challenged subcutaneously with a lethal dose of the serotype Ia/c GBS strain C388/90. Mortality of the pups was monitored for the next 7 days.

GBS strain C388/90. None of the nineteen pups from the control groups survived the challenge compared to 24 out of 25 pups (96%) whose dams had received the semi purified rabbit antibodies (Fig. 10). The presence of circulating rabbit Sip-specific antibodies in the sera collected from these pups was confirmed by immunoblots.[27] These results clearly demonstrated that Sip-specific antibodies produced in an other animal species can efficiently cross the placental barrier to get to the fetus blood circulation and then confer protection to the newborn pups against GBS infection.

To demonstrate that maternal immunization with the Sip protein could also provide cross-protective immunity, female CD-1 mice were immunized with purified rSip protein. At the end of the immunization period, the mice were mated and the newborn pups were challenged with one of the following serotypes Ia/c, Ib, II, III or V GBS strains. From 75% up to 98% of the pups born from dams immunized with the rSip protein survived the challenge with these five serologically different GBS strains compared to < 12% for the control groups (Fig. 11). When pooled together, the protection data indicated 90% of the pups born from Sip-immunized dams survived the GBS challenge, compared to only 3% of the pups born from control dams. In all cases, the number of surviving pups in the immunized groups was shown to be significantly different ($P<0.001$, Fisher's exact test) from the number of survivors recorded in the control groups. ELISA and immunoblots indicated that maternal Sip-specific antibodies crossed the placental barrier and were found in the pups sera.[27] ELISA results indicated that there were still Sip-specific antibodies present in the sera of pups born from rSip-immunized dams 43 days after challenge (Fig. 12). This result suggests that maternal Sip-specific antibodies generated after vaccination could be present long enough in the blood circulation of newborns to confer protection against early and late onset GBS diseases.

In this section, we have presented results that clearly demonstrate that Sip protein can induce the development of a cross-reactive and protective immune response that protects against lethal GBS infection. This protein could be developed as a stand-alone vaccine or as a useful carrier protein for carbohydrate antigens from other encapsulated pathogens.

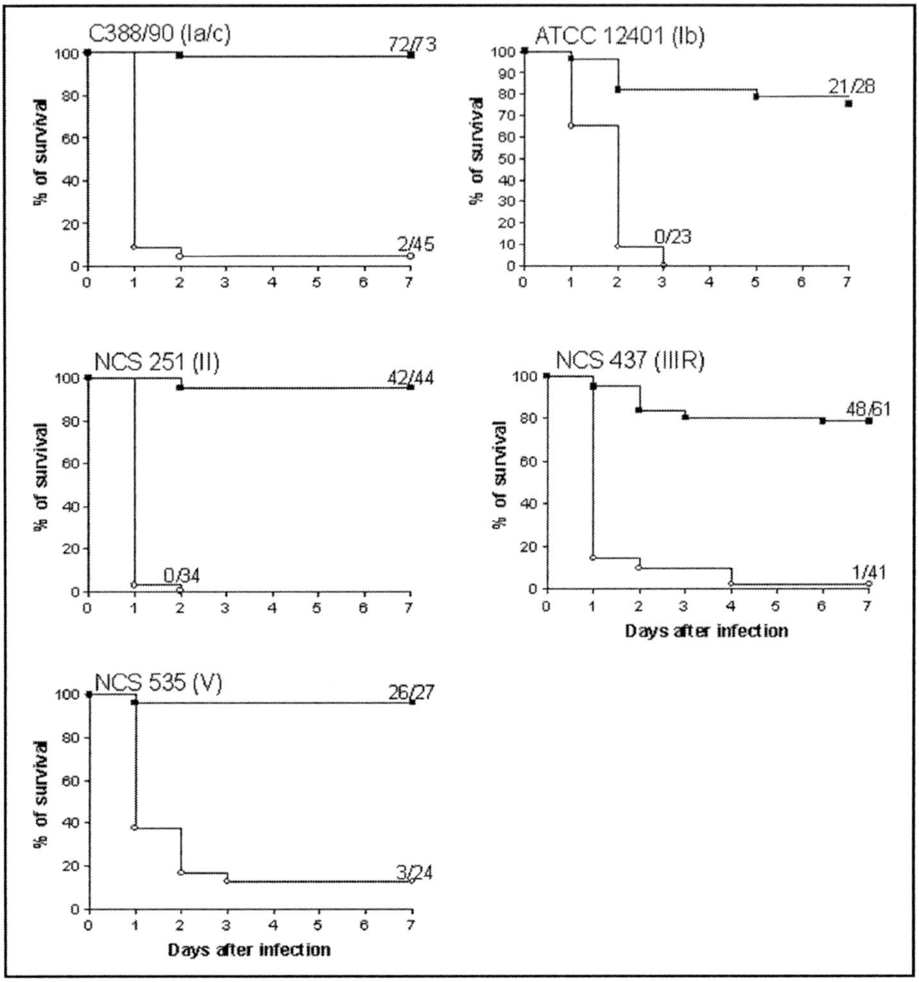

Figure 11. Protection of neonates born from female CD-1 mice immunized with purified recombinant Sip protein against lethal challenge with five different GBS strains. The pregnant mice were immunized three times with 20 μg of rSip protein (closed square) or adjuvant only (open circle) and were mated at the end of the immunization period. The pups were challenged subcutaneously with 50 μL of a GBS culture. The bacterial challenge doses were respectively adjusted to $4x10^4$, $8x10^5$, $6x10^4$, $6x10^4$ and $8x10^5$ CFU for the GBS strains C388/90 (Ia/c), ATCC12401 (Ib), NCS 251 (II), NCS 437 (IIIR) and NCS 535 (V). Number of survivors was evaluated for 7 days after challenge. The numbers of survivors in the Sip-immunized groups were shown to be statistically different from the number of survivors in the control groups with a $P<0.001$ using the Fisher's exact test.

Pneumococcal BVH Proteins

The chapter on *S. pneumoniae* vaccines presents in detail the challenges associated with this important pathogen. Emergence of antibiotic-resistant strains, poor protection in infants conferred by Ps vaccines, or serotype replacement induced by Ps conjugate vaccines emphasize the need for protein-based vaccines. Recently, our laboratory discovered antigenically conserved and protective surface-exposed proteins.[28]

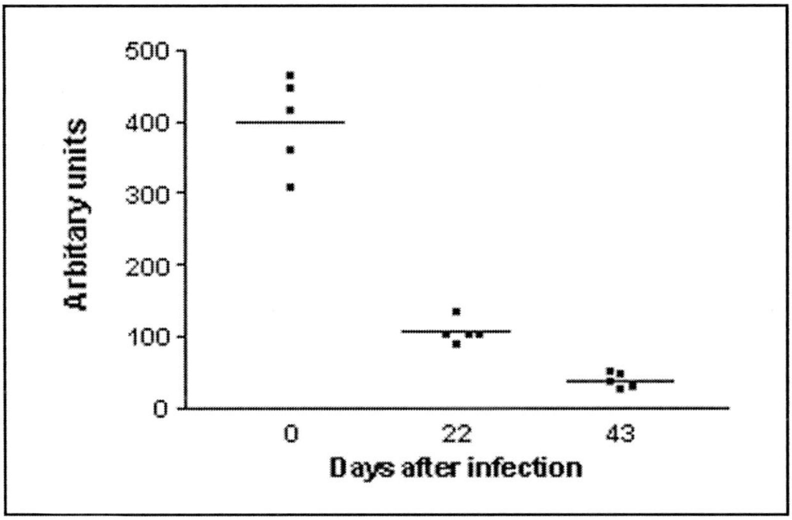

Figure 12. Evaluation of the persistence of the anti-Sip antibodies in the sera collected from certain pups born from Sip-immunized mice. Results are expressed in arbitrary units. Each square represents the ELISA value determined for an individual pup and the line represents the median ELISA value determined for every pup of the same litter. ELISA values < 1 arbitrary unit were recorded for sera collected from pups born from a control mouse injected with adjuvant only. These pups were not challenged with GBS. Maternal Sip-specific antibodies were still present 43 days after challenge.

Two previously unknown pneumococcal proteins, designated BVH-3 and BVH-11, were identified by immunoscreening of a serogroup 6 genomic expression library using human sera that were highly reactive against *S. pneumoniae.*[28] Nucleotide sequencing of the DNA inserts revealed ORFs of 3120 and 2523 bp encoding polypeptides of 1039 (BVH-3) and 840 (BVH-11) amino acid residues respectively. The calculated molecular weights are 114.6 kDa for BVH-3 and 94.4-kDa for BVH-11. Both proteins contained a predicted signal sequence typical of bacterial lipoproteins, with a cysteine as a putative cleavage and lipid attachment site. Comparison of BVH-3 protein sequences obtained from strains of different serogroups revealed 99-100% identity. Comparison of the predicted BVH-11 protein sequences revealed that they were 75% identical and 82% homologous.

To evaluate the immunogenicity and protective ability of both proteins, the genes were cloned and overexpressed in *E. coli* and the recombinant proteins purified. BALB/c mice were immunized subcutaneously with either recombinant protein two or three times at 3-week intervals. Good antibody responses were observed in ELISA, and immunoblots revealed that antibodies raised to recombinant BVH-3 and BVH-11 proteins recognized the native *S. pneumoniae* antigens. Moreover, cytofluorometry studies on live bacterial cells using mouse sera indicated that both proteins are exposed at the surface of homologous and heterologous strains.

A first protection assay was performed using an experimental sepsis model. Mice were challenged intravenously (i.v.) with 50 x LD_{50} of a heterologous serogroup 3 pneumococcal strain fourteen days following the last immunization. Mice immunized with either recombinant protein survived the challenge over a 2-week observation period. Another protection assay was then performed using an experimental pneumonia model. Fourteen days following the last injection, mice were challenged intra-nasally with 2000 x LD_{50} of a different serogroup 3 pneumococcal strain. Once again, all mice immunized with either recombinant protein survived the challenge over the 2-week observation period.

To monitor the presence of bacteria in blood and lung homogenates, some animals were sacrificed three days after an intranasal challenge. Pneumococci were not detected in blood or lung samples collected from 9 out of 10 BVH-3- and BVH-11-vaccinated mice. In contrast, bacteria were recovered in hemocultures and lung homogenates of all control-immunized mice. These results indicate that vaccination promoted the ability of mice to clear pneumococci from the lower respiratory tract and prevented septicemia and death. Overall, these assays demonstrate that both BVH-3 and BVH-11 proteins are immunogenic and provide protection in bacteremia and pneumonia animal models.[28]

In order to emphasize the importance of the humoral immune response in pneumoccal protection, rabbits were immunized with BVH-3 and BVH-11 recombinant proteins. A specific antibody response was detectable in the serum of each rabbit. Semi-purified rabbit antibodies were passively transfered to naïve mice 4 h before an i.v. challenge with 20 X LD_{50} of a serogroup 3 heterologous strain. Antibodies from animal vaccinated with either protein passively protected mice, whereas mice that received twice the amount of semi-purified antibodies from a pre-immune serum were all dead by day 2.[29]

Overall, extensive studies on BVH proteins performed in our laboratory indicate the high potential of these antigens as part of a new pneumococcal protein-based vaccine.

Conclusions

Within the next decade, many new vaccines to prevent and control all forms of infectious diseases will surely appear. Future success will be based on the development and application of new strategies such as those summarized here as well as those presented in many of the chapters of this book. In spite of many difficulties facing the future of vaccines, it is realistic to assume that, because vaccination has prevented more premature deaths and sufferings than any other medical discovery, lifelong protection will eventually be conferred against most vaccine preventable diseases.

References

1. Plotkin SA, Orenstein WA. Preface. In: Plotkin SA, Orenstein WA, eds. Vaccines. 3rd ed. Philadelphia: W B Sanders Co., 1999.
2. Hoiseth S.Vaccines, Bacterial. In: Lederberg J, ed. Encyclopedia of Microbiology. 2nd ed. San Diego: Academic Press, 2000:767-778
3. Hayrinen J, Jennings H, Raff HV et al. Antibodies to polysialic acid and its N-propyl derivative: binding properties and interaction with human embryonal brain glycopeptides. J Infect Dis 1995 ; 171:1481-1490.
4. Finne J, Bitter-Suermann D, Goridis C et al. An IgG monoclonal antibody to group B meningococci cross-reacts with developmentally regulated polysialic acid units of glycoproteins in neural and extraneural tissues. J Immunol 1987; 138:4402-4407.
5. Martin D, Cadieux N, Hamel J et al. Highly conserved Neisseria meningitidis surface protein confers protection against experimental infection. J Exp Med 1997; 185:1173-1183.
6. Cadieux N, Plante M, Rioux CR et al. Bactericidal and cross-protective activities of a monoclonal antibody directed against Neisseria meningitidis NspA outer membrane protein. Infect Immun 1999; 67:4955-4959.
7. Martin D, Brodeur BR, Hamel J et al. Candidate Neisseria meningitidis NspA vaccine. J Biotechnol 2000 ; 83:27-31.
8. Plante M, Cadieux N, Rioux CR et al. Antigenic and molecular conservation of the gonococcal NspA protein. Infect Immun 1991; 67:2855-2861.
9. Moe GR, Tan S, Granoff DM. Differences in surface expression of NspA among Neisseria meningitidis group B strains. Infect Immun 1999; 67:5664-5675.
10. Moe GR, Zuno-Mitchell P, Lee SS et al. Functional activity of anti-Neisserial surface protein A monoclonal antibodies against strains of Neisseria meningitidis serogroup B. Infect Immun 2001; 69:3762-3771.
11. Maslanka SE, Gheesling LL, Libutti, DE. Standardization and a multilaboratory comparison of Neisseria meningitidis serogroup A and C serum bactericidal assays. Clin Diagn Lab Immunol 1997; 4:156-167.

12. Jansen C, Kuipers B, van der Biezen J et al. Immunogenicity of in vitro folded outer membrane protein PorA of Neisseria meningitidis. FEMS Immunol Med Microbiol 2000; 27:227-233.
13. Peeters CC, Claassen IJ, Schuller M et al. Immunogenicity of various presentation forms of PorA outer membrane protein of Neisseria meningitidis in mice. Vaccine 1999; 17:2702-2712.
14. Niebla O, Alvarez A, Martin A et al. Immunogenicity of recombinant class 1 protein from Neisseria meningitidis refolded into phospholipid vesicles and detergent. Vaccine 2001; 19:3568-3574.
15. Carnemate T, Mesa C, Menéndez T et al. Recombinant Opc protein from Neisseria meningitidis reconstitued into liposomes elicits opsonic antibodies following immunization. Biotechnol Appl Biochem 2001; 34:63-69.
16. Kasper DL, Paoletti LC, Wessels MR et al. Immune response to type III group B streptococcal polysaccharide-tetanus toxoid conjugate vaccine. J Clin Investig 1996; 98:2308-2314.
17. Lachenauer CS, Kasper DL, Shimada J et al. Serotypes VI and VIII predominate among group B streptococci isolated from pregnant Japanese women. J Infect Dis 1999; 179:1030-1033.
18. Brodeur BR, Boyer M, Charlebois I et al. Identification of group B streptococcal Sip protein, which elicits cross-protective immunity. Infect Immun 2000; 68:5610-5618.
19. Birkeland NK. Cloning, molecular characterization, and expression of the genes encoding the lytic functions of lactococcal bacteriophage phi LC3: a dual lysis system of modular design. Can J Microbiol 1994; 40:658-665.
20. Gravekamp C, Kasper DL, Paoletti LC et al. Alpha C protein as a carrier for type III capsular polysaccharide and as a protective protein in group B streptococcal vaccines. Infect Immun 1999; 67:2491-2496.
21. Stålhammar-Carlemalm M, Stenberg L, Lindahl G. Protein Rib: a novel group B streptococcal cell surface protein that confers protective immunity and is expressed by most strains causing invasive infections. J Exp Med 1993; 177:1593-1603.
22. Ferrieri P, Flores AE. Surface protein expression in group B streptococcal invasive isolates. Adv Exp Med Biol 1997; 418:635-637.
23. Larsson,C, Stålhammar-Carlemalm M, Lindahl G. Experimental vaccination against group B streptococcus, an encapsulated bacterium, with highly purified preparations of cell surface proteins Rib and α. Infect Immun 1996; 64:3518-3523.
24. Baker CJ, Kasper DL. Correlation fo maternal antibody deficiency with susceptibility to neonatal group B streptococcal infection. N Engl J Med 1976; 294:753-756
25. Baker CJ, Rench MA, Edwards MS et al. Immunization of pregnant women with a polysaccharide vaccine of group B Streptococcus. N Engl J Med 1988; 319:1180-1185.
26. Madoff LC, Paoletti LC, Tai JY et al. Maternal immunization of mice with group B streptococcal type III polysaccharide-beta C protein conjugate elicits protective antibody to multiple serotypes. J Clin Invest 1994; 94:286-292.
27. Martin D, Rioux S, Gagnon E et al. Protection from Group B streptococcal infection in neonatal mice by maternal immunization with recombinant Sip protein. Infect Immun 2002; 70:4897-4901
28. Hamel J, Charland N, Pineau I et al. Vaccination with newly identified pneumococcal conserved surface proteins confers protection against experimental pneumonia. Poster E-65. 2001. American Society for Microbiology 101st General Meeting, Orlando, FL.
29. Charland N, Martin D, Brodeur BR et al. Passive transfer of antibodies to pneumococcal BVH-3 and BVH-11 surface proteins prevented lethal experimental infection. Poster E-39. 2002. American Society for Microbiology 102nd General Meeting, Salt Lake City, UT.
30. Pautsch A, Schulz, GE. High-resolution structure of the OmpA membrane domain, J Mol Biol 2000; 298:273-282.
31. Guex N, Peitsch MC. SWISS-MODEL and the Swiss-Pdb viewer: An environment for comparative protein modeling. Electrophoresis 1997; 18:2714-2723.

Chapter 3

DNA Vaccines

John J. Donnelly

Summary

DNA vaccines have been used widely in laboratory animals and nonhuman primates over the last decade to induce antibody and cellular immune responses. This approach has shown some promise in models of infectious diseases of both bacterial and viral origin as well as in tumor models. Clinical trials of DNA vaccines have shown that DNA vaccines need to be made much more potent to be candidates for preventive immunization of humans. This review summarizes recent work using DNA vaccines in infectious disease and tumor challenge models. This review also describes recent work to improve the delivery of plasmid DNA vaccines and also to increase the immunogenicity of antigens expressed from the DNA vaccine plasmids, including formulations, molecular adjuvants, and the use of attenuated *Salmonella* and *Shigella* bacteria to deliver plasmid to mucosal surfaces. If potency can be improved, plasmid DNA vaccines offer advantages in speed, simplicity, and breadth of immune response that may be useful for the immunization of humans against infectious diseases and cancers.

Elements of the Technology

It has been approximately 10 years since the first publications reported that immune responses could be induced by the injection into vertebrate animals of bacterial plasmids containing foreign genes driven by promoters active in eukaryotic cells (reviewed in ref. 1).[2,7] This approach to immunization has generated sustained interest because of its speed, simplicity, ability to elicit immune responses against native protein antigens with complex structures, and ability to elicit both humoral and cellular immune responses, without the need for live vectors or complex biochemical techniques.

Since the first few publications, a wide range of methods have been used to deliver plasmids including needle injection, fluid jet injection, injection followed by electroporation, bombardment with gold particles coated with DNA, and topical administration to various mucosal sites including the gut, respiratory tract, skin, and eye.[8,15] The design of the plasmids themselves has been less diverse. The most commonly used plasmids employ a minimal backbone containing a selectable marker, an origin of replication active in *E. coli*, a strong viral promoter such as CMVintA, and a transcriptional chain terminator or polyadenylation signal sequence.[16] The major exception to the trend toward small plasmids is the addition of alphavirus replicon elements. These elements comprise the replicase proteins of an alphavirus in tandem with the antigen gene of interest, which allows the alphavirus replicase to produce a large number of copies of the subgenomic mRNA encoding the antigen from the original full-length RNA that encodes both the replicase and the antigen gene.[17,18]

The potential of a DNA vaccine plasmid to induce an effective immune response is directly related to the level of expression of the encoded protein in eukaryotic cells.[16] In the case of viral

New Bacterial Vaccines, edited by Ronald W. Ellis and Bernard R. Brodeur.

antigens, alteration of codon usage to remove regulatory sequences and deletion of functional sequence elements has proven to be important for maximizing the immunogenicity of DNA vaccines.[19,22] For bacterial, protozoal, and fungal antigens, compactly folded, secreted single polypeptides that express well in eukaryotic cells may be more likely to be successful than integral membrane proteins or large heteromultimers.[23,27] The sequence composition of the plasmid itself also may play some role in immunogenicity. Oligonucleotides having the sequence purine-purine-CG-pryimidine-pyrimidine, in which the CpG sequence is unmethylated, can activate antigen-presenting cells in vitro and exert immune stimulating effects in vivo.[28,32] The presence of such sequences in bacterial plasmids may serve to increase the immunogenicity of DNA vaccines.[33]

Bacterial Vaccines

Immunization against bacteria presents a particular challenge for DNA vaccines. Unlike viral antigens, the target antigens are proteins that have not necessarily been selected through evolution for efficient expression in eukaryotic cells, and in some instances are not proteins at all. Potentially protective immune responses targeted against surface-expressed antigens have been demonstrated for DNA vaccines against *Streptococcus pneumoniae*, *Escherichia coli*, *Borrelia burgdorferi*, *Mycoplasma pulmonis*, and *Pseudomonas aeruginosa*. A DNA vaccine encoding the α-helical domain of PspA of *S. pneumoniae* induced anti-PspA antibodies.[34] This vaccine conferred protection in mice against different *S. pneumoniae* strains with distinct capsule types and serotypes of PspA.[34] Immunization by gene gun (dry powder injectors that deliver DNA intradermally, complexed to gold microbeads) with a DNA vaccine encoding a peptide mimotope of Pn type 4 capsular polysaccharide induced anti-capsular antibodies in mice.[35] This unique approach demonstrates the potential of DNA vaccines to induce immune responses against nonprotein antigens. Candidate DNA vaccines against Lyme disease have been developed that express OspA alone and also OspA and OspC as a single fusion protein.[36,37] OspC DNA vaccines were not immunogenic unless expressed as a fusion protein with OspA, illustrating the difficulty of expressing some bacterial surface proteins as DNA vaccines.[38] Both the OspA and OspA-OspC vaccine protected mice from challenge infection with *B. burgdorferi*.[38]

Immunization of mice by gene gun with a random genomic library from *M. pulmonis* also conferred protection against challenge.[39,40] A further refinement of this approach used unligated complexes comprising PCR products hybridized to a promoter and a terminator sequence.[41] These approaches, termed expression library immunization or ELI, offer a potentially useful way to screen for protective immunogens from complex pathogens. A candidate DNA vaccine against *P. aeruginosa*, expressing the major outer membrane porin OprF, induced opsonophagocytic antibodies when administered by gene gun. Mice given 3 immunizations with this DNA vaccine had lower bacterial counts and milder severity of lesions compared with control mice 8 days after pulmonary challenge with *Pseudomonas* bacteria.[42] Immunization of mice with a DNA vaccine encoding the CFA/I fimbria protein of enterotoxigenic *E. coli* (ETEC) induced serum antibodies capable of blocking the adhesion of CFA/I positive ETEC with red blood cells.[43] These studies indicate that even complex bacterial surface proteins can be expressed in vertebrates with a sufficiently native structure to induce antibodies that react with the bacteria and that have the potential to provide a protective immune response.

DNA vaccines also have been used successfully to immunize against bacterial toxins. A DNA vaccine encoding fragment C of tetanus toxoid was shown to induce antibodies in mice that were able to neutralize wild-type toxin.[44] The immunogenicity of this candidate vaccine in mice was increased substantially by modifying the codon usage to improve the quantity of protein produced in eukaryotic cells.[45] Anthrax toxin is unusual among A-B type bacterial toxins in that the B subunit (Protective Antigen or PA) is secreted separately from the two A subunits (Edema Factor or EF and Lethal Factor or LF). Final assembly of the toxin complex occurs on the surface of the target cell after the B subunit has bound to its ligand. Gene-gun immunization of mice with a combination of two plasmids encoding amino acids 175-764 of PA and 10-254 of LF induced antibodies at higher antibody titer than either component plasmid given separately. Mice given either the individual components or the combination vaccine were protected from intravenous challenge with a lethal dose of *B. anthracis* lethal toxin.[46]

DNA vaccines induce both $CD4^+$ and $CD8^+$ T-cell-mediated immune responses against viral antigens very efficiently in laboratory animals. Therefore, the ability of DNA vaccines to protect against intracellular bacteria and protozoa, where CMI is thought to play an important role in protection, has been studied extensively. Tuberculosis was the first intracellular bacterium to be studied as a target for DNA vaccines. Initially DNA vaccines against the heat shock protein HSP65 were shown to protect mice from challenge with MTb.[47,49] Immunization with DNA encoding HSP65 induced $CD4^+$ and $CD8^+$ antigen-specific T cells, with $CD8^+$ T-cell responses being best correlated with protective responses.[50] In contrast, the heat shock proteins HSP60 and HSP70 were immunogenic but did not confer protection.[51]

The antigen 85 complex (Ag85A, B and C) also has been studied extensively.[52,53] DNA vaccines encoding Ag85A were able to protect C57BL/6 mice but not BALB/c mice from challenge with MTb.[54] The protective ability of the Ag85A DNA vaccine was associated with a strong Th1 response in the C57BL/6 mice.[54] The frequency of IFN-γ-producing $CD4^+$ T cells and the protective efficacy of the vaccine was increased by boosting with recombinant Ag85A protein after a priming with intramuscular injections of Ag85A DNA vaccines.[55] Others have reported that the protective response to the MTb 63-kD protein can be increased if priming with a DNA vaccine is followed by boosting with recombinant MVA.[56] The Ag85A protein is well conserved between *M. bovis* BCG and *Mycobacterium ulcerans*, which causes Buruli ulcer, and mice immunized with DNA vaccines encoding Ag85A from *M. bovis* also were protected from intradermal challenge with *M. ulcerans*.[57] Other MTb antigens that have been used in DNA vaccines include ESAT-6, 38-kD protein, Mtb 8.4, the glycosylated surface proteins Rv1796 and Rv1860, and the culture-filtrate protein MPT64.[58-63] A DNA vaccine encoding the *M. bovis* antigen MBP83 is being studied for its ability to protect cattle from *M. bovis* infection.[64] Plasmid encoding the *M. leprae* 35-kD protein, which is common to *M. leprae* and *M. avium* but not MTb, protected mice against *M leprae* footpad challenge when given as a DNA vaccine.[65] Thus the ability of DNA vaccines to give potent Th1-type $CD4^+$ T-cell responses and to prime CTL responses may make them useful in future vaccines against tuberculosis.

DNA vaccines against *Chlamydia*, *Leishmania*, and *Brucella* also have been studied. A DNA vaccine encoding the HSP-60 gene of *C. pneumoniae* was able to protect C57BL/6 mice from intranasal challenge and the 5-to 20-fold reduction in bacterial burden seen in immunized mice was enhanced when DNA encoding IL-12 was coadministered intranasally.[66] Intradermal immunization did not protect, and IFN-γ-/- mice were not protected, indicating that a local IFN-γ response was important for the protective response.[66] BALB/c mice showed comparable reductions in lung bacterial counts following intranasal challenge after intramuscular immunization with either HSP-60 or Omp2 given as DNA vaccines.[67] A DNA vaccine encoding MOMP from serovar A *C. psittaci*, given either intramuscularly and intranasally, or intradermally by gene gun, protected turkeys from challenge with the same serovar.[68,70] Immunization of BALB/c mice by 3 intramuscular injections of DNA vaccines encoding bacterioferritin or P39 protein of *B. abortus* induced strong proliferative and IFN-γ $CD4^+$ T-cell responses and provided some protection from challenge.[71] A DNA vaccine comprised of multiple plasmids encoding the *Leishmania* antigens LACK, LmSTI1, and TSA protected C57BL/6 mice from low dose (100 promastigotes) intradermal challenge.[72] Immunized mice were unable to transmit the *L major* infection to sandfly vector fed on infected skin.[72] Where strong $CD4^+$, IFN-γ-producing T-cell responses are important for protection, DNA vaccines may be useful either alone or in combination with recombinant proteins.

Results of Initial Clinical Studies

Since 1993 many studies have been published showing that injection of plasmid DNA can elicit immune responses and protection from infectious disease and tumor challenges in a variety of laboratory animal models (reviewed in refs.1,73). A partial but by no means inclusive list comprises viruses such as influenza, herpes simplex, rabies, ebola, hantaan, and S/HIV; bacteria such as *Mycobacterium tuberculosis*, *Clostridium tetani*, *Streptococcus pneumoniae* and *Bacillus anthracis*; protozoa such as *Plasmodium yoelii* and *Leishmania manor*; and both transplanted and endogenously arising tumors expressing immunogenic oncogenes such as Her-2/neu.[3,6,24,47,52,74,81] Both antibody and cell-mediated mechanisms of protection were demonstrated in the various models, a consequence of the potent antibody, Th1, and CTL responses evoked by DNA vaccines in mice, rabbits, and nonhuman primates.

Studies to evaluate the safety and immunogenicity of DNA vaccination in humans began within two years of the first published reports of protective immune responses against infectious diseases in animals, and many studies are still ongoing. Among the first clinical studies initiated were evaluations of intramuscular injection of DNA plasmid encoding single-chain immunoglobulin variable regions (Fv's) derived from the surface immunoglobulins of B-cell lymphomas from individual patients for therapy of B-cell lymphoma;[23,82,83] intratumoral injection of plasmid encoding an MHC alloantigen, formulated in cationic lipids, for treatment of melanoma,[84,85] and intramuscular injection of HIV gp160/rev, formulated in bupivicaine, in asymptomatic HIV-positive patients.[86,88] Later, studies of the gp160/rev construct were extended to healthy subjects not infected with HIV.[89,90] A plasmid encoding circumsporozoite protein from the malaria parasite *Plasmodium falciparum*, formulated in a saline solution, was tested by intramuscular injection in healthy adult volunteers.[91,92]

In all of the clinical studies reported so far, preliminary results indicate that the DNA vaccines are generally well tolerated at doses of up to 2.5 mg of plasmid over 3^+ injections when given intramuscularly or intradermally. Intramuscular injection of plasmid DNA by needle or fluid jet injector and intradermal injection by fluid jet injector were given at doses of up to 2.5 mg per immunization.[93] In an open-label, uncontrolled, study of intratumoral injection of plasmid encoding the alloantigen HLA-B7 formulated in cationic lipids in patients with late-stage melanoma, although tumor infiltration with $CD3^+$ T cells were observed in 6/7 patients evaluated, and tumor-infiltrating CTL were found in 2/2 subjects evaluated, increases in CTL were not detected in peripheral blood of 3 subjects given 30, 100 and 300 micrograms of plasmid, respectively.[85] In an open-label, uncontrolled study of HIV gp160/rev in healthy HIV seropositives, the antibody responses seen to doses of up to 300 micrograms of plasmid encoding gp120 were minimal and 1/11 subjects exhibited a possible rise in CTL activity.[86] Robust CTL responses were seen to a DNA vaccine encoding *P. falciparum* circumsporozoite protein in 4/6 subjects after 3 doses of 2.5 mg each in an open-label dose-escalation study.[92-94] In a second study 13/14 subjects responded at this dose level.[93] Multiple epitope peptides from circumsporozoite protein were recognized in the context of both MHC Class I and II antigens by immunized subjects.[93]

In the first clinical trial of immunization by gene gun, healthy young adult volunteers were given 3 immunizations with DNA encoding hepatitis B preS2 plus S antigens.[95] Seroprotective titers of antibody against hepatitis B surface antigen (considered to be 10 mIU/mL) were seen after 3 immunizations in 11/11 healthy young adult (< 40 years of age) volunteers.[95-96] For purposes of comparison, seroprotection rates among healthy adults over 40 (a more difficult group to immunize against hepatitis B) can reach 96% after 2 immunizations (with 40 and 20 mcg, respectively) with a conventional recombinant hepatitis B vaccine plus aluminum adjuvant.[97]

Combining DNA vaccines as a priming immunization with a different modality, such are recombinant protein or a recombinant viral vector, as a boost is being studied extensively both in animal models and in humans, particularly in malaria and HIV. In malaria, priming with DNA encoding epitopes from *P. falciparum* followed by boosting with modified vaccinia Ankara (MVA) encoding the same epitopes induced strong CTL responses in animals. In a clinical study, increased CTL responses and a delay in onset of parasitemia were seen (reference in press). In HIV and SIV challenge models, boosting with MVA or adenovirus after DNA priming increased CTL responses and provided control of viremia after SIV or SHIV challenge.[98-99] Clinical studies of DNA prime/MVA and adenovirus boosts are planned. Boosting with recombinant HIV envelope protein after DNA priming induces strong neutralizing antibody responses in both rabbits and macaques and provides very effective control of viremia after challenge with a related SHIV.[100-101]

A recurring observation in the DNA vaccine clinical studies reported in the literature so far is that antibody responses induced by DNA vaccination are relatively low compared with those induced by direct injection of proteins with adjuvants. These observations are consistent with studies in which recombinant virus-like particles (VLP) and DNA vaccines comprising the L1 major capsid protein of cottontail rabbit papilloma virus were evaluated in rabbits,[102-103] but differ from reports comparing the immunogenicity of influenza HA DNA versus protein in ferrets and nonhuman primates.[104] Significant CTL responses have been reported in clinical studies, particularly when higher doses of plasmid (≥2.5 mg per immunization) were used.[91] Thus although it appears possible to induce substantial CTL responses in humans with DNA vaccines, relatively high doses of DNA may be required depending on the antigen of interest. Therefore, the development of adjuvants and excipients to increase immune responses to DNA vaccines has become an active area of research.

Adjuvants and Delivery Vehicles for DNA Vaccines

Adjuvants

Studies of methods of enhancing immune responses to the proteins expressed by DNA vaccines also have been ongoing since early in the development of this technology. Various cytokines have been used both as recombinant proteins and as cotransfected genes to stimulate immune responses to foreign proteins after intramuscular injection of plasmid DNA.[105-107] GM-CSF has shown a consistent ability to increase immune responses in a number of laboratories, while other cytokines and chemokines such as SLC, IFN-gamma, IL-2, IL-4, IL-12, and IL-18 also have been reported to modulate immune responses to DNA vaccines.[107-115] Cotransfection of accessory molecules such as CD154 and CD80 also has been reported to increase immune responses.[116-119] Modifications of intra- and extracellular trafficking including ubiquitination, lysosomal targeting, CTLA-4 and L-selectin targeting have been reported to increase different aspects of the immunogenicity of DNA vaccines. Ubiquitination increased $CD8^+$ responses while lysosomal targeting increased $CD4^+$ T-cell responses.[120-122] CTLA-4 and L-selectin fusion proteins elicited substantially increased antibody responses.[123]

Of particular interest has been the ability of the DNA itself to act as an adjuvant through the immune-stimulating effects of nonmethylated DNA sequences containing the sequence purine-purine-cytosine-guanosine-pyrimidine-pyrimidine, also known as CpG's.[28] Although bacterial DNA has long been known to activate innate mechanisms of immunity, recent work has shown that oligonucleotides containing CpG sequences are mitogenic for B cells and can act as adjuvants for protein antigens.[124] These oligonucleotides are thought to act through toll-like receptor 9 and DNA-protein kinase to activate antigen-presenting cells.[125-126] Plasmid DNA containing similar sequences can show enhanced immunogenicity,[33] while coadministration of CpG-containing oligonucleotides with DNA vaccines appears to have a negative effect.[127] CpG-containing sequences have the potential to be useful adjuvants both for protein antigens and for DNA vaccines.[32]

Delivery Vehicles

Early work in DNA vaccines included various strategies to increase the amount of protein produced after intramuscular injection of DNA. Muscle that had undergone necrosis and repair was suggested to support higher levels of expression of reporter genes. Cardiotoxin, local anesthetics such as bupivicaine, and metal salts such as barium chloride were used initially and are still used in animals in some laboratories (reviewed in refs. 1,128). Bupivicaine was used both in preclinical and clinical studies (see above), although formulations with and without bupivicaine have not been compared directly (reviewed in ref. 1).[86]

Recent work on improving the immunogenicity of DNA vaccines has focused on 3 primary areas of investigation: increasing the efficiency of transfection; stimulating the immune responses to the antigen produced; and maximizing the ability of the antigen to be presented by dendritic cells. Application of electric currents after injection of naked DNA in saline has been shown to substantially increase both the efficiency of transfection of muscle cells in vivo as well as the immune responses to the encoded antigens.[129,131] Increased immune responses have been seen in both mice and nonhuman primates. Cationic lipids have been shown to increase expression of reporter genes from DNA plasmids in various tissues, including airway epithelium and liver.[132,135] Cationic lipids also have been reported to increase the immunogenicity of DNA vaccines.[136,138] Poly (N-vinyl pyrrolidone) (PVP) has been used to formulate DNA and has been found to have some ability to increase expression and resulting immune responses in laboratory animals.[139] Ionic interactions of DNA plasmids with polymers such as poly-L-lysine, polyethyleneimine, and chitosan have been used to collapse DNA strands into microparticles and to attach targeting ligands to the resulting complexes.[140,146] These formulations have demonstrated enhanced transfection in liver and epithelial cells in vivo.[147] Addition of conventional adjuvants such as aluminum phosphate to DNA vaccines has been shown to increase their immunogenicity in laboratory animals.[148] The activity of the adjuvant was dependent on the negatively-charged DNA remaining unbound to the negatively charged adjuvant; the use of positively-charged alum adjuvants such as aluminum hydroxide ablated the immune response to the DNA vaccines.[148]

Recent work on dendritic cells (DC) has shown that presentation of antigens by DC is a potent stimulus to immune responses, particularly to cell-mediated immunity and the development of CTL. DC pulsed with peptides derived from tumor antigens or transfected ex vivo with genes encoding tumor antigens elicit highly potent antitumor immune responses in laboratory animals,[149-150] and this approach is now being attempted in clinical studies of cancer immunotherapy. Studies of DNA vaccines have shown that bone marrow-derived antigen-presenting cells play a pivotal role in the induction of CTL responses by both intramuscular and gene gun delivery.[151,156] The extent to which DCs are transfected directly by intramuscular injection of plasmid DNA is undetermined at present and may depend on the excipients used in the particular formulation of the plasmid. In gene-gun immunization, it appears that Langerhans cells (LC), the resident antigen-presenting cells (APCs) of the skin, may become directly transfected when gold particles coated with DNA are introduced by bombardment of the epidermis.[157] Thus, responses to gene gun vaccination are likely to include a component related to antigen presented directly by transfected LC. The potency of antigens presented directly by DC and LC in inducing CTL responses have made targeting of these cell types a research priority for DNA vaccination against both infectious diseases and cancer. Various ligands for DC are being evaluated as potential methods for targeting DNA vaccines directly to DC.[158]

A growing appreciation of the potential importance of transfection of APCs has led to increased interest in the formulation of DNA vaccines in or on phagocytosable particles. The biodegradable polymer, poly-lactide-coglycolide (PLG) has been widely used in medical devices and for sustained-release delivery of drugs. Several groups have investigated the entrapment of DNA in PLG microparticles as well as adsorption of DNA to PLG microparticles with modified surfaces. Initial studies of DNA entrapped in PLG focused on entrapping DNA in large particles as had been done previously for drug delivery.[159] In contrast to DNA in saline, which is largely ineffective in inducing immune responses when applied to mucosal surfaces, mucosal administration of DNA entrapped in PLG microparticles was able to induce immune responses in mice.[159] Injection of DNA entrapped in PLG microparticles resulted in prolonged persistence of the DNA with evidence for transfection of antigen-presenting cells.[160]

Entrapment of DNA in PLG microparticles prepared by homogenization subjects the DNA to shear forces and encapsulates the DNA with limited efficiency. An alternative approach that has been used is to prepare PLG microparticles with a surface charge by incorporating a charged detergent into the water/oil/water emulsion, in place of the neutral detergents such as polyvinyl alcohol that are used to make conventional PLG microparticles.[161] When a cationic detergent was used, the resulting positively-charged particles bound the negatively-charged DNA by adsorption with very high efficiency, in much the same way as alum adjuvants bind charged antigens.[162] Unlike adsorption to alum, the immunogenicity of DNA vaccines was substantially increased by adsorption to PLG.[163] The structural integrity of the DNA was very well preserved in microparticles prepared by adsorption.[162] Small (1 μm) charged PLG microparticles were shown to be transported efficiently to the regional lymph node after intramuscular injection.[164] In cell culture, DNA that had been adsorbed to charged PLG microparticles transfected immature mouse DCs much more efficiently than other agents such as lipofectin.[164] Formulation of DNA vaccines on charged microparticles significantly increased their ability to induce antibody and CTL responses in mice and nonhuman primates.[163-165]

Bacterial Delivery of DNA

A number of laboratories are seeking to exploit the ability of intracellular bacteria to deliver genes as a means of immunization. By using auxotrophic mutants that invade host cells and then lyse to liberate plasmid into the cytosol, it potentially is possible to immunize mucosally with high efficiency.[166] Such vaccines could be produced at very low cost, as purification of the DNA would not be required. Principally being studied are the Gram negative *Salmonella typhimurium* and *typhi*, *Shigella flexneri*, invasive *E. coli*, and the Gram positive *Listeria monocytogenes*. *S. flexneri* strain CVD1203 has the *aroA* auxotrophic mutation and the *iscA* mutation that prevents cell-to-cell spread.[167,168] Intranasal immunization of BALB/c mice intranasally with 10^4 CFU of *S. flexneri* containing a plasmid encoding *env* from the MN strain of HIV-1 induced $CD8^+$, IFN-γ-secreting *env*-specific T cells in the spleen 10 days later.[169] Intraperitoneal challenge of immunized mice 28 days later with 10^8 PFU of vaccinia-*env* resulted in a 3-log reduction of vaccinia titers, a similar response to that seen in mice injected IM with the plasmid.[169] The frequency of splenic IFN-γ spot-forming $CD8^+$ T cells after vaccinia-*env* challenge in the mice that received the *Shigella* vaccine was equivalent to the response in those that received the plasmid DNA IM.[169]

Immunization of *Salmonella*-susceptible BALB/c mice orally with the aroA- SL7237 strain of *S. typhimurium* harboring plasmids encoding the LLO or ActA genes of *Listeria monoctyogenes* induced $CD4^+$ and $CD8^+$ T-cell responses in spleen and serum antibodies against the *Listeria* antigens.[170] The mice also were protected from challenge with 10 LD_{50}s of wild type *L. monocytogenes* bacteria.[170] In studies using an *aroA* mutant SL7207 *S. typhimurium* strain containing a plasmid encoding HIV-1 *env*, IFN-γ spot-forming $CD8^+$ T cells were present in Peyer's patch mononuclear cells in mice that received the *Shigella* vaccine 3 times intragastrically but not in mice that received the plasmid DNA IM.[171]

Attenuated *L. monocytogenes* stably transfected with genes encoding various antigens and secreting the proteins of interest have been used to deliver protein antigens intracellularly for processing and presentation on MHC Class I molecules.[172] Recently, *Listeria* vectors have been developed based on the delta2 mutant strain that also express a *Listeria*-specific phage lysin.[173] These bacteria lyse in infected cells and can release plasmids into the cytosol.[174] This approach has been used successfully to deliver plasmids encoding GFP to mouse, cotton rat, and fish macrophages in cell culture.[173-175] Future studies will determine whether this approach can be applied successfully for immunization in vivo.

Conclusions

The early reports of the immunogenicity of plasmid DNA vaccines in laboratory animals sparked interest because of the simplicity of preparing them and their ability to deliver protein antigens with native conformational structures and to induce $CD8^+$ T cell responses. Their relevance to bacterial vaccines was not immediately obvious with the exception of mycobacterial infections, where cell-mediated immunity has long been thought to have an important role in host defense. In practice DNA vaccines have provided useful laboratory tools for studying immune responses to a wide variety of bacteria and eukaryotes. It is yet to be determined whether the mechanical problems of delivering plasmid DNA vaccines effectively to humans can be solved to enable future clinical application of this technology.

Acknowledgment

The author is grateful to Suzanne Stevenson and Nelle Cronen for their expert assistance in preparing the manuscript.

References

1. Donnelly JJ, Ulmer JB, Shiver JW et al. DNA vaccines. Annu Rev Immunol 1997; 15:617-648.
2. Tang DC, De Vit M, Johnston SA, Genetic immunization is a simple method for eliciting an immune response. Nature 1992; 356(6365):152-154.
3. Ulmer JB, Donnelly JJ, Parker SE et al. Heterologous protection against influenza by injection of DNA encoding a viral protein. Science 1993; 259(5102):1745-1749.
4. Robinson HL, Hunt LA, Webster RG. Protection against a lethal influenza virus challenge by immunization with a haemagglutinin-expressing plasmid DNA. Vaccine 1993; 11(9):957-960.
5. Wang B, Ugen KE, Srikantan V et al. Gene inoculation generates immune responses against human immunodeficiency virus type 1. Proc Natl Acad Sci USA 1993; 90(9):4156-4160.
6. Cox G, Zamb TJ, Babiuk LA. Bovine herpesvirus-1 - immune-responses in mice and cattle injected with plasmid dna. J Virol 1993; 67(9):5664-5667.
7. Fynan EF, Webster RG, Fuller DH et al. DNA vaccines: protective immunizations by parenteral, mucosal, and gene-gun inoculations. Proc Natl Acad Sci USA 1993; 90(24):11478-11482.
8. Davis HL, Michel ML, Mancini M et al. Direct gene transfer in skeletal muscle: plasmid DNA-based immunization against the hepatitis B virus surface antigen. Vaccine 1994; 12(16):1503-1509.
9. Gramzinski RA, Millan CL, Obaldia N et al. Immune response to a hepatitis B DNA vaccine in Aotus monkeys: a comparison of vaccine formulation, route, and method of administration. Mol Med 1998; 4(2):109-118.
10. Pertmer TM, Eisenbraun MD, McCabe D et al. Gene gun-based nucleic-acid immunization - elicitation of humoral and cytotoxic t-lymphocyte responses following epidermal delivery of nanogram quantities of dna. Vaccine 1995; 13(15):1427-1430.
11. Daheshia M, Kuklin N, Manickan E et al. Immune induction and modulation by topical ocular administration of plasmid DNA encoding antigens and cytokines. Vaccine 1998; 16(11-12):1103-1110.
12. Fan H, Lin Q, Morrissey GR et al. Immunization via hair follicles by topical application of naked DNA to normal skin. Nat Biotechnol 1999; 17(9):870-872.
13. Klavinskis LS, Gao L, Barnfield C et al. Mucosal immunization with DNA-liposome complexes. Vaccine 1997; 15(8):818-820.
14. Jones DH, Corris S, McDonald S et al. Poly(DL-lactide-coglycolide)-encapsulated plasmid DNA elicits systemic and mucosal antibody responses to encoded protein after oral administration. Vaccine 1997; 15(8):814-817.
15. Selby M, Goldbeck C, Pertile T et al. Enhancement of DNA vaccine potency by electroporation in vivo. In; 1999;
16. Montgomery DL, Donnelly JJ, Shiver JW et al. Protein expression in vivo by injection of polynucleotides. Curr Opin Biotechnol 1994; 5(5):505-510.
17. Dubensky TW Jr, Driver DA, Polo JM et al. Sindbis virus DNA-based expression vectors: utility for in vitro and in vivo gene transfer. J Virol 1996; 70:508-519.
18. Hariharan MJ, Driver DA, Townsend K et al. DNA immunization against herpes simplex virus: enhanced efficacy using a Sindbis virus-based vector. J Virol 1998; 72(2):950-958.

19. Haas J, Park EC, Seed B. Codon usage limitation in the expression of HIV-1 envelope glycoprotein. 1996; 6(3):315-324.
20. Shiver J, Ulmer J, Donnelly J. Humoral and cellular immunities elicited by DNA vaccines: Application to the human immunodeficiency virus and influenza. Adv Drug Del Rev 1996; 21:19-31.
21. Andre S, Seed B, Eberle J et al. Increased immune response elicited by DNA vaccination with a synthetic gp120 sequence with optimized codon usage. J Virol 1998; 72(2):1497-1503.
22. zur Megede J Chen MC, Doe B et al. Increased expression and immunogenicity of sequence-modified human immunodeficiency virus type 1 gag gene [In Process Citation]. J Virol 2000; 74(6):2628-2635.
23. King CA, Spellerberg MB, Zhu D et al. DNA vaccines with single-chain Fv fused to fragment C of tetanus toxin induce protective immunity against lymphoma and myeloma. Nat Med 1998; 4(11):p1281-1286.
24. Saikh KU, Sesno J, Brandler P et al. Are DNA-based vaccines useful for protection against secreted bacterial toxins? Tetanus toxin test case. Vaccine 1998; 16(9-10):1029-1038.
25. Lopez-Macias C, Lopez-Hernandez MA, Gonzalez CR et al. Induction of antibodies against Salmonella typhi OmpC porin by naked DNA immunization. Ann N Y Acad Sci 1995; 772:285-288.
26. Silva CL, Bonato VL, Lima VM. DNA encoding individual mycobacterial antigens protects mice against tuberculosis. Braz J Med Biol Res 1999; 32(2):231-234.
27. Weiss R, Durnberger J, Mostbock S et al. Improvement of the immune response against plasmid DNA encoding OspC of Borrelia by an ER-targeting leader sequence. Vaccine 1999; 18(9-10):815-824.
28. Krieg AM, Yi AK, Matson S et al. CpG motifs in bacterial DNA trigger direct B-cell activation. Nature 1995; 374(6522):546-549.
29. Davis HL, Weeratna R, Waldschmidt TJ et al. CpG DNA is a potent enhancer of specific immunity in mice immunized with recombinant hepatitis B surface antigen [published erratum appears in J Immunol 1999 Mar 1;162(5):3103]. J Immunol 1998; 160(2):870-876.
30. McCluskie MJ, Davis HL. CpG DNA is a potent enhancer of systemic and mucosal immune responses against hepatitis B surface antigen with intranasal administration to mice. J Immunol 1998; 161(9):4463-4466.
31. Klinman DM, Barnhart KM, Conover J. CpG motifs as immune adjuvants. Vaccine 1999; 17(1):19-25.
32. Krieg AM. CpG oligonucleotides as immune adjuvants. Ernst Schering Res Found Workshop 2000; (30):105-118.
33. Sato Y, Roman M, Tighe H et al. Immunostimulatory DNA sequences necessary for effective intradermal gene immunization. Science 1996; 273(5273):352-354.
34. Bosarge JR, Watt JM, McDaniel DO et al. Genetic immunization with the region encoding the alpha-helical domain of PspA elicits protective immunity against Streptococcus pneumoniae. Infect Immun 2001; 69(9):5456-5463.
35. Lesinski GB, Smithson SL, Srivastava N et al. A DNA vaccine encoding a peptide mimic of Streptococcus pneumoniae serotype 4 capsular polysaccharide induces specific anti-carbohydrate antibodies in Balb/c mice. Vaccine 2001; 19(13-14):1717-1726.
36. Simon MM, Gern L, Hauser P et al. Protective immunization with plasmid DNA containing the outer surface lipoprotein A gene of Borrelia burgdorferi is independent of an eukaryotic promoter. Eur J Immunol 1996; 26(12):2831-2840.
37. Zhong W, Wiesmuller KH, Kramer MD et al. Plasmid DNA and protein vaccination of mice to the outer surface protein A of Borrelia burgdorferi leads to induction of T helper cells with specificity for a major epitope and augmentation of protective IgG antibodies in vivo. Eur J Immunol 1996; 26(11):2749-2757.
38. Wallich R, Siebers A, Jahraus O et al. DNA vaccines expressing a fusion product of outer surface proteins A and C from Borrelia burgdorferi induce protective antibodies suitable for prophylaxis but Not for resolution of Lyme disease. Infect Immun 2001; 69(4):2130-2136.
39. Barry MA, Lai WC, Johnston SA. Protection against mycoplasma-infection using expression-library immunization. Nature 1995; 377(6550):632-635.
40. Lai WC, Bennett M, Johnston SA et al. Protection against Mycoplasma pulmonis infection by genetic vaccination. DNA Cell Biol 1995; 14(7):643-651.
41. Sykes KF, Johnston SA. Linear expression elements: a rapid in vivo method to screen for gene functions [see comments]. Nat Biotechnol 1999; 17(4):355-359.
42. Price BM, Galloway DR, Baker NR et al. Protection against Pseudomonas aeruginosa chronic lung infection in mice by genetic immunization against outer membrane protein F (OprF) of P. aeruginosa. Infect Immun 2001; 69(5):3510-3515.

43. Alves AM, Lasaro MO, Almeida DF et al. DNA immunisation against the CFA/I fimbriae of enterotoxigenic Escherichia coli (ETEC). Vaccine 2000; 19(7-8):788-795.
44. Anderson R, Gao XM, Papakonstantinopoulou A et al. Immunization of mice with DNA encoding fragment C of tetanus toxin. Vaccine 1997; 15(8):827-829.
45. Stratford R, Douce G, Zhang-Barber L et al. Influence of codon usage on the immunogenicity of a DNA vaccine against tetanus. Vaccine 2000; 19(7-8):810-815.
46. Price BM, Liner AL, Park S et al. Protection against anthrax lethal toxin challenge by genetic immunization with a plasmid encoding the lethal factor protein. Infect Immun 2001; 69(7):4509-4515.
47. Lowrie DB, Tascon RE, Colston MJ et al. Towards a DNA vaccine against tuberculosis. Vaccine 1994; 12(16):1537-1540.
48. Lowrie DB. DNA vaccines against tuberculosis. Curr Opin Mol Ther 1999; 1(1):30-33.
49. Silva CL. The potential use of heat-shock proteins to vaccinate against mycobacterial infections. Microbes Infect 1999; 1(6):429-435.
50. Lima KM, Bonato VL, Faccioli LH et al. Comparison of different delivery systems of vaccination for the induction of protection against tuberculosis in mice. Vaccine 2001; 19(25-26):3518-3525.
51. Turner OC, Roberts AD, Frank AA et al. Lack of protection in mice and necrotizing bronchointerstitial pneumonia with bronchiolitis in guinea pigs immunized with vaccines directed against the hsp60 molecule of Mycobacterium tuberculosis. Infect Immun 2000; 68(6):3674-3679.
52. Huygen K, Content J, Denis O et al. Immunogenicity and protective efficacy of a tuberculosis DNA vaccine. Nat Med 1996; 2(8):893-898.
53. Ulmer JB, Montgomery DL, Tang A et al. DNA vaccines against tuberculosis. 1998; 217:239-246.
54. Tanghe A, Denis O, Lambrecht B et al. Tuberculosis DNA vaccine encoding Ag85A is immunogenic and protective when administered by intramuscular needle injection but not by epidermal gene gun bombardment. Infect Immun 2000; 68(7):3854-3860.
55. Tanghe A, D'Souza S, Rosseels V et al. Improved immunogenicity and protective efficacy of a tuberculosis DNA vaccine encoding Ag85 by protein boosting. Infect Immun 2001; 69(5):3041-3047.
56. McShane H, Brookes R, Gilbert SC et al. Enhanced immunogenicity of CD4(+) t-cell responses and protective efficacy of a DNA-modified vaccinia virus Ankara prime-boost vaccination regimen for murine tuberculosis. Infect Immun 2001; 69(2):681-686.
57. Tanghe A, Content J, Van Vooren JP et al. Protective efficacy of a DNA vaccine encoding antigen 85A from Mycobacterium bovis BCG against Buruli ulcer. Infect Immun 2001; 69(9):5403-5411.
58. Kamath AT, Feng CG, Macdonald M et al. Differential protective efficacy of DNA vaccines expressing secreted proteins of Mycobacterium tuberculosis. Infect Immun 1999; 67(4):1702-1707.
59. Mollenkopf HJ, Groine-Triebkorn D, Andersen P et al. Protective efficacy against tuberculosis of ESAT-6 secreted by a live Salmonella typhimurium vaccine carrier strain and expressed by naked DNA. Vaccine 2001; 19(28-29):4028-4035.
60. Fonseca DP, Benaissa-Trouw B, van Engelen M et al. Induction of cell-mediated immunity against Mycobacterium tuberculosis using DNA vaccines encoding cytotoxic and helper T-cell epitopes of the 38-kilodalton protein. Infect Immun 2001; 69(8):4839-4845.
61. Coler RN, Campos-Neto A, Ovendale P et al. Vaccination with the T cell antigen Mtb 8.4 protects against challenge with Mycobacterium tuberculosis. J Immunol 2001; 166(10):6227-6235.
62. Garapin A, Ma L, Pescher P et al. Mixed immune response induced in rodents by two naked DNA genes coding for mycobacterial glycosylated proteins. Vaccine 2001; 19(20-22):2830-2841.
63. Delogu G, Howard A, Collins FM et al. DNA vaccination against tuberculosis: expression of a ubiquitin-conjugated tuberculosis protein enhances antimycobacterial immunity. Infect Immun 2000; 68(6):3097-3102.
64. Chambers MA, Vordermeier H, Whelan A et al. Vaccination of mice and cattle with plasmid DNA encoding the Mycobacterium bovis antigen MPB83. Clin Infect Dis 2000; 30(Suppl 3):S283-287.
65. Martin E, Roche PW, Triccas JA et al. DNA encoding a single mycobacterial antigen protects against leprosy infection. Vaccine 2001; 19(11-12):1391-1396.
66. Svanholm C, Bandholtz L, Castanos-Velez E et al. Protective DNA immunization against Chlamydia pneumoniae. Scand J Immunol 2000; 51(4):345-353.
67. Penttila T, Vuola JM, Puurula V et al. Immunity to Chlamydia pneumoniae induced by vaccination with DNA vectors expressing a cytoplasmic protein (Hsp60) or outer membrane proteins (MOMP and Omp2). Vaccine 2000; 19(9-10):1256-1265.
68. Vanrompay D, Vanloock M, Cox E et al. Genetic immunization for Chlamydia psittaci. Verh K Acad Geneeskd Belg 2001; 63(2):177-188; discussion 188-191.

69. Vanrompay D, Cox E, Vandenbussche F et al. Protection of turkeys against Chlamydia psittaci challenge by gene gun-based DNA immunizations. Vaccine 1999; 17(20-21):2628-2635.
70. Vanrompay D, Cox E, Volckaert G et al. Turkeys are protected from infection with Chlamydia psittaci by plasmid DNA vaccination against the major outer membrane protein. Clin Exp Immunol 1999; 118(1):49-55.
71. Al-Mariri A, Tibor A, Mertens P et al. Induction of immune response in BALB/c mice with a DNA vaccine encoding bacterioferritin or P39 of Brucella spp. Infect Immun 2001; 69(10):6264-6270.
72. Mendez S, Gurunathan S, Kamhawi S et al. The potency and durability of DNA- and protein-based vaccines against Leishmania major evaluated using low-dose intradermal challenge. J Immunol 2001; 166(8):5122-5128.
73. Dubensky Jr TW, Liu MA, Ulmer JB. Delivery systems for gene-based vaccines. Mol Med 2000; 6(9):723-732.
74. Xiang ZQ, Spitalnik SL, Cheng J et al. Immune responses to nucleic acid vaccines to rabies virus. Virology 1995; 209(2):569-579.
75. Vanderzanden L, Bray M, Fuller D et al. DNA vaccines expressing either the GP or NP genes of Ebola virus protect mice from lethal challenge. Virology 1998; 246(1):134-144.
76. Kamrud KI, Hooper JW, Elgh F et al. Comparison of the protective efficacy of naked DNA DNA-based Sindbis replicon and packaged Sindbis replicon vectors expressing Hantavirus structural genes in hamsters. Virology 1999; 263(1):209-219.
77. Letvin NL, Montefiori DC, Yasutomi Y et al. Potent protective anti-HIV immune responses generated by bimodal HIV envelope DNA plus protein vaccination. Proc Natl Acad Sci USA 1997; 94(17):9378-9383.
78. McDaniel LS, Loechel F, Benedict C et al. Immunization with a plasmid expressing pneumococcal surface protein A (PspA) can elicit protection against fatal infection with Streptococcus pneumoniae. Gene Ther 1997; 4(4):375-377.
79. Sedegah M, Hedstrom R, Hobart P et al. Protection against malaria by immunization with plasmid DNA encoding circumsporozoite protein. Proc Natl Acad Sci USA 1994; 91(21):9866-9870.
80. Xu D, Liew FY. Protection against leishmaniasis by injection of dna encoding a major surface glycoprotein gp63 of l-major. Immunol 1995; 84(2):173-176.
81. Amici A, Smorlesi A, Noce G et al. DNA vaccination with full-length or truncated neu induces protective immunity against the development of spontaneous mammary tumors in HER-2/neu transgenic mice. Gene Ther 2000; 7(8):703-706.
82. Spellerberg MB, Zhu D, Thompsett A et al. DNA vaccines against lymphoma: promotion of anti-idiotypic antibody responses induced by single chain Fv genes by fusion to tetanus toxin fragment C. J Immunol 1997; 159(4):1885-1892.
83. Stevenson FK, Zhu D, Spellerberg MB et al. DNA vaccination against cancer antigens. Ernst Schering Res Found Workshop 2000; (30):119-136.
84. Nabel GJ, Yang ZY, Nabel EG et al. Direct gene transfer for treatment of human cancer. Ann N Y Acad Sci 1995; 772:227-231.
85. Nabel GJ, Gordon D, Bishop DK et al. Immune response in human melanoma after transfer of an allogeneic class I major histocompatibility complex gene with DNA-liposome complexes. Proc Natl Acad Sci USA 1996; 93(26):15388-15393.
86. MacGregor RR, Boyer JD, Ugen KE et al. First human trial of a DNA-based vaccine for treatment of human immunodeficiency virus type 1 infection: safety and host response. J Infect Dis 1998; 178:92-100.
87. Ugen KE, Nyland SB, Boyer JD et al. DNA vaccination with HIV-1 expressing constructs elicits immune responses in humans. Vaccine 1998; 16(19):p1818-1821.
88. Boyer JD, Chattergoon MA, Ugen KE et al. Enhancement of cellular immune response in HIV-1 seropositive individuals: A DNA-based trial. Clin Immunol 1999; 90(1):100-107.
89. Boyer JD, Cohen AD, Vogt S et al. Vaccination of seronegative volunteers with a human immunodeficiency virus type 1 env/rev DNA vaccine induces antigen-specific proliferation and lymphocyte production of beta-chemokines. J Infect Dis 2000; 181(2):476-483.
90. MacGregor RR, Boyer JD, Ciccarelli RB et al. Safety and immune responses to a DNA-based human immunodeficiency virus (HIV) type I Env/Rev vaccine in HIV-infected recipients: follow-up data [In Process Citation]. J Infect Dis 2000; 181(1):406.
91. Wang R, Doolan DL, Le TP et al. Induction of antigen-specific cytotoxic T lymphocytes in humans by a malaria DNA vaccine. Science 1998; 282(5388):476-480.
92. Le TP, Coonan KM, Hedstrom RC et al. Safety tolerability and humoral immune responses after intramuscular administration of a malaria DNA vaccine to healthy adult volunteers. Vaccine 2000; 18(18):1893-1901.

93. Wang R, Epstein J, Baraceros FM et al. Induction of CD4(+) T cell-dependent CD8(+) type 1 responses in humans by a malaria DNA vaccine. Proc Natl Acad Sci USA 2001; 98(19):10817-10822.
94. Wang R, Doolan DL, Le TP et al. Induction of antigen-specific cytotoxic T lymphocytes in humans by a malaria DNA vaccine. Science 1998; 282:476-480.
95. Tacket CO, Roy MJ, Widera G et al. Phase 1 safety and immune response studies of a DNA vaccine encoding hepatitis B surface antigen delivered by a gene delivery device. Vaccine 1999; 17(22):2826-2829.
96. Roy MJ, Wu MS, Barr LJ et al. Induction of antigen-specific CD8+ T cells T helper cells and protective levels of antibody in humans by particle-mediated administration of a hepatitis B virus DNA vaccine. Vaccine 2000; 19(7-8):764-778.
97. Gellin BG, Greenberg RN, Hart RH et al. Immunogenicity of two doses of yeast recombinant hepatitis B vaccine in healthy older adults. J Infect Dis 1997; 175(6):1494-1497.
98. Amara RR, Villinger F, Altman JD et al. Control of a mucosal challenge and prevention of AIDS by a multiprotein DNA/MVA vaccine. Science 2001; 292(5514):69-74.
99. Barouch DH, Craiu A, Santra S et al. Elicitation of high-frequency cytotoxic T-lymphocyte responses against both dominant and subdominant simian-human immunodeficiency virus epitopes by DNA vaccination of rhesus monkeys. J Virol 2001; 75(5):2462-2467.
100. Barnett SW, Lu S, Srivastava I et al. The ability of an oligomeric human immunodeficiency virus type 1 (HIV-1) envelope antigen to elicit neutralizing antibodies against primary HIV-1 isolates is improved following partial deletion of the second hypervariable region. J Virol 2001; 75(12):5526-5540.
101. Cherpelis S, Srivastava I, Gettie A et al. DNA vaccination with the human immunodeficiency virus type 1 SF162DeltaV2 envelope elicits immune responses that offer partial protection from simian/human immunodeficiency virus infection to CD8(+) T-cell-depleted rhesus macaques. J Virol 2001; 75(3):1547-1550.
102. Jansen KU, Rosolowsky M, Schultz LD et al. Vaccination with yeast-expressed cottontail rabbit papillomavirus (CRPV) virus-like particles protects rabbits from CRPV-induced papilloma formation. Vaccine 1995; 13(16):1509-1514.
103. Donnelly JJ, Martinez D, Jansen KU et al. Protection against papillomavirus with a polynucleotide vaccine. J Infect Dis 1996; 173(2):314-320.
104. Donnelly JJ, Friedman A, Martinez D et al. Preclinical efficacy of a prototype DNA vaccine: enhanced protection against antigenic drift in influenza virus. Nat Med 1995; 1(6):583-587.
105. Xiang Z, Ertl HC. Manipulation of the immune response to a plasmid-encoded viral antigen by coinoculation with plasmids expressing cytokines. Immunity 1995; 2(2):129-135.
106. Conry RM, Widera G, Lobuglio AF et al. Selected strategies to augment polynucleotide immunization. Gene Ther 1996; 3(1):67-74.
107. Iwasaki A, Stiernholm BJ, Chan AK et al. Enhanced CTL responses mediated by plasmid DNA immunogens encoding costimulatory molecules and cytokines. J Immunol 1997; 158(10):4591-4601.
108. Barouch DH, Craiu A, Kuroda MJ et al. Augmentation of immune responses to HIV-1 and simian immunodeficiency virus DNA vaccines by IL-2/Ig plasmid administration in rhesus monkeys. Proc Natl Acad Sci USA 2000; 97(8):4192-4197.
109. Barouch DH, Santra S, Schmitz JE et al. Control of viremia and prevention of clinical AIDS in rhesus monkeys by cytokine-augmented DNA vaccination. Science 2000; 290(5491):486-492.
110. Chow YH, Huang WL, Chi WK et al. Improvement of hepatitis B virus DNA vaccines by plasmids coexpressing hepatitis B surface antigen and interleukin-2. J Virol 1997; 71(1):169-178.
111. Garren H, Ruiz PJ, Watkins TA et al. Combination of gene delivery and DNA vaccination to protect from and reverse Th1 autoimmune disease via deviation to the Th2 pathway. Immunity 2001; 15(1):15-22.
112. Kim JJ, Yang JS, Manson KH et al. Modulation of antigen-specific cellular immune responses to DNA vaccination in rhesus macaques through the use of IL-2 IFN-gamma or IL-4 gene adjuvants. Vaccine 2001; 19(17-19):2496-2505.
113. Hanlon L, Argyle D, Bain D et al. Feline leukemia virus DNA vaccine efficacy is enhanced by coadministration with interleukin-12 (IL-12) and IL-18 expression vectors. J Virol 2001; 75(18):8428-8433.
114. Billaut-Mulot O, Idziorek T, Loyens M et al. Modulation of cellular and humoral immune responses to a multiepitopic HIV-1 DNA vaccine by interleukin-18 DNA immunization/viral protein boost. Vaccine 2001; 19(20-22):2803-2811.
115. Eo SK, Lee S, Kumaraguru U et al. Immunopotentiation of DNA vaccine against herpes simplex virus via codelivery of plasmid DNA expressing CCR7 ligands. Vaccine 2001; 19(32):4685-4693.

116. Xiang R, Primus FJ, Ruehlmann JM et al. A dual-function DNA vaccine encoding carcinoembryonic antigen and CD40 ligand trimer induces T cell-mediated protective immunity against colon cancer in carcinoembryonic antigen-transgenic mice. J Immunol 2001; 167(8):4560-4565.
117. Burger JA, Mendoza RB, Kipps TJ. Plasmids encoding granulocyte-macrophage colony-stimulating factor and CD154 enhance the immune response to genetic vaccines. Vaccine 2001; 19(15-16):2181-2189.
118. Barber BH. The immunotargeting approach to adjuvant-independent subunit vaccine design. 1997; 9(5):293-301.
119. Agadjanyan MG, Kim JJ, Trivedi N et al. CD86 (B7-2) can function to drive MHC-restricted antigen-specific CTL responses in vivo. J Immunol 1999; 162(6):3417-3427.
120. Fu TM, Guan L, Friedman A et al. Induction of MHC class I-restricted CTL response by DNA immunization with ubiquitin-influenza virus nucleoprotein fusion antigens. Vaccine 1998; 16(18): 1711-1717.
121. Rodriguez F, An LL, Harkins S et al. DNA immunization with minigenes: low frequency of memory cytotoxic T lymphocytes and inefficient antiviral protection are rectified by ubiquitination. J Virol 1998; 72(6):5174-5181.
122. Rodriguez F, Zhang J, Whitton JL. DNA immunization: ubiquitination of a viral protein enhances cytotoxic T-lymphocyte induction and antiviral protection but abrogates antibody induction. J Virol 1997; 71(11):8497-8503.
123. Drew DR, Boyle JS, Lew AM et al. The comparative efficacy of CTLA-4 and L-selectin targeted DNA vaccines in mice and sheep. Vaccine 2001; 19(31):4417-4428.
124. Brazolot Millan CL, Weeratna R, Krieg AM et al. CpG DNA can induce strong Th1 humoral and cell-mediated immune responses against hepatitis B surface antigen in young mice. Proc Natl Acad Sci USA 1998; 95(26):15553-15558.
125. Chu W, Gong X, Li Z et al. DNA PKcs is required for activation of innate immunity by immunostimulatory DNA. Cell 2000; 103:909-918.
126. Hemmi H, Takeuchi O, Kawai T et al. A Toll-like receptor recognizes bacterial DNA. Nature 2000; 408(6813):740-745.
127. Weeratna R, Brazolot MC, Krieg AM et al. Reduction of antigen expression from DNA vaccines by coadministered oligodeoxynucleotides. 1998; 8(4):351-356.
128. Wells DJ, Maule J, McMahon J et al. Evaluation of plasmid DNA for in vivo gene therapy: factors affecting the number of transfected fibers. J Pharm Sci 1998; 87(6):763-768.
129. Bachy M, Boudet F, Bureau M et al. Electric pulses increase the immunogenicity of an influenza DNA vaccine injected intramuscularly in the mouse. Vaccine 2001; 19(13-14):1688-1693.
130. Selby M, Goldbeck C, Pertile T et al. Enhancement of DNA vaccine potency by electroporation in vivo. J Biotechnol 2000; 83(1-2):147-152.
131. Widera G, Austin M, Rabussay D et al. Increased DNA vaccine delivery and immunogenicity by electroporation in vivo. J Immunol 2000; 164(9):4635-4640.
132. Logan JJ, Bebok Z, Walker LC et al. Cationic lipids for reporter gene and CFTR transfer to rat pulmonary epithelium. Gene Ther 1995; 2(1):38-49.
133. Parker SE, Ducharme S, Norman J et al. Tissue distribution of the cytofectin component of a plasmid-DNA/cationic lipid complex following intravenous administration in mice. Hum Gene Ther 1997; 8(4):393-401.
134. McCluskie MJ, Chu Y, Xia JL et al. Direct gene transfer to the respiratory tract of mice with pure plasmid and lipid-formulated DNA. Antisense Nucleic Acid Drug Dev 1998; 8(5):401-414.
135. Mahato RI, Anwer K, Tagliaferri F et al. Biodistribution and gene expression of lipid/plasmid complexes after systemic administration. Hum Gene Ther 1998; 9(14):2083-2099.
136. Gregoriadis G, Saffie R, de Souza JB. Liposome-mediated DNA vaccination. FEBS Lett 1997; 402(2-3):107-110.
137. Hartikka J, Bozoukova V, Ferrari M et al. Vaxfectin enhances the humoral immune response to plasmid DNA-encoded antigens. Vaccine 2001; 19(15-16):1911-1923.
138. Perrie Y, Frederik PM, Gregoriadis G. Liposome-mediated DNA vaccination: the effect of vesicle composition. Vaccine 2001; 19(23-24):3301-3310.
139. Mumper RJ, Duguid JG, Anwer K et al. Polyvinyl derivatives as novel interactive polymers for controlled gene delivery to muscle. Pharm Res 1996; 13(5):701.
140. Wu GY, Wilson JM, Shalaby F et al. Receptor-mediated gene delivery in vivo Partial correction of genetic analbuminemia in Nagase rats. J Biol Chem 1991; 266(22):14338-14342.
141. Perales MA, Schwartz DH, Fabry JA et al. A vaccinia-gp160-based vaccine but not a gp160 protein vaccine elicits anti-gp160 cytotoxic T lymphocytes in some HIV-1 seronegative vaccinees. J Acquir Immune Defic Syndr Hum Retrovirol 1995; 10(1):27-35.

142. Nishikawa M, Takemura S, Takakura Y et al. Targeted delivery of plasmid DNA to hepatocytes in vivo: optimization of the pharmacokinetics of plasmid DNA/galactosylated poly(L-lysine) complexes by controlling their physicochemical properties. J Pharmacol Exp Ther 1998; 287(1):408-415.
143. Adami RC, Collard WT, Gupta SA et al. Stability of peptide-condensed plasmid DNA formulations. J Pharm Sci 1998; 87(6):678-683.
144. MacLaughlin FC, Mumper RJ, Wang J et al. Chitosan and depolymerized chitosan oligomers as condensing carriers for in vivo plasmid delivery. J Control Release 1998; 56(1-3):259-272.
145. Orson FM, Kinsey BM, Hua PJ et al. Genetic immunization with lung-targeting macroaggregated polyethyleneimine-albumin conjugates elicits combined systemic and mucosal immune responses. J Immunol 2000; 164(12):6313-6321.
146. Erbacher P, Bettinger T, Belguise-Valladier P et al. Transfection and physical properties of various saccharide poly(ethylene glycol) and antibody-derivatized polyethylenimines (PEI). J Gene Med 1999; 1(3):210-222.
147. Cui Z, Mumper RJ. Chitosan-based nanoparticles for topical genetic immunization. J Control Release 2001; 75(3):409-419.
148. Ulmer JB, DeWitt CM, Chastain M et al. Enhancement of DNA vaccine potency using conventional aluminum adjuvants. Vaccine 1999; 18(1-2):18-28.
149. Fields RC, Shimizu K, Mule JJ. Murine dendritic cells pulsed with whole tumor lysates mediate potent antitumor immune responses in vitro and in vivo. Proc Natl Acad Sci USA 1998; 95(16):9482-9487.
150. Shimizu K, Fields RC, Giedlin M et al. Systemic administration of interleukin 2 enhances the therapeutic efficacy of dendritic cell-based tumor vaccines. Proc Natl Acad Sci USA 1999; 96(5):2268-2273.
151. Fu TM, Ulmer JB, Caulfield MJ et al. Priming of cytotoxic T lymphocytes by DNA vaccines: requirement for professional antigen presenting cells and evidence for antigen transfer from myocytes. Mol Med 1997; 3:362-371.
152. Ulmer JB, Deck RR, DeWitt CM et al. Generation of MHC class I-restricted cytotoxic T lymphocytes by expression of a viral protein in muscle cells: antigen presentation by nonmuscle cells. Immunol 1996; 89(1):59-67.
153. Huang AY, Golumbek P, Ahmadzadeh M et al. Role of bone marrow-derived cells in presenting MHC class I restricted tumor antigens. Science 1994; 264:961-965
154. Condon C, Watkins SC, Celluzzi CM et al. DNA-based immunization by in vivo transfection of dendritic cells. Nat Med 1996; 2(10):1122-1128.
155. Manickan E, Kanangat S, Rouse RJ et al. Enhancement of immune response to naked DNA vaccine by immunization with transfected dendritic cells. J Leukoc Biol 1997; 61:125-132.
156. Doe B, Selby M, Barnett S et al. Induction of cytotoxic T lymphocytes by intramuscular immunization with plasmid DNA is facilitated by bone marrow-derived cells. Proc Natl Acad Sci USA 1996; 93(16):8578-8583.
157. Porgador A, Irvine KR, Iwasaki A et al. Predominant role for directly transfected dendritic cells in antigen presentation to CD8+ T cells after gene gun immunization. J Exp Med 1998; 188(6):p1075-1082.
158. Barry MA, Johnston SA. Biological features of genetic immunization. Vaccine 1997; 15(8):788-791.
159. Barnes AG, Barnfield C, Brew R et al. Recent developments in mucosal delivery of pDNA vaccines. Curr Opin Mol Ther 2000; 2(1):87-93.
160. Lunsford L, McKeever U, Eckstein V et al. Tissue distribution and persistence in mice of plasmid DNA encapsulated in a PLGA-based microsphere delivery vehicle. J Drug Target 2000; 8(1):39-50.
161. Singh M, Briones M, Ott GS et al. Cationic microparticles: a potent delivery system for DNA vaccines. Proc Natl Acad Sci USA 2000.
162. Briones M, Singh M, Ugozzoli M et al. The preparation, characterization and evaluation of cationic microparticles for DNA vaccine delivery. Pharm Res 2001; 18(5):709-711.
163. O'Hagan D, Singh M, Ugozzoli M et al. Induction of potent immune responses by cationic microparticles with adsorbed HIV DNA vaccines. J Virol 2001; 75(19):9037-9043.
164. Denis-Mize KS, Dupuis M, MacKichan ML et al. Plasmid DNA adsorbed onto cationic microparticles mediates target gene expression and antigen presentation by dendritic cells. Gene Ther 2000; 7(24):2105-2112.
165. Otten GR, Chen M, Doe B et al. Delivery Technologies Enhance Plasmid DNA Vacccination in a Rhesus Macaque Model for HIV. In: 8th Conference on Retroviruses and Opportunistic Infections; 2001. Chicago: Illinois, 2001:
166. Mollenkopf H, Dietrich G, Kaufmann SH. Intracellular bacteria as targets and carriers for vaccination. Biol Chem 2001; 382(4):521-532.

167. Sizemore DR, Branstrom AA, Sadoff JC. Attenuated Shigella as a DNA delivery vehicle for DNA-mediated immunization. Science 1995; 270(5234):299-302.
168. Shata MT, Stevceva L, Agwale S et al. Recent advances with recombinant bacterial vaccine vectors. Mol Med Today 2000; 6(2):66-71.
169. Shata MT, Hone DM. Vaccination with a Shigella DNA vaccine vector induces antigen-specific CD8(+) T cells and antiviral protective immunity. J Virol 2001; 75(20):9665-9670.
170. Darji A, zur Lage S, Garbe AI et al. Oral delivery of DNA vaccines using attenuated Salmonella typhimurium as carrier. FEMS Immunol Med Microbiol 2000; 27(4):341-349.
171. Shata MT, Reitz Jr MS, DeVico AL et al. Mucosal and systemic HIV-1 Env-specific CD8(+) T-cells develop after intragastric vaccination with a Salmonella Env DNA vaccine vector. Vaccine 2001; 20(3-4):623-629.
172. Frankel FR, Hegde S, Lieberman J et al. Induction of cell-mediated immune responses to human immunodeficiency virus type 1 Gag protein by using Listeria monocytogenes as a live vaccine vector. J Immunol 1995; 155(10):4775-4782.
173. Spreng S, Dietrich G, Niewiesk S et al. Novel bacterial systems for the delivery of recombinant protein or DNA. FEMS Immunol Med Microbiol 2000; 27(4):299-304.
174. Gentschev I, Dietrich G, Spreng S et al. Recombinant attenuated bacteria for the delivery of subunit vaccines. Vaccine 2001; 19(17-19):2621-2628.
175. Dietrich G, Kolb-Maurer A, Spreng S et al. Gram-positive and Gram-negative bacteria as carrier systems for DNA vaccines. Vaccine 2001; 19(17-19):2506-2512.

Chapter 4

Live, Attenuated *Salmonella* Vaccine Vectors

Sims K. Kochi and Kevin P. Killeen

Introduction

There were few effective means available for preventing human infectious diseases prior to the beginning of the 19th century, and millions of people succumbed to smallpox, cholera, diphtheria, typhoid fever, and influenza. In the late 1700s, Edward Jenner conceived the notion to vaccinate humans with a naturally attenuated virus to protect against smallpox infection. More than a century later, Louis Pasteur established the basis of modern live, attenuated vaccine technology by intentionally attenuating a microorganism and using it to vaccinate humans against infection1. The number of vaccines available in 21st century industrialized countries has increased considerably since the times of Jenner and Pasteur (Fig. 1). The ease with which people travel today from one country to another has increased to an estimated 2.5 billion travelers per year. Virtually any place in the world can be reached within 36 hours, less than the incubation period for most infectious diseases. Thirty million people alone trek to regions every year where Hepatitis A is endemic, and many others face potential exposure to diarrhea-causing bacteria, typhoid and yellow fever, and malaria. Vaccines for many of these diseases are inadequate or do not exist. There also continues to be a pressing need for similar types of vaccines in developing countries and particularly those ravaged by natural disaster or civil war. These needs are accentuated by an increasing polarization between the standards of living of rich and poor nations and make issues of vaccine cost and availability plainly evident.

The early vaccines produced by Pasteur and others were attenuated through methods such as repeated passaging in culture. It was soon evident, however, that the use of empirical approaches like these was associated with health risks due to residual pathogenicity. During the past decade, advances in recombinant DNA technology and in the structural and functional analyses of genomes and gene products from a wide variety of microorganisms have made it possible to design a new generation of rationally attenuated vaccines against bacterial infections. Attenuated bacteria are an attractive means of delivering recombinant antigens for a number of reasons: 1) they are inexpensive to manufacture; 2) they are practical for large-scale distribution; 3) antigen delivery is simple (e.g., oral), facilitating a high level of patient compliance; 4) the natural tissue tropism of the vector targets recombinant antigens to inductive sites of immunity; and 5) attenuated vectors can be genetically engineered to express more than one antigen, generating potential protection against multiple diseases with a limited dosing regimen.

It has been estimated that 90% of human infectious diseases are initiated at mucosal surfaces.[2] For this reason, new strategies for developing vaccines intended to prevent infection of the mucosa are actively being pursued. Many of these strategies exploit the advantages of live, attenuated bacterial vectors to express protective antigens of heterologous microorganisms. The applicability of these methods has been studied most extensively with attenuated mutants of *Salmonella enterica* serovar Typhi (*S. typhi*) and *S. enterica* serovar Typhimurium

New Bacterial Vaccines, edited by Ronald W. Ellis and Bernard R. Brodeur.

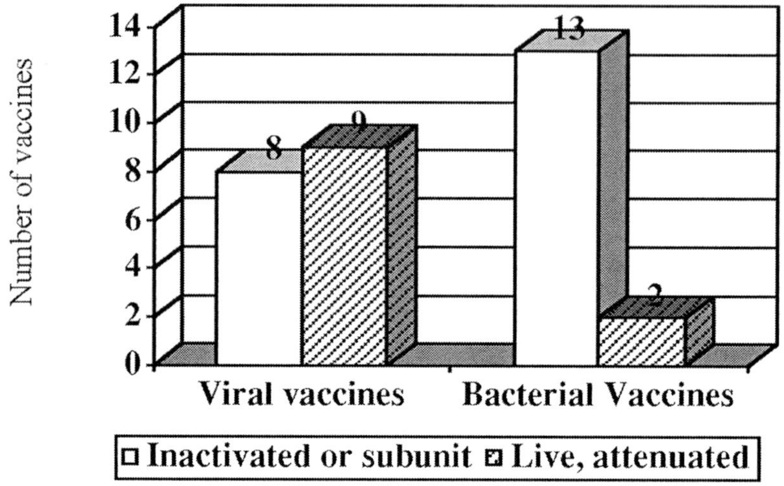

Figure 1. Comparison of the number of viral and bacterial vaccines commercially available in the U.S. in 1994 distributed according to vaccine type.

(*S. typhimurium*) and evaluated using more than 50 different bacterial, viral, and protozoan antigens in both animal models and humans.[2,3] The development of new *S. typhi*-based vectors has been limited by the narrow host range of *S. typhi* and a paucity of appropriate animal models. Since humans are the only known natural host for *S. typhi*, many of the strategies for producing attenuated mutants were initially identified as attenuating in *S. typhimurium*, as discussed below (see Section *Live, Attenuated Salmonella Vaccines and Vectors; Evolution of Attenuated Salmonella Vaccine Vectors; Alternative S. typhi Pre-Clinical Models* in this chapter). It is beyond the scope of this chapter to survey the extensive preclinical efforts that have led to the current state of development of *Salmonella* vectors or to examine the importance of mucosal immunity in vaccine development. Rather, we will limit our review to the more recent advances made in the evaluation and development of safer and more effective attenuated *Salmonella* vectors for use in humans. We will begin by examining the methods used to produce attenuated *Salmonella* vector strains and the effect of these methods on vector immunogenicity and protective efficacy. In addition, we will discuss expressions systems that show promise for enhancing the efficiency of attenuated *Salmonella* to deliver foreign or heterologous antigens. Finally, we will discuss the potential of attenuated *Salmonella* vectors as delivery systems for new vaccine technologies such as plasmid DNA immunization and for novel vaccines in health care areas including cancer and bioterrorism.

Live, Attenuated *Salmonella* Vaccines and Vectors

Pathogenic salmonellae are highly host restricted and invade by crossing the intestinal mucosa via specialized microfold (M) cells and colonizing gut-associated lymphoid tissues (GALT). Eventually, the bacteria pass through the draining mesenteric lymph nodes into the bloodstream and spread to other tissues like the spleen and liver where they replicate and grow in macrophages and other niches of the reticulo-endothelial system.[4] Therefore, a critical requirement in the development of clinically useful *Salmonella* vectors is the production of mutants that are highly attenuated for invasiveness. Immunization with attenuated strains of *Salmonella* primes the host to produce antigen-specific immune responses, including the production of MHC class I-restricted $CD8^+$ and class II-restricted $CD4^+$ T lymphocytes. Oral vaccination with the live, attenuated typhoid fever vaccine, *S. typhi* Ty21a, elicits production of anti-*Salmonella* mucosal secretory immunoglobulin A (sIgA)[5] and systemic (serum IgG) antibody responses as well as $CD8^+$ T cells.[6-9] The ability of attenuated *Salmonella* strains to induce cytotoxic T-lymphocyte (CTL) responses is an interesting property of a bacterium generally believed to reside in phagolysosomal compartments of infected cells. As we will discuss below, this feature has facilitated the development of attenuated *Salmonella* strains as a broad-based vaccine delivery platform.

Evolution of Attenuated Salmonella *Vaccine Vectors*

S. typhi Ty21a

Salmonella typhi Ty21a is the only live, attenuated typhoid fever vaccine currently licensed in the United States for use in humans. The basis for the attenuation of Ty21a is a mutation in *galE*, but the strain carries additional mutations that undoubtedly contribute to its avirulence.[10] The first report of an avirulent *Salmonella* strain expressing a foreign antigen described Ty21a transformed with the *Shigella sonnei* virulence plasmid and expressing the *S. sonnei* cell surface form I antigen (lipopolysaccharide [LPS])[11]. Animal studies demonstrated that Ty21a expressing *S. sonnei* LPS (rTy21a) induced the production of protective anti-vector and anti–*Shigella* antibodies following challenge. The safety of rTy21a was confirmed in several human studies as well as the ability to stimulate detectable IgA immune responses to *S. sonnei* O-antigen.[12,13] However, the inability to show reproducible immunogenicity in volunteers with five subsequent lots of vaccine prevented the further clinical development of rTy21a.[14] Subsequent studies in humans using Ty21a and its derivatives to deliver other heterologous antigens supported the limited applications of Ty21a as a vaccine vector.[15,16] The reasons for the ineffectiveness of Ty21a as a vaccine vector were not determined in these studies but may have been due to low antigen expression in vivo, poor antigen presentation, or the weak immunogenicity of the vector.[15-17] The lessons learned from the development of Ty21a have nevertheless contributed greatly to subsequent efforts to develop safe and immunogenic *Salmonella* vaccines and vectors.

S. typhi Aromatic Amino Acid Biosynthesis Mutants

S. typhi CVD 908

The typhoid fever vaccine candidate, *S. typhi* 541Ty, was derived from a *S. typhi* Ty2 parental strain and was one of the first *S. typhi*-based vaccines to be created by the targeted deletion of genes with known function. *Salmonella typhi* 541Ty was constructed with precise deletions in genes involved in the biosynthesis of aromatic amino acids (*aroA)* and purines (*purA*).[18] The subsequent evaluation of 541Ty in human volunteers showed that, while the vaccine was well tolerated, it was less immunogenic than Ty21a,[19] and therefore not considered for further development. The over-attenuation of 541Ty, a probable result of having mutations in two distinct biosynthetic pathways, suggested that a strain with a mutation in a single biosynthetic pathway might result in a more viable vaccine candidate. An attenuated strain based on this idea was created by disrupting the function of AroC and AroD, gene products required for aromatic amino acid biosynthesis in *S. typhi* Ty2.[20] The resulting vaccine strain, *S. typhi* CVD 908, carried targeted deletions in two separate genes as a safety measure to limit the effect that reversion of one of the mutations would have on the overall virulence of the vaccine strain.[21] *Salmonella typhi* CVD 908 was shown to be well-tolerated and immunogenic in volunteers given single, oral doses of the vaccine, and ~90% of vaccinees developed antibodies to *S. typhi* specific antigens.

Based on its promising immunogenicity profile, CVD 908 expressing a protozoan antigen was evaluated for its ability to elicit a productive immune response against an intracellular parasite, *Plasmodium falciparum*. In preclinical testing, an attenuated *S. typhimurium* mutant expressing an immunogenic fragment from the *P. falciparum* circumsporozite protein (CSP) was shown to induce CSP-specific cell-mediated immunity and to protect mice against sporozoite challenge.[22] *Salmonella typhi* CVD 908 expressing the same CSP fragment (CVD 908Ω) provoked no serious adverse events when administered in a single, oral dose to 10 volunteers.[23] Most of the volunteers shed the vector over a period of several days and developed serologic responses to the *S. typhi* O and H antigens. However, only two of the volunteers developed detectable anti-sporozoite antibody responses, and only one vaccinee responded with a CSP-specific $CD8^+$ CTL response. The results of this study were important in that they were the first to show that attenuated *S. typhi* could be used as a vector in humans to induce serological or cellular immune responses against a heterologous antigen.

S. typhi CVD 908-*htrA*

In spite of the limited success of CVD 908 Ω, a propensity to cause bacteremia in volunteers receiving moderately high doses limited the clinical development of the vaccine. To address this issue, CVD 908 was further attenuated by deleting *htrA* (CVD 908-*htrA*), a heat shock response-associated protease that produced a phenotype in *S. typhimurium* that was more susceptible to oxidative stress than the parent strain.[24] CVD 908-*htrA* was evaluated in human clinical studies and did not cause bacteremia, although a few volunteers receiving the higher vaccine dose reported mild diarrhea.[25] Anti-LPS IgA antibody-secreting cells were detected in 90-100% of vaccinees, and about one-half of the volunteers developed serologic anti-LPS IgG responses. An evaluation of CVD 908-*htrA* as a vaccine vector was originally tested using the well-characterized and highly immunogenic nontoxic, fragment C of tetanus toxin (tetanus toxoid).[26] Volunteers were given a single, oral dose of the recombinant CVD 908-*htrA* strain, and the safety and immune responses to *S. typhi*-specific antigens and tetanus toxoid were evaluated. Results from this study confirmed the safety of the recombinant vaccine and no incidents of bacteremia or fever were reported at any dose. However, only three of the nine vaccinees who received doses containing 10^8 or 10^9 colony-forming units (cfu) developed any increase in serum anti-tetanus toxoid levels. Moreover, only one of the three patients who seroconverted began the study with a preimmune anti-tetanus toxoid titer at a level considered naive. The increase in post-immunization anti-tetanus toxoid titers of the other two volunteers was most likely due to boosting pre-existing immunity. Interestingly, the expression of fragment C also negatively impacted the ability of CVD 908-*htrA* to induce effective anti-vector antibody and cellular immune responses, which were less frequent than those previously observed in volunteers who were given the vector only. This observation highlights the difficulty of balancing antigen expression sufficient to induce an adequate immune response without adversely affecting vector fitness.

S. typhi Mutants Bearing Mutations in Regulatory Genes

S. typhi chi^{4073}

The elucidation of microbial metabolic pathways and the identification of the gene products involved were events that directly contributed to the development of improved *Salmonella* vectors attenuated by deficiencies in aromatic amino acid biosynthesis. Similar revelations led to the development of attenuated *Salmonella* strains bearing mutations involved in the transcriptional regulation of gene expression. Preclinical studies with *S. typhimurium* demonstrated that deletions in the *cya* (adenylate cyclase) and the *crp* (cyclic AMP receptor protein) genes resulted in significantly reduced virulence in mice.[27] *S. typhimurium* mutants bearing these deletions were very stable and, unlike *aro* or *gal* mutants, were less capable of colonizing the spleens of infected animals. A deletion in the *cdt* gene was shown to diminish further the ability of mutants to reach and persist in deep tissues.[28] Based on results in both animal models and in humans, a triple-deletion mutant, chi^{4073}(*ΔcyaΔcrpΔcdt*), was developed that did not cause bacteremia when initially tested as a single oral-dose vaccine in adult volunteers.[29] Furthermore, chi^{4073} was immunogenic and induced seroconversion to *S. typhi* LPS and stimulated the production of IgA secreting lymphocytes.

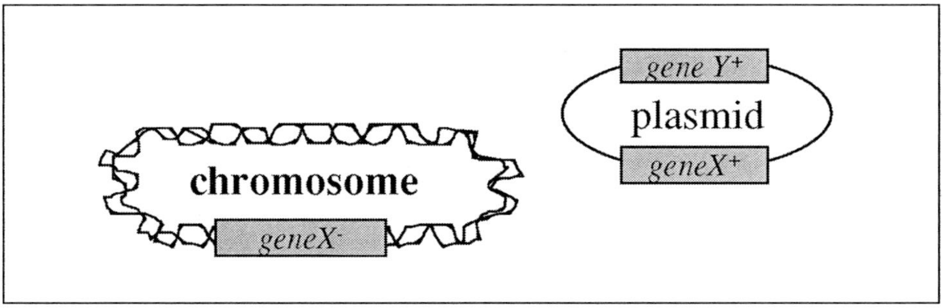

Figure 2. Diagrammatic representation of a balanced-lethal plasmid-host expression system. Gene "X" encodes an essential cellular metabolic function; gene "Y" encodes a heterologous antigen.

S. typhi chi^{4632}

The development of chi^{4073} as a vaccine vector introduced the concept of a balanced-lethal plasmid expression system (Fig. 2).[30] At the time that chi^{4632} ((*ΔcyaΔcrp-cdt*) *Δasd*) was created,[29] methods for expressing heterologous antigens in *Salmonella* were generally based on recombinant plasmids carrying antibiotic resistance markers to facilitate identification and select against plasmid loss. While this strategy generally worked in vitro, these plasmids tended to be unstable in vivo in the absence of selective antibiotic pressure.[31] An alternative approach—chromosomal integration of a single-copy foreign gene—also proved unsatisfactory, since higher gene copy numbers were shown generally to result in more vigorous host immune responses.[17,32,33] *Salmonella typhi* chi^{4632} utilized a balanced-lethal plasmid to allow stable, high-level expression of heterologous antigens in the absence of drug selection. *Salmonella* bearing mutations in *asd* (aspartate semi-aldehyde dehydrogenase) grow only in the presence of an exogenous source of diaminopimelic acid or when transformed with a complementing Asd$^+$ balanced-lethal plasmid.

The efficiency of chi^{4632} as a vaccine vector was evaluated in volunteers receiving a single, oral dose of chi^{4632} carrying plasmid pYA3167, an Asd$^+$ balanced-lethal plasmid expressing a hepatitis B virus core/preS1 hybrid fusion protein. Six of the seven volunteers immunized orally and one of six volunteers vaccinated rectally seroconverted against *S. typhi* LPS, and several volunteers developed anti-LPS sIgA responses. However, only one LPS seropositive vaccinee developed a serum anti-preS1 antibody response.[29] In a second study, *S. typhi* chi^{4632} (pYA3167) was given orally to 10 human volunteers. While most of the volunteers developed *S. typhi*-specific serum antibody responses and produced anti-*S. typhi* specific antibody secreting cells, none of the vaccinees developed serum antibody to the HBV preS1 envelope protein.[34]

S. typhi Bearing Mutations in Virulence-Associated Genes

S. typhi Ty445

Strain Ty445 was the first typhoid fever vaccine candidate produced based on the concept of attenuating two different cell functions: amino acid biosynthesis and virulence.[35] The idea of attenuating virulence is predicated on the notion that genes required for virulence generally encode nonessential or dispensable functions. Therefore, the deletion of such genes should not significantly compromise growth in vivo or the ability to induce an immune response. Ty445 was originally based on an *aroA* mutant of *S. typhi* Ty2. Previous studies including those with CVD 908 suggested that an *aroA S. typhi* mutant could potentially be reactogenic in humans. To further attenuate Ty2Δ*aroA*, additional deletions were introduced into *phoP* and *phoQ*. The *phoPQ* regulon was first identified in *S. typhimurium* as a prototypical bacterial two-component regulatory system, comprised of a membrane-associated sensor kinase (PhoQ) and a cytoplasmic transcriptional regulator (PhoP).[36,37] The *phoPQ* locus was shown to regulate multiple, unlinked *phoP*-activated and -repressed genes necessary for *Salmonella* virulence, and *phoP/Q* null mutants were markedly attenuated in mice.[36] *S. typhi* Ty445 was well tolerated when it was evaluated in a one- or two-dose oral regimen in humans.[35] However, only 2 of 14 volunteers given two doses of the vaccine produced significant serum IgG responses to *S. typhi* whole-cell lysates or LPS O-antigen. Based on its limited immunogenicity, the clinical development of Ty445 was discontinued.

S. typhi Ty800

The observation that very large doses of *S. typhi* Ty445 were well-tolerated, but only modestly immunogenic, catalyzed the development of Ty800, a *S. typhi* Ty2 derivative carrying a deletion mutation only in *phoPQ*. In a limited phase I clinical study, Ty800 was shown to be well tolerated and immunogenic after single, oral doses ranging from ~10^7-10^{10} cfu.[38] Furthermore, the majority of vaccinees who seroconverted also developed large numbers of IgA-secreting cells, suggesting vigorous mucosal immune responses.

The evaluation of Ty800 as a suitable vaccine vector in humans was initially performed in four volunteers given single, oral doses of a *S. typhi* Ty800 *asd* mutant carrying plasmid pYA3167, an Asd^+ balanced lethal plasmid encoding a hybrid hepatitis B virus fusion protein. Three of four volunteers given the vaccine seroconverted against the vector, but none developed serologic immune responses to the hybrid fusion protein (K. Killeen and E. Hohmann, unpublished observations). Further evaluation of Ty800 as a vector was conducted using the enzymatically inactive structural subunits of *Helicobacter pylori* urease (UreA/B) as a model antigen.[39] Preclinical studies evaluating immune responses to *H. pylori* UreA/B in mice, had shown previously that animals orally immunized with a *ΔphoPQ* strain of *S. typhimurium* expressing UreA/B developed strong serological and mucosal anti-UreA/B immune responses.[40,41] Based on these results, a recombinant Ty800 *purB* mutant carrying a $PurB^+$ balanced-lethal plasmid encoding UreA/B (Ty1033) was constructed and evaluated in humans. In a phase I inpatient study, eight volunteers were given a single, oral dose of the vaccine and the safety and immune responses to *S. typhi*-specific antigens and UreA/B were evaluated.[42] The results from this study confirmed the safety of the vector and showed that immunized volunteers developed strong serologic responses to *S. typhi* antigens. However, none of the vaccinees developed a detectable mucosal or humoral immune response to either urease subunit proteins.

Alternative *S. typhi* Preclinical Models

The development of new *S. typhi*-based vectors has been limited by the narrow host range of the organism and the lack of a suitable animal model. Since humans are the only known natural host for *S. typhi*, many of the strategies for producing attenuated mutants were initially identified as attenuating for *S. typhimurium* in mice.[43,44] The extrapolation of attenuation data from *S. typhimurium* to *S. typhi* was based on the recognition that *S. typhimurium* produces disease symptoms in mice similar to those caused by *S. typhi* in humans.[45] Aside from this model, the only other accepted method for evaluating attenuated *S. typhi* mutants employs the intraperitoneal coinjection of the organism with hog gastric mucin to enhance virulence. While the level of virulence observed by *S. typhimurium* given to mice via the oral route is thought to closely parallel the pathogenesis of *S. typhi* in humans, differences between the two serovars are compounded by the physical and genetic differences between inbred mice and humans. Nevertheless, support for the isogenic *S. typhimurium* murine model comes from the repeated demonstration that *S. typhi* strains bearing mutations proven to attenuate *S. typhimurium* have in most cases also been attenuated in humans, although not always as effective at inducing immune responses.[35,43,44]

The recent discovery that intranasal rather than oral vaccination of mice may be more efficient at inducing humoral responses to *S. typhi* provides an additional in vivo model for evaluating attenuation, immunogenicity, and protective efficacy.[46] The potential utility of this model was originally supported by studies showing that CVD 908-*htrA* colonized the mucosa-associated lymphoid tissue, Peyer's patches, and lungs of immunized mice.[47,48] More recently, we used this model to evaluate the immunogenicity of derivatives of *S. typhi* Ty800. Experience from many studies has highlighted the prudence of having alternative vaccine candidates ready for clinical evaluation in the event that deficiencies or reactogenicity are observed in later stage trials. The Ty800 derivative strains carry additional deletions in a variety of genes, including *crp* (a global regulator of growth),[27] *pmr* (polymyxin B/antimicrobial peptide resistance),[49] *poxA* (a regulator of pyruvate oxidase),[50] *aroA* (aromatic amino acid synthesis),[51] and *pmi* (LPS biosynthesis).[52] All of these gene mutations were identified from experiments showing the limited impact they had on *S. typhimurium* virulence in mice. Based on the results from animal studies, isogenic mutations were introduced in *S. typhi* Ty800 to create new vaccines and vectors that were intended to be as immunogenic as Ty800 and potentially better tolerated. In preliminary experiments, mice were immunized intranasally with a priming and booster dose of ~5 x 10^8 cfu of Ty800 or derivatives of Ty800. Many of the derivatives of Ty800 colonized mice and were found in Peyer's Patches following immunization. However, the degree of host colonization by the derivative strains was significantly less than that shown by Ty800 suggesting, as anticipated, the derivative strains were more attenuated than the parental strain. Several of the Ty800 derivatives also induced detectable antibody titers to *S. typhi* LPS, although to lesser degrees than that elicited by Ty800. Interestingly, a Ty800 derivative that did not colonize well and did not induce a significant immune response was a Ty445, a *ΔphoPQ ΔaroA* mutant. These results are consistent with those from human clinical studies showing that Ty800 is safe and immunogenic[38] while Ty445 is safe but over-attenuated[35] and supports the utility of the intranasal immunization of mice as a valuable model for identifying potential attenuating mutations in *S. typhi.*

S. typhimurium Attenuated by Mutations in Virulence-Associated Genes

S. typhimurium LH1160

Investigators have recently taken an innovative approach to develop the potential of live, attenuated *Salmonella* vectors. This strategy is based on the notion that the more prolonged intestinal phase of nontyphoidal salmonellosis may induce a qualitatively and/or quantitatively different immunological stimulation of the gastrointestinal immune system than *S. typhi*-based vector. This concept was tested in volunteers who were given a single, oral dose of a recombinant *S. typhimurium* strain bearing mutations in the *phoPQ* regulon and in *purB.*[53] The resulting strain, *S. typhimurium* LH1160, was a purine auxotroph transformed with a $PurB^+$ balanced-lethal plasmid expressing the *H. pylo*ri *ureAB* genes. The amount of UreA/B produced by LH1160 in vitro was shown to be roughly equivalent to that produced by *S. typhi* Ty1033. Most of the subjects vaccinated with LH1160 developed *S. typhimurium*–specific anti-LPS and anti-flagella mucosal and humoral immune responses. More significantly, 50% of the volunteers also developed specific antibody responses to UreA/B, in direct contrast to volunteers immunized with *S. typhi* Ty1033. The vaccine was generally well tolerated with no reports of bacteremia or serious diarrhea, although a few subjects developed elevated temperatures.

The volunteer study with LH1160 was the first to demonstrate that an attenuated *S. typhimurium* vaccine vector could elicit an immune response in humans against a heterologous antigen. The differences between the apparent success of *S. typhimurium* LH1160 and the failure of *S. typhi* Ty1033[42] to deliver urease antigens in humans may be related to a number of factors, including the increased ability of *S. typhimurium* to invade and colonize the host GALT. Additionally, balanced-lethal plasmid stability was enhanced in LH1160 and resulted in volunteers who were colonized longer than those immunized with Ty1033. This presumably resulted in a larger antigen load being received by patients immunized with LH1160, a notion supported by the observation that LH1160 vaccinees were given about a 100-fold lower dose than those vaccinated with Ty1033.

The mild reactogenicity associated with LH1160 or any other Δ*phoPQ* strain of *S. typhimurium* will need to be addressed before the full potential of *S. typhimurium* can be explored further in clinical trials. Based on the experience with derivatives of Ty800, derivatives of LH430 (a *S. typhimurium* Δ*phoPQ* mutant virtually identical to LH1160) carrying additional gene deletions, including *crp* (global growth regulator) *pmr* (polymyxin B/antimicrobial peptide resistance), and *poxA* (pyruvate oxidase regulator) were produced. These vectors ideally would be more attenuated than LH1160/LH430 and could elicit immune responses at higher doses and with fewer adverse events. Colonization and immunogenicity were evaluated in preliminary experiments of mice given a single, intragastric dose of 10^9 cfu of LH430 or a LH430 derivative. LH430 derivatives with additional gene deletions in *pox* and *pmr* colonized the spleen and Peyer's patches of immunized animals at levels suggesting they were only marginally less fit than LH430. The immunogenicity of these strains was diminished to varying degrees compared to the parental strain, but colonizing strains elicited significant serologic immune responses to *S. typhimurium* LPS. The development of alternative vaccine strains derived from LH430 should provide new vaccine vectors with enhanced safety profiles and only a limited compromise in fitness.

Expression Systems Adapted for Use in Attenuated *Salmonella*

A variety of systems for expressing heterologous antigens in *Salmonella* vectors have been developed.[54] The development of these systems has shown that a number of factors influence efficient protein expression, including improper protein folding (e.g., inclusion body formation), differences in codon usage between *Salmonella* and the heterologous gene, foreign protein sequences that are hydrophobic and/or toxic for *Salmonella*, or degradation of vaccine antigens by endogenous bacterial proteases. Confounding issues of expression are factors influencing the magnitude of an immune response such as where the antigen is localized in the vector (periplasmic, cytosolic) and in the host (intra- or extracellular).[55] The development of new approaches to address these factors are beginning only now to be tested in attenuated *Salmonella* vectors and are based on mounting experimental evidence showing that antigens presented on the cell surface or extracellularly are more efficiently recognized by the host immune system than those that remain in the cytosol.

Ice Nucleation Fusion Protein

The display of antigens on bacterial cell surfaces is a promising new approach for vaccine development. Surface display has been adapted for use in a number of Gram negative bacterial systems and is based on a variety of lipoproteins and outer membrane and cell surface structural proteins.[56] The applicability of many of these systems for vaccine use, however, is limited by the allowable size of the vectored antigen. For example, the display of chimeric fusion proteins longer than 60 amino acids appears to perturb many outer membrane structures and results in significantly diminished growth of the host strain.[57] A surface display system based on the ice nucleation protein (INP) of *Pseudomonas syringae* has recently been described and suggests several potential advantages over other display systems adapted from Gram negative bacteria.[58,59] INP is a glycosylphosphatidylinositol-anchored outer membrane protein that catalyzes the formation of ice crystals in supercooled water.[60] The genetic fusion of heterologous vaccine antigens to INP has a number of features that make it attractive for vaccine applications. For example, the expression of even large INP fusion proteins, e.g., HIV gp120 (60 kD) does not appreciably inhibit cell growth or cause perturbations in outer membrane architecture.[59] In addition, it was reported recently that a recombinant *Escherichia coli* strain was able to stably express an immunologically reactive *Bacillus anthracis* Protective Antigen (83 kD)-INP fusion, demonstrating that truly high molecular weight antigens can be effectively displayed.[61]

The adaptation of the INP display system for use in attenuated *Salmonella* followed logically from observations that extracellularly accessible antigens were more effective at eliciting immune responses than cytosolically localized antigens. The use of INP to support this concept was shown with a hybrid fusion protein consisting of INP genetically fused to the major surface antigen of hepatitis B virus (HBsAg) and the hepatitis C virus core protein (HCcAg).[62] The fusion protein was stably displayed on the surface of recombinant *S. typhi* Ty21a, and elicited production of high-titer serum antibody to HBsAg and HCcAg in mice immunized by intranasal or intraperitoneal inoculation. The anti-HBsAg and anti-HCcAg antibody titers were significantly higher in mice immunized with recombinant *Salmonella* displaying the INP-viral antigen fusion protein on their surfaces than those retaining the antigen in the cytosol. Interestingly, surface display of the hybrid protein was observed when expression was induced at 25° C prior to immunization but not 37° C. The investigators suggested that expression at the lower temperature might have prevented the premature folding of the fusion protein during export. The effectiveness of the INP display system in attenuated *Salmonella* vectors, however, awaits the results from additional studies evaluating the in vivo kinetics and duration of heterologous antigen display on the bacterial cell surface.

Antigen Secretion

The secretion of a foreign antigen into the extracellular environment by *Salmonella* vectors is a method that has several potential applications to live, attenuated vaccine development. Alpha-hemolysin (HlyA) is secreted by a multi-component type I secretion system of *E. coli*.[63] In addition to HlyA, the α-hemolysin export system includes HlyB, HlyD, and TolC, proteins that are localized in the bacterial periplasm and outer membrane. The TolC protein, which is not part of the *hly* operon, has a putative homologue on the *Salmonella* chromosome.[64] Secretion of HlyA is dependent on the carboxyl-terminal 27 amino acids of the protein ($HlyA_S$) that are recognized by the HlyB-HlyD-TolC secretion machinery.[65]

The α-hemolysin export system was originally adapted for use in attenuated *Salmonella* to deliver two proteins naturally secreted by *Listeria monocytogenes*, p60 (a murein hydrolase involved in host-cell invasion) and listerolysin O (a hemolysin required for egress into the cytosol; LLO).[66] There is strong evidence to suggest that immunity to listeriosis is due in large part to a specific $CD8^+$ T-cell response elicited by listerial antigens such as LLO and p60 that are secreted into the host cell cytoplasm and routed to the MHC Class I processing pathway for appropriate presentation.[67-69] Listerolysin O or p60 were expressed from a recombinant *S. typhimurium aroA* mutant as either somatic (cytosolic) or secreted proteins genetically fused to $HlyA_S$.[66] Oral immunization induced protection against listeriosis in mice when animals were given *Salmonella aroA* mutants secreting $HlyA_S$-LLO or $HlyA_S$-p60, but not when immunized with attenuated *Salmonella* expressing unsecreted forms of LLO or p60. Interestingly, the expression of $HlyA_S$-p60 by attenuated *Salmonella* elicited protective $CD4^+$ and $CD8^+$ T lymphocyte responses, even though the vector remained in phagolysosomes. The ability of HlyA fusions to render immunogenic proteins that are normally cytosolic was explored further using superoxide dismutase (SOD), a protein that is normally localized in the cytosol of *L. monocytogenes*.[55] Mice immunized intravenously with a *S. typhimurium aroA* mutant secreting the $HlyA_S$-SOD fusion protein elicited protective host immune responses to lethal listeriosis. In this study, the participation of both $CD4^+$ and $CD8^+$ T lymphocytes was inferred, based upon potent protection against virulent *Listeria* infection.

More recently, the application of HlyA secretion technology to potential vaccines against bioterrorism was reported. Recent attacks in the U.S. using anthrax have stimulated efforts to develop effective, new vaccines that could confer rapid protective immunity to civilians and military personnel at potential risk of exposure. Using anthrax as a model, investigators were successful in producing an attenuated strain of *S. typhimurium* expressing the native (83 kD) or mature (63 kD) forms of *B. anthracis* Protective Antigen genetically fused to HlyA.[70] This finding supports the vaccine potential of attenuated *Salmonella* vectors expressing HlyA-fusions to a variety of heterologous proteins, including those not naturally secreted.

Salmonella-Based Type III Secretion Systems

Much of the emphasis on developing attenuated strains of *Salmonella* for vaccine use has focused on optimizing serum antibody responses, and relatively few studies have been conducted to evaluate the potential of attenuated *Salmonella* mutants to induce heterologous cellular immune responses to vectored antigens. One possible reason for this lack of attention may be an inability to show consistent induction of MHC Class I-restricted immune responses,[71] an important feature for attenuated *Salmonella* vectors directed against intracellular infections. While a hybrid expression system like HlyA can be used to elicit cell-mediated immunity, its use in *Salmonella* requires the presence of additional *E. coli* accessory genes whose expression may have undesirable consequences on the fitness of the vector. To address this potential shortcoming, some investigators are developing alternative strategies for using attenuated *Salmonella* to elicit the production of CD8$^+$ T lymphocytes. One approach is the modification of a homologous *S. typhimurium* type III secretion system that is required for host cell invasion. The type III secretion system is independent from the *sec*-dependent pathway and functions by injecting effector proteins into the cytosol of a target cell and activating cellular transcription factors and inducing cytoskeletal reorganization.[4] *Salmonella* protein tyrosine phosphatase (SptP), an effector protein transported into the host cell by the type III secretion system, was modified by genetically fusing it to murine-restricted CTL epitopes from nucleoproteins of influenza virus or lymphocytic choriomeningitis virus (LCMV).[72] Mice orally immunized with a *S. typhimurium ΔaroAΔspt* mutant expressing either hybrid fusion protein developed MHC class-I-restricted CTL that were epitope-specific and recognized endogenously processed antigen. Furthermore, immunized mice were protected against lethal LCMV infection. The development of homologous type III secretion systems like SptP may find a particular application in *Salmonella* vectors such as Ty800 that have been attenuated by impeding the bacterium's ability to escape from phagolysosomes and entering the cytosol of antigen presenting cells (APCs).

One of the limitations often encountered when creating fusion proteins to functional proteins is the size of the heterologous insert that can be accommodated. In many cases where in-frame fusions to functional domains are employed, insert sizes are limited to epitopes or small protein fragments. The SptP protein, for example, apparently can accept inserts of about 45-55 amino acids without significantly comprising protein function.[72] To address this limitation, hybrid type III secretion systems composed of heterologous elements have been developed for use in *Salmonella*. In one such example, defined secretion and translocation domains of *Yersinia* outer protein E (YopE) were genetically fused to one of two large, antigenic fragments derived from *L. monocytogenes* LLO and p60.[73-75] Mice immunized with a single, oral dose of a *Salmonella ΔaroAΔspt* mutant expressing either of the YopE-LLO or YopE-p60 hybrid proteins elicited CD8$^+$ T lymphocytes that protected mice against lethal *L. monocytogenes* infection.

Delivery of Plasmid DNA by Attenuated Strains of *Salmonella*

Genetic immunization is a promising new vaccine approach, and it has been demonstrated that several attenuated bacterial vectors are capable of delivering plasmid DNA.[74, 75] The use of attenuated bacterial vectors takes advantage of the natural ability of organisms like *Shigella* and *Listeria*, which that are normally highly invasive to grow and subsequently escape from endocytic or phagocytic vacuoles of APCs. The release of the vector from vacuoles into the host cell cytoplasm has been shown to be a viable method for delivering plasmid DNA.[74,76] The ability of attenuated *Salmonella* mutants to deliver nucleic acid-based vaccines is, therefore, an unexpected property of a bacterium that resides in phagolysosomal compartments and does not normally enter the cytosol.

In early proof of concept studies, a *S. typhimurium aroA* mutant was engineered to deliver a plasmid encoding a model antigen, β-galactosidase, constitutively expressed by a CMV promoter (pCMVβ).[77] Experiments conducted in vitro showed that cultures of peritoneal macrophages infected with *S. typhimurium* (pCMVβ) expressed functional β-galactosidase. Subsequently, mice were orally immunized with a single dose of the same recombinant *Salmonella* vector and shown to produce significant levels of antibody and antigen-specific CTLs against β-galactosidase. These results are supported by recent studies from another group using a *S. typhimurium aroA* mutant to express β-galactosidase as a model tumor-associated antigen. This study showed that orally vaccinated mice produced both antigen-specific humoral and cell-mediated immune responses and were highly protected against tumor growth when challenged with a transfected *lacZ*-expressing fibrosarcoma cell line.[78]

The precise mechanism by which *Salmonella* can deliver DNA vaccines is unclear. It has been proposed that DNA released from macrophages or other APCs undergoing apoptosis may be taken up by neighboring dendritic cells.[75,79,80] Regardless of the mechanism involved, the use of attenuated *Salmonella* as a delivery vehicle has several advantages over the direct injection of naked DNA, including oral administration, a natural tropism for APCs, and the presence of recognized immunomodulatory components like LPS that may enhance the host's immune response to the plasmid-encoded foreign antigen.[77]

Novel Applications of Attenuated Salmonella *Vectors*

Biowarfare and Bioterrorism

At the end of the19th century, field studies conducted by Pasteur on vaccinating against anthrax were directed against a malady that was largely a disease of livestock. More than a century later, it is once again necessary to focus on anthrax, along with other pathogenic microorganisms, only this time as agents of biological warfare and bioterrorism against both military personnel and civilian populations. The U.S. Centers for Disease Control and Prevention (CDC) have designated certain microorganisms, including *B. anthracis* (anthrax), *Yersinia pestis* (bubonic and pneumonic plague), and *Francisella tularensis* (tularemia) as disease agents that pose a risk to national security. All of the potential biological warfare agents on the CDC list can be spread easily by aerosolization, and vaccines against these and other potential biowarfare agents are either outdated or do not exist.

Anthrax

The apparent ease with which anthrax-based bioterrorist attacks could be launched against U. S. civilians, together with the high mortality rate of inhalation anthrax, has made *B. anthracis* one of the most feared agents of biological warfare and terrorism. The standard anthrax vaccine (AVA; anthrax vaccine adsorbed) is routinely administered to people at risk for the disease and may also be given to patients to combat latent spores that may germinate after the cessation of antibiotic treatment.[81]

The AVA vaccine is often painful upon administration, requires a lengthy dosing regimen (6 injections over the course of 18 months with annual booster injections) and is expensive to manufacture. For these reasons, there is considerable promise in the development of live, attenuated *Salmonella* delivery systems to vaccinate against anthrax. The potential of such a vaccine was originally evaluated in an attenuated *S. typhimurium aroA* recombinant expressing the *B. anthracis* gene for Protective Antigen (PA) (SL3261 (pORF1)).[82] The recombinant full-length product (rPA) was localized almost exclusively to the *Salmonella* periplasm. Mice given two oral doses of SL3261(pORF1) were partially protected against lethal spore challenge, although a serum anti-PA antibody response was not detected. However, all mice given three intravenous injections of the same vaccine died from infection. The investigators concluded that partial protection against aerosol anthrax challenge was likely to have been mediated by local immune responses in the lungs and on other mucosal surfaces.

Plague

Y. pestis is the etiologic agent of bubonic and pneumonic plague. During the Cold War, the U.S. and Soviet biological weapons programs developed techniques to directly aerosolize plague particles, a technique that leads to pneumonic plague, a highly lethal and potentially contagious form of the infection. There is currently no commercially available vaccine against plague. A formaldehyde-killed *Y. pestis* whole-cell vaccine was available until recently, but was reactogenic and offered little protection against pneumonic plague; it was discontinued in 1999.[83]

Efforts to attenuate *Y. pestis* using mutations identified in other pathogens including *Salmonella* and *Shigella* e.g., *aroA* have been unsuccessful. Accordingly, new approaches have been devised to use attenuated, bacterial vectors to deliver *Y. pestis* vaccine antigens. There have been several reports of the expression of the F1 antigen in attenuated *S. typhimurium*. Immunity to plague has been correlated with the presence of antibody to the capsular F1 antigen (Caf1[84]), and immunization of mice with Cafl induced protection against infectious challenge.[85-87] Oral immunization of mice with a *S. typhimurium aroA* mutants expressing either F1 from in vivo-induced promoters or genes from the entire *caf* operon elicited production of protective levels of antibody to high dose (10^7 LD50) challenge with virulent *Y. pestis*.[88] In addition, sIgA was detected in the lungs and gut of mice immunized with recombinant *Salmonella* expressing F1 on its surface, suggesting the potential of this vaccine in providing protection against ingested or inhalational exposure to *Y. pestis*. It is worth noting that mice immunized similarly with a *S. typhimurium aroA* mutant expressing an intracellularly localized form of F1 developed significantly lower anti-F1 immune responses that provided only partial protection to a lower challenge dose (10^5 LD50). These results support previous observations that heterologous antigens expressed on the surface of recombinant *Salmonella* are more effective, at least in animal models of infection, at inducing protective immune responses than expression of the same antigen in somatic form. More recently, mice immunized with an attenuated strain of *Sallmonella* expressing F1 genetically fused to *Y. pestis* V antigen were shown to elicit protective immune responses against virulent plague challenge.[88b] This type of vaccine has the potential to provide effective protection against a wide range of virulent *Y. pestis* strains, including those that are unencapsulated.

Tularemia

Tularemia is a normally zoonotic disease caused by the bacterium *F. tularensis*. Primary pneumonic tularemia results from the inhalation of *F. tularensis* and is the most severe clinical form of tularemia, with a mortality rate as high as 60 percent in the absence of treatment. Tularemia was one of several biological weapons that were stockpiled by both the U.S. and Soviet military during the height of the Cold War, because of the bacterium's extreme infectivity, ease of dissemination, and substantial capacity to cause illness and death.[89]

The nature of protective immunity to tularemia, and as such correlates of protection, is not well defined. The most effective vaccine developed for stimulating protective immune responses against tularemia is a live, attenuated vaccine derived from avirulent *F. tularensis* LVS. Strain LVS was created to protect laboratory workers and other personnel at risk to *F. tularensis* exposure, but is not available to the general public.[90]

The natural ability of attenuated *Salmonella* to induce specific T-lymphocyte responses makes it attractive as a potential vaccine vector to protect against tularemia. There have been few reports of the expression of *F. tularensis* antigens by *Salmonella*. An early study used *S. typhimurium* chi4072 (pTUL4-15), an attenuated Δ*cya*Δ*crp* mutant, to express the 17 kD *F. tularensis* TUL4 outer membrane lipoprotein.[91] TUL4 was shown in previous studies to stimulate the proliferation of T lymphocytes from *F. tularensis*-infected humans. Mice that were orally immunized with chi4072 (pTUL4-15) and subsequently challenged with virulent *F. tularensis* had a lower bacterial load in liver and spleen than animals immunized with the non-recombinant strain. In a second study, a *S. typhimurium aroA* mutant expressing FopA, a major *F. tularensis* outer membrane protein failed to induce significant protection against a virulent *Francisella* challenge.[92] In contrast, mice immunized with *F. tularensis* LPS did seroconvert and were protected against lethal challenge. It is notable that mice in both of the studies described above were immunized by injection, a route of administration that would not be expected to take full advantage of the ability of *Salmonella* to colonize the GALT and other tissues of the reticulo-endothelial system. As such, recent successes in cloning and expressing LPS genes in a number of heterologous vaccine vectors should serve as an impetus to explore the feasibility of expressing the appropriate *F. tularensis* LPS genes in attenuated *Salmonella*.

Therapeutic Use of Attenuated *Salmonella* for Cancer Treatment

S. typhimurium VNP20009

It has been known for some time that *Salmonella* has a natural tropism for solid tumors and can selectively replicate to as high as 10^9 cfu per gram of tumor mass. *Salmonella typhimurium* VNP20009 was originally developed to exploit this tropism to deliver potential therapeutic proteins like prodrug-converting enzymes to a tumor site. VNP20009 was created by chromosomal deletion of two genes, *purI* (purine biosynthesis) and *msbB* (LPS biosynthesis) and was attenuated at least 10,000-fold in mice compared to the parental wild-type stain. Preclinical evaluation of VNP20009 unexpectedly showed that VNP20009 by itself induced tumoricidal effects in mice, inhibiting tumor growth by 94% compared to untreated mice bearing subcutaneously implanted melanoma.[93]

In a phase I human study designed to evaluate safety and potential efficacy, VNP20009 was given as a single, intravenous bolus infusion to 24 patients with metastatic melanoma and one with metastatic renal cell carcinoma. Tumor colonization was observed in two patients receiving 10^9 cfu/m^2, but none of the patients showed signs of tumor regression.[94] In another study, eight of eleven patients receiving direct, intratumoral injections of VNP20009 showed signs of persistent colonization lasting for at least two weeks.[95] While neither of these studies demonstrated any vaccine-related anti-tumor effects, they did show that high-doses of VP20009 could be safely administered to humans and provided impetus for the further development of the strain.

S. typhimurium VNP20029

The safety and colonization profiles of VNP20009 supported the continued development of attenuated *Salmonella* as a vector for delivering anti-tumor therapeutics such as prodrug-converting enzymes. The local, intratumoral conversion of relatively nontoxic compounds (prodrugs) into highly cytotoxic metabolites offers the potential for eradicating tumors in the absence of systemic toxicity. Current methods for delivering prodrug-converting enzymes have a number of limitations, including a lack of tumor specificity and an inability to administer the agent systemically.[96] To address these limitations, new approaches such as tumor-amplified protein expression therapy (TAPET) have been adapted for use in attenuated *Salmonella*. Development of this technology is based on expressing cytosine deaminase (CD), an enzyme that converts 5-fluorocytosine (5-FC) to 5-fluorouracil (5-FU). 5-FC (the prodrug) is generally nontoxic for eukaryotic cells but 5-FU is highly cytotoxic. *Salmonella typhimurium* VNP20009 expressing CD, (strain VNP20029) displayed safety and efficacy profiles similar to those of VNP20009.[95] Preclinical studies showed that tumor-bearing mice immunized with VNP20029 had a >90% reduction in tumor growth in several murine tumor models and that reduction corresponded to the presence of high levels of 5-FU in animals injected post-immunization with 5-FC. The effectiveness of VNP20029 as a human therapeutic is currently being evaluated in expanded Phase I clinical trials.

Summary

Early advances in producing safe and protective live attenuated bacterial vaccines like *S. typhi* Ty21a facilitated the development of safe vaccine vectors. During the last quarter century, however, the development of new vectors has progressed from an empirical science employing attenuation strategies producing undefined mutations to the generation of rationally attenuated strains with precise gene deletions. The result is the creation of vaccines and vectors like Ty800, CVD 908-*htrA*, and LH1160 that are well-tolerated and immunogenic in humans. The recent sequencing and annotation of the entire genomes of *S. typhi*[97] and *S. typhimurium*[98] promise to provide additional insights into the virulence, metabolic, and growth mechanisms of the salmonellae. Comparisons of the *Salmonella* genomes have already identified specific gene clusters in *S. typhimurium* that are absent in *S. typhi*, suggesting the roots of host adaptation and specificity. As previously unknown genes and their functions continue to be elucidated, safer and more effective vector strains of *Salmonella* will emerge.

The continuing development of attenuated *Salmonella* vectors opens an exciting new realm of potential therapies, including applications to cancer treatment and the protection of military personnel and civilian populations against the threat of biological weapons attack. The evolution of *Salmonella* vectors for use in these applications will be driven by efforts to improve heterologous immune responses; the challenge remains to develop clinically useful attenuated *Salmonella* vectors that stimulate heterologous immune responses after a single oral vaccination. Given our increased ability to analyze and compare the genetic contents and organization of bacterial pathogens and the availability of new tools like DNA microarrays, the next generation of attenuated *Salmonella* vectors appears very promising.

References

1. Pasteur L, Roux E, Chamberland C. De la possibilit de rendre les moutons r fractaires au charbon par la m thod des inoculations pr ventives. C R Acad Sci 1881; 152.
2. Kraehenbuhl JP, Neutra MR. Defense of mucosal surfaces: pathogenicity, immunity and vaccines. Curr Top Microbiol Immunol. New York: Springer-Verlag New York Inc., 1998; 236:306.
3. Sirard J-C, Niedergang F, Kraehenbuhl J-P. Live attenuated Salmonella: a pardigm of mucosal vaccines. Immunol Rev 1999; 171:5-26.
4. Ohl ME, Miller SI. Salmonella a model for bacterial pathogenesis. Annu Rev Med 2001; 52:259-274.
5. Cancellieri V, Fara GM. Demonstration of specific IgA in human feces after immunization with live Ty21a Salmonella typhi vaccine. J Infect Dis 1985; 151:482-484.
6. Tagliabue A, Nencioni L, Caffarena A et al. Cellular immunity against Salmonella typhi after live oral vaccine. Clin Exp Immunol 1985; 62:242-247.
7. Bumann D, Metzger W, Mansouri E et al. Safety and immunogenicity of live recombinant Salmonella enterica serovar Typhi Ty21a expressing urease A and B from Helicobacter pylori in human volunteers. Vaccine 2001; 20:845-852.
8. Levine MM, Ferreccio C, Black RE et al. Progress in vaccines against typhoid fever. Rev Infect Dis 1989; 11:S552-567.
9. Viret J-F, Favre D, Wegmüller B et al. Mucosal and systemic immune responses in humans after primary and booster immunizations with orally administered invasive and noninvasive live attenunated bacteria. Infect Immun 1999; 67:3680-3685.
10. Germanier R, Furer E. Isolation asnd characterization of galE mutant Ty21a of Salmonella typhi: a candidate strain for a live oral typhoid vaccine. J Infect Dis 1975; 141.
11. Formal SB, Baron LS, Kopecko DJ et al. Construction of a potential bivalent vaccine strain:introduction of Shigella sonnei form I antigen genes into the galE Salmonella typhi Ty21a typhoid vaccine strain. Infect Immun 1981; 34:746-750.
12. Tramont EC, Chung R, Berman S et al. Safety and antigenicitgy of typhoid-Shigella sonnei vaccine (strain 5076-1C). J Infect Dis 1984; 149:133-136.
13. Van de Verg L, Herrington DA, Murphy JR et al. Specific immunoglobulin A-secreting cells in peripheral blood of humans following oral immunization with a bivalent Salmonella typhi-Shigella sonnei vaccine or infection by pathogenic S sonnei. Infect Immun 1990; 58:2002-2004.
14. Herrington DA, Verg LVd, Formal SB et al. Studies in volunteers to evaluate candidate Shigella vaccines: further experience with a bivalent Salmonella typhi-Shigella sonnei vaccine and protection conferred by previous Shigella sonnei disease. Vaccine 1990; 8:353-357.
15. Forrest B, LaBrooy J, Attridge SR et al. Immunogenicity of a candidate live oral typhoid/cholera hybrid vaccine in humans. J Infect Dis 1989; 159:145-146.
16. Tacket CO, Forrest B, Morona R et al. Safety, Immunogneicity and efficacy against cholera challenge in humans of a typhoid-cholera hybrid vaccine derived from Salmonella typhi Ty21a. Infect Immun 1990; 58:1620-1627.
17. Cárdenas L, Clements JD. Oral immunization using live attenuated Salmonella spp as carriers of foreign antigens. Clin Microbiol Rev 1992; 5:328-342.
18. Edwards MF, Stocker BA. Construction of ΔaroAhis Δpur strains of Salmonella typhi. J Bacteriol 1988; 170:3991-3995.

19. Levine MM, Ferreccio C, Black RE et al. Large-scale field trial of Ty21a live oral typhoid fever vaccine in enteric-coated capsule formulation. Lancet 1987; 1:1049-1052.
20. Hone DM, Harris AM, Chatfield S et al. Construction of genetically defined double aro mutants of Salmonella typhi. Vaccine. 1991; 9:810-816.
21. Tacket CO, Hone DM, R.C.III et al. Comparison of the safety and immunogenicity of ΔaroC ΔaroD and Δcya Δcrp Salmonella typhi strains in adult volunteers. Infect Immun 1992; 60:536-541.
22. Aggarwal A, Kumar S, Jaffe R et al. Oral Salmonella: malaria circumsporozite recombinants induce specific CD8+ cytotoxic T cells. J Exp Med 1990; 172:1083-1090.
23. González C, Hone D, Noriega FR et al. Salmonella typhi vaccine strain CVD 908 expressing the circumsporozoite protein of Plasmodium falciparum: strain construction and safety and immunogennicity in humans. J Infect Dis 1994; 13:927-931.
24. Johnson KI, Charles I, Dougan G et al. The role of a stress-response protein in Salmonella typhimurium virulence. Mol Microbiol 1991; 5:104-107.
25. Tacket CO, Sztein MB, Wasserman SS et al. Phase 2 clinical trial of attenuated Salmonella enterica serovar Typhi oral live vector vaccine CVD 908-htrA in US volunteers. Infect Immun 2000; 68:1196-1201.
26. Tacket CO, Galen J, Sztein MB et al. Safety and immune responses to attenuated Salmonella enterica serovar Typhi oral live vector vaccines expressing tetanus toxin fragment C. Clin Immunol 2000; 97:146-153.
27. Curtiss R III, Kelly SM. Salmonella typhimurium deletion mutant lacking adenylate cyclase and cyclic AMP receptor protein are avirulent and immunogenic. Infect Immun 1987; 55:3035-3043.
28. Kelly SM, Bosecker BA, RC 3rd. Characterization and protective properties of attenuated mutants of Salmonella cholerasuis. Infect Immun 1992; 60:4881-4890.
29. Nardelli-Haefliger D, Kraehenbuhl JP, Curtiss R III et al. Oral and rectal immunization of adult femal volunteers with a recombinant attenuated Salmonella typhi vaccine. Infect Immun 1996; 64:5219-5224.
30. Nakayama K, Kelly SM, RC 3rd. Construction of an Asd+ expression-cloning vector: stable maintenance and high-level expression of cloned genes in a Salmonella vaccine strain. Bio/technology 1988; 6.
31. Tijhaar EJ, Zheng-Xin Y, Karlas JA et al. Construction and evaluation of an expression vector allowing the stable expression of foreign antigens in a Salmonella typhimurium vaccine strain. Vaccine 1994; 12:1004-1011.
32. Hone D, Attridge S, Bosch Lvd et al. A chromosomal integration system for stabilization of heterologous genes in Salmonella based vaccine strains. Microb Pathog 1988; 5:407-418.
33. Cieslak PR, Zhang T, Stanley JSL. Expression of a recombinant Entamoeba histolytica antigen in a Salmonella typhimurium vaccine strain. Vaccine 1993; 11:773-776.
34. Tacket CO, Kelly SM, Sch del F et al. Safety and immunogenicity in humans of an attenuated Salmonella typhi vaccine vector strain expressing plasmid-encoded Hepatitis B antigens stabilized by the Asd-balanced lethal vector system. Infect Immun 1997; 65:3381-3385.
35. Hohmann EL, Oletta CA, Miller SI. Evaluation of a phoP/phoQ-deleted, aroA-deleted live oral Salmonella typhi vaccine strain in human volunteers. Vaccine 1996; 14:19-24.
36. Miller SI, Kukral AM, Mekalanos JJ. A two-component regulatory system (phoP phoQ) controls Salmonella typhimurium virulence. Proc Natl Acad Sci USA 1989; 86:5054-5058.
37. Gálan J, RC III. Virulence and vaccine potential of phoP mutants of S. typhimurium. Microb Pathog 1989; 6:422-443.
38. Hohmann EL, Oletta CA, Killeen KP et al. phoP/phoQ-deleted Salmonella typhi (Ty800) is a safe and immunogenic single-dose typhoid fever vaccine in volunteers. J Infect Dis 1996; 173:1408-1414.
39. Lee CK, Weltzin R, Thomas Jr WD et al. Oral immunization with recombinant Helicobacter pylori urease induces secretory IgA antibodies and protects mice from challenge with Helicobacter felis. J Infect Dis 1995; 172:161-172.
40. Corthesy-Theulaz I, Hopkins S, Bachmann D et al. Mice are protected from Helicobacter pylori infection by nasal immunization with attenuated Salmonella typhimurium expressing urease A and B subunits. Infect Immun 1998; 66:581-586.
41. Gómez-Duarte OG, Lucas B, Yan ZX et al. Protection of mice against gastric colonization by Helicobacter pylori by single oral dose immunization with attenuated Salmonella typhimurium producing urease subunits A and B. Vaccine 1998; 16:460-471.
42. Dipetrillo MD, Tibbetts T, Kleanthous H et al. Safety and immunogenicity of phoP/phoQ-deleted Salmonella typhi expressing Helicobacter pylori urease in adult volunteers. Vaccine 2000; 18:449-459.
43. Stocker BA. Auxotrophic Salmonella typhi as live vaccine. Vaccine 1988; 6:141-145.

44. Levine MM, Tacket CO, Herringtton D et al. The current status of typhoid vaccine development and clinical trials with typhoid vaccines. Southeast Asian J Trop Med Public Health 1988; 19:459-469.
45. Killeen K, DiRita V. Live attenuated bacterial vaccines in New Vaccine Technologies. In: Ellis R, ed. Texas: Landes Bioscience, Georgetown, 2000:151-185.
46. Gálen JE, G—mez-Duarte OG, Losonsky GA et al. A murine model of intranasal immunization to assess the immunogneicity of attenuated Salmonella typhi live vector vaccines in stimulating serum antibody responses to foreing antigens. Vaccine 1997; 15:700-708.
47. Pickett TE, Pasetti MF, Galen JE et al. In vivo characterization of the murine intranasal model for assessing the immunogenicity of attenuated Salmonella enterica serovar Typhi strains as live mucosal vaccines and as live vectors. Infect Immun 2000; 68:205-213.
48. Pasetti MF, Pickett TE, Levine MM et al. A comparison of immunogenicity and in vivo distribution of Salmonella enterica serovar typhi and typhimurium live vector vaccines delivered by mucosal routes in the murine model. Vaccine 2000; 18:3208-3213.
49. Gunn JS, Miller SI. PhoP/PhoQ activates transcription of pmrA/B, encoding a two-componenet system involved in Salmonella typhimurium antimicrobial peptide resistance. J Bacteriol 1996; 178:6857-6864.
50. Kaniga K, Compton MS, R.C.III et al. Molecular and functional characterization of Salmonella enterica serovar Typhimurium poxA gene:effect on attenuation of virulence and protection. Infect Immun 1998; 66:5599-5606.
51. Chatfield SN, Strahan K, Pickard D et al. Evaluation of Salmonella typhimurium strains harbouring defined mutations in htrA and aroA in the murine salmonellosis model. Microb Pathog 1991; 12:145-151.
52. Collins LV, Attridge S, Hackett J. Mutations at rfc or pmi attenuate Salmonella typhimurium virulence for mice. Infect Immun 1991; 59:1079-1085.
53. Angelakopoulos H, Hohmann EL. Pilot study of phoP/phoQ-deleted Salmonella enterica serovar Typhimurium expressing Helicobacter pylori urease in adult volunteers. Infect Immun 2000; 68:2135-2141.
54. Kochi SK, Killeen KP. Live attenuated bacterial vectors in New Vaccine Technologies. In: Ellis R, ed. Georgetown: Landes Bioscience, 2000:171-185.
55. Hess J, Dietrich G, Gentschev I et al. Protection against murine listeriosis by an attenuated recombinant Salmonella typhimurium vaccine strain that secretes the naturallly somatic antigen superoxide dismutase. Infect Immun 1997; 65:1286-1292.
56. Georgiou G, Stathopoulos C, Daugherty PS et al. Display of heterologous proteins on the surface of microorganisms: from the screening of combinatorial libraries to live recombinant vaccines. Nat Biotechnol 1997; 15:29-34.
57. Hofnung M. Expression of foreign polypeptides at the Escherichia coli cell surface. Methods Cell Biol 1991; 34:77-105.
58. Jung H-C, Lebeault J-M, Pan J-G. Surface display of Zymomonas mobilis levan sucrase by using the ice-nucleation protein of Pseudomonas syringae. Nat Biotechnol 1998; 16:576-580.
59. Kwak Y-D, Yoo S-K, Kim E-J. Cell surface display of human immunodeficiency virus type 1 gp120 on Escherichia coli by using ice nucleation protein. Clin Diagn Lab Immunol 1999; 6:499-503.
60. Orser C, Staskawicz BJ, Panopoulos NJ et al. Cloning and expression of bacterial ice nucleation genes in Escherichia coli. J Bacteriol 1985; 164:359-366.
61. Kim S, Kim H, Chai Y. Cell surface display of Bacillus anthracis Protective Antigen on Escherichia coli by using ice nucleation protein. In: Abstracts of the Fourth International Conference on Anthrax. Board 36A. Saint John's College, Andover, MD, 2001.
62. Lee J-S, Shin K-S, Pan J-G et al. Surface-displayed viral antigens on Salmonella carrier vaccine. Nat Biotechnol 2000; 18:645-648.
63. Blight MA, Holland IB. Heterologous protein secretion and the versatile Escherichia coli haemolysin translocator. Trends Biotechnol 1994; 12:450-453.
64. Stone BJ, Miller VL. Salmonella enteriditis has a homologue of tolC that is required for virulence in BALB/c mice. Mol Microbiol 1995; 17:701-712.
65. Gentschev I, Hess J, Goebel W. Change in the cellular localization of alkaline phosphatase by alteration of its carboxy-terminal sequence. Mol Gen Genet 1990; 222:211-216.
66. Hess J, Gentschev I, Miko D et al. Superior efficacy of secreted over somatic antigen display in recombinant Salmonella vaccine induced protection against listeriosis. Proc Natl Acad Sci USA 1996; 93:1458-1463.
67. Berche P, Gaillard J-L, Sansonetti PJ. Intracellular growth of Listeria monocytogenes as a prerequisite for in vivo induction of T cell-mediated immunity. J Immunol 1987; 138:2266-2271.

68. Harty JT, Bevan MJ. CD8 T cells specific for a single nonamer epitope of Listeria monocytogenes are protective in vivo. J Exp Med 1992; 175:4642-4650.
69. Harty JT, Pamer EG. CD8 lymphocytes specific for the secreted p60 antigen protect against Listeria monocytogenes. J Immunol 1995; 1564:4642-4650.
70. Beyer W, Griffin KE, Garmory HS et al. Improvements in the development of live Salmonella vectors for the delivery of vaccine candidates against B anthracis. In: Abstracts of the Fourth International Conference on Anthrax. Board 39B. Saint John's College, Andover, MD, 2001.
71. Franchini G, Robert-Guroff M, Tartaglia J et al. Highly attenuated HIV type 2 recombinant poxviruses, but not HIV-2 recombinant Salmonella vaccines, induce long-lasting protection in rhesus macaques. AIDS Res Hum Retroviruses 1996; 11:909-920.
72. Rüssmann H, Shams H, Poblete F et al. Delivery of epitopes by the Salmonella type III secretion system for vaccine development. Science 1998; 281:565-568.
73. Rüssmann H, Igwe EI, Sauer J et al. Protection against murine listeriosis by oral vaccination with recombinant Salmonella expressing hybrid Yersinia type III proteins. J Immunol 2001; 167:357-365.
74. Grillot-Courvalin C, Goussard S, Courvalin P. Wild-type intracellular bacteria deliver DNA into mammalian cells. Cell Microbiol 2002; 4:177-186.
75. Shata MT, Stevceva L, Agwale S et al. Recent advances with recombinant bacterial vaccine vectors. Mol Med Today 2000; 6:66-71.
76. Dietrich G, Gentschev I, Hess J et al. Delivery of DNA vaccines by attenuated intracellular bacteria. Immunol Today 1999; 20:251-253.
77. Darji A, Guzman CA, Gerstel B et al. Oral somatic transgene vaccination using attenuated S typhimurium. Cell 1997; 91:765-775.
78. Paglia P, Medina E, Arioli I et al. Gene transfer in dendritic cells, induced by oral DNA vaccination with Salmonella typhimurium, results in protective immunity against a murine fibrosarcoma. Blood 1998; 92:3172-3176.
79. Albert ML, Sauer B, Bhardwaj N. Dendritic cells acquire antigen from apoptotic cells and induce class I-restricted CTLs. Nature 1998; 392:86-89.
80. Monack DM, Raupach B, Hromockyj AE et al. Salmonella typhimurium invasion induces apoptosis in infected macrophages. Proc Natl Acad Sci USA 1996; 93:9833-9838.
81. Dixon TC, Meselson M, Guillemin J et al. Anthrax. N Engl J Med 1999; 341:815-825.
82. Coulson NM, Fulop M, Titball RW. Bacillus anthracis protective antigen, expressed in Salmonella typhimurium SL 3261, affords protection against anthrax spore challenge. Vaccine 1994; 12:1395-401.
83. Titball RW, Williamson ED. Vaccination against bubonic and pneumonic plague. Vaccine 2001; 19:4175-4184.
84. Williams JE, Arntzen L, Tyndal GL et al. Application of enzyme immunoassays for the confirmation of clinically suspect palgue in Namibia, 1982. Bull World Health Organ 1986; 64:745-752.
85. Williamson ED, Eley SM, Griffin KF et al. A new improved sub-unit vaccine for plague: the basis of protection. FEMS Immunol Med Microbiol 1995; 12:223-230.
86. Meyer KF, Hightower JA, McCrumb FR. Plague immunization VI Vaccination with the fractional antigen of Yersinia pestis. J Infect Dis 1974; 129:S41-S45.
87. Simpson WJ, Thomas RE, Schwan TG. Recombinant capsular antigen (fraction 1) from Yersinia pestis induces a protective antibody response in Balb/c mice. American Journal of Tropical Medicine and Hygiene 1990; 43:389-396.
88. Titball RW, Howells AM, Oyston PCF et al. Expression of the Yersinia pestis capsular antigen (F1 antigen) on the surface of an aroA mutant of Salmonella typhimurium induces high levels of protection against plague. Infect Immun 1997; 65:1926-1930.
88b. Leary SEC, Griffin KF, Garmory HS et al. Expression of an [sic] F1/V fusion protein in attenuated Salmonella typhimurium and protection of mice against plague. Vaccine 1997; 23:167-179.
89. Dennis DT, Inglesby TV, Henderson DA et al. Tularemia as a biological weapon: medical and public health management. JAMA 2001; 285:2763-2773.
90. Burke DS. Immunization against tularemia: analysis of the effectiveness of live Francisella tularensis vaccine in prevention of laboratory-acquired tularemia. J Infect Dis 1977; 135:55-60.
91. Sjöstedt A, Sandström G, Tärnvik A. Humoral and cell-mediated immunity in mice to a 17-kilodalton lipoprotein of Francisella tularensis expressed by Salmonella typhimurium. Infect Immun 1992; 60:2855-2862.
92. Fulop M, Manchee R, Titball R. Role of lipopolysaccharide and a major outer membrane protein from Francisella tularensis in the induction of immunity against tularemia. Vaccine 1995; 13:1220-1225.
93. Low KB, Ittensohn M, Le T et al. Lipid A mutant Salmonella with suppressed virulence and TNF-a induction retain tumor-targeting in vivo. Nat Biotechnol 1999; 17:37-41.

94. Toso JF, Gill VJ, Hwu P et al. Phase I study of the intravenous administration of attenuated Salmonella typhimurium to patients with metastatic melanoma. J Clin Oncol 2002; 20:142-152.
95. Cunningham C, Nemunaitis J. A phase I trial of genetically modified Salmonella typhimurium expressing cytosine deaminase (TAPET-CD, VNP20029) administered by intratumoral injection in combination with 5-fluorocytosine for patients with advanced or metastatic cancer. Protocol no:CL-17 Version: April 9, 2001. Human Gene Therapy 2001; 12:1594-1596.
96. Zheng L-M, Luo X, Feng M et al. Tumor amplified protein expression therapy: Salmonella as a tumor-selective protein delivery vector. Oncol Res 2000; 12:127-135.
97. Parkhill J, Dougan G, James KD et al. Complete genome sequence of a multiple drug resistant Salmonella enterica serovar Typhi CT18. Nature 2001; 413:848-852.
98. McClelland M, Sanderson KE, Spieth J et al. Complete genome sequence of Salmonella enterica serovar Typhimurium LT2. Nature 2001; 413:852-856.

Chapter 5

Mucosal Immunity

Michael W. Russell

Introduction

A perceptive reader scanning the *Contents* of this volume will notice that of 16 bacterial infections covered, only one (*Borrelia burgdorferi*) is normally delivered transcutaneously by arthropod bite; the remaining 15 either directly afflict, or normally invade across a mucosal surface. There is nothing unusual about this, as it applies to the great majority of human bacterial and viral infections, with malaria (a protozoal infection) being numerically the most important exception. The immune system counters this threat by deploying the majority of its resources at the mucosae (Fig.1), so that IgA is produced in quantities that exceed all other immunoglobulin isotypes combined (Table 1), most of this being secretory IgA (S-IgA). There also are more lymphocytes present in the intestinal tract than in all lymphoid organs combined.[1,2] Viewed from this standpoint, mucosal protection is the predominant preoccupation of the entire immune system. Therefore, one may ask why there has not been a greater emphasis on developing vaccines that would elicit protection at the portal of entry of pathogens; the oral polio vaccine remains the only human mucosally delivered vaccine that has been widely adopted, although several others are at various stages of development. Part of the reason must be the undoubted success of many vaccines that have been developed for parenteral administration, although most of those in routine use are against invasive viral or toxigenic bacterial diseases, and they work largely by inducing serum neutralizing antibodies. Perhaps as a consequence of this success, immunologists have been slow to recognize the role of mucosal immunity in protection against infection despite the evidence dating back to the time of Besredka,[3] and understanding of the mucosal immune system has emerged comparatively recently. However, several circumstances now combine to focus attention on the exploitation of mucosal immunity and mucosal vaccine delivery. These include pragmatic and logistical considerations as well as the scientific rationale of inducing protective immunity at the first site of pathogen encounter (Table 2).

Furthermore, it has become increasingly evident that the default mode of response within the mucosal immune system is essentially muted. The well-known concept of 'oral tolerance' refers to the abrogation of systemic responses to a parenterally administered immunogen by the prior feeding of the same antigen.[4] Even in the absence of such demonstrable suppression, the response to enteric immunization by the repeated administration of most soluble or nonviable antigens in large doses, as measured in terms of S-IgA antibodies, is generally modest at best and of short duration. Moreover, in early experiments using such simple approaches, immunological memory, one of the cardinal attributes of immunity, was usually not evident as detected by greater, more rapid, or longer lasting antibody responses to a subsequent administration of the same immunogen. As a result, the concept arose that there was little or no memory within the mucosal immune system. However, viable organisms such as attenuated enteric pathogens, as well as certain bacterial toxins (most notably cholera and related enterotoxins) can induce very strong mucosal IgA as well as circulating IgG antibodies that persist for several months

New Bacterial Vaccines, edited by Ronald W. Ellis and Bernard R. Brodeur.

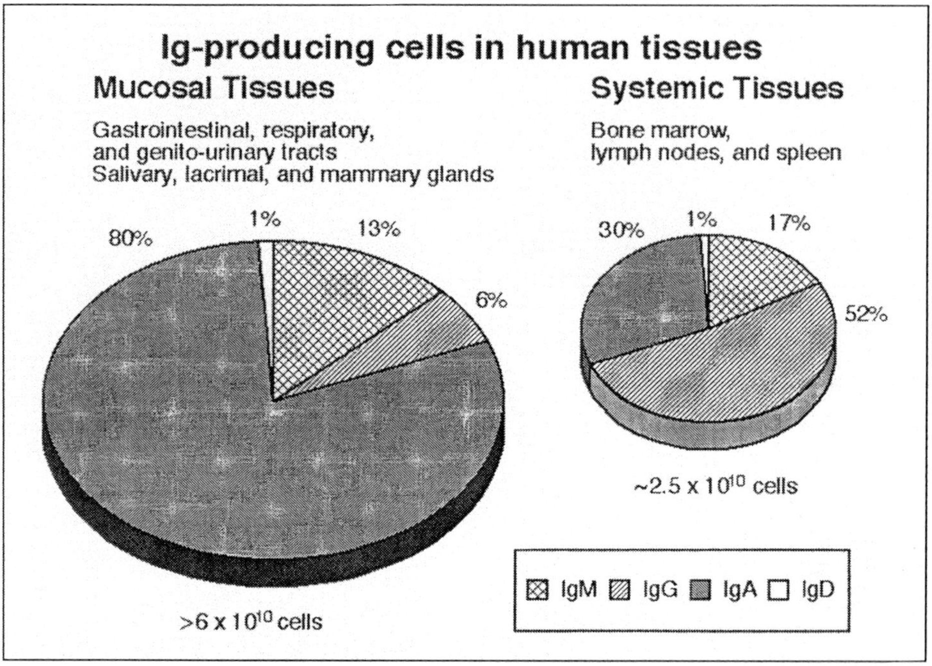

Figure 1. The distribution and isotype of immunoglobulin-producing cells in human tissues.

and that can be recalled with the typical features of anamnestic responses by booster immunization.[5-7] Thus, given a sufficiently strong stimulus, particularly with an immunogen that has characteristics of an aggressive pathogen or noxious toxin, the mucosal immune system can respond vigorously and furthermore can induce responses also in the systemic compartment. Such responses contrast markedly with the muted or even tolerant response to a huge variety of nonthreatening antigens comprising food components and inhaled dust particles, as well as the

Table 1. Production rates of IgA and IgG in adult humans (mg/day)*

Tissue/Fluid	IgA	IgG
Circulation	1300 – 2100	2100
Saliva	100 – 200	1 – 2
Tears	1 – 5	? †
Bile	50 – 400	160
Intestine, small	2100 – 5200	600
Intestine, large	1200	140
Urine	1 – 3	1 – 3
Nasopharynx	45	15
Genital tract, female	? †	? †
Genital tract, male	? †	? †
TOTAL	4800 – 9000	3000

* Data compiled from various sources (see ref. 19; J. Mestecky, pers. comm.)
† No data available

Table 2. Advantages of mucosal immunization

- Syringes and needles not required
  — avoids hazards in supply, use, and disposal of devices
- Reduced risk of transmission of infections between individuals
- Fewer trained personnel needed for administration
  — cheaper to administer
- Applicable to mass community immunization
- Less stringent requirements for sterility and non-reactogenicity?
  — less dependence on cold chain
- Response developed at site of challenge
- May also generate systemic responses
- May suppress mucosal carriage as well as invasive infection
- Reduced systemic complications?

normal commensal microbiota. Thus, the mucosal immune system appears able to distinguish not only between self and nonself, but also between essentially harmless microbes and antigens, and potentially dangerous pathogens. The 'danger hypothesis' of Matzinger[8] may be most applicable in the context of mucosal immunity.

Exploitation of mucosal immunity for future vaccine development therefore involves numerous strategies[9] that have been developed to overcome the inherent tolerance of the mucosal immune system and to harness its responsiveness to dangerous stimuli in a safe and acceptable way (Table 3); these will be discussed below.

Distinct Features of the Mucosal Immune System

The concept of mucosal immunity developed initially as one of *local* immunity, in which antigen applied to a mucosal surface or secretory gland induced a response in the underlying tissues that resulted in the secretion of antibodies (generally S-IgA) restricted to the immediate vicinity. For example, antigen applied to the conjunctiva in one eye led to the appearance of specific antibodies in the lacrimal secretion of that eye but not the opposite one, nor in other secretions such as saliva.[10] More recent demonstrations of a similar nature include the induction of genital tract IgA antibody responses by intravaginal instillation of soluble antigens: the responses are largely confined to the genital tract and not disseminated to remote sites.[11] However, the findings that milk and other secretions such as saliva contain IgA antibodies to enteric bacteria or food antigens, and that enteric administration of antigens induces S-IgA antibodies not only in the gut but also in other secretions, led to the concept of the *common* mucosal immune system, whereby responses induced at one site (the gut) could be expressed as specific antibodies in most other mucosae.[12]

Both the intestinal and upper respiratory tracts contain organized immune inductive tissues, collectively referred to as mucosa-associated lymphoid tissue (MALT), which can disseminate T and B cells, after antigenic stimulation, via the circulation to populate remote mucosal tissues with predominantly polymeric IgA-secreting plasma cells and supportive T-helper cells (Fig. 2). MALT typically consists of nonencapsulated lymphoid follicles having distinct T- and B-cell areas with germinal centers, as well as dendritic cells, and it is overlaid by a specialized follicle-associated epithelium (FAE) that includes M (membranous or microfold) cells.[13] M cells are distinct from adjacent columnar epithelial cells and take up soluble and microparticulate materials which they pass by transcytosis to underlying immunocompetent cells. Efferent lymphatics drain cells emigrating from MALT follicles to the local lymph nodes (mesenteric lymph nodes in the case of intestinal Peyer's patches) and thence via the thoracic duct into the circulation. The naïve B cells in MALT express surface IgM, but upon antigen stimulation and passage into germinal centers these B cells switch to the expression of surface

Table 3. Selected strategies for enhancing mucosal immune responses

Strategy and Examples	Advantages	Disadvantages
Mucosal adjuvants:	Stimulate responding cells	May be toxic
Enterotoxins (CT, LT), lipid A derivatives, muramyl dipeptide derivatives	Chemical/genetic modifications to eliminate/reduce toxicity	Adjuvanticity related to toxicity?
Coupling to carriers:	Targets antigen to cells	Chemical coupling is cumbersome
Enterotoxin B subunits	Safe (non-toxic)	Loss of binding activity?
-chemically conjugated	May promote Th2 responses	May require adjuvant
-peptide fusions	Peptides limited to linear epitopes	
-chimeric proteins	Chimeric proteins require assembly	
Microparticles, microvesicles:	Conceptually simple	Loss of immunogenicity in preparation
Biodegradable polymers, liposomes, cochleates	Protect against digestion	Inefficient uptake
	Surface modifications to promote uptake	
ISCOMs	ISCOMs promote Th1 responses	
Live bacterial vectors:	Simple production	Response to vector may preclude further use
Attenuated *Salmonella* etc., BCG	Multiple antigens possible	Weak expression of antigens
		Attenuation diminishes immunogenicity
Commensals: lactobacilli, oral streptococci	*Salmonella* and BCG promote Th1 responses	Weak response to commensal bacteria
Live viral vectors:	Based on effective vaccines	Response to vector may preclude further use
Vaccinia, adenovirus, influenza virus, rotavirus,	Genetically simpler than bacteria	Reversion to virulence?
poliovirus replicons	Multiple antigens possible	Limited room for multiple insertions
	May promote CTL responses	Production requires cell culture
Edible plant vectors:		
Potatoes, bananas, tomatoes	Potentially inexpensive	Protein expression low,or in inaccessible location
	Simple to administer	Antigens destroyed in cooking
	Multiple antigens possible	Low immunogenicity of food?

IgA and will ultimately differentiate into polymeric IgA-secreting plasma cells.[14] Stimulated B and T cells that emigrate from MALT (especially from Peyer's patches) express the integrin $\alpha4\beta7$ by which they recognize the mucosal addressin MAdCAM-1 which is strongly expressed on vascular endothelial cells within intestinal lamina propria and lactating mammary glands,

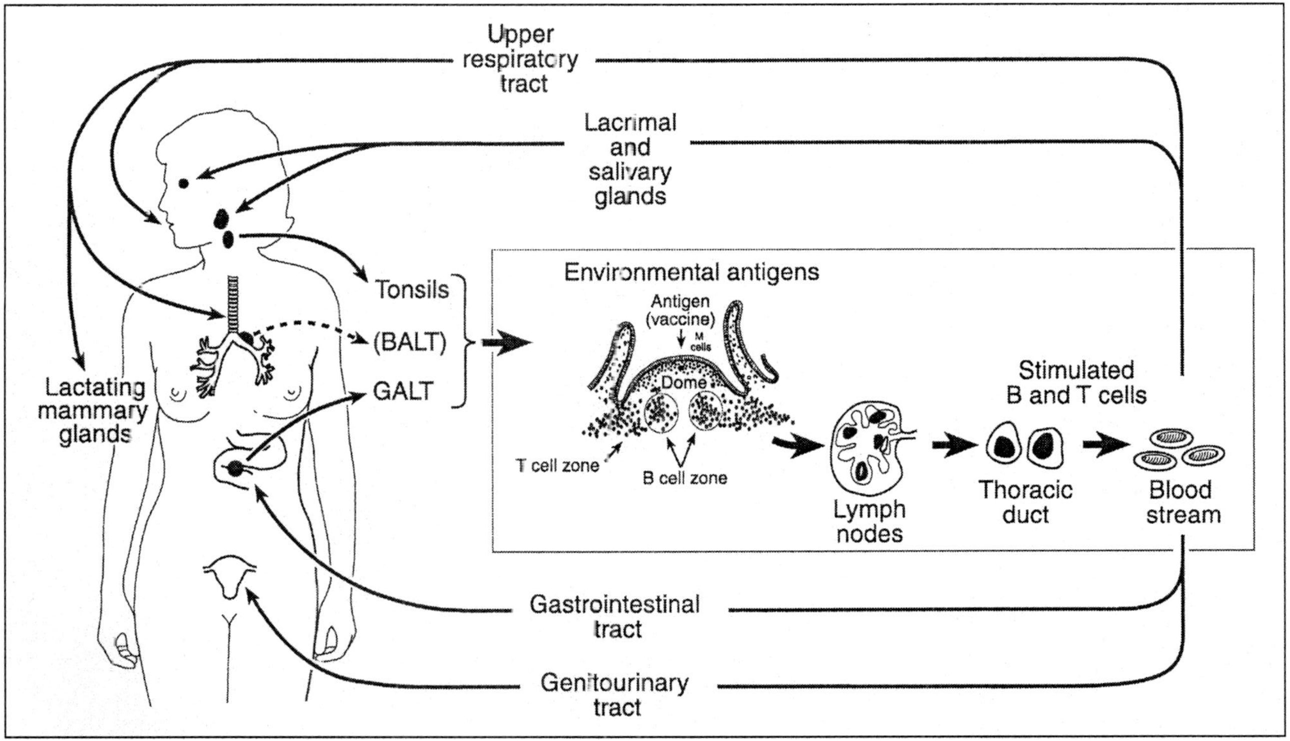

Figure 2. The common mucosal immune system: illustrating the origin of antigen-stimulated, IgA-committed B cells and cognate T cells in inductive sites, mainly the organized MALT of the intestinal and respiratory tracts; trafficking of the cells through draining lymph nodes and efferent lymphatics into the circulation; and homing of the cells into the lamina propria of intestinal, respiratory, and genital tracts and stroma of salivary, lacrimal, and lactating mammy glands, etc. Terminal differentiation of B cells into polymeric IgA-secreting plasma cells occurs in these effector sites with help from T cells and locally produced cytokines, and S-IgA is formed by the pIgR-mediated epithelial transport of this IgA into the secretions. Homing of cells into different effector sites is not uniform, but varies according to the display of vascular endothelial addressins and corresponding lymphocyte integrins. (Modified from ref. 12, with permission.)

but not normally in other mucosae.[15] Cells stimulated in respiratory tract MALT (e.g., tonsils or rodent nasal lymphoid tissue—NALT) express less α4β7 but also L-selectin and have a greater propensity to home to nonintestinal mucosae, including the respiratory and genital tracts.[16,17] The vascular addressins responsible for this have not been conclusively determined but may include VCAM-1 and ICAM-1. Other tracts and glands that lack organized MALT may be able to mount local immune responses, but not to disseminate them throughout the common mucosal immune system.

Once located in mucosal subepithelial spaces, IgA-committed B cells terminally differentiate into plasma cells secreting polymeric IgA which is taken up by epithelial cells through the polymeric Ig receptor (pIgR) expressed on their basolateral surfaces.[18] During transcytosis the extracellular domains of pIgR become covalently linked (through disulfide bridges) to the Fc of the pIgA and are cleaved from the transmembrane segment, so that S-IgA is released from the apical surface into the lumen or secretion.[19] The reader is referred elsewhere for the full cellular and molecular details of the operation of the CMIS.[2,20]

Less well understood are the cell-mediated aspects of mucosal immunity, for example, the generation and role of cytotoxic T cells. The intestinal and probably most other epithelia contain huge numbers of intra-epithelial lymphocytes (IEL) which are T cells predominantly of $CD8^+$ phenotype, many of them expressing the CD8αα dimer or TCRγδ instead of the usual TCRαβ.[21] These cells have a limited repertoire of receptor specificities, many do not undergo thymic selection, and some recognize MHC-like molecules that may enable them to respond to and possibly kill abnormal epithelial cells.[22] Other IEL that recognize nonclassical MHC molecules such as CD1c may be able to respond to lipid or glycolipid antigens presented by CD1c. However, it remains uncertain whether IEL have a role in mucosal defense against bacterial infections.

The intimate relationship between immune cells and epithelium is a distinctive feature of the mucosal immune system that extends beyond physical contact between IEL and epithelial cells.[23] The latter cells are a source of numerous cytokines involved in the influx, activation, and differentiation of myeloid and lymphoid cells (e.g., IL-1, IL-6, IL-7, IL-8, IL-10, and TGF-β); indeed the pattern of cytokines present in the mucosal environment may be responsible for the selective differentiation of pIgA-secreting cells. Conversely the expression of pIgR and transport of S-IgA by epithelial cells are regulated by cytokines (IL-4, IFN-γ, TGF-β and TNF-α) secreted by lymphocytes.[24] Moreover, expression of MHC class II molecules by epithelial cells (also regulated by these cytokines) supports the possibility that they may be able to process and present antigens to T cells,[25] though whether the outcome of this is tolerance or active immunity has been debated.

The challenge for mucosal vaccine development therefore is to determine routes and strategies of immunization that will elicit the desired response in the appropriate location to combat the particular infection.

Strategies and Routes of Mucosal Immunization

Undoubtedly the simplest route for administering a vaccine is by mouth. This requires minimal supervision by trained personnel and can be accomplished without the need for sterile devices such as syringes and needles and without the problems inherent in their provision and disposal as well as cost. Oral vaccination is clearly applicable to mass immunization and so may be readily instituted in under-developed regions where a need for large-scale immunization is greatest, or in community emergency situations posed, for example, by the deployment of biological warfare agents. However, most vaccines as normally prepared for parenteral use are completely unsuitable for enteric administration for two main reasons: they are inactivated by digestive processes including stomach acid, proteolytic enzymes, and possibly also the activities of the commensal microbiota; and they have little or no propensity for uptake by the MALT. Thus protection against digestion and targeting to the MALT-FAE are important goals for development. Furthermore, it is necessary to provoke the mucosal inductive site tissues in such a way that the default response of tolerance is overcome and an appropriate active response is generated. Considerable attention has been given to the development of mucosal adjuvants that can substantially enhance the mucosal IgA antibody response,[26] chief among these being the use of bacterial enterotoxins and their nontoxic derivatives,[27] and to the packaging of vaccines in a variety of microparticulate or microvesicular formulations that would protect the vaccine components against digestion, promote uptake by MALT-FAE, and in some instances exert an adjuvant effect on immune processing.[28] Live attenuated bacteria themselves have also been proposed as mucosal vaccines, and some have been developed for human use.[29] Viruses that target epithelial cells, including poliovirus, rotavirus, influenza, and adenovirus have also been exploited in analogous fashion, to varying extents.

Alternative approaches include the exploitation of other routes of administration, among which the intranasal route is probably the most readily acceptable, though intra-rectal or intra-vaginal instillation could be considered in certain applications. Intranasal immunization would substantially avoid exposing the vaccine to the harsh digestive environment of the gut, and likely bring the vaccine components into more immediate contact with the presumed sites of uptake, whether these are Waldeyer's ring (tonsils and adenoids) or the general nasal epithelium. A large body of experimental evidence attests to its effectiveness in animal models, (e.g. refs. 30-33), and data from human trials are accumulating.[34-36] At least one human intranasally applied vaccine has been extensively evaluated: an attenuated influenza virus vaccine for use in infants.[37]

Selected Approaches to Mucosal Immunization

Detoxified Enterotoxin Adjuvants

Cholera toxin (CT) has become recognized as a 'gold standard' mucosal immunogen, at least in experimental rodents that are resistant to its diarrheagenic effects. Enteric or intranasal administration of microgram doses induces strong mucosal IgA antibody responses in most external secretions and also strong circulating IgG (and IgA) antibodies. These have been shown to persist for prolonged periods and to be recallable by booster immunization several months later, with features typical of anamnestic responses.[38,39] Although CT is far too toxic to be administered to humans, the B subunit alone possesses a similar degree of immunogenicity to the holotoxin and is well-tolerated and "safe": a 'first-generation' oral cholera vaccine therefore consists of the nontoxic B subunit of CT plus killed *Vibrio cholerae* organisms.[40] The closely homologous type I heat-labile enterotoxin of *Escherichia coli* (LT-I) and its B subunit have very similar (but not identical) properties.[41]

In addition to being highly immunogenic, CT and LT-I have adjuvant properties such that they promote strong mucosal IgA and circulatory IgG antibodies against protein antigens with which they are coadministered either orally or intranasally.[42,43] Controversy, however, has issued over the extent to which adjuvanticity is associated with toxicity and the ADP-ribosylating activity of the A subunit, and whether the B subunits alone or nontoxic mutants of the holotoxins have adjuvant activity. Different results have been reported by various investigators depending upon such variables as the contamination of B subunit with intact holotoxin, the inherent immunogenicity and other properties of the coadministered protein antigen, the route of administration (oral or intranasal), and the animal species studied.[44-47] One of the complicating factors is that minor contamination of B subunit with holotoxin is sufficient to reveal synergy between the two;[45,48] thus residual enzyme activity in detoxified mutants could have a similar effect. However, recombinant CTB subunit, and apparently completely nontoxic mutants of CT or LT-I have been shown by some investigators to have mucosal adjuvant activity in mice, although so far trials in humans have been disappointing. Resolving the apparent trade-off between toxicity and adjuvanticity will probably depend upon greater understanding of the mechanisms by which enterotoxins and their A and B subunits exert their immunological properties. These include a variety of effects on antigen-presenting cells, T and B cells, the expression of MHC and costimulatory molecules, secretion of cytokines, and even the permeability of mucosal epithelia.[49]

One new development arises out of reports that type II heat-labile enterotoxins (LT-IIa and LT-IIb) that are produced by rare animal strains of *E. coli* also possess adjuvant activity.[50] These toxins contain B subunits having weak homology to type I enterotoxin B subunits and different ganglioside receptor specificities, but are much less toxic for humans than CT or LT-I. Moreover, initial findings suggest that LT-IIb in particular may be able to drive the immune response more towards type 1 help than the type 2 bias which is usually reported for CT.[51]

Enterotoxin adjuvants have usually been examined for their effects on antibody production, but a few reports have demonstrated elevated cytotoxic T-cell responses.[52,53] In general, the generation and role of cell-mediated immunity in the mucosal immune system are poorly understood, and are therefore areas deserving closer attention.

Recently, concern has arisen over the uptake of enterotoxins or their B subunits by neurons which express ganglioside receptors and their consequent retrograde transmission into the central nervous system.[54,55] Although CTB has a considerable track-record of safety upon intragastric administration in humans, it is uncertain whether potential uptake from nasal passages by the olfactory nerve, which is directly connected to the brain without an intervening synapse, could lead to neurological side-effects.

Enterotoxin B Subunits As Carriers

Given that the potent immunogenicity of enterotoxins depends upon their receptor-binding B subunits for uptake by mucosal inductive sites, an alternative approach to exploiting their immunological properties is to couple a vaccine antigen to the toxin B subunit. This has been elaborated in three different ways: by chemically conjugating protein or polysaccharide antigens to B subunit;[56] by genetically fusing peptides to either terminus or into a surface-exposed loop of B subunit;[57,58] or by genetically constructing chimeric proteins in which a protein antigen is coupled to B subunit pentamer using the A2 subunit, thereby replacing the toxic A1 subunit of the holotoxin by the antigen of choice.[59] All three have been demonstrated to work in principle, but with different limitations. Chemical conjugation is a laborious procedure requiring the purification first of the two components, it yields a somewhat variable and incompletely defined product, and care must be taken to preserve the receptor-binding property of the B subunit. Peptide fusion to B subunits is limited by the finding that peptides longer than approximately 12-20 residues tend to interfere with the assembly of B subunit monomers into pentamers that are necessary for high-affinity receptor binding, as well as by whether linear peptides represent protein antigen epitopes with sufficient fidelity. Construction of holotoxin-like chimeric proteins has been accomplished in recombinant *E. coli* using several different protein antigen partners,[59-61] but success depends on whether the antigen-A2 fusion protein can be expressed in soluble form to be exported to the periplasm for assembly with B subunit.

As with the use of enterotoxin B subunits as adjuvants, controversy exists as to whether antigen-B subunit constructions of whatever form are immunogenic and under what conditions. Coadministration of intact holotoxin as an adjuvant may be necessary but this requirement depends on both the species and the route of immunization.[30,59,62] Furthermore, enteric immunization with antigen chemically conjugated to CTB without any intact holotoxin has been shown to induce profound T-cell tolerance and even to reverse previously induced T cell-mediated immunity[63]—a finding that may have considerable practical application against autoimmune diseases. The extent to which this depends on the inherent properties of the coupled antigen, or to which T-cell tolerance can be induced concomitantly with a mucosal IgA antibody response (or the balance between these two outcomes) has not been fully elucidated. Although impressive data have been obtained in experimental animals immunized with numerous CTB-coupled immunogens, in terms of either responses and protection against infection or tolerance and suppression of autoimmunity, equivalent results from trials of such immunogens in humans have not yet been reported.

Microparticulate and Adhesive Delivery Systems

A large variety of microparticulate or microvesicular formulations of antigens have been developed, many by commercial enterprises, as delivery systems for mucosal vaccines. These include incorporation of antigens into microspheres of biocompatible-biodegradable polymers such as poly(lactide-coglycolide; PLG), liposomes, cochleates, or even emulsions and bioadhesive polymers.[28] The properties of these systems depend upon the physical and biochemical properties of the diverse materials used in their construction, and full consideration of these is not possible within the scope of this chapter. The rationale for this approach is two-fold: particulate antigen is generally more immunogenic than soluble forms of the same material; and enclosing an antigen within a particle or membrane affords protection against digestion and the deleterious conditions that often prevail at mucosal surfaces. In some instances, e.g., ISCOMs ("immuno-stimulating complexes") formed by compounding proteins with certain plant-derived saponins, the resulting particles also enhance immune responses by stimulating antigen-presenting cells.[64] Incorporation of antigens into emulsions or bioadhesive polymers may promote uptake, and while these strategies alone may not afford protection from intestinal digestion they may be applicable in less harsh environments such as the respiratory tract.[65] Limitations of microparticulate delivery systems include the generally low efficiency of uptake of the material by the MALT and the stability of the vaccine antigen to the formulation process, which may involve exposure to heat or organic solvents. However, these systems are amenable to combination with other strategies, such as the use of mucosal adjuvants or by coupling to targeting agents.[66]

Live Bacteria As Carriers

The original forms of live bacterial vectors for mucosal vaccines were enteric pathogens that had been attenuated by the targeted deletion of multiple genes.[67] Numerous species and strains have been developed for delivering cloned vaccine antigens enterically or even intranasally,[29] and most of these exploit the ability of enteropathogens to colonize intestinal mucosae, especially MALT, which is the main portal of invasion for organisms such as *Salmonella* or *Shigella*.[68] However, realizing the potential of this otherwise attractive strategy has been a much more complicated task than originally foreseen. Because antibiotic pressure cannot be applied in vivo, other means of maintaining plasmids have had to be developed, such as the "balanced lethal" *asd*⁻ system, in which deletion of the chromosomal *asd* gene (essential for the synthesis of diaminopimelic acid to make peptidoglycan in *Salmonella*) is compensated by inserting it into the plasmid.[69] Frequently, the level of expression of the cloned vaccine antigen is low, or the antigen is not efficiently translocated to the bacterial surface where most protective antigens are displayed. Consequently, the response to the cloned antigen is often much weaker than the response to the carrier organism. In turn, this can lead to another problem, that a potent response to the carrier may preclude its further use either for boosting or for delivering another antigen, although the extent of this difficulty varies between different reports.[70,71] In addition, gram negative enteric bacteria tend to drive Th1-biased responses, which depending upon the nature of the disease against which protection is required may not be desirable.[72] One potential solution to this could be to coexpress the antigen with CTB in order to exert a Th2 drive.[73] Because high-level expression of a cloned antigen often interferes with growth and metabolism, most recombinant clones are designed to suppress expression of the plasmid containing the gene for the cloned antigen under in vitro growth conditions (e.g., at 30°C) but to turn it on under in vivo conditions (e.g., at 37°C). However, a high burst of expression of the antigen usually curtails survival of the organism in vivo, so that antigen production cannot be sustained. Alternative cloning strategies that permit sustained antigen production, albeit at a low level but still compatible with the persistence of the organism within the MALT may then be more successful.[74] In essence, a central problem seems to be that too much attenuation for the sake of safety diminishes immunogenicity that requires some degree of aggressiveness on the part of the carrier. Thus balancing all these requirements is a major task even when dealing with an inbred experimental animal model, and further development for use in outbred human populations will add another dimension of challenge.

An alternative approach therefore has been to consider developing human commensal strains as vaccine carriers, with the idea that such organisms already possess the attributes that enable them to colonize human mucosae safely. Lactobacilli and oral streptococci (such as *S. gordonii*) have been proposed for this purpose.[75,76] In the latter case, for example, vaccine antigen protein sequences have been inserted into segments of the group A streptococcal M proteins from which potentially harmful regions have been deleted, so that the chimeric protein is anchored into the cell wall and displayed at the surface. Such recombinant organisms have been shown to colonize experimental animals and induce significant mucosal IgA antibody responses to the cloned antigen. Questions remain, however, as to how successful this attractive strategy will be in humans, for several reasons. Once the natural microbiota is established (probably early in infancy and childhood) it is usually difficult to introduce another commensal strain that persists for any length of time. Furthermore, commensal organisms have typically evolved an intimate relationship with their host species in which they provoke minimal immune responses.[77] Whether cloning a foreign antigen into the commensal is sufficient to overcome this without affecting its ability to persistently colonize the host, or whether including another immunostimulatory molecule such as an enterotoxin or its B subunit would improve the response, remain to be seen. The relationships between commensals and their specific hosts are poorly understood at present, so that results from experiments in which nonnatural hosts are colonized with recombinant commensals do not necessarily predict outcomes in natural hosts (humans); these can be determined only by experiment.

Edible Plant Vaccines

An interesting approach to large-scale mucosal immunization at low cost and therefore of great potential significance is the expression of vaccine antigens in edible plant materials.[78] The basic proof of concept has been demonstrated, for example, by cloning CTB or hepatitis B virus surface antigen into potatoes which, when consumed by mice, result in the development of serum and mucosal antibody responses.[79,80] Limitations, however, include the level of expression of the cloned protein antigen and whether the antigen is available to the host's immune system or conversely destroyed by digestion or by cooking procedures. The use, for example, of tomatoes or bananas as vehicles, which have the advantage that they can be eaten raw, has so far been disappointing because either protein production is low or the protein is predominantly produced in the seeds that pass intact through the intestine. As with the use of commensal carriers, an issue may be whether vaccine antigens disguised as food will stimulate an active immune response or induce tolerance unless additional immuno-stimulatory molecules are also included. However, the practical advantage of edible plant vaccines is that, once appropriate plant varieties have been developed, huge quantities might be grown at low cost, possibly even close to the locations where they would be required.

DNA Vaccines for Mucosal Use

DNA vaccines have attracted considerable attention because of the ease with which appropriate plasmids can be constructed, the high stability of DNA, and the avoidance of problems associated with protein antigen expression in recombinant microorganisms. Significant responses especially with respect to cell-mediated immunity have been reported in experimental animals when DNA vaccines have been administered parenterally using the 'gene gun' to inject DNA-coated gold particles subcutaneously or by intramuscular injection of DNA.[81] One report has described the use of the gene gun to administer a DNA vaccine to the female reproductive tract exposed by laparotomy, but responses were modest and this procedure is not generally practicable.[82] Otherwise, attempts at mucosal immunization with DNA vaccines have been few and disappointing, but some interesting strategies have been devised. Among these are the use of adenoviruses, similar to those proposed for gene therapy, to insert vaccine

DNA into mucosal epithelia,[83] and the development of a suicidal strain of *asd⁻ Shigella* carrying a plasmid bearing the vaccine gene that would be released intramucosally upon death of the organism.[84] A recent paper describes the use of reovirus $\sigma 1$ protein to target DNA complexed with poly-L-lysine to nasal mucosa and thereby enhance the ensuing responses.[85] Further effort will be required to develop these and other strategies of mucosal DNA immunization for eventual human use.

Synthetic oligodeoxynucleotides containing immunostimulatory CpG motifs have been applied orally or intranasally as adjuvants with some success, particularly in generating Th1-governed responses in mice.[86] However, these have not yet been evaluated in humans.

Selected Applications of Mucosal Immunization

Most current efforts in mucosal vaccine development concentrate on immunity to enteric pathogens, some of which are discussed elsewhere in this work. However, through the operation of the common mucosal immune system and the distinct properties of IgA antibodies, mucosal immunization might find interesting application in other situations. It should be noted that potent methods of mucosal immunization, particularly exploiting enterotoxins, induce strong circulating IgG as well as mucosal IgA antibodies.

Respiratory Pathogens

Most vaccine efforts to date against *Streptococcus pneumoniae* and *Neisseria meningitidis* have focused on the provision of systemic immunity by inducing circulating antibodies especially to the capsular polysaccharides, although new developments involve either polysaccharide-protein conjugates or surface protein antigens again for parenteral application. An alternative approach might be the development of mucosal immunity aimed at suppressing colonization by the induction of S-IgA antibody in the nasopharyngeal secretions. The principle of this has been demonstrated in a mouse model of nasal colonization by *S. pneumoniae*, in which animals immunized intranasally with a protein antigen (PspA) together with CTB as an adjuvant developed mucosal IgA and circulatory IgG antibodies to PspA and were protected against nasal carriage as well as against lethal intratracheal or intraperitoneal challenge.[87] If this principle could be applied to humans, it might diminish pneumococcal infections by suppressing the carriage rate of *S. pneumoniae*, thereby protecting not only those who are immunized but indirectly also those who are not or cannot be effectively immunized.

Otitis media in infants usually arises when bacteria such as *S. pneumoniae, Haemophilus influenzae*, or *Moraxella catarrhalis* ascend into the middle ear from the nasopharynx via the eustachian tube. Since the middle ear appears to be lined with a mucosal epithelium that is capable of transporting S-IgA from underlying pIgA-secreting plasma cells, mucosal immunization with relevant antigens applied to an inductive site that would generate responses in the upper respiratory tract and its associated passages might be an appropriate means of delivering antibodies to the infected area.[88] Presumably such immunization would suppress nasopharyngeal colonization that is the likely proximate source of infection. An underappreciated bonus of this strategy could be that IgA is a noninflammatory isotype of immunoglobulin, in contrast to IgG. Although the generation of IgG antibodies by systemic immunization might eliminate the infection by opsonophagocytic or complement-dependent mechanisms, some evidence has indicated that IgG antibodies can provoke further immune-mediated inflammation within the middle ear.[89] It is possible that noninflammatory IgA antibodies could help to ameliorate this effect.

Sexually Transmitted Diseases

Despite the general success of antibiotic therapy, the classic bacterial STDs, including gonorrhea, chlamydia, and syphilis, continue to exert a considerable toll on human health especially in regions where modern medical practice is poorly developed, and no vaccines exist to control these infections.[90] Reasons for this include the complicated nature of the organisms concerned, but in addition, comparatively little attention has been paid to how immune protection might be induced in the reproductive tracts. While the genital tracts comprise effector sites of the mucosal immune system, they also include components of circulating immunity.[91] A remarkable finding, repeated in many laboratories in the past decade, is that intranasal immunization is effective in generating antibody responses in the genital tract, although the cellular and molecular mechanisms responsible remain uncertain.[30,92] Although demonstrated initially in mice, similar findings have been reported in primates, and even in small-scale human trials.[32,93] While most efforts have concentrated on the female tract (in which the burden of morbidity is generally greater) limited evidence suggests that the male tract may be similarly responsive.[94] Local (intravaginal) immunization has also been successfully performed in experimental animals with potent stimuli such as live attenuated viruses or CT.[11,95] Exploitation of these findings in the development of vaccines against STDs is sorely lacking, but if successful could have a major impact on human health.

Therapeutic Immunization Against Infection-Driven Inflammatory Diseases

The stomach normally does not display the characteristics of typical mucosal inductive or effector sites: in healthy conditions there are no organized MALT follicles, the epithelium does not normally express pIgR, and there are few IgA-secreting plasma cells in the lamina propria. Given these conditions, it would seem unlikely that prophylactic immunization designed to elicit protective S-IgA antibodies could be successfully developed, for example to prevent colonization by *Helicobacter pylori*. However, when gastritis develops, foci of lymphocytes and plasma cells appear, and S-IgA can be produced and transported through the gastric epithelium.[96,97] Experimental effort has therefore been directed at intragastric immunization with antigens derived from *H. pylori* often using enterotoxins or their B subunits as adjuvants, and some degree of success has been reported in murine models of infection.[98,99] As the natural response to *H. pylori* infection is predominantly Th1-governed, mucosal immunization could have multiple effects,[100] such as helping to eliminate the causative organism by S-IgA antibody-dependent mechanisms, promoting a Th2 bias, or promoting a noninflammatory environment dominated by IgA antibodies. Whether any or all of these mechanisms are instrumental in the observed beneficial effect remains to be determined.

Similar considerations could apply in other instances of infection-driven inflammatory disease, for example, periodontitis, in which chronic infection of the gingivae with certain species of gram negative anaerobes leads to inflammatory destruction of the tissues supporting the teeth and resorption of alveolar bone.[101] Bacterial antigens such as lipopolysaccharides and fimbriae as well as potent proteases have all been implicated in provoking inflammatory responses involving an array of cytokines and other mediators. However, although the gingival mucosa is bathed with saliva that contains abundant S-IgA, it is not an effector site of the CMIS, and the lymphoid aggregates that appear in advanced disease contain cells secreting IgM, IgG, and IgA reflecting the systemic arm of immunity. Most current vaccine efforts are aimed at inducing serum antibodies that would eliminate the bacterial infection.[102,103] Circumstantial evidence associating increased gingival IgA levels with a favorable outcome to treatment suggests the possibility that strategies designed to enhance an IgA component in the response might be beneficial in reducing the inflammation,[104,105] but this remains a speculative idea.

The Future for Mucosal Immunization

While mucosal immunization offers the prospect of major advantages (Table 2) especially in application to large communities, significant problems apart from scientific development need to be overcome before it can become widely adopted. Among these is one of attitude, on the part of scientists and physicians as much as on the part of the public, and a willingness to think "outside the box" of conventional approaches to immunization by parenteral injection. Indeed, the words "immunization" and "vaccine" have become indelibly associated in the public mind with the hypodermic syringe, and aversion to this device still poses an obstacle for some individuals. Moreover, syringes are expensive, sometimes more so than the vaccine material itself, and their use requires trained personnel as well as secure procedures for safe handling, storage, and disposal.

Moreover, the guidelines for regulatory approval of vaccines are focused on efficacy criteria such as seroconversion, which depends upon the development of serum antibody, usually IgG. This is not necessarily accomplished by mucosal immunization, or if so may not accurately reflect the status of immunity at the mucosal site where protection against initial infection is manifested. There is a need for improved methods and standards of assessing immunity in mucosal secretions that can be recommended to regulatory authorities. Secretions are inherently more variable in their composition than serum, and their concentration may be altered by the methods used for their collection, for example by administering secretagogues or the use of lavage procedures, or even inadvertently through unintended and inapparent neuro-endocrine stimuli. Such effects must be accounted for in reporting secretory antibody data, for example by measuring total IgA concentration as well as specific IgA antibody levels. Other strategies that have been proposed include measures of total protein or other constituents, and comparative data on their utility need to be obtained. Improper methods of collection can result in contamination of secretions with blood or tissue fluids. Furthermore, since immunoglobulin concentrations in secretions are low (typically ~1% of those found in serum), and since assay procedures and reagents for IgA are often less sensitive than those for IgG, there are severe limits on both the accuracy and sensitivity of measuring antibodies in secretions. These practical considerations, together with a lack of uniformity in data reporting and the absence of any agreed standard in assay calibration, accentuate the problems of comparing mucosal and systemic antibody responses on an equal basis. The greater statistical variance that can result from all of these factors in estimates of mucosal antibody responses, in comparison to estimates of serum antibodies, may lead to weaker correlations with measures of protection against infection, and consequently could result in erroneous conclusions being drawn concerning the causes of protective immunity.

Nevertheless, the principle of mucosal immunization has been demonstrated by the development of oral or intranasal vaccines against polio, cholera, typhoid, influenza, and rotavirus for human use, as well as numerous others for veterinary applications. Some of these vaccines need further improvement to increase efficacy or to avoid side-effects (as have unfortunately occurred with the oral rotavirus vaccine). Many more are in various stages of development.

Acknowledgments

Studies in the author's laboratory are supported by US-PHS grants DE06746, DE09691, and AI46561 from the National Institutes of Health.

References

1. Brandtzaeg P. Overview of the mucosal immune system. Curr Topics Microbiol Immunol 1989; 146:13-25.
2. Mestecky J, McGhee JR. Immunoglobulin A (IgA): Molecular and cellular interactions involved in IgA biosynthesis and immune response. Adv Immunol 1987; 40:153-245.
3. Mestecky J, Bienenstock J, McGhee JR et al. Historical aspects of mucosal immunology. In: Ogra PL, Mestecky J, Lamm ME, eds. Mucosal Immunology. 2nd Edition. San Diego: Academic Press, 1999:xxiii-xliii.
4. Mowat AM, Weiner HL. Oral tolerance. Physiological basis and clinical applications. In: Ogra PL, Mestecky J, Lamm ME, eds. Mucosal Immunology. 2nd ed. San Diego: Academic Press, 1999:587-618.
5. Harrod T, Martin M, Russell MW. Long-term persistence and recall of immune responses in aged mice after mucosal immunization. Oral Microbiol Immunol 2001; 16:170-177.
6. Harokopakis E, Hajishengallis G, Greenway TE et al. Mucosal immunogenicity of a recombinant Salmonella typhimurium-cloned heterologous antigen in the absence or presence of coexpressed cholera toxin A2/B subunits. Infect Immun 1997; 65:1445-1454.

7. Kohler JJ, Pathangey L, Hasona A et al. Long-term immunological memory induced by recombinant oral Salmonella vaccine vectors. Infect Immun 2000; 68:4370-4373.
8. Matzinger P. Tolerance, danger, and the extended family. Annu Rev Immunol 1994; 12:991-1045.
9. Ogra PL, Faden H, Welliver RC. Vaccination strategies for mucosal immune responses. Clin Microbiol Rev 2001; 14:430-445.
10. Mestecky J, McGhee JR, Michalek SM et al. Concept of the local and common mucosal immune response. Adv Exp Med Biol 1978; 107:185-192.
11. Wu HY, Abdu S, Stinson D et al. Generation of female genital tract antibody responses by local or central (common) mucosal immunization. Infect Immun 2000; 68:5539-5545.
12. Mestecky J. The common mucosal immune system and current strategies for induction of immune response in external secretions. J Clin Immunol 1987; 7:265-276.
13. Kraehenbuhl J-P, Neutra MR. Molecular and cellular basis of immune protection of mucosal surfaces. Physiol Rev 1992; 72:853-879.
14. Fagarasan S, Kinoshita K, Muramatsu M et al. In situ class switching and differentiation to IgA-producing cells in the gut lamina propria. Nature 2001; 413:639-643.
15. Butcher EC. Lymphocyte homing and intestinal immunity. In: Ogra PL, Mestecky J, Lamm ME, eds. Mucosal Immunology. 2nd ed. San Diego: Academic Press, 1999:507-522.
16. Quiding-Järbrink M, Nordström I, Granström G et al. Differential expression of tissue-specific adhesion molecules on human circulating antibody-forming cells after systemic, enteric, and nasal immunizations. A molecular basis for the compartmentalization of effector B cell responses. J Clin Invest 1997; 99:1281-1286.
17. Johansson EL, Rudin A, Wassén L et al. Distribution of lymphocytes and adhesion molecules in human cervix and vagina. Immunology 1999; 96:272-277.
18. Mostov K, Kaetzel CS. Immunoglobulin transport and the polymeric immunoglobulin receptor. In: Ogra PL, Mestecky J, Lamm ME, eds. Mucosal Immunology. 2nd ed. San Diego: Academic Press, 1999:181-211.
19. Mestecky J, Lue C, Russell MW. Selective transport of IgA: cellular and molecular aspects. Gastroenterol Clin N Amer 1991; 20:441-471.
20. McGhee JR, Lamm ME, Strober W. Mucosal immune responses. An overview. In: Ogra PL, Mestecky J, Lamm ME, eds. Mucosal Immunology. 2nd ed. San Diego: Academic Press, 1999: 485-506.
21. Lefrancois L, Puddington L. Basic aspects of intraepithelial lymphocyte immunobiology. In: Ogra PL, Mestecky J, Lamm ME, eds. Mucosal Immunology. 2nd ed. San Diego: Academic Press, 1999:413-428.
22. Aranda R, Sydora BC, Kronenberg M. Intraepithelial lymphocytes: function. In: Ogra PL, Mestecky J, Lamm ME, eds. Mucosal Immunology. 2nd ed. San Diego: Academic Press, 1999:429-437.
23. Fujihashi K, Ernst PB. A mucosal internet. Epithelial cell-immune cell interactions. In: Ogra PL, Mestecky J, Lamm ME, eds. Mucosal Immunology. 2nd ed. San Diego: Academic Press, 1999:619-630.
24. Norderhaug IN, Johansen FE, Schjerven H et al. Regulation of the formation and external transport of secretory immunoglobulins. Crit Rev Immunol 1999; 19:481-508.
25. Mayer L, Blumberg RS. Antigen-presenting cells. Epithelial cells. In: Ogra PL, Mestecky J, Lamm ME, eds. Mucosal Immunology. 2nd ed. San Diego: Academic Press, 1999:365-379.
26. O'Hagan DT, MacKichan ML, Singh M. Recent developments in adjuvants for vaccines against infectious diseases. Biomol Eng 2001; 18:69-85.
27. Pizza M, Giuliani MM, Fontana MR et al. Mucosal vaccines: non toxic derivatives of LT and CT as mucosal adjuvants. Vaccine 2001; 19:2534-2541.
28. Michalek SM, O'Hagan DT, Gould-Fougerite S et al. Antigen delivery systems. Nonliving microparticles, liposomes, cochleates, and ISCOMS. In: Ogra PL, Mestecky J, Lamm ME, eds. Mucosal Immunology. 2nd ed. San Diego: Academic Press, 1999:759-778.
29. Hantman MJ, Hohmann EL, Murphy CG et al. Antigen delivery systems. Development of recombinant live vaccines using viral or bacterial vectors. In: Ogra PL, Mestecky J, Lamm ME, eds. Mucosal Immunology. 2nd ed. San Diego: Academic Press, 1999:779-791.
30. Wu H-Y, Russell MW. Induction of mucosal immunity by intranasal application of a streptococcal surface protein antigen with the cholera toxin B subunit. Infect Immun 1993; 61:314-322.
31. Gallichan WS, Johnson DC, Graham FL et al. Mucosal immunity and protection after intranasal immunization with recombinant adenovirus expressing herpes simplex virus glycoprotein B. J Infect Dis 1993; 168:622-629.
32. Russell MW, Moldoveanu Z, White PL et al. Salivary, nasal, genital, and systemic antibody responses in monkeys immunized intranasally with a bacterial protein antigen and the cholera toxin B subunit. Infect Immun 1996; 64:1272-1283.

33. Staats HF, Montgomery SP, Palker TJ. Intranasal immunization is superior to vaginal, gastric, or rectal immunization for the induction of systemic and mucosal anti-HIV antibody responses. AIDS Res Hum Retroviruses 1997; 13:945-952.
34. Hashigucci K, Ogawa H, Ishidate T et al. Antibody responses in volunteers induced by nasal influenza vaccine combined with Escherichia coli heat-labile enterotoxin B subunit containing a trace amount of the holotoxin. Vaccine 1996; 14:113-119.
35. Haneberg B, Dalseg R, Wedege E et al. Intranasal administration of a meningococcal outer membrane vesicle vaccine induces persistent local mucosal antibodies and serum antibodies with strong bactericidal activity in humans. Infect Immun 1998; 66:1334-1341.
36. Rudin A, Johansson E-L, Bergquist C et al. Differential kinetics and distribution of antibodies in serum and nasal and vaginal secretions after nasal and oral vaccination of humans. Infect Immun 1998; 66:3390-3396.
37. Belshe RB, Mendelman PM, Treanor J et al. The efficacy of live attenuated, cold-adapted, trivalent, intranasal influenzavirus vaccine in children. N Engl J Med 1998; 338:1405-1412.
38. Vajdy M, Lycke N. Stimulation of antigen-specific T- and B-cell memory in local as well as systemic lymphoid tissues following oral immunization with cholera toxin adjuvant. Immunology 1993; 80:197-203.
39. Jertborn M, Svennerholm AM, Holmgren J. Immunological memory after immunization with oral cholera B subunit-whole-cell vaccine in Swedish volunteers. Vaccine 1994; 12:1078-1082.
40. Sack DA, Clemens JD, Huda S et al. Antibody responses after immunization with killed oral cholera vaccines during the 1985 vaccine field trial in Bangladesh. J Infect Dis 1991; 164:407-411.
41. Klipstein FA, Engert RF, Clements JD. Arousal of mucosal secretory immunoglobulin A antitoxin in rats immunized with Escherichia coli heat-labile enterotoxin. Infect Immun 1982; 37:1086-1092.
42. Clements JD, Hartzog NM, Lyon FL. Adjuvant activity of Escherichia coli heat-labile enterotoxin and effect on the induction of oral tolerance in mice to unrelated protein antigens. Vaccine 1988; 6:269-277.
43. Elson CO. Cholera toxin and its subunits as potential oral adjuvants. Curr Topics Microbiol Immunol 1989; 146:29-33.
44. Lycke N, Tsuji T, Holmgren J. The adjuvant effect of Vibrio cholerae and Escherichia coli heat-labile enterotoxins is linked to their ADP-ribosyltransferase activity. Eur J Immunol 1992; 22:2277-2281.
45. Tamura S, Yamanaka A, Shimohara M et al. Synergistic action of cholera toxin B subunit (and Escherichia coli heat-labile toxin B subunit) and a trace amount of cholera whole toxin as an adjuvant for nasal influenza vaccine. Vaccine 1994; 12:419-426.
46. de Haan L, Verweij WR, Feil IK et al. Mutants of the Escherichia coli heat-labile enterotoxin with reduced ADP-ribosylation activity or no activity retain the immunogenic properties of the native holotoxin. Infect Immun 1996; 64:5413-5416.
47. Wu HY, Russell MW. Induction of mucosal and systemic immune responses by intranasal immunization using recombinant cholera toxin B subunit as an adjuvant. Vaccine 1998; 16:286-292.
48. Wilson AD, Clarke CJ, Stokes CR. Whole cholera toxin and B subunit act synergistically as an adjuvant for the mucosal immune response of mice to keyhole limpet haemocyanin. Scand J Immunol 1990; 31:443-451.
49. Elson CO, Dertzbaugh MT. Mucosal adjuvants. In: Ogra PL, Mestecky J, Lamm ME, eds. Mucosal Immunology. 2nd ed. San Diego: Academic Press, 1999:817-838.
50. Martin MH, Metzger DJ, Michalek SM et al. Comparative analysis of the mucosal adjuvanticity of the type II heat-labile enterotoxins, LT-IIa and LT-IIb. Infect Immun 2000; 68:281-287.
51. Martin MH, Metzger DJ, Michalek SM et al. Distinct cytokine regulation by cholera toxin and the type II heat-labile enterotoxins involves differential regulation of CD40 ligand on $CD4^+$ T cells. Infect Immun 2001; 69:4486-4492.
52. Porgador A, Staats HF, Itoh Y et al. Intranasal immunization with cytotoxic T-lymphocyte epitope peptide and mucosal adjuvant cholera toxin: Selective augmentation of peptide-presenting dendritic cells in nasal mucosa-associated lymphoid tissue. Infect Immun 1998; 66:5876-5881.
53. Belyakov IM, Ahlers JD, Clements JD et al. Interplay of cytokines and adjuvants in the regulation of mucosal and systemic HIV-specific CTL. J Immunol 2000; 165:6454-6462.
54. Van Ginkel FW, Jackson RJ, Yuki Y et al. Cutting edge: The mucosal adjuvant cholera toxin redirects vaccine proteins into olfactory tissues. J Immunol 2000; 165:4778-4782.
55. Hagiwara Y, Iwasaki T, Asanuma H et al. Effects of intranasal administration of cholera toxin (or Escherichia coli heat-labile enterotoxin) B subunits supplemented with a trace amount of the holotoxin on the brain. Vaccine 2001; 19:1652-1660.
56. Russell MW, Wu H-Y. Distribution, persistence, and recall of serum and salivary antibody responses to peroral immunization with protein antigen I/II of Streptococcus mutans coupled to the cholera toxin B subunit. Infect Immun 1991; 59:4061-4070.

57. Dertzbaugh MT, Peterson DL, Macrina FL. Cholera toxin B-subunit gene fusion: structural and functional analysis of the chimeric protein. Infect Immun 1990; 58:70-79.
58. Jagusztyn-Krynicka EK, Clark-Curtiss JE, Curtiss R. Escherichia coli heat-labile toxin subunit B fusions with Streptococcus sobrinus antigens expressed by Salmonella typhimurium oral vaccine strains: importance of the linker for antigenicity and biological activities of the hybrid proteins. Infect Immun 1993; 61:1004-1015.
59. Hajishengallis G, Hollingshead SK, Koga T et al. Mucosal immunization with a bacterial protein antigen genetically coupled to cholera toxin A2/B subunits. J Immunol 1995; 154:4322-4332.
60. Jobling MG, Holmes RK. Fusion proteins containing the A2 domain of cholera toxin assemble with B polypeptides of cholera toxin to form immunoreactive and functional holotoxin-like chimeras. Infect Immun 1992; 60:4915-4924.
61. Sultan F, Jin LL, Jobling MG et al. Mucosal immunogenicity of a holotoxin-like molecule containing the serine-rich Entamoeba histolytica protein (SREHP) fused to the A2 domain of cholera toxin. Infect Immun 1998; 66:462-468.
62. Hajishengallis G, Russell MW, Michalek SM. Effectiveness of an adherence domain in comparison to a structural domain of Streptococcus mutans antigen I/II in protection against dental caries in rats after intranasal immunization. Infect Immun 1998; 66:1740-1743.
63. Sun JB, Holmgren J, Czerkinsky C. Cholera toxin B subunit: An efficient transmucosal carrier-delivery system for induction of peripheral immunological tolerance. Proc Natl Acad Sci USA 1994; 91:10795-10799.
64. Grdic D, Smith R, Donachie A et al. The mucosal adjuvant effects of cholera toxin and immune-stimulating complexes differ in their requirement for IL-12, indicating different pathways of action. Eur J Immunol 1999; 29:1774-1784.
65. Gizurarson S. Optimal delivery of vaccines: clinical pharmacokinetic considerations. Clin Pharmacokinet 1996; 30:1-15.
66. Harokopakis E, Hajishengallis G, Michalek SM. Effectiveness of liposomes possessing surface-linked recombinant B subunit of cholera toxin as an oral antigen delivery system. Infect Immun 1998; 66:4299-4304.
67. Curtiss R, Kelly SM, Gulig PA et al. Selective delivery of antigens by recombinant bacteria. Curr Topics Microbiol Immunol 1989; 146:35-49.
68. Carter PB, Collins FM. The route of enteric infection in normal mice. J Exp Med 1974; 139:1189-1203.
69. Galan JE, Nakayama K, Curtiss R. Cloning and characterization of the asd gene of Salmonella typhimurium: use in stable maintenance of recombinant plasmids in Salmonella vaccine strains. Gene 1990; 94:29-35.
70. Roberts M, Bacon A, Li JL et al. Prior immunity to homologous and heterologous Salmonella serotypes suppresses local and systemic anti-fragment C antibody responses and protection from tetanus toxin in mice immunized with Salmonella strains expressing fragment C. Infect Immun 1999; 67:3810-3815.
71. Kohler JJ, Pathangey LB, Gillespie SR et al. Effect of preexisting immunity to Salmonella on the immune response to recombinant Salmonella enterica serovar Typhimurium expressing a Porphyromonas gingivalis hemagglutinin. Infect Immun 2000; 68:3116-3120.
72. Klimpel GR, Asuncion M, Haithcoat J et al. Cholera toxin and Salmonella typhimurium induce different cytokine profiles in the gastrointestinal tract. Infect Immun 1995; 63:1134-1137.
73. Hajishengallis G, Harokopakis E, Hollingshead SK et al. Construction and oral immunogenicity of a Salmonella typhimurium strain expressing a streptococcal adhesin linked to the A2/B subunits of cholera toxin. Vaccine 1996; 14:1545-1548.
74. Huang Y, Hajishengallis G, Michalek SM. Construction and characterization of a Salmonella enterica serovar Typhimurium clone expressing a salivary adhesin of Streptococcus mutans under control of the anaerobically inducible nirB promoter. Infect Immun 2000; 68:1549-1556.
75. Medaglini D, Pozzi G, King TP et al. Mucosal and systemic immune responses to a recombinant protein expressed on the surface of the oral commensal bacterium Streptococcus gordonii after oral colonization. Proc Natl Acad Sci USA 1995; 92:6868-6872.
76. Shaw DM, Gaerthé B, Leer RJ et al. Engineering the microflora to vaccinate the mucosa: serum immunoglobulin G responses and activated draining cervical lymph nodes following mucosal application of tetanus toxin fragment C-expressing lactobacilli. Immunology 2000; 100:510-518.
77. Shroff KE, Meslin K, Cebra JJ. Commensal enteric bacteria engender a self-limiting humoral mucosal immune response while permanently colonizing the gut. Infect Immun 1995; 63:3904-3913.
78. Palmer KE, Arntzen CJ, Lomonossoff GP. Antigen delivery systems.Transgenic plants and recombinant plant viruses. In: Ogra PL, Mestecky J, Lamm ME, eds. Mucosal Immunology. 2nd ed. San Diego: Academic Press, 1999:793-807.

79. Thanavala Y, Yang YF, Lyons P et al. Immunogenicity of transgenic plant-derived hepatitis B surface antigen. Proc Natl Acad Sci USA 1995; 92:3358-3361.
80. Mason HS, Haq TA, Clements JD et al. Edible vaccine protects mice against Escherichia coli heat-labile enterotoxin (LT): potatoes expressing a synthetic LT-B gene. Vaccine 1998; 16:1336-1343.
81. Fynan EF, Webster RG, Fuller DH et al. DNA vaccines: protective immunizations by parenteral, mucosal, and gene-gun inoculations. Proc Natl Acad Sci USA 1993; 90:11478-11482.
82. Livingston JB, Lu S, Robinson H et al. Immunization of the female genital tract with a DNA-based vaccine. Infect Immun 1998; 66:322-329.
83. Van Ginkel FW, Liu C, Simecka JW et al. Intratracheal gene delivery with adenoviral vector induces elevated systemic IgG and mucosal IgA antibodies to adenovirus and beta-galactosidase. Hum Gene Ther 1995; 6:895-903.
84. Sizemore DR, Branstrom AA, Sadoff JC. Attenuated Shigella as a DNA delivery vehicle for DNA-mediated immunization. Science 1995; 270:299-302.
85. Wu Y, Wang X, Csencsits KL et al. M cell-targeted DNA vaccination. Proc Natl Acad Sci USA 2001; 98:9318-9323.
86. McCluskie MJ, Weeratna RD, Krieg AM et al. CpG DNA is an effective oral adjuvant to protein antigens in mice. Vaccine 2000; 19:950-957.
87. Briles DE, Ades E, Paton JC et al. Intranasal immunization of mice with a mixture of the pneumococcal proteins PsaA and PspA is highly protective against nasopharyngeal carriage of Streptococcus pneumoniae. Infect Immun 2000; 68:796-800.
88. Russell MW, Martin MH, Wu H-Y et al. Strategies of immunization against mucosal infections. Vaccine 2001; 19 (Suppl.1):S122-S127.
89. Suzuki M, Kawauchi H, Mogi G. Immune-mediated otitis media with effusion. Am J Otolaryngol 1988; 9:199-209.
90. Sparling PF, Elkins C, Wyrick PB et al. Vaccines for bacterial sexually transmitted infections: A realistic goal? Proc Natl Acad Sci USA 1994; 91:2456-2463.
91. Mestecky J, Russell MW. Induction of mucosal immune responses in the genital tract. FEMS Immunol Med Microbiol 2000; 27:351-355.
92. Gallichan WS, Rosenthal KL. Specific secretory immune responses in the female genital tract following intranasal immunization with a recombinant adenovirus expressing glycoprotein B of herpes simplex virus. Vaccine 1995; 13:1589-1595.
93. Johansson E-L, Wassen L, Holmgren J et al. Nasal and vaginal vaccinations have differential effects on antibody responses in vaginal and cervical secretions in humans. Infect Immun 2001; 69:7481-7486.
94. Rudin G, Riise GC, Holmgren J. Antibody responses in the lower respiratory tract and male urogenital tract in humans after nasal and oral vaccination with cholera toxin B subunit. Infect Immun 1999; 67:2884-2890.
95. Parr EL, Parr MB. Immune responses and protection against vaginal infection after nasal or vaginal immunization with attenuated herpes simplex virus type-2. Immunology 1999; 98:639-645.
96. Valnes K, Brandtzaeg P, Elgjo K et al. Quantitative distribution of immunoglobulin-producing cells in gastric mucosa: relation to chronic gastritis and glandular atrophy. Gut 1986; 27:505-514.
97. Ahlstedt I, Lindholm C, Lönroth H et al. Role of local cytokines in increased gastric expression of the secretory component in Helicobacter pylori infection. Infect Immun 1999; 67:4921-4925.
98. Czinn SJ, Nedrud JG. Oral immunization against Helicobacter pylori. Infect Immum 1991; 59:2359-2363.
99. Weltzin R, Guy B, Thomas Jr WD et al. Parenteral adjuvant activities of Escherichia coli heat-labile toxin and its B subunit for immunization of mice against gastric Helicobacter pylori infection. Infect Immun 2000; 68:2775-2782.
100. Hatzifoti C, Wren BW, Morrow WJW. Helicobacter pylori vaccine strategies - triggering a gut reaction. Immunol Today 2000; 21:615-619.
101. Loesche WJ, Grossman NS. Periodontal disease as a specific, albeit chronic, infection: diagnosis and treatment. Clin Microbiol Rev 2001; 14:727-752.
102. Moritz AJ, Cappelli D, Lantz MS et al. Immunization with Porphyromonas gingivalis cysteine protease: Effects on experimental gingivitis and ligature-induced periodontitis in Macaca fascicularis. J Periodontol 1998; 69:686-697.
103. Houston LS, Lukehart SA, Persson GR et al. Function of anti-Porphyromonas gingivalis immunoglobulin classes in immunized Macaca fascicularis. Oral Microbiol Immunol 1999;14:86-91.
104. Grbic JT, Lamster IB, Fine JB et al. Changes in gingival crevicular fluid levels of immunoglobulin A following therapy: Association with attachment loss. J Periodontol 1999; 70:1221-1227.
105. Russell MW, Sibley DA. IgA as an anti-inflammatory regulator of immunity. Oral Dis 1999; 5:55-56.

Chapter 6

New Technologies for Bacterial Vaccines

Ronald W. Ellis

Introduction

Vaccines represent one of the two most effective health-care interventions of the past century. As was the case with the introduction of supplies of clean water, vaccinations with billions of doses during the 20th century are estimated to have contributed an additional 10-15 years to the average human life-span, in addition to preventing much disease and suffering. Moreover, vaccinations have been generally highly cost-effective, sparing tens of billions of dollars in health-care costs. New vaccine technologies offer the prospect for the development of many new vaccines that could prevent even more diseases.

There are two broad categories of vaccines and vaccination, active and passive. Active vaccination stimulates the host's immune system to produce specific antibodies or cellular immune responses or both, which would protect against or eliminate a disease. Passive vaccination uses a preparation of antibodies that neutralizes the bacterial infectivity and is administered before or around the time of known or potential exposure. The term vaccine generally refers to active vaccines, which are the object of the majority of research and development activities in the field. Almost all work in the field of bacterial vaccines has been for prophylactic vaccines, since relatively few bacteria (e.g., *Helicobacter pylori*) establish chronic infections and disease. This chapter summarizes the major technologies for making different kinds of prophylactic bacterial vaccines. The status of development of major vaccines made by each approach is identified as licensed or in clinical or preclinical evaluations (Table 1). The technologies and examples presented should provide a strong framework for appreciating the diverse approaches to the research and development of new bacterial vaccines.

There are three general categories of bacterial vaccines. A live vaccine is a bacteria that can replicate in the host, thereby functioning as an immunogen without causing its natural disease. A subunit or inactivated vaccine is an immunogen that cannot replicate in the host. A DNA-based vaccine is taken up by cells, in which it directs the synthesis of bacterial vaccine antigen(s).

The strategic decision for developing a live, subunit/inactivated, or DNA-based bacterial vaccine should be made after considering the epidemiology, pathogenesis and immunobiology of the disease in question as well as the technical feasibility of each approach. Epidemiology indicates the target population, which may favor certain strategies as more appropriate for eliciting protective immunity. For example, safety is very important for a vaccine intended for healthy infants, yet polysaccharide vaccines are useless for infants because they do not elicit protective immunity. Knowledge of immunobiology should aid in identifying the nature of protective immunity that should be elicited by the vaccine. Certain immune responses may be protective, while others may be useless to the prevention of a particular infection. For example, the clearance of the natural infection may correlate with the appearance of specific antibodies against the bacteria; the antigen that elicits such antibodies would be a candidate vaccine immunogen. The study of immunobiology is greatly facilitated or enabled by developing an experimental animal model, the availability of which enables candidate vaccines to be tested and optimized for efficacy before development for clinical evaluation.

New Bacterial Vaccines, edited by Ronald W. Ellis and Bernard R. Brodeur.

Table 1. Status of development of bacterial vaccines made by different technologies

Type of Vaccine*	Status of Development** Preclinical Evaluation***	Clinical Evaluation[§]	Licensed Product[§§]	Example[#]	References
I. Live					
A. Classical strategies			x	Tuberculosis (*Bacille Calmette-Guérin (BCG)*)	1
			x	Typhoid fever (*Salmonella typhi*)	3
B. Recombinant bacteria			x	Cholera (*Vibrio cholerae)*	4
		x		*Shigella sonnei*	5
C. Recombinant bacterial vector		x		*Salmonella typhi*[a]	6,7
		x		*Vibrio cholerae*[a]	8
	x			*Shigella flexneri*[a]	9
	x			*Streptococcus gordoni*	10
II. Subunit/inactivated Vaccines					
A. Whole bacteria			x	Pertussis (*Bordetella pertussis*)	11
			x	Cholera	12,14
		x		Enterotoxigenic *Escherichia coli*	13
B. Protein-based					
1. Natural			x	Meningococcal (*Neisseria meningitidis)*	17
			x	Pertussis	18-20
2. Chemically inactivated			x	Tetanus (*Clostridium tetani*)	21
			x	Diphtheria (*Corynebacterium diphtheriae*)	22
			x	Pertussis	23
3. Genetically inactivated			x	Pertussis	24
		x		Diphtheria	25
4. Recombinant polypeptide			x	Lyme disease (*Borrelia burgdorferi*)	26
			x	Cholera[b]	14
		x		Pneumococcal (*Streptococcus pneumoniae*)	27
		x		Meningococcal	28,29

Continued on next page

Table 1. Status of development of bacterial vaccines made by different technologies (continued)

Type of Vaccine*	Status of Development** Preclinical Evaluation***	Clinical Evaluation§	Licensed Product§§	Example#	References
C. Peptide based					
1. Conjugate		x		*Pseudomonas aeruginosa*[c]	31
		x		Malaria[c]	32
2. Fusion protein		x		Malaria[d]	33
D. Polysaccharide-based					
1. Plain polysaccharide			x	*Haemophilus influenza type b* (Hib)	34
			x	Meningococcal	35
			x	Pneumococcal	36
2. Conjugate			x	Hib[e]	37
			x	Pneumococcal[f]	38,39
			x	Meningococcal serogroup C[c,f]	40
		x		*P. aeruginosa*[c]	41
III. DNA-based					
A. DNA- naked	x			Tuberculosis	44
B. Facilitated DNA	x			Malaria	48
C. Bacterial delivery	x			*S. flexneri*	49
	x			*Salmonella typhimurium*	50

* These categories are presented in the same outline as in the text.
** This denotes the single most advanced status achieved by each example.
*** Not yet evaluated in a human clinical trial.
§ In clinical trial but not yet licensed.
§§ Licensed in one or more major countries in the world.
# These are representative examples for each vaccine strategy, with one or two key illustrative references.

a Examples of foreign polypeptides include toxoids from *E. coli, V. cholerae, and C. tetani.*
b Mixed with whole-cell cholera to constitute final vaccine.
c Conjugate carrier is TT.
d Fusion partner is hepatitis B surface antigen.
e Conjugate carriers are TT, DT, CRM_{197} and OMPC.
f Conjugate carrier is CRM_{197}

Live Vaccines

Live vaccines consist of bacterial strains that replicate in the host, so that the vaccine may elicit an immune response similar to that elicited by the natural infection. The live vaccine is attenuated, meaning that its disease-causing capacity is eliminated by biological or technical manipulations. It is critical to ensure that the live vaccine is neither underattenuated, i.e., retaining even limited pathogenicity, nor overattenuated, being no longer infectious enough to be an effective vaccine). Live vaccines usually elicit both humoral immunity (antibodies) as well as cellular immunity [e.g., cytotoxic T-lymphocytes (CTL)]. Although these properties per se make live vaccines highly desirable, such vaccines are not technically feasible for most targets under development. The window for attenuation may be too narrow: the vaccine strain may be incompletely attenuated and consequently causing its natural disease at a low frequency, or completely attenuated and incompletely immunogenic. Because a live vaccine can replicate, reversion to its more naturally pathogenic form may be possible. Live vaccine strains can be transmitted from the vaccinee to an unvaccinated individual, which can be quite serious if the recipient is immunodeficient or is undergoing cancer chemotherapy. In some cases, the natural bacterial infection per se fails to produce a protective immune response, such that an attenuated bacterial strain would not be expected to elicit a protective response. Given these challenges, there are only three live bacterial vaccines that have been approved for routine use.

Classical Strategies

The term *classical* refers to technical strategies that do not utilize recombinant DNA (rDNA) technology. One would anticipate that the techniques of rDNA technology would be applied to attenuating a new bacterial strain. Therefore, by current technical and regulatory standards, it seems highly unlikely that a *new* live bacterial vaccine attenuated by a classical strategy alone will be developed.

Attenuation in Vitro

It has not been readily possible to develop live attenuated bacterial vaccines by classical strategies, because there has been relatively little success with the in vitro cultivation of bacteria for attenuation while maintaining their immunogenic properties. There also may be little competitive or selective pressure for bacteria to become less virulent during in vitro passage; bacteria could stop expressing virulence factors in vitro, then turn their expression back on in vivo. The one widely available live bacterial vaccine based on serial in vitro passage is for tuberculosis. This vaccine consists of a live attenuated strain of *Mycobacterium bovis*, known as Bacille Calmette-Guérin (BCG),[1] which was attenuated by 231 successive in vitro subculturings. Having been inoculated into more than 3 billion people worldwide, available BCG vaccines vary in immunogenicity and in rate of protective efficacy in clinical trials.

Chemical Mutagenesis

Another technique for creating an attenuated strain has been chemical mutagenesis followed by selection. The Ty21a strain of *Salmonella typhi* was derived in this fashion[2] and licensed for preventing typhoid fever.[3]

Recombinant Bacteria

The engineering of bacteria for attenuation is complex, given the large size of bacterial genomes. The strategy is to identify the gene(s) responsible for virulence, colonization and/or survival and to either eliminate the gene(s) (preferred) or to abolish or modulate its in vivo expression. There is a balance between virulence and activity as a vaccine. In order to assure attenuation by reducing the probability of reversion, it is desirable to delete two or more independent genes or genetic loci that contribute to virulence. A licensed *V. cholerae* vaccine is based on a strain produced by deleting genes that encode virulence factors [e.g., cholera toxin (CT)].[4] *Shigella* strains have been developed by mutating particular plasmid or chromosomal genes to reduce pathogenicity.[5]

Recombinant Vectors

The second application of rDNA technology to the development of live vaccines has been the engineering of bacteria as vectors for expressing foreign polypeptides from other pathogens. The goal of creating such vectors is to present the foreign antigen to the immune system in the context of a live bacterial infection so that the immune system responds to the antigen as a live immunogen and thereby develops broader immunity to the corresponding pathogen. This strategy also has the potential advantage of amplification of the immunogenic signal following replication. For bacteria that replicate intracellularly, the recombinant polypeptide would be expressed within the infected cell; the polypeptide then either is transported to the cell surface to stimulate antibody production or is broken down into peptide fragments that are transported to the cell surface where they elicit CTL responses. For the majority of bacteria, which do not infect cells, the recombinant polypeptide should be expressed at the bacterial cell surface, where the polypeptide would elicit the production of antibodies. The most common applications have been to engineer enteric pathogens so that they can induce mucosal immunity against the foreign polypeptide upon oral delivery.

In the field of live bacterial vectors, *S. typhi* has been the focus of the most effort in terms of strain development, immunology, molecular development, and clinical testing. Applications of *Salmonella* vectors as oral vaccines have included malaria[6] and bioterrorism agents such as anthrax.[7] *V. cholerae*,[8] and *S. flexneri*[9] also have been engineered into oral recombinant vectors and have undergone clinical evaluations.

The challenge for these live attenuated vectors is both to retain sufficient virulence for replication in the gut and expression of appropriate levels of foreign polypeptides as well as to be attenuated. The ability of some of these bacterial species to replicate intracellularly may augment the ability of expressed foreign polypeptides to elicit cellular immune responses.

Another live vector strategy has employed strains of commensal bacteria for the presentation of foreign antigens. Commensal bacteria, e.g., *Streptococcus gordonii*, are naturally attenuated and able to persist for years, if not for life, in bodily compartments such as the oral mucosa. It has been shown that oral immunization with *S. gordonii* can elicit protective immunity to a foreign pathogen whose antigen is being vectored.[10]

Subunit/Inactivated Vaccines

Such vaccines have advantages that relate to their inability to multiply within the host. Generally they are well tolerated, especially for the majority of such vaccines that undergo purification to remove other bacterial macromolecules. Given the broad range of available technical approaches, it also is generally more feasible to produce a subunit or inactivated vaccine. The immunogen in such vaccines may be inactivated bacteria, purified protein or mixture of proteins, peptides or polysaccharides (Ps). Immunogenicity may be enhanced by administration with an adjuvant or delivery system (see Section on *Formulation of Antigens* in this chapter). Nevertheless, multiple doses of such vaccines, including boosters, are necessary for attaining long-term protective immunity against bacterial disease. These vaccines usually function by stimulating humoral immune responses as well as by priming for immunological memory; this is appropriate to bacteria in that most bacterial vaccines are effective through the induction of antibody responses. In certain cases, especially when administered with appropriate adjuvants and delivery systems, such vaccines may stimulate cell-mediated immunity, which may be useful for preventing diseases caused by bacteria that replicate intracellularly.

Whole Bacteria

Inactivated vaccines based on the use of whole bacteria elicit antibodies to multiple antigens; some of these antibodies would neutralize the pathogen. These vaccines are prepared by cultivating the bacteria, collecting the cells, and inactivating them with heat or chemical agents, e.g., thimerosal or phenol.[11] The vaccine does not undergo purification. Given their biochemically highly crude nature, which includes virtually all bacterial cellular components, the reactogenicity of such vaccines when given parenterally (e.g., *Bordetella pertussis*) is greater than that of most other types of vaccines. In contrast, inactivated whole-cell *V. cholerae*[12] and enterotoxigenic *Escherichia coli* (ETEC)[13] vaccines are well tolerated by the oral route. Orally administered inactivated whole-cell cholera (WCC) vaccine, which lacks CT and its toxic effects, has been shown to be very well tolerated and efficacious.[12] The recombinant B subunit of CT (rCTB), which lacks toxin activity, has been independently expressed, purified, and added back to the WCC vaccine. This combined WCC + rCTB vaccine was shown to have a somewhat higher rate of efficacy than WCC vaccine alone.[14] Since CTB is immunologically cross-reactive with the B subunit of *E. coli* heat-labile toxin (LT), the combined vaccine also elicits some protection against ETEC infections.

Protein-Based

Developing a protein-based vaccine is a preferred strategy for many pathogens. Protein-based approaches have relied on immunological, genetic, and biochemical techniques to identify protective epitopes and their corresponding polypeptides as candidate vaccine antigens. A common biochemical technique has been the purification of bacterial surface proteins, followed by the assessment of their protective potential in an animal model of infection. Sera from humans or animals infected with the particular bacteria can be used to screen for reactivity to bacterial proteins, which then can be purified for evaluations in animal models. More recently, genomics technology has enabled the identification of new vaccine antigens in lieu of prior available biochemical or antigen data. Open reading frames (ORFs) are identified based on the genomic DNA sequence. The derived amino acid sequence of each ORF can be inspected for structural features, such as a hydrophobic N-terminal sequence that suggests surface localization or homologies with proteins that are vaccine candidates from other related pathogens. The genes are expressed in recombinant *E. coli*, and the recombinant polypeptide is purified and used to immunize animals to derive polyclonal antibodies for identifying whether the protein is produced by most/all strains of the bacteria, especially on the surface. Antisera also are used in biological assays (opsonization, bacteriolysis) to see whether the protein may be an attractive vaccine candidate. The new protein also can be used for immunization and challenge in an animal model. The genomic approach was applied to *Neisseria meningitidis* (meningococcus); >400 proteins were screened, from which 7 candidate vaccine antigens were defined based on biological assays.[15] Likewise, sequencing and analyzing the complete *Streptococcus pneumoniae* (pneumococcus) genome resulted in the identification of novel candidate vaccine antigens.[16]

Natural 1

Outer membrane vesicles (OMVs) have formed the basis for a meningococcal vaccine.[17] *N. meningitidis* cells are grown to early stationary phase, and OMVs are extracted with deoxycholate, followed by further physical and chromatographic enrichment. This vaccine has been shown to elicit protective immunity in field trials; however, the protection is subtype-specific and therefore not useful for routine vaccinations.

Proteins purified from cultures of *B. pertussis* are combined to formulate acellular pertussis ($_{a}$P) vaccines, which have replaced whole-cell pertussis ($_{w}$P) vaccine for routine pediatric vaccinations in most developed countries. Based on the number of different protein antigens, these $_{a}$P vaccines are referred to as one-, two-, three-, four-, or five-component vaccines.[18-20] These vaccines all contain pertussis toxoid (PT) as a component, whose preparation is described below.

Chemical Inactivation

Many bacteria produce toxins that are responsible for the pathogenesis of infection. It had been recognized that, when a toxin was the pathogenic mechanism after infection, antisera enriched in toxin-specific antibodies that were effective in neutralizing toxin activity in vivo could prevent or ameliorate symptoms of certain bacterial infections. This precedent established the basis for bacterial toxins to be formulated as active vaccines. The toxin molecules are purified from bacterial cultures [e.g., *Corynebacterium diphtheriae* (D), *Clostridium tetani* (T), *B. pertussis* (P)] and then chemically detoxified by incubation with formalin or glutaraldehyde. Detoxified toxins, i.e., *toxoids,* represent two of the vaccines (D,T) in the diphtheria, tetanus, and pertussis (DTP) combination vaccine.[21,22] Pertussis toxin (PT)[23] combined with other *B. pertussis* antigens comprise the $_a$P vaccines.

Genetic Inactivation

The chemical toxoiding procedure has potential disadvantages, including the alteration of protective epitopes with ensuing reduced immunogenicity and potential reversion to an active toxin. To produce a stable PT molecule, codons for amino acids required for toxin bioactivity [adenosine diphosphate (ADP) ribosyl transferase] were mutated; two mutations were introduced into PT to assure the lack to reversion.[24] The altered gene was substituted for the native gene in *B. pertussis,* which then produces immunogenic and stably inactivated PT. A double-mutant PT (which also is treated with formalin under milder conditions to improve its immunogenicity or stability) is a component of an $_a$P vaccine.[18] In a related application, mutated cultures of *C. diphtheriae* were screened for the secretion of enzymatically inactive yet antigenic diphtheria toxins (DT). Subsequent cloning and sequencing of one such mutated toxin gene identified a single amino acid mutation at the enzymatic active site (also an ADP-ribosyl transferase). This genetic toxoid (CRM_{197})[25] is the protein carrier for licensed *Haemophilus influenzae* type b (Hib) and pneumococcal conjugate vaccines (see Section *Subunit/Inactivated Vaccines; Polysaccharide-Based; Conjugate*). This technology also has been applied to CT and LT to produce candidate mucosal adjuvants (see Section *Formulation of Antigens; Adjuvants*).

Recombinant Polypeptides

There are innumerable ongoing research and development applications of rDNA technology to produce proteins as vaccine candidates. The major *Borrelia burgdorferi* surface protein (OspA), expressed in *E. coli* as a recombinant lipoprotein,[26] has been licensed as a vaccine for Lyme disease. As mentioned above, rCTB is part of a licensed WCC vaccine. Purified recombinant *E. coli*-expressed proteins from *S. pneumoniae*[27] and *N. meningitidis*[28] have been evaluated in clinical trials.

A uniquely-derived meningococcal PorA vaccine has been evaluated clinically.[29] This highly type-specific antigen requires up to 6 different PorA proteins to provide for group-common immunity. Therefore, 3 different PorA genes were transformed into each of 2 Ps^- *N. meningitidis* strains, and the 6 recombinant PorA molecules were copurified from these strains.

Peptide-Based

In many cases, it has been possible to identify B-cell epitopes within a polypeptide against which neutralizing antibodies are directed. Some B-cell epitopes are conformational, being formed by the three-dimensional juxtaposition of amino acid residues from different parts of the polypeptide, which means that such epitopes require the full polypeptide for their proper immunogenic presentation. In contrast, other peptide epitopes are linear in nature, being fully antigenic as short linear sequences in the range of ~4-20 consecutive amino acid residues in the polypeptide. Many linear epitopes are only weakly immunogenic in the context of the full polypeptide; such natural peptides would be effective vaccine antigens if they were rendered sufficiently immunogenic. Linear B-cell epitopes of this type have been defined for the malarial circumsporzoite (CS) protein (repetitive 4-amino acid sequence)[30] and for the *Pseudomonas aeruginosa* pilus protein.[31] These polypeptides contain linear epitopes that are recognized by antibodies that neutralize the respective pathogens, yet the whole polypeptides elicit such antibodies only weakly. It is interesting to speculate that this may represent a mechanism by which pathogens escape immunological surveillance through rendering their neutralization epitopes less immunogenic. The peptide can be chemically conjugated to a carrier protein in order to increase immunogenicity. The peptide sequence is synthesized chemically with a reactive amino acid residue through which conjugation occurs to the carrier protein. The most commonly used carriers are bacterial proteins that humans commonly encounter, e.g., tetanus toxoid (TT), for which a conjugate with the malarial CS epitope has been tested clinically.[32] CS peptide also has been fused genetically to hepatitis B surface antigen as a vaccine candidate.[33]

Polysaccharide-Based

There are many bacteria with an outer polysaccharide (Ps) capsule. In many if not most of the encapsulated bacteria studied, antibodies directed against capsular Ps are protective against infection. These observations have established capsular Ps as effective vaccine antigens. However, the multiple serotypes of capsular Ps of many bacteria create the need for multivalent vaccines, including conjugates, which are technically more complicated to produce and analyze. Components of lipopolysaccharide (LPS) also are candidate antigens, given their abundance on the surface of Gram negative bacteria.

Plain Ps

Native capsular Ps contain up to hundreds of repeat units distinctive for each bacterial species and antigenic subtype, in which each monomer repeat unit consists of a combination of monosaccharides, phosphate groups, and small organic moieties. The Ps is shed by the organism during its growth and is harvested from the culture medium. These Ps preparations are immunogenic in adults and children over 2 years of age and elicit antibodies that may mediate the opsonization or bacteriolysis, thereby protecting against bacterial infection. Ps vaccines have been licensed for Hib[34] (monovalent for serotype b), meningococcus[35] (quadrivalent), and pneumococcus[36] (23-valent). The shortcoming of these vaccines is that Ps, being T-cell–independent (TI) immunogens, are poorly immunogenic or nonimmunogenic in children younger than 2 years and do not elicit immunological memory in older children and adults.

Conjugate

Although infants and children younger than 2 years old do not recognize TI immunogens efficiently, they can respond immunologically to T-cell–dependent (TD) immunogens such as proteins. The chemical conjugation of Ps to a carrier protein converts the Ps from a TI to a TD immunogen. As a consequence, conjugate vaccines can elicit protective IgG and immunological memory in infants and young children. This strategy is particularly important for encapsulated bacteria such as Hib and pneumococcus owing to the frequency of invasive diseases caused by these bacteria in children younger than 2 years old, in which Ps vaccine is ineffective. There are four different licensed Hib conjugate vaccines,[37] all with different carrier proteins (TT, DT, CRM_{197}, and an outer membrane protein complex from meningococcal Group B) of different sizes and immunological character, distinct Ps chain lengths, and different conjugation chemistries. Given these differences, the four vaccines display one or more differences in the following immunological properties: response of 2-month-old infants to the first dose of vaccine, responses of 4- and 6-month-old infants to the second and third doses, response of children older than 1 year to a booster dose, kinetics of decay of antibody levels, peak of antibody titer, and age at which protection from clinical disease first can be shown.

Pneumococcal bacteria consist of >90 serotypes, as reflected in distinct capsular Ps structures. For designing a pediatric conjugate vaccine, 7 serotypes have been recognized as responsible for ~60-75% of the major pediatric pneumococcal diseases (meningitis, acute otitis media). On that basis, 7 individual conjugate vaccines were produced and mixed, and the resultant heptavalent conjugate vaccine has been developed and licensed.[38] Other conjugate vaccines in advanced clinical trials consist of a mixture of up to 11 different conjugates.[39]

A meningococcal serogroup C conjugate vaccine has been licensed,[40] with other serogroup conjugate vaccines in development.

An LPS conjugate vaccine has been evaluated for preventing *P. aeruginosa* disease.[41] This octavalent conjugate vaccine is based on the type-specific O-Ps antigens derived from *P. aeruginosa* LPS, such that the vaccine elicits an anti-LPS antibody response.

DNA

It was shown that, after cells in vivo take up DNA encoding vaccine antigen(s), the antigens can be secreted or can be associated with the cell surface in a way that would trigger a humoral or cellular immune response. Furthermore, the uptake of DNA can be facilitated by chemical formulation or delivery by bacteria. The latter approaches fit the definition of a DNA-based vaccine as one that cannot replicate in humans.

Naked DNA

Following intramuscular injection of DNA encoding a vaccine antigen,[42] cells take up and transcribe the plasmid DNA to synthesize the antigen, which may be processed in a similar way to that in a live bacterial infection. The advantages of using DNA are the relative technical ease of preparation and the ability to direct the synthesis of multiple copies of mRNA, hence amplification of both antigen synthesis and the consequent immune response. Such vaccines are effective in many animal models of infection.[43] In addition to eliciting the production of specific antibodies, DNA vaccines may be particularly effective at stimulating Th1-type immune responses (cell-mediated). Given that protective immunity to *Mycobacterium tuberculosis* infections may be cell-mediated, a DNA vaccine for tuberculosis has shown promise in animal studies.[44]

As a novel route of delivery, naked DNA has been applied to mouse skin, from which it is taken up by hair follicles to stimulate an immune response.[45]

Formulated DNA

Facilitation of cellular uptake, expression, or immunological activation can increase the immunogenicity of DNA vaccines. One strategy has been the incorporation of DNA into microprojectiles that then are "fired" into cells, which produce the encoded antigen. This "gene gun" technique has been reported to be potent at eliciting antibody responses.[46] For improving the efficiency of uptake, DNA has been coated with cationic lipids, lipospermines or other molecules that neutralize their charge and have lipid groups for facilitating membrane transfer.[47] Such formulations also are being researched for alternate administration routes (e.g., oral, nasal) that may elicit mucosal immunity. The base composition of the DNA may affect its potency, in that unmethylated CpG dinucleotides can adjuvant responses to DNA vaccines.[48]

Bacterial Delivery

Bacteria that replicate intracellularly can be engineered to deliver plasmid DNA into cells for the expression of recombinant proteins. *S. flexneri* has been attenuated by making a deletion mutant in an essential gene (*asd*). While such a strain can be grown in vitro in the presence of diaminopimelic acid (DAP), it cannot replicate in vivo, where DAP is not available. A *S. flexneri* strain harboring a plasmid with a eukaryotic promoter and recombinant gene was shown to be able to invade mammalian cells in vitro and to express the plasmid-encoded protein as a potential vaccine antigen.[49] Since *S. flexneri* replicates in the intestine and stimulates mucosal immunity, this vector may be administered orally for delivering DNA to cells where mucosal immunity is stimulated. Other attenuated strains of bacterial species, e.g., *Salmonella*,[50] that can invade mammalian cells but not divide also can deliver recombinant plasmids orally for expressing recombinant proteins as vaccine antigens.

Formulation of Antigens

The immunological effectiveness of vaccines (other than live) may be enhanced by their formulation, which refers to the final form of the vaccine to be administered in vivo. In addition to the "active substance" (antigen or DNA), the formulation may contain an adjuvant and/or delivery system plus other excipients. The adjuvant is a substance that stimulates an increased humoral and/or cellular immune response to a coadministered antigen or antigen expressed by a DNA vaccine. The delivery system is a vehicle that assures the presentation of the vaccine to cells of the immune system or for stabilizing and releasing the antigen over an extended time-period. There may be overlap in structure and function between adjuvants and delivery systems. Gaining clinical and pharmaceutical experience with new delivery systems and adjuvants remains a key goal in the field. There is a range of potential benefits and challenges accompanying the use of adjuvants and delivery systems[51,52] that have been evaluated preclinically and clinically.

Adjuvants

Aluminum salts, e.g., hydroxide or phosphate, are currently the only adjuvants widely licensed for human use. This adjuvant has been used for decades in vaccines injected into more than 1 billion people worldwide, e.g., DT_wP. The vaccine antigen binds stably to the aluminum salt by ionic interactions and forms a macroscopic suspension.[53] This adjuvant preferentially promotes a Th2-type immune response and thus is not useful in applications where inducing a cell-mediated immune response is needed for protection. While aluminum salts have been useful for certain vaccines, they are not potent enough for other vaccine antigens in eliciting antibody responses that are high enough to be optimally effective. Aluminum salts have not been shown to be useful for presentation of vaccines by the oral or intranasal routes. Therefore, many chemicals, biochemicals from natural sources, and proteins with immune-modulating activity (cytokines) have been researched as potential adjuvants. The adjuvanticity of virtually all known formulations is associated with local or systemic side-effects, which may be mechanism-based or nonspecific. The ideal adjuvant needs to achieve a balance between degree of side-effects and immune-enhancement. The only new adjuvant that has been developed as part of a licensed vaccine is MF59, an oil-in-water emulsion.[54]

Several bacterial proteins have received considerable attention as mucosal adjuvants. CT was shown to be active as a mucosal adjuvant for a coadministered antigen[55] when presented by the oral, nasal, vaginal or rectal routes, as was shown subsequently for LT. These toxins are composed of a catalytic A subunit and a pentameric B subunit that binds to GM1 ganglioside on the surface of many cell types. However, both CT and LT are toxic in humans by the oral route, through which they induce diarrhea. To dissociate the toxicity and adjuvanticity of CT and LT, point mutations have been made that result in reduced or eliminated ADP-ribosylating activity, reduced toxicity, and the apparent retention of adjuvanticity in mice.[56] Antigen given together CT or LT or their mutant toxoids and applied to the skin can stimulate transcutaneous immunization.[57] An alternative CT-based design substitutes (instead of the B subunit) a synthetic dimeric peptide, derived from *Staphylococcus aureus* Protein A (DD), that binds to immunoglobulin (Ig). The fusion of the CTA subunit with the DD domain binds to Ig^+ cells, is devoid of apparent toxicity in mice, retains ADP-ribosylating activity, and is active as a mucosal adjuvant in mice.[58] The fibronectin-binding protein of *Streptococcus pyogenes*, which lacks a known enzymatic activity, also is active as a mucosal adjuvant.[59] OMVs[17] also have been shown to have adjuvant activity.

Delivery Systems

Besides presenting an antigen or DNA to cells of the immune system, a delivery system may perform other key functions, e.g., a depot effect whereby the antigen is maintained in an appropriate in vivo site for continual immune stimulation, or an enhancement of vaccine stability in vivo. For mucosally-delivered vaccines, the delivery system may enable efficient presentation and uptake by M cells, followed by transcytosis into Peyer's patches and presentation to lymphocytes for the induction of mucosal immunity.[60] For certain formulations, the vaccine may be maintained inside a physical structure in vivo for a significant period of time, during which it is released slowly or in pulsatile fashion such that it may function as a 1-dose vaccine. Delivery systems also are being developed for DNA vaccines.[61] However, no delivery systems have been licensed for any type of vaccine.

Conclusion

Technological developments in the past two decades have rapidly expanded the number of strategies for making new bacterial vaccines. Over the next decade, the number of approaches should continue to expand and technical aspects should be further refined, such that many antigens should be able to be presented in a highly immunogenic form in the context of a live or subunit vaccine. Protein antigens alternatively can be expressed through a DNA-based vaccine. Further understanding of gene function in bacterial pathogens should enable live vaccines to be more stably and predictably attenuated as vaccines and as live vectors for immunizing against other bacteria. Adjuvant technologies should advance to the point where new formulations that are more potent than aluminum salts, yet as well tolerated, may gain widespread use for subunit/inactivated vaccines. It is also possible that oral delivery of purified proteins for immunization becomes technically feasible. Similarly, new formulations may improve the potency of DNA vaccines and their ability to be delivered by routes that elicit mucosal immunity.

As all these technological advances proceed, the rate-limiting factor in developing new vaccines for human use likely will continue to be a more comprehensive understanding of immunology. Some areas in which increased knowledge would have a practical payoff for vaccine development are the immunobiology of bacteria, the type and specificity of immune response required for persistent protection against disease, the attainment of durable mucosal immunity, and the optimal vaccination strategies to achieve this protection.

References

1. Bloom BR, Fine PEM. The BCG experience: implications for future vaccines against tuberculosis. In: Bloom BR, ed. Tuberculosis: Pathogenesis, Prevention and Control. Washington DC: ASM Press, 1994:531-58.
2. Germanier R, Furer E. Isolation and characterization of galE mutant Ty21a of Salmonella typhi: A candidate strain for a live, oral typhoid vaccine. J Infect Dis 1975; 131:553-558.
3. Levine MM, Black RE, Ferreccio C et al. Clinical Typhoid Committee. Large-scale field trial of Ty21a live oral typhoid vaccine in enteric-coated capsule formulation. Lancet 2: 1987; 1049-1052.
4. Tacket CO, Losonsky G, Nataro JP et al. Onset and duration of protective immunity in challenged volunteers after vaccination with live oral cholera vaccine CVD 103-HgR. J Infect Dis 1992; 166:837-841.
5. Kotloff KL, Taylor DN, Sztein MB et al. Phase 1 evaluation of DvirG Shigella sonnei live, attenuated, oral vaccine strain WRSS1 in healthy adults. Infect Immun 2002; 70:2016-21.
6. Gonzalez C, Hone D, Noriega FR et al. Salmonella typhi vaccine strain CVD 908 expressing the circumsporozoite protein of Plasmodium falciparum: Strain construction and safety and immunogenicity in humans. J Infect Dis 1994; 169:927-931.
7. Coulson NM, Fulop M, Titball RW. Bacillus anthracis protective antigen, expressed in Salmonella typhimurium SL 3261, affords protection against anthrax spore challenge. Vaccine 1994; 12:1395-401.
8. Butterton JR, Beattie DT, Gardel CL et al. Heterologous antigen expression in Vibrio cholerae vector strains. Infect Immunol 1995; 63:2689-2696.
9. Noriega FR, Losonsky G, Wang JY et al. Further characterization of DaroA DvirG Shigella flexneri as a mucosal Shigella vaccine and a live-vector vaccine for delivering antigens of enterotoxigenic Escherichia coli. Infect Immunol 1996; 64:23-27.
10. Fischetti VA, Medaglini D, Pozzi G. Gram-positive bacteria for mucosal vaccine delivery. Current Opinion Biotechnol 1996; 7:659-666.
11. Cherry JD, Brunell PA, Golden GS et al. Report of the task force on pertussis and pertussis immunization—1988. Pediatrics 1988; 81:939.
12. Clemens JD, Sack DA, Harris JR et al. Field trial of oral cholera vaccines in Bangladesh: Results from three-year follow-up. Lancet 1990; 355:270-273.
13. Svennerholm A-M, Holmgren J, Sack DA. Development of oral vaccines against enterotoxigenic Escherichia coli diarrhoea. Vaccine 1989; 7:196-198.
14. Clemens JD, Sack DA, Harris JR et al. Impact of B subunit killed whole-cell and killed whole-cell-only oral vaccines against cholera upon treated diarrheal illness and mortality in an area endemic for cholera. Lancet 1:1988; 1375-1379.
15. Pizza M, Scarlato V, Masignani V et al. Identification of vaccine candidates against serogroup B Meningococcus by whole-genome sequencing. Science 287:1816-20.

16. Rosen CA, Masure HR, Tuomanen E et al. Use of a whole genome approach to identify vaccine molecules affording protection against Streptococcus pneumoniae infection. Infection and Immunity Mar:2001; 1593-1598.
17. Perez O, Lastre M, Lapinet J et al. Immune response induction and new effector mechanisms possibly involved in protection conferred by the Cuban anti-meningococcal BC vaccine. Infection and Immunity July:2001; 4502-4508.
18. Greco D, Salmaso S, Mastrantonio P et al. A controlled trial of two acellular vaccines and one whole-cell vaccine against pertussis. New Engl J Med 1996; 334:341-348.
19. Gustafson L, Hallander HO, Olin P et al. A controlled trial of a two-component acellular, a five-component acellular, and a whole-cell pertussis vaccine. New Engl J Med 1996; 334:349-355.
20. Schmitt H-J, Wirsing von König, Neiss A et al. Efficacy of acellular pertussis vaccine in early childhood after household exposure. J Am Med Assoc 1996; 275:37-41.
21. Jones FG, Moss JM. Studies on tetanus toxoid. I. The antitoxic titer of human subject following immunization with tetanus toxoid and tetanus alum precipitated toxoid. J Immunol 1936; 30:115–125.
22. Ramon G. Sur le pouvoir floculant et sur les proprietes immunisantes d'une toxin diphterique rendue anatoxique (anatoxine). Compt Rend Acad Sci 1923; 177:1338–1340.
23. Chazono M, Yoshida I, Konobe T. The purification and characterization of an acellular pertussis vaccine. J Biol Stand 1988; 16:83–89.
24. Nencioni L, Pizza MG, Bugnoli M et al. Characterization of genetically inactivated pertussis toxin mutants: Candidates for a new vaccine against whooping cough. Infect Immunol 1990; 58:1308–1315.
25. Giannini G, Rappuoli R, Ratti G. The amino-acid sequence of two nontoxic mutants of diphtheria toxin: CRM_{45} and CRM_{197}. Nucleic Acids Res 1984; 12:4063–4069.
26. Van Hoecke C, Comberbach M, De Grave D et al. Evaluation of the safety, reactogenicity and immunogenicity of three recombinant outer surface protein (OspA) Lyme vaccines in healthy adults. Vaccine 1996; 14:1620-1626.
27. Briles DE, Hollingshead SK, King J et al. Immunization of humans with recombinant pneumococcal surface protein A (rPspA) elicits antibodies that passively protect mice from fatal infection with Streptococcus pneumoniae bearing heterologous PspA. J Infec Dis 2000; 182:694-701.
28. Martin D, Brodeur BR, Hamel J et al. Candidate Neisseria meningitides NspA vaccine. J Biotechnology 2000; 83:27-31.
29. de Kleijn E, van Eijndhoven L, Vermont C et al. Serum bactericidal activity and isotype distribution of antibodies in toddlers and schoolchildren after vaccination with RIVM hexavalent PorA vesicle vaccine. Vaccine 2002; 20:352-358.
30. Zavala F, Cochrane AH, Nardin EH et al. Circumsporozoite proteins of malaria parasites contain a single immunodominant region with two or more identical epitopes. J Exp Med 1983; 157:1947–1957.
31. Cachia PJ, Glasier LM, Hodgins RR et al. The use of synthetic peptides in the design of a consensus sequence vaccine for Pseudomonas aeruginosa. J Pept Res 1998; 52:289-99.
32. Herrington DA, Clyde DF, Losonsky G et al. Safety and immunogenicity in man of a synthetic peptide in malaria vaccine against Plasmodium falciparum sporozoites. Nature 1987; 328:257–259.
33. Vreden SGS, JP, Oettinger T et al. Phase I clinical trial of a recombinant malaria vaccine consisting of the circumsporozoite repeat region of Plasmodium falciparum coupled to hepatitis B surface antigen. Am J Trop Med Hyg 1991; 45:533–538.
34. Rodrigues LP, Schneerson R, Robbins JB. Immunity to H. influenzae type b I. The isolation, and some physicochemical, serologic and biologic properties of the capsular polysaccharide of H. influenzae type b. J Immunol 1971; 107:1071–1080.
35. Gotschlich EC, Liu TY, Artenstein MS. Human immunity to the meningococcus. III. Preparation and immunochemical properties of the group A, group B and group C meningococcal polysaccharides. J Exp Med 1969; 129:1349–1365.
36. Kass EG. Assessment of the pneumococcal polysaccharide vaccine. Rev Infect Dis 1981; 3:S1 S197.
37. Kniskern PJ, Marburg S, Ellis RW. Haemophilus influenzae type b Conjugate Vaccines. In: M. Powell, M. Newman, eds. Vaccine Design. The Subunit Approach. New York Plenum Publishing Corporation, 1995:673-694.
38. Black S, Shinefeld H, Fireman B et al. Efficacy, safety and immunogenicity of heptavalent pneumococcal conjugate vaccine in children. Ped Infect Dis J 2000; 19:187-95.
39. Wuorimaa T, Kayhty H, Leroy O et al. Tolerability and immunogenicity of an 11- valent pneumococcal conjugate vaccine in adults. Vaccine 2001; 19:1863-1869.

40. Slack MH, Schapira D, Thwaites RJ et al. Immune response of premature infants to meningococcal serogroup C and combined diphtheria-tetanus toxoids-acellular pertussis-Haemophilus influenzae type b conjugate vaccines. J Infect Dis 2001; 184:1617-20.
41. Lang AB, Schaad UB, Rudeberg A et al. Effect of high-affinity anti-Pseudomonas aeruginosa lipopolysaccharide antibodies induced by immunization on the rate of Pseudomonas aeruginosa infection in patients with cystic fibrosis. J Pediatrics 1995; 127:711-717.
42. Wolff JA, Malone RW, Williams P et al. Direct gene transfer into mouse muscle in vivo. Science 1990; 247:1465–1468.
43. Leitner WW, Ying H, Restifo NP. DNA- and RNA-based vaccines: principles, progress and prospects. Vaccine 2000; 18:765-77.
44. Huygen K, Content J, Denis O et al. Immunogenicity and protective efficacy of a tuberculosis DNA vaccine. Nature Med 1996; 2:893-7.
45. Fan H, Lin Q, Morrissey GR et al. Immunization via hair follicles by topical administration of naked DNA to normal skin. Nature Biotechnol 1999; 17:870-2.
46. Tacket CO, Roy MJ, Widera G et al. Phase 1 safety and immune response studies of a DNA vaccine encoding hepatitis B surface antigen delivered by a gene delivery device. Vaccine 1999; 17:2826-9.
47. Scherman D, Bossodes M, Cameron B et al. Application of lipids and plasmid design for gene delivery to mammalian cells. Current Opinion Biotechnol 1998; 9:480-5.
48. Jones TR, Obaldia N, Gramzinski RA et al. Synthetic oligodeoxynucleotides containing CpG motifs enhance immunogenicity of a peptide malaria vaccine in Aotus monkeys. Vaccine 1999; 17:3065-71.
49. Sizemore DR, Branstrom AA, Sadoff JC. Attenuated Shigella as a DNA delivery vehicle for DNA-mediated immunization. Science 1996; 270:299-302.
50. Darji A, Guzman CA, Gerstel B et al. Oral somatic transgene vaccination using attenuated S. typhimurium. Cell 1997; 91:765-75.
51. Cox JC, Coulter AR. Adjuvants—a classification and review of modes of action. Vaccine 1997; 15:248-256.
52. Singh M, O'Hagan D. Advances in vaccine adjuvants. Nature Biotech 1999;17:1075-81.
53. Shirodkar S, Hutchinson RL, White JL et al. Aluminum compounds used as adjuvants in vaccines. Pharm Res 1990; 7:1282-1288.
54. De Donato S., Granoff D, Minutello M et al. Safety and immunogenicity of MF59-adjuvanted influenza vaccine in the elderly. Vaccine 1999; 17:3094-3101.
55. Elson CD, Falding W. Generalized systemic and mucosal immunity in mice after mucosal stimulation with cholera toxin. J Immunol 1984; 132:2736-2744.
56. Douce G, Turcottee C, Cropley I et al. Mutants of Escherichia coli heat-labile toxin lacking ADP-ribosylating activity act as nontoxic mucosal adjuvants. Proc Natl Acad Sci USA 1995; 92: 1644-1648.
57. Glenn GM, Scharton-Kersten T, Vassell R et al. Transcutaneous immunization using bacterial ADP-ribosylating exotoxins as antigens and adjuvants. Infect Immun 1999; 67:1100-6.
58. Agren LC, Ekman L, Lowenadler B et al. A genetically-engineered nontoxic vaccine adjuvant that combines B-cell targeting with immunomodulation by cholera toxin A1 subunit. J Immunol 1997; 158:3936-3946.
59. Medina E, Talay SR, Chhatwal GS et al. Fibronectin-binding protein 1 of Streptococcus pyogenes is a promising adjuvant for antigens delivered by the mucosal route. Eur J Immunol 1998; 28:1069-77.
60. Mestecky J, Moldoveanu Z, Michalak SM et al. Current options for vaccine delivery systems by mucosal routes. J Controlled Release 1997; 48:243-57.
61. Luo D, Saltzman WM. Synthetic DNA delivery systems. Nature Biotechnol 2000; 18:33-7.

CHAPTER 7

Chlamydia trachomatis and *Chlamydia pneumoniae* Vaccines

Svend Birkelund and Gunna Christiansen

Summary

Chlamydia spp. are obligate intracellular Gram negative bacteria with a unique biphasic developmental cycle. *C. trachomatis* and *C. pneumoniae* most frequently cause human infections. *C. trachomatis* strains of the trachoma biovar (serovar A, B and C) are mucosal pathogens that cause the ocular infection trachoma, the leading cause of preventable blindness in developing countries. The remaining serovars (D-K) of the trachoma biovar cause genital infections being the leading cause of sexually transmitted bacterial infections in the Western world with sequelae such as tubal factor infertility and ectopic pregnancy. There exists no vaccine against human *Chlamydia* infections. Clinical trials for vaccination against trachoma were initiated more than 3 decades ago. Inactivated whole-cell *C. trachomatis* EB preparations were used for immunization. Good but short-lived protection was observed. All *Chlamydia* species have highly homologous major outer membrane proteins (MOMP) that are immunogenic. This molecule has been studied in detail with respect to humoral and cellular immunity. In a mouse model a vaccine consisting of MOMP extracted from purified *C. trachomatis* gave protection. However, MOMP shows variable immunogenic domains. Therefore, other components are being sought for vaccine development. Genomics, molecular and cellular immunology, and nucleic acid immunizations are among the techniques used to exploit the immune response to develop component vaccines.

Chlamydia Biology and Diseases

Chlamydia are obligate intracellular Gram negative bacteria with a unique biphasic developmental cycle. The genus *Chlamydia* contains four species of which *C. trachomatis* and *pneumoniae* most frequently causes human infections, but also *C. psittaci* occasionally is transmitted from infected birds to humans, often causing severe pneumonia. Common for all species of *Chlamydia* are the unique biphasic developmental cycle and the species-specific lipopolysaccharide (LPS). During the biphasic developmental cycle, the infectious but metabolically inactive elementary bodies (EB) attach to susceptible host cells, where they mediate their own uptake by phagocytosis. Shortly after the uptake, the EB transform to the metabolically active, replicating reticulate bodies (RB) which divide by binary fission within the phagosome. EB differ structurally from RB by being small (0.3-μm diameter) and having a condensed nucleoid and disulfide-cross-linked rigid cell wall. During transformation to RB, the disulfide bridges are reduced, the cells are enlarged (1 μm), and the nucleoid is decondensed. Replication continues for 48-72 hours, with the chlamydiae being surrounded during the entire developmental cycle by the phagosomal membrane forming the chlamydial inclusion. Late in the developmental cycle, the RB transform to EB and the inclusion bursts, releasing infectious EB to the extracellular environment (Fig. 1). For review see ref. 1.

New Bacterial Vaccines, edited by Ronald W. Ellis and Bernard R. Brodeur.

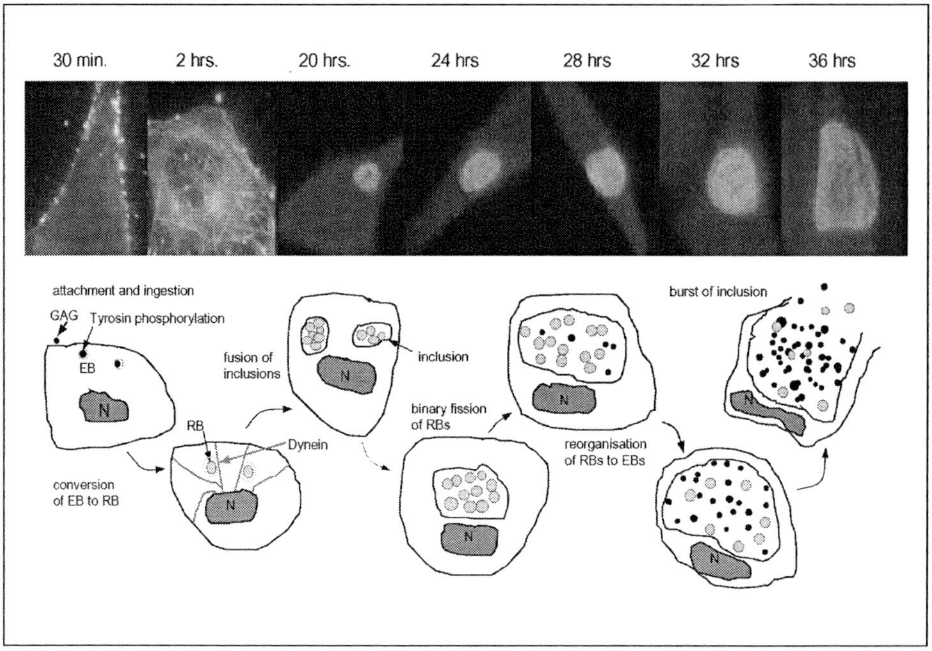

Figure 1. The developmental cycle of *Chlamydia*: Immunofluorescence microscopy of *C. trachomatis* L2 infected HeLa cells 30 min, and 2, 20, 24, 32 and 36 hrs post infection. A schematic drawing shows steps in the developmental cycle.

C. trachomatis consists of two biovars: the trachoma biovar contains the serovars A, B, Ba, C, D, E, F, G, H, I, J, and K; the lymphogranuloma venereum (LGV) biovar contains serovar L1, L2 and L3. The biological basis for division of *C. trachomatis* into serovars is variations within the four surface-exposed variable sequence (VS1-4) domains of the MOMP (Fig. 2). Strains of the trachoma biovar (serovar A, B and C) are mucosal pathogens causing the ocular infection trachoma, a chronic follicular conjunctivitis that can lead to conjunctival scarring, eyelid deformation and blindness. It is the leading cause of preventive blinding in third-world countries. The remaining serovars (D-K) cause genital infections and are the leading cause of sexually transmitted bacterial infections in the Western world. The organism can cause urethritis in men and cervical infections in women. The infections may be asymptomatic but persistent if untreated, leading to pelvic inflammatory disease, the sequelae of which are tubal factor infertility and ectopic pregnancy.[1] Even the ascending infections may be asymptomatic.[2,3] Passage through an infected birth canal can cause lung and eye infections in newborns.

C. pneumoniae is a human respiratory pathogen.[4] It can cause acute respiratory tract infections, e.g., bronchitis, pneumonia and sinusitis,[5] and it is associated with a number of chronic conditions such as asthma and atherosclerosis.[6,7,8] Compared to *C. trachomatis, C. pneumoniae* MOMP is antigenically invariable, with only small variations observed among the 3 fully sequenced genomes.[9,10,11]

Diagnosis, Treatment and Prevention

Chlamydia infections are diagnosed by cultivation in tissue culture, or by noncultivation techniques such as immunofluorescence staining of patient sample smear. Diagnosis can also be done by polymerase chain reaction (PCR) or by other specific nucleic acid detection methods.[12] Finally infection can be determined by the presence of specific antibodies.[13,14]

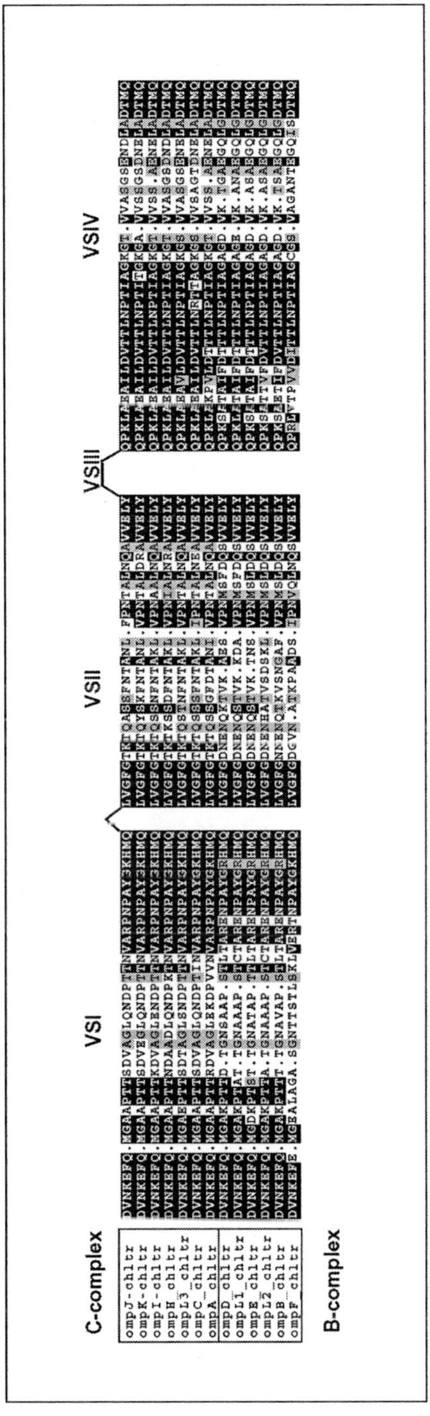

Figure 2. Multiple alignment of MOMP VSI, VSII and VSIV performed with pileup from the GCG package. Differences between the C-complex and B-complex are seen in VSI and VSII, but variation is also present in VSIV.

Chlamydia infections can be treated with antibiotics (tetracyclins or macrolides), but it is unclear whether persistent infections are susceptible to antibiotic treatment.[15]

There is no vaccine for human *Chlamydia* infections, and it is a question whether natural immunity develops following human chlamydial infection. If this prove to be the case, then understanding which immune mechanisms contribute to the resolution of intracellular infection leading to protection may elucidate what is required for successful vaccine development.

Chlamydia Surface-Exposed Components

Microbial surface components are of interest for vaccine development because they are the targets for antibody responses and are responsible for contact with host cells and for protection of the microorganism. Surface components are often specific for a given microbial species and are also some of the most variable structures. Electron microscopy has been used to study the morphology of the *Chlamydia* surface.[16] The cell wall of purified *C. psittaci* EB and RB was seen as a granular outer layer and an inner layer composed of hexagonal arrayed structures with a periodicity of 10-20 nm. Purified inclusions showed the presence of cylindrical surface projections on RB and EB connecting the *Chlamydia* with the inclusion membrane.[17] Spike-like rods also have been seen on the surface of *C. trachomatis* L2 and on *C. pneumoniae*.[18,19]

Purification of the sarkosyl-insoluble chlamydial outer membrane complex (OMC)[20] and determination of its protein content by sodium dodecyl sulfate-polyacrylamide gel electrophoresis (SDS-PAGE) and immunoblotting identified components responsible for its structural appearance. The analyses revealed that all *Chlamydia* OMC contained LPS, MOMP, Omp2 and Omp3 and proteins 90-100 kD in size.[21,22,23] The 90- to 100-kD proteins have been identified as members of a family of proteins named Pomps or Pmps (putative OMPs/ polymorphic membrane proteins).[21,23,24] Physical localization of the components showed that LPS is surface-localized both on EB and RB.[19,25] MOMP is also surface-localized on *C. psittaci* and *C. trachomatis*, where it is associated closely with LPS.[26] Conformation-dependent, but not linear, epitopes of *C. pneumoniae* MOMP were surface-localized on EB and immunogenic based on reactivity with human sera by micro-IF (immunofluorescence).[27] Omp2 and Omp3 are cysteine-rich proteins synthesized late in the developmental cycle. Omp3 is a 12-kD highly cysteine-rich membrane lipoprotein forming a disulfide cross-linked layer within the periplasmic space and cross-linked to Omp2. It has been debated whether a part of Omp2 is surface-exposed at EB. It was suggested that Omp2 is the structural element for the hexagonal-arrayed structures seen at the inner surface outer membrane of the cell wall;[28] Stephens et al[29] showed that the most N-terminal part (aa 51-70) of the molecule is surface-localized and binds heparin (Fig. 3).

In each of the three *Chlamydia* genomes a family of distantly related Pomp/Pmp genes encoding the 90-100 kD proteins were found. The highest number of such genes (21) was found in the *C. pneumoniae* genome;[9] 16 of the 21 genes are full-length, while one lacks its C-terminal portion. Four of the genes had small insertions or deletions that caused the open reading frames to be disrupted and thus provided the genes with a premature stop. Two of the genes (Pmp10 and Pmp11)[24] differed from the others by having a cleavage site for signal peptidase II indicating that these proteins probably were lipid-modified, as shown for Pmp11 expressed in *E. coli*.[30] Expression of Pmp10 and Pmp11 was analyzed by immunofluorescence microscopy of *C. pneumoniae*-infected Hep2 cells reacted with polyclonal rabbit-antibodies generated to the recombinant proteins.[24] The results showed that antibodies to Pmp11 stained all inclusions, whereas antibodies to Pmp10 only stained part of the inclusions.[31] Double-IF staining with monoclonal antibodies (MAbs) reacting with the surface of *C. pneumoniae* EB and anti-Pmp10 antibodies showed identical reaction patterns.[31] Due to weak reaction in immunoblotting with micro-IF positive patient sera, it has been debated whether Pmps were immunogenic and surface-exposed, but identity in IF reactivity of anti-Pmp10 and MAbs that reacted with the surface of *C. pneumoniae* EB strongly suggested Pmp10 to be surface-exposed.

In the *C. trachomatis* genome 9 Pmp genes were found by Stephens et al[32] and PmpG and H are present in the *C. trachomatis* L2 OMC.[23] Their surface localization and function are unknown.

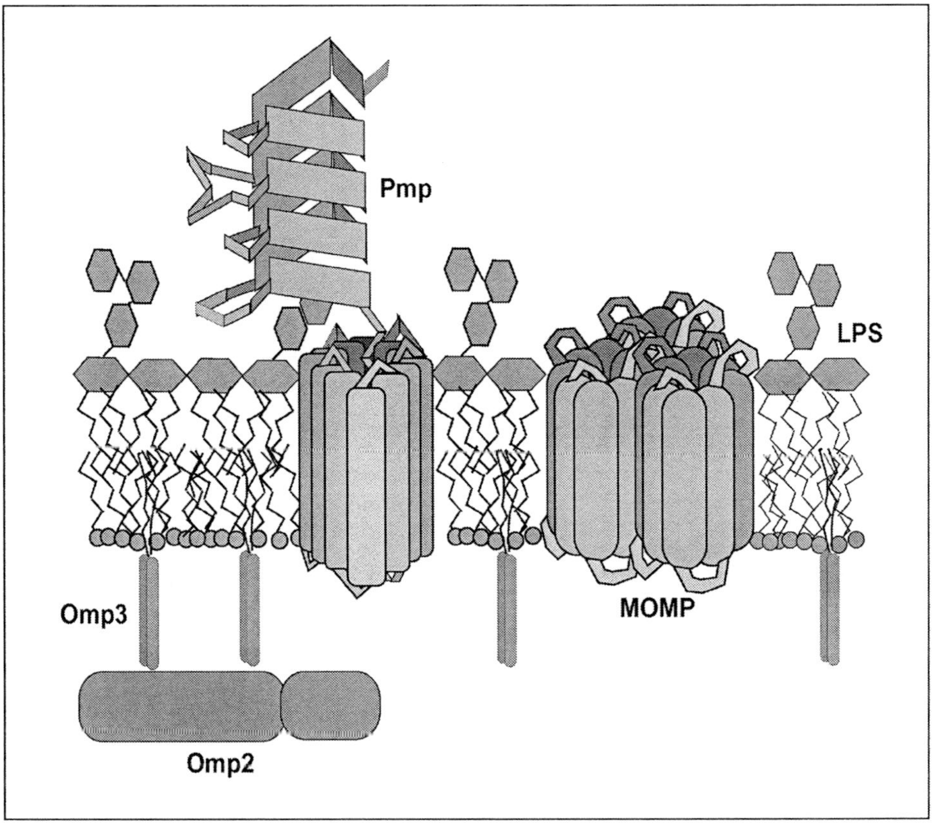

Figure 3. Model of *Chlamydia* outer membrane. Omp2 is in the periplasmic space cross-linked to Omp3 (28). MOMP is present as a trimeric porin in close relation to the LPS (26). MOMP forms b-sheets in the membrane, and the variable sequences (VS) are exposed on the surface. The Pmps form a b-barrel with the C-terminal part in the membrane (35). The N-terminal part of the protein is likely to from a b-tube (36). Depending on the *Chlamydia* species, the amount and number of polymorphic OMPs varies.

The *C. psittaci* genome has not been fully sequenced, such that the number of Pomp genes is unknown. The 4 Pomp genes sequenced thusfar are found in two clusters, Pomp 90A and 91A, and Pomp 91B and 90B according to the molecular size of the deduced amino acid sequences.[21] Pomp 90A and B are completely identical, and this is the first example of the presence of two identical *Chlamydia* genes in the same genome. By use of immunoelectron microscopy Longbottom et al[33] showed Pomp 90 proteins to be surface localized. The Pomps constitute only a minor fraction of the *C. psittaci* OMC. However, they are among the major immunogens as seen in immunoblotting with post-abortion ovine sera.

The rapidly expanding genome databases provide the option to search for sequence similarities among proteins from a wide variety of species. The presence of sequence similarity is the simplest and most commonly used method for predicting the structure and function of uncharacterized proteins. Generation of more sophisticated algorithms has increased the search options. Chlamydial Pmp genes are heterogeneous, with some common characteristics. The majority of the genes have the capacity to encode 90- to 100-kD proteins. Most of the putative proteins have an N-terminal leader sequence with a predicted cleavage site for signal peptidase I, characteristic of proteins transported across the plasma membrane. Another characteristic is the presence of repeats of the amino acid motif GGAI in the N-terminal part of the proteins. Analysis of the most C-terminal part of the proteins showed that all full-length proteins ended with an amphipathic β-sheet and a terminal phenylalanine residue characteristic of OMPs of Gram negative bacteria. In addition to this the program AMPHI predicted the C-terminal part of the proteins to have the capacity to form a transmembrane β-barrel .[34,35] Such a structure could be used for translocation of the N-terminal part of the protein to the chlamydial surface (type IV secretion). This is in agreement with the finding that it is the N-terminal part of the *C. psittaci* Pomp molecules that are surface-exposed.[33] Due to similarity in the predicted structure this also may be the case in *C. pneumoniae*. A new sophisticated search algorithms (BetaWrap by Bradley et al[36]) predicted the N-terminal part of the chlamydial Pmps to be members of the b-helix family, a family of proteins that contains parallel right-handed β-helix strands (Fig. 3). The folded proteins are characterized by a repeated pattern of parallel β-strands connected by turns. Therefore amino acids that are close in the folded protein can be distantly apart in the primary amino acid sequence, in agreement with the presence of conformational epitopes in these proteins.[24,31] Analysis of the *C. pneumoniae* proteome by 2-D gel electrophoresis and mass spectrometry revealed that 10 Pmp genes are expressed.[37] The GGAI domain of 2 of the proteins are cleaved, but both fragments are localized within the EB.[37] This is similar to the *E. coli* type IV secreted autotransporter molecule AIDA, which also is synthesized as a larger precursor molecule that is cleaved between the β-barrel part and the surface-exposed external domain.[38]

The components comprising the surface projections have not been determined, but physically they resemble the type III secretion apparatus found in other bacteria. Since genes with homology to such structures have been found in both the *C. trachomatis* and *C. pneumoniae* genomes [9,32] and are expressed,[37] it was speculated that the projections represent a type III secretion system.[39] The function of the surface projections may be to provide contact to the outside of the inclusion.

During most of the developmental cycle, *Chlamydia* are surrounded by the phagosomal membrane; thus, contact to the environment is limited to the phase in which the infectious EB are localized extracellularly and to components that are secreted from the phagosome to the outside of the *Chlamydia*. Inclusion membrane proteins (Inc) probably are secreted through the type III secretion apparatus and incorporated into the phagosome membrane.[40] These proteins may provide contact with the host cell, but whether they are of importance for development of immunity remains to be elucidated. Only one protein (CPAF) has been found to be secreted into the host cell cytoplasm.[41] CPAF is a protease or proteasome-like activity factor that degrades the host transcription factors RFX5 and upstream stimulation factor 1 (USF-1). CPAF is thus responsible for *Chlamydia*'s escape from T-lymphocyte immune recognition by degrading the host' transcription factors required for major histocompatibility complex (MHC) antigen expression.[41]

Humoral Immune Response to *C. trachomatis*

The immune response to *Chlamydia* infections has been intensively studied. During infection both the humoral and cellular immune response are activated. The main targets for the humoral immune response during *C. trachomatis* infections are the major surface localized components LPS and MOMP, but antibodies to other components like Omp2 and the heat shock homologues GroEL (Hsp60) and DnaK (Hsp70) are also found.[42]

To investigate the humoral immune response to *C. trachomatis*, Wang and Grayston developed the micro-IF technique, which uses acetone fixed *C. trachomatis* EB spots on a slide.[44] *C. trachomatis* first was cultivated in the yolk sac. Later the method was modified to use tissue-cultivated *Chlamydia* that are formaldehyde-fixed and mixed with egg yolk before being spotted to the slide.[43] For measuring human antibodies, serial dilutions of patient serum samples were added to the spots, and the binding of antibodies was detected with human immunoglobulin class-specific FITC-conjugated antibodies.[43] This technique can be used for all *Chlamy-*

dia species and for serotypes of *C. trachomatis*. The advantage of the technique is that it measures antibodies primarily directed against the surface of the microorganism, hence possibly also neutralizing antibodies. The disadvantage is that the genus-specific LPS is present in the preparations and thereby cross-reactions can occur. However, the technique gives no information on which components are immunogenic. Newhall et al[45] found MOMP, the 62/60-kD antigen and a 29-kD antigen as dominant immunogens, but MOMP also bound antibodies from patients known not to have had infections by *C. trachomatis*. Serum antibodies from patients with postabortal *C. trachomatis* salpingitis can mediate C'-dependent neutralization of *C. trachomatis*-infected host cells in vivo, but there was not a good correlation between micro-IF titers and neutralization.[42] When the sera were analyzed by immunoblotting, women who were protected against the postabortal salpingitis had more antibodies to antigen of 75-, 60-, and 57-kD proteins, and antibodies to the 100-, 32- and 28-kD proteins were only present in this group. The investigators used only *C. trachomatis* serovar D as antigen for immunoblotting, and therefore the reactivity to MOMP was inconclusive. The identity of the immunogens migrating at 75 kD was determined to be either the *C. trachomatis* DnaK homolog [46,47] or the comigrating ribosomal protein S1.[48] DnaK is the predominant cytosolic antigen in *C. trachomatis* EB.[46] Two different immunogenic proteins are present in the 62/60-kD protein dyad; the *C. trachomatis* GroEL/heat shock protein (HSP) 60 homolog and Omp2. Both antigens have a high homology between the *Chlamydia* species. Antibodies to Omp2 are specific for *Chlamydia* infections but cannot be differentiated between *C. trachomatis* and *C. pneumoniae* species.[49] Antibodies to *C. trachomatis* GroEL are correlated to tubal-factor infertility, but they are not specific for *Chlamydia* infection due to the high phylogenetic conservation of GroEL.[50,51]

The nature of the 100- and 29-kD antigens were not known, and several immunogens were identified within these size-ranges by two-dimensional gel electrophoresis.[48] The 100-kD antigen comprises members of the family of Pomp/Pmp described as immunogens for *C. psittaci* and *C. pneumoniae*.[33,35] Whether the products of the Pmp genes found in the *C. trachomatis* D genome are immunogenic has not been determined, even though two of the genes are expressed as 100-kD antigens in *C. trachomatis* L2.[32,23]

Mapping of Neutralizing Epitopes on MOMP with Mouse MAbs

MOMP is the best characterized *C. trachomatis* antigen. *C. trachomatis* can be divided serologically into B-complex (B, D, E, F, L1, L2) and C-complex serotypes (A, C, H, I, J, K, L3).[44] This is reflected in the amino acid sequence of MOMP where the B- and C-complexes differ with variations in VSI, VSII and VSIV. VSI of the C-complex is two amino acids longer than in the B-complex, and VSI in the B-complex is less variable than the C-complex (Figs. 2 and 4). The opposite is the case for VSII, where there is variation in the B-complex, being one amino acid longer than in the conserved C-complex (Figs. 2 and 4). Hayes et al[52] showed that VSI of the C-complex group contained the serotype-specific epitopes, whereas for the B-complex organisms the serotype-specific epitopes were localized in VSIV.

Of mapped MAbs to MOMP it was clear that VSII is immunogenic when B-complex serotypes were used as antigens (see **Table** 1).[52-60] When a C-complex serotype as serotype C was used, VSI was immunogenic.[56,57] All neutralizing antibodies mapped either with VSI or VSIV; none mapped with VSII or VSIII. The B-complex contains the serovars D and E that are commonly isolated from genital tract infections (Table 1). Therefore the small, conserved VSI of the B-complex may be of advantage due to the lack of neutralizing antibodies to this region.

Humoral Immune Response to *C. pneumoniae*

The humoral immune response to *C. pneumoniae* is dsetermined by micro-IF.[61] By this method it has been clearly shown that seropositivity increases with age and that the individual levels of antibodies are kept constant over time.

The micro-IF technique functions well with *C. pneumoniae*, but few antigens are seen by immunoblotting.[43] As for the *C. trachomatis* infections, Omp2 is a major immunogen in

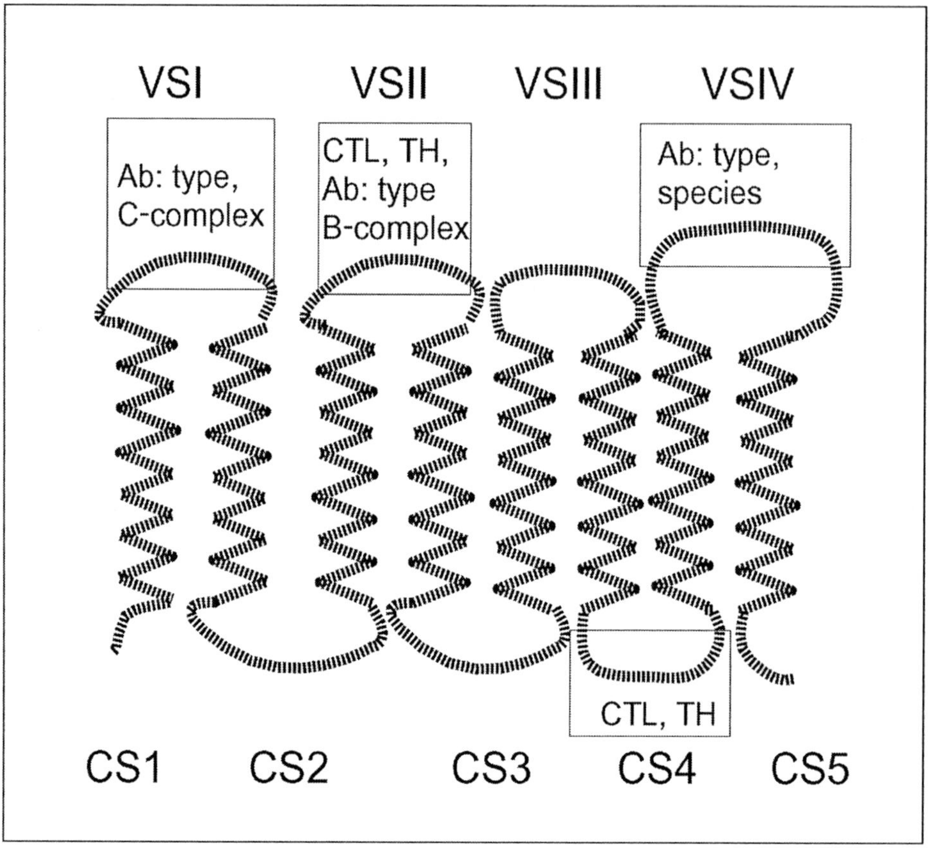

Figure 4. Schematic view of the variable (VS) and constant sequences (CS) of *C. trachomatis* MOMP with marked B-cell epitopes (Ab) (VSI is immunogenic in the B-complex group and VSII is immunogenic in the C-complex group), CD8$^+$ T-cell epitopes (CTL) and CD4$^+$ T-cell epitopes (TH).

patient sera that are micro-IF positive for *C. pneumoniae* but negative for *C. trachomatis.*[49] The antibodies to GroEL cannot be unraveled due to the conserved epitopes to both *C. trachomatis* GroEL and to other bacterial GroEL proteins. When micro-IF sera positive only for *C. pneumoniae* were used for immunoblotting, the reaction to a 98-kD band was *C. pneumoniae*-specific, but the reactions to MOMP, GroEL and Omp2 were not species-specific.[62]

There is a clear discrepancy between the reaction in micro-IF of sera and the reaction in immunoblotting. This can be due to the fact that the proteins are denatured under the separation by SDS-PAGE, and only limited refolding is obtained when the proteins are transferred to nitrocellulose. The 98-kD protein in the outer membrane of *C. pneumoniae* is composed of the Pmp.[24,62] After treatment of *C. pneumoniae* with SDS-sample buffer but without boiling, the Pmp proteins migrates as ~75-kD bands, and by using this condition it is a major immunogen reacting with patient sera positive by micro-IF.[35] There is a variable reaction to MOMP in immunoblotting that may be explained by the presence of conformational epitopes.[27] A 54-kD protein also has been described as an immunogen, and the reaction to it is species-specific.[63] In addition, MAbs to a 54-kD protein were neutralizing in a cell-culture test, but the identity of this protein has not been determined.

Table 1. Mapped monoclonal antibody epitopes on MOMP

MAb	Antigen for Immunization	Isotype	Sequences	Domain	Serotype/[Complex]	Protection	Ref.
J50	B	IgM	VSL	VDIV +	Genus	?	53
5F9	L1	IgG2a	DAVP	VDII	L1 [B]	?	53
L2/27/1bB1/G7	L2		DAVP	VDII	L1 [B]	?	53
10Eii	L1	IgG2b	IFDT	VDIV	B, Ba, D, E, L1, L2 [B]	?	53
6E	L1	IgG2b	LNPTIA	VDIV	C. trachomatis	?	53
2C1	(B,C, L2)		DVTTLNPTIAG	VDIV	C. trachomatis	?	54
2G3	(B,C, L2)		DVTTLNPTIAG	VDIV	H, K, L3, L1, L2, B, Ba; E, D	?	54
2IIE3	(B,C, L2)		ATTVFDVTTLNPTIAG	VDIV	L1, L2, B, Ba;E, D	?	54
IVF1	(B,C, L2)		DNENHATVSDSKLV	VDII	L2 [B]	?	54
1B7	(B,C, L2)		NNENQTKVSNGAFV	VDII	B [B]	?	54
2B1	(B,C, L2)		TKTQSSSFNTAKLI	VDII	C, J [C]	?	54
KK12, 5C2			TLNPTI	VDIV	Species	?	55
6E, 6Ciii, E21			LNPTIA	VDIV	Species	?	55
LV21, E4			LNPTI	VDIV	Species	?	55
L1/2C5/B8, DP10			NPTI	VDIV	Species	?	55
BD11, BB11			TAIGAGD	VDIV	B-complex	?	55
L2/57B1/2A			IAGAG	VDIV	B-compex	?	55
F22/4C11			FPLD(L/I)T	VDIII	Species -B, Ba	?	55
F2/3G8			FPLDLT	VDII	B, Ba, D, F, L1 (B)	?	55
C10	C		VAGLQNDPT	VDI	C,J,I,L3,K, H (C)	Yes, in vivo	58
L3-1	L3		AEFPLDIT	VDIII	A, H, I, J, K, L3	No, in vitro No, in vivo	59

Continued on next page

Table 1. Mapped monoclonal antibody epitopes on MOMP (continued)

MAb	Antigen for Immunization	Isotype	Sequences	Domain	Serotype/[Complex]	Protection	Ref.
C1.1 -C1.5	C	IgG3, IgG3, IgG1, IgG2b, IgG1	AGLQND	VDI	C (C)	Yes, in vitro	56
C1.6	C	IgG1	LQND	VDI	A, C (C)	Yes, in vitro	56
C1.7 -C1.8		IgG3, IgG3	LQND	VDI	C (C)	Yes, in vitro	56
PD10	K	I	LDVTTLNPTI	VDIV	Species	Yes, in vitro	57
9F12	K		SDVEGLQNDP	VDI	K (C)	Yes, in vitro	57
4A1	K		VEFPLDITAG	VDIII		No	57
11A12	K		LQNDPTTNVA	VDI		Yes, in vitro	57
2D7	K		LQNDPTTNVA	VDI	L3, K, J, H, C (C)	Yes, in vitro	57
3F6	K		VEFPLDITAG	VDIII	?	No, in vitro	57
5C2	K		LDVTTLNPTI	VDIV	L3, L2, K, J, I,H, F, C, Ba, B, A	Yes, in vitro	57
E4			LNPTI	VDIV	L1,L2, L3, B, D, E ,F, MoPn	Yes, in vitro	60
L1-4			LNPTI	VDIV	L1, L3, B, D, E, MoPn	Yes, in vitro	60
L1-24			LNPT	VDIV	L1, L2, L3, B, D, E, MoPn	Yes, in vitro	60
A36			EKD	VDI	A (C)	?	52
A30			VAGL	VDI	A,C (C)	?	52

Cellular Immunity to *C. trachomatis*, T-Helper Cell Response

During infection *Chlamydia* are taken up by antigen-presenting cells (APCs) as dendritic cells (DC) or macrophages. In contrast to what is the case in infected cells, the *Chlamydia* antigens are degraded when phagosomes in these cells fuse with lysosomes. A peptide fragment will eventually be presented in the groove of HLA class II to stimulate a T-helper response. The human response to MOMP during *C. trachomatis* infection has been investigated.[64-66] The authors analyzed T-cell epitopes on MOMP. They mixed APCs and T cells from patients with known infections and added purified MOMP to select clones; epitopes subsequently were determined by stimulation with synthetic peptides. The T-helper epitopes were localized to the constant sequence 4 (CS4) of MOMP as well as to the surface exposed VSII, which also contains B-cell epitopes.[64,66] These are the only human T-helper epitopes so far mapped.

Cytotoxic T-Cell Response

Cytotoxic T-cells mediate the lysis of infected cells by recognizing specific microbial peptide sequences (8-9 amino acids in length) presented to the $CD8^+$ cells by HLA Class I of the infected cell. It is possible to computer predict epitopes *in silico* and then test the epitopes for response in vitro.[67] Because *Chlamydia* grow in an inclusion in the cytoplasm, there is no obvious way for *Chlamydia* proteins to be exposed to the host cell cytoplasmic proteasomes, transported to the endoplasmic reticulum (ER) by the TAP complex, and eventually be presented in the groove of the HLA class I molecule on the cell surface. To determine whether MOMP contained $CD8^+$ T-cell epitopes, epitopes were predicted for HLA-A2 and HLA-B71, synthesized and tested by in vitro stimulation of purified $CD8^+$ cells from *C. trachomatis*-infected patients. The positive epitopes were localized to VSII and CS4. The epitopes in CS4 could be detected by flow cytometry with and without stimulation from STD patients using tetrameric HLA-A2 molecules with bound epitopes.[68] The stimulated $CD8^+$ T-cells lysed peptide-treated target cells as well as *C. trachomatis*-infected cells. This indicated that MOMP peptides were present in the HLA Class I groove, even though MOMP is a molecule that is tightly bound in the outer membrane of *Chlamydia* within the inclusion. A possible explanation for this could be that the host cell could inhibit the growth of *Chlamydia* in the presence of γ-interferon. This may lead to liberation of MOMP and thereby proteasome degradation followed by recognition by specific $CD8^+$ cells. The clustering of both B-cell, $CD4^+$ and $CD8^+$ cell epitopes in VSII and the presence of several CD4 and CD8 epitopes in CS4 is unique for MOMP,[69] which makes MOMP an excellent vaccine candidate. A DNA vaccine with the *C. trachomatis* mouse pneumonitis (MoPn) *momp* gene protected mice against pneumonia.[70] No human trials have been performed yet.

Proteins that are secreted to the *Chlamydia* inclusion membrane or to the host cell cytoplasm will contact the cytoplasmic proteasomes and therefore are more likely to be presented by HLA Class I. The inclusion membrane protein (Inc) A, B and C has been identified; there are 46 more candidates in the *C. trachomatis* genome found *in silico* with the predicted presence of a common hydrophobic β-sheet.[71] However, by screening a *Chlamydia*-specific $CD8^+$ T-cell line with a *C. trachomatis* genomic DNA library in a retroviral vector transformed into eukaryotic cells, Fling et al[72] succeeded only in identifying a CD8 epitope in the *C. trachomatis* CT529 protein. They named the protein Cap1 for class I accessible protein-1. The protein was localized to the inclusion membrane but did not contain the motif predicted from the Inc proteins. The CPAF protein is the first identified protein localized in the cytoplasm of the host cell, but it is not known whether it processes CD8 epitopes.

Vaccines

There exists no vaccine against human *Chlamydia* infections even though there is a need to prevent both *C. trachomatis* and *C. pneumoniae* infections.[73,74] Clinical trials with vaccination against trachoma were initiated more than 3 decades ago. Dhir et al[75] conducted vaccine trials in an area of high trachoma prevalence in Northern India. Two inactivated whole-cell *C.*

trachomatis EB preparations were used for immunization and compared with placebo. Good protection was found, but the protection was short-lived. In a long-term follow-up study twelve years later an equal number of children in each of the three groups had signs of mostly minimally active trachoma, and in addition 6-10% in each group had signs of potentially blinding sequelae.[76] Thus the initial observation of protection had been reversed, and there was no long-term protection. There was, however, no evidence of adverse effects from the vaccines. This was in contrast to what was found in monkey vaccine trials where higher attack rates and aggravated eye disease were found in the vaccinated animals challenged with heterologous strains.[77] Further evidence for a possible hypersensitivity reaction came with the discovery by Morrison et al[78] that the 57-kD hypersensitivity antigen was identified as the homolog to the *E. coli* GroEL/Hsp60, which is present both in prokaryotic and eukaryotic cells. The role of this protein was further analyzed by Patton et al[79] who in an animal model demonstrated that recombinant chlamydial Hsp60 was able to induce delayed hypersensitivity in animals sensitized with live *C. trachomatis* organisms. These early trials thus pointed out two problems: short-lasting protection and potential development of delayed hypersensitivity when whole-cell vaccines were used.

Animal Vaccines and Vaccine Studies

There are currently three vaccines produced to protect sheep from *C. psittaci* infections. Two are live attenuated vaccines, and one is an inactivated preparation of *C. psittaci*. These vaccines offer adequate protection against ovine infections with *C. psittaci*. To avoid mass cultivation of *Chlamydia* and to obtain a more standardized vaccine, the immunogenic components in the vaccines were determined. Since an experimental vaccine based on the OMC of *C. psittaci* provided protection, it was assumed that MOMP, which constituted ~90% of the protein content, was the major immunogen conferring immunity.[80] Therefore a vaccine based on recombinant MOMP was tested, but the results were disappointing in that the efficacies were variable and not as good as with the OMC preparations.[81] It was speculated that the reason for this could be either that MOMP needed a proper folding that was not obtained when produced in *E. coli* or that other components present in the OMC preparations were required for complete protection. For review on immune control of chlamydial infection in sheep, see Entrican et al.[82]

Vaccine Development

The development of methods to produce recombinant proteins has made it possible to study reactions to individual components in detail and to dissect how the immune system deals with such components. The major question for vaccine development is to determine what is required to produce long lasting resistance to reinfection. The major themes have been the analysis of protective antibodies and the identification of a protective T-cell response. Due to its high expression level, surface localization and immunogenicity, MOMP have been the major protective antigens investigated.

Zhang et al[83] first reported in 1989 that monoclonal antibodies (MAb) to serovar- or serogroup specific MOMP epitopes were protective and thus useful as a recombinant subunit *C. trachomatis* vaccine. Further studies confirmed MOMP as an attractive candidate, since both IgG and IgA anti MOMP MAbs could reduce the incidence of infection upon vaginal challenge; however, the MAb had marginal effect in preventing chlamydial colonization.[84] These observations led to vaccine studies where oligopeptides or recombinant full-length or fragments of MOMP were used, but at best only partial protective immunity was observed (reviewed by Beagley and Timms).[85] More promising results were obtained by Pal et al,[86] who purified and refolded MOMP extracted from *C. trachomatis* MoPn and mixed the preparation with Freund's adjuvant by vortexing or sonication. The two preparations differed by SDS-PAGE, the vortexed preparation probably consisting primarily of homopolymers of MOMP while the sonicated preparation contained monomeric MOMP. BALB/c mice were immunized and subsequently challenged with live *C. trachomatis* MoPn in the upper genital tract. Better protection in terms of less vaginal shedding and higher levels of fertility was observed when the vortexed MOMP vaccine was used. Both vaccines produced a strong humoral immune response, but only using the vortexed MOMP vaccine did a strong cellular response develop. These results illustrate the importance of correct presentation of the proteins to the immune system to obtain protection based on stimulation of both humoral and cellular immune responses. The results also indicate that MOMP still may be the only required component in a protective vaccine when *C. trachomatis* MoPn is used. Whether this is also the case for other *Chlamydia* species remains to be determined. The results are in agreement with results obtained by Igietseme and Murdin[87] who prepared a MOMP-ISCOM vaccine based on MOMP extracted from *C. trachomatis* serovar D for immunization of mice. This vaccine was able to produce a Th1 antigen-specific immune response. Immunized mice cleared a vaginal challenge within one week, and immunity was still present 8 weeks after primary infection.

The dendritic cell (DC) is one of the most potent antigen-presenting cells (APC). Bone marrow-derived DC can be obtained from mice and have the capability to phagocytose antigens, secrete interleukine and present antigens to sensitized T-cells. Su et al[88] used DC pulsed ex vivo with killed *C. trachomatis* MoPn for vaccination of C57BL/10 mice. The mice produced specific antibodies and a CD4$^+$ T-cell response. DC vaccination could reduce shedding of *C. trachomatis* MoPn and protected mice against genital tract obstructive disease upon intravaginal challenge with live *C. trachomatis* MoPn. In all three examples of potentially protective immunizations, the vaccine was based on cultivated *Chlamydia*, as was also the case for the available animal vaccines. Such vaccines provide excellent tools for analysis of the immune response required for protection against reinfections but are not optimal for human vaccine production.

A different but attractive vaccine candidate is a MOMP-DNA vaccine, since DNA immunization provides for stable and long-lived production of the immunogenic protein.[89] Vanrompay et al constructed a DNA plasmid capable of expressing *C. psittaci* MOMP and used this plasmid in vaccine trials of turkeys. Both T-helper and B-cell memory were primed even though only a limited increase in antibody titer was obtained. In spite of the rather weak antibody response the vaccine was able to protect turkeys against a generalized *C. psittaci* challenge.[89]

Conclusion and Perspectives

Whether MOMP is the most attractive component for human vaccines against chlamydial infections is questionable. MOMP is a variable protein, and both B- and T-cell epitopes are mapped to VS regions. There also are several serovars responsible for both trachoma and genital tract infections. Therefore, other approaches as the use of genomics for vaccine discovery are attractive.[90] With the publication of the genomes of both *C. trachomatis* and *C. pneumoniae* knowledge has been gained concerning all possible open reading frames, and this knowledge can be used to exploit how the immune system deals with each of these components. Of course some components are more attractive than others with regard to their potential of having a protective capability. As stimulators of antibody responses, surface-exposed components are still the most attractive candidates, but they need to be correctly folded. Only very few membrane proteins have been crystallized, and thus the precise structure remains unknown for most of these proteins. Careful analysis of the immune response to native components is crucial for determining whether recombinant proteins will be effective vaccines. As stimulators of cellular immune responses, secreted proteins or proteins present in the phagosomal membrane are attractive candidates because they may be able to contact the host cell cytoplasm for processing. Mixed vaccine strategies probably should be used in concert: DNA vaccine, synthetic peptides and recombinant proteins could be used in combination to elicit protective immunity.

References

1. Pearce JH, Gaston JSH. Chlamydia. In: Susmann M, ed. Molecular Medical Microbiology. San Diego: Acad Press, 2001:1825-64.
2. Westrom LR. Incidence, prevalence and trends of acute pelvic inflammatory disease and its consequences in industrialised countries. Am. J Obstet Gynecol 1980; 138:880-892.
3. Cates W, Wasserheit JN, Marchbanks PA. Pelvic inflammatory disease and tubla infertility - the preventable conditions. Ann. N Y Acad Sci 1994; 709:179-195.
4. Grayston JT, Kuo C-C, Wang S-P et al. A new Chlamydia psittaci strain, TWAR, isolated in acute respiratory tract infections. N Engl J Med 1986; 315:161-168.
5. Grayston JT, Campbell LA, Kuo C-C et al. A new respiratory tract pathogen: Chlamydia pneumoniae strain TWAR. J Infect Dis 1990; 161:618-625.
6. Hahn DL, Dodge RW, Glubjatnikov R. Association of Chlamydia pneumoniae (strain TWAR) infection with wheezing, asthmatic bronchitis and adult onset asthma. JAMA 1991; 266:225-230.
7. Johnston SL. Is Chlamydia pneumoniae important in asthma? The first controlled trialof therapy leaves the question unanswered. Am J Respir Crit Care Med 2001; 164:536-541.
8. Campbell LA, Rosenfeld M, Kuo C-C. The role of Chlamydia pneumoniae in atherosclerosis - recent evidence from animal models. Trends Microbiol 2000; 8:255-257.
9. Kalman S, Mitchell W, Marathe R et al. Comparative genomes of Chlamydia pneumoniae and C. trachomatis. Nature Genet 1999; 21:385-389.
10. Read TD, Brunham RC, Shen C et al. Genome sequences of Chlamydia trachomatis MoPn and Chlamydia pneumoniae AR39. Nucleic Acids Res 2000; 28:1397-1406.
11. Shirai M, Hirakawa H, Kimoto M et al. Comparison of whole genome sequences of Chlamydia pneumoniae J138 from Japan and CWL029 from USA. Nucleic Acids Res 2000; 28:2311-2314.
12. Barnes RC. Laboratory diagnosis of human chlamydial infections. Clin Microbiol Rev 1989; 2; 119-136.
13. Wang SP, Grayston JT. Human serology in Chlamydia trachomatis infection with microimmunofluorescence. J Infect Dis 1974; 130:388-397
14. Kuo CC, Jackson LA, Campbell LA et al. Chlamydia pneumoniae (TWAR). Clin Microbiol Rev 1995; 8:451-461.
15. Ridgway GL. Advances in the antimicrobial therapy of chlamydial genital infections. J Infect 1992; 25: 51-59.
16. Manire GP. Structure of purified cell walls of dense forms of meningopneumonitis organisms. J Bacteriol 1966; 91:409-413.
17. Matsumoto A. Electron microscopic observations of surface projections on Chlamydia psittaci reticulate bodies. J Bacteriol 1982; 150:358-364.
18. Nichols BA, Setzer PY, Pang F et al. New view of the surface projections of Chlamydia trachomatis. J Bacteriol 1985; 164:344-349.
19. Miyashita N, Matsumoto A. Establishment of a particle-counting method for purified elementary bodies of chlamydiae and evaluation of sensitivities of the IDEIA Chlamydia kit and DNA probe by using the purified elementary bodies. J Clin Microbiol 1992; 30:2911-2916.
20. Caldwell HD, Kromhout J, Schachter J. Purification and partial characterization of the major outer membrane protein of Chlamydia trachomatis. Infect Immun 1981; 31:1161-1176.
21. Longbottom D, Russell M, Dunbar SM et al. Molecular cloning and characterization of the genes coding for the highly immunogenic cluster of 90-kilodalton envelope proteins from the Chlamydia psittaci subtype that causes abortion in sheep. Infect Immun 1998; 66:1317-1324.
22. Melgosa MP, Kuo C-C, Campbell LA. Outer membrane complex proteins of Chlamydia pneumoniae. FEMS Microbiol Lett 1993; 112:199-204.
23. Mygind PH, Christiansen G, Roepstorff P et al. Membrane proteins PmpG and PmpH are major constituents of Chlamydia trachomatis L2 outer membrane complex. FEMS Microbiol Lett 2000; 186:163-169.
24. Knudsen K, Madsen AS, Mygind P et al. Identification of two novel genes encoding 97- to 99-kilodalton outer membrane proteins of Chlamydia pneumoniae. Infect Immun 1999; 67:375-383.
25. Birkelund S, Lundemose AG, Christiansen G. Immunoelectron microscopy of lipopolysaccharide in Chlamydia trachomatis. Infect Immun 1989; 57:3250-3253.
26. Birkelund S, Lundemose AG, Christiansen G. Chemical cross-linking of Chlamydia trachomatis. Infect Immun 1988; 56:654-659.
27. Wolf K, Fischer E, Mead D et al. Chlamydia pneumoniae major outer membrane protein is a surface-exposed antigen that elicits antibodies primarily directed against conformation-dependent determinants. Infect Immun 2001; 69:3082-3091.

28. Mygind P, Christiansen G, Birkelund S. Topological analysis of Chlamydia trachomatis L2 outer membrane protein 2. J Bacteriol 1998; 180:5784-5787.
29. Stephens RS, Koshiyama K, Lewis E et al. Heparin-binding outer membrane protein of chlamydiae. Mol Microbiol 2001; 40:691-699.
30. Vandahl B, Christiansen G, Birkelund S. Expression of lipid modification of a polymorphic membrane protein in Chlamydia pneumoniae. In: Saikku P, ed. Proceedings of the Fourth Meeting of the European Society for Chlamydia Research. Helsingi: Universitas Helsingiensis, 2000:54.
31. Pedersen AS, Christiansen G, Birkelund S. Differential expression of Pmp10 in cell culture infected with Chlamydia pneumoniae CWL029. FEMS Microbiol Lett 2001; 203:153-159.
32. Stephens RS, Kalman S, Lammel C et al. Genome sequence of an obligate intracellular pathogen of humans: Chlamydia trachomatis. Science 1998; 282:754-759.
33. Longbottom D, Findlay J, Vretou E et al. Immunoelectron microscopic localisation of the OMP90 family on the outer membrane surface of Chlamydia psittaci. FEMS Microbiol Lett 1998; 164:111-117
34. Jahnig F. Structure predictions of membrane proteins are not that bad. Trends Biochem Sci 1990; 15:93-95.
35. Christiansen G, Pedersen AS, Hjerno K et al. Potential relevance of Chlamydia pneumoniae surface proteins to an effective vaccine. J Infect Dis 2000; 181:S528-37.
36. Bradley P, Cowen L, Menke M et al. Predicting the Beta-Helix Fold from Protein Sequence Data. In: Zimmer R, ed. Proceedings of the Fifth Annual International Conference on Computational Molecular Biology. New York: ACM Press, 2001:59-67
37. Vandahl B, Birkelund S, Christiansen G. Proteome analysis of the Chlamydia pneumoniae elementary body. Electrophoresis 2001; 22:1204-1223.
38. Benz I, Schmidt MA. AIDA-I, the adhesin involved in diffuse adherence of the diarrhoeagenic Escherichia coli strain 2787 (O126:H27), is synthesized via a precursor molecule. Mol Microbiol 1992; 6:1539-1546.
39. Bavoil PM, Hsia RC. Type III secretion in Chlamydia: a case of deja vu? Mol Microbiol 1998; 28:860-2.
40. Hackstadt T, Scidmore-Carlson MA, Shaw EI et al. The Chlamydia trachomatis IncA protein is required for homotypic vesicle fusion. Cell Microbiol 1999; 1:119-130.
41. Zhong G, Fan P, Ji H et al. Identification of a chlamydial protease-like activity factor responsible for the degradation of host transcription factors. J Exp Med 2001; 193:935-942.
42. Brunham RC, Peeling R, Maclean I et al. Postabortal Chlamydia trachomatis salpingitis: correlating risk with antigen-specific serological responses and with neutralization. J Infect Dis 1987; 155:749-755.
43. Wang SP. The microimmunofluorescence test for Chlamydia pneumoniae infection: technique and interpretation. J Infect Dis 2000; 181:S421-5.
44. Wang SP, Grayston JT. Immunologic relationship between genital TRIC, lymphogranuloma venereum, and related organisms in a new microtiter indirect immunofluorescence test. Am J Ophthalmol 1970; 70:367-374.
45. Newhall WJ, Batteiger B, Jones RB. 1982. Analysis of the human serological response to proteins of Chlamydia trachomatis. Infect Immun 38:1181-1189.
46. Birkelund S, Lundemose AG, Christiansen G. Characterization and identification of early proteins in Chlamydia trachomatis serovar L2 by two-dimensional gel electrophoresis. Infect Immun 1990; 58:2478-2486.
47. Birkelund S, Lundemose AG, Christiansen G. The 75-kilodalton cytoplasmic Chlamydia trachomatis L2 polypeptide is a DnaK-like protein. Infect Immun 1990; 58:2098-2104.
48. Sanchez-Campillo M, Bini L, Comanducci M et al. Identification of immunoreactive proteins of Chlamydia trachomatis by Western blot analysis of a two-dimensional electrophoresis map with patient sera. Electrophoresis 1999; 20:2269-2279.
49. Mygind P, Christiansen G, Persson K et al. Analysis of the humoral immune response to Chlamydia outer membrane protein 2. Clin Diagn Lab Immunol 1998; 5:313-318.
50. Persson K, Osser S, Birkelund S et al. Antibodies to Chlamydia trachomatis heat shock proteins in women with tubal factor infertility are associated with prior infection by C. trachomatis but not by C. pneumoniae. Hum Reprod 1999; 14:1969-1973.
51. LaVerda D, Albanese LN, Ruther PE et al. Seroreactivity to Chlamydia trachomatis Hsp10 correlates with severity of human genital tract disease. Infect Immun 2000; 68:303-309.
52. Hayes LJ, Pickett MA, Conlan JW et al. The major outer-membrane proteins of Chlamydia trachomatis serovars A and B: intra-serovar amino acid changes do not alter specificities of serovar- and C subspecies-reactive antibody-binding domains. J Gen Microbiol 1990; 136:1559-1566.

53. Conlan JW, Clarke IN, Ward ME. Epitope mapping with solid-phase peptides: identification of type-, subspecies-, species- and genus-reactive antibody binding domains on the major outer membrane protein of Chlamydia trachomatis Mol Microbiol 1988; 2:673-679.
54. Stephens RS, Wagar EA, Schoolnik GK. High-resolution mapping of serovar-specific and common antigenic determinants of the major outer membrane protein of Chlamydia trachomatis. J Exp Med 1988; 167:817-831.
55. Batteiger BE. The major outer membrane protein of a single Chlamydia trachomatis serovar can possess more than one serovar-specific epitope. Infect Immun 1996; 64:542-547.
56. Zhong G, Berry J, Brunham RC. Antibody recognition of a neutralization epitope on the major outer membrane protein of Chlamydia trachomatis. Infect Immun 1994; 62:1576-1583.
57. Villeneuve A, Brossay L, Paradis G et al. Determination of neutralizing epitopes in variable domains I and IV of the major outer-membrane protein from Chlamydia trachomatis serovar K. Microbiology 1994; 140:2481-2487.
58. Qu Z, Cheng X, de la Maza LM et al. Characterization of a neutralizing monoclonal antibody directed at variable domain I of the major outer membrane protein of Chlamydia trachomatis C-complex serovars. Infect Immun 1993; 61:1365-1370.
59. Pal S, Cheng X, Peterson EM et al. Mapping of a surface-exposed B-cell epitope to the variable sequent 3 of the major outer-membrane protein of Chlamydia trachomatis. J Gen Microbiol 1993; 139:1565-1570.
60. Peterson EM, Cheng X, Markoff BA et al. Functional and structural mapping of Chlamydia trachomatis species-specific major outer membrane protein epitopes byuse of neutralizing monoclonal antibodies. Infect Immun 1991; 59:4147-4153.
61. Dowell SF, Peeling RW, Boman J et al. Standardizing Chlamydia pneumoniae assays: recommendations from the Centers for Disease Control and Prevention (USA) and the Laboratory Centre for Disease Control (Canada). Clin Infect Dis 2001; 33:492-503.
62. Campbell LA, Kuo CC, Grayston JT. Structural and antigenic analysis of Chlamydia pneumoniae. Infect Immun 1990; 58:93-97
63. Wiedmann-Al-Ahmad M, Schuessler P et al. Reactions of polyclonal and neutralizing anti-p54 monoclonal antibodies with an isolated, species-specific 54-kilodalton protein of Chlamydia pneumoniae. Clin Diagn Lab Immunol 1997; 4:700-704.
64. Arno JN, Xie C, Jones RB et al. Identification of T cells that respond to serovar-specific regions of the Chlamydia trachomatis major outer membrane protein in persons with serovar E infection. J Infect Dis 1998; 178:1713-1718.
65. Ortiz L, Angevine M, Kim SK et al.T-cell epitopes in variable segments of Chlamydia trachomatis major outer membrane protein elicit serovar-specific immune responses in infected humans. Infect Immun 2000; 68:1719-23.
66. Ortiz L, Demick KP, Petersen JW et al. Chlamydia trachomatis major outer membrane protein (MOMP) epitopes that activate HLA class II-restricted T cells from infected humans. J Immunol 1996; 157:4554-4567.
67. Lauemoller SL, Holm A, Hilden J et al. Quantitative predictions of peptide binding to MHC class I molecules using specificity matrices and anchor-stratified calibrations. Tissue Antigens 2001; 57:405-414.
68. Kim SK, Devine L, Angevine M et al. Direct detection and magnetic isolation of Chlamydia trachomatis major outer membrane protein-specific CD8+ CTLs with HLA class I tetramers. J Immunol 2000; 165:7285-7292.
69. Kim SK, DeMars R. Epitope clusters in the major outer membrane protein of Chlamydia trachomatis. Curr Opin Immunol. 2001; 13:429-436.
70. Brunham RC, Zhang D. Transgene as vaccine for Chlamydia. Am Heart J 1999; 138:S519-522.
71. Bannantine JP, Griffiths RS, Viratyosin W et al. A secondary structure motif predictive of protein localization to the chlamydial inclusion membrane. Cell Microbiol 2000; 2:35-47.
72. Fling SP, Sutherland RA, Steele LN et al. CD8+ T cells recognize an inclusion membrane-associated protein from the vacuolar pathogen Chlamydia trachomatis. Proc Natl Acad Sci USA 2001; 98:1160-1165.
73. Stagg AJ. Vaccines against Chlamydia: approaches and progress. Mol Med Today 1998; 4:166-173.
74. Murdin AD, Gellin B, Brunham RC et al. Collaborative multidisciplinary workshop report: progress toward a Chlamydia pneumoniae vaccine. J Infect Dis 2000; 181:S552-557.
75. Dhir SP, Agarwal LP, Detels R et al. Field trial of two bivalent trachoma vaccines in children of Punjab Indian villages. Am J Ophtalmol 1967; 63:1639-1644
76. Clements C, Dhir SP, Grayston JT et al. Long term follow-up study of a trachoma vaccine trial in villages of Northern India. Am J Ophtalmol 1979; 87:350-353

77. Wang SP, Grayston JT, Alexander ER. Trachoma vaccine studies in Monkeys. Am J Ophtalmol 1967; 63:1615-1630.
78. Morrison RP, Belland RJ, Lyng K et al. Chlamydial disease pathogenesis. The 57-kD chlamydial hypersensitivity antigen is a stress response protein. J Exp Med 1989; 170:1271-1283.
79. Patton DL, Sweeney YT, Kuo C-C. Demonstration of delayed hypersensitivity in Chlamydia trachomatis in monkeys: a pathogenic mechanism of tubal damage. J Infect Dis 1994; 169:680-683.
80. Tan TW, Herring AJ, Anderson IE et al. Protection of sheep against Chlamydia psittaci infection with a subcellular vaccine containing the major outer membrane protein. Infect Immun 1990; 58:3101-3108.
81. Herring, AJ, Jones GE, Dunbar SM et al. Recombinant vaccines against Chlamydia psittaci - an overview of results using bacterial expression and a new approach using plant virus "overcoat" system. In: Stephens RS, Byrne, GI, Christinsen, eds. Diseases of Sheep. Bologna: Sicieta Editrice Esculpio, 1998:434-437.
82. Entrican G, Buxton D, Longbottom D. Chlamydial infection in sheep: immune control versus fetal pathology. J R Soc Med 2001; 94:273-277.
83. Zhang YX, Stewart SJ, Caldwell HD. Protective monoclonal antibodies to Chlamydia trachomatis serovar- and serogroup-specific major outer membrane protein determinants. Infect Immun 1989; 57:636-638.
84. Cotter TW, Meng Q, Shen ZL et al. Protective efficacy of major outer membrane protein-specific immunoglobulin A (IgA) and IgG monoclonal antibodies in a murine model of Chlamydia trachomatis genital tract infection. Infect Immun 1995; 63:4704-4714.
85. Beagley KW, Timms P. Chlamydia trachomatis infection: incidence, health cost and prospects for vaccine development. J Reprod Immunol 2000; 48:47-68.
86. Pal S, Theodor I, Peterson EM et al. Immunization with the Chlamydia trachomatis mouse pneumonitis major outer membrane protein can elicit a protective immune response against a genital challenge. Infect Immun 2001; 69:6240-6247.
87. Igietseme JU, Murdin A. Induction of protective immunity against Chlamydia trachomatis genital infection by a vaccine based on major outer membrane protein-lipophilic immune response-stimulating complexes. Infect Immun 2000; 68:6798-806.
88. Su H, Messer R, Whitmire W et al. Vaccination against chlamydial genital tract infection after immunization with dendritic cells pulsed ex vivo with nonviable Chlamydiae. J Exp Med 1998; 188:809-818.
89. Vanrompay D, Cox E, Volckaert G et al. Turkeys are protected from infection with Chlamydia psittaci by plasmid DNA vaccination against the major outer membrane protein. Clin Exp Immunol 1999; 118:49-55.
90. Stephens RS. Chlamydial genomics and vaccine antigen discovery. J Infect Dis 2000; 181:S521-3.

Chapter 8

Escherichia coli Vaccines

Myron M. Levine and Michael S. Donnenberg

Summary

Escherichia coli is a component of the normal intestinal flora where it performs physiological functions. However, in immunocompromised hosts or in normal hosts whose anatomical barriers have been disrupted (as by trauma), *E. coli* can cause invasive septicemic disease. Moreover, there exist subsets of *E. coli* that possess arrays of virulence properties allowing them to behave as primary pathogens causing urinary tract infections, meningitis in neonates, or various forms of diarrheal disease. At least six distinct categories of diarrheagenic *E. coli* are recognized: enteropathogenic *E. coli* (EPEC), a cause of young infant diarrhea in developing countries; enterotoxigenic *E. coli* (ETEC), the most common cause of travelers' diarrhea and a main agent of infant diarrhea in developing countries; enteroinvasive *E. coli* (EIEC), a cause of dysentery as well as watery diarrhea; enterohemorrhagic *E. coli* (EHEC), which can cause hemorrhagic colitis and hemolytic uremic syndrome (HUS); enteroaggregative *E. coli* (EAggEC), the most frequent agent responsible for persistent diarrhea in children in developing countries; and diffuse adherence *E. coli* (DAEC), a cause of diarrhea in preschool children in developing countries. Candidate vaccines in clinical trials include a parenteral subunit vaccine against uropathogenic *E. coli* (UPEC) and several vaccines to prevent ETEC diarrhea. One EHEC vaccine has also entered clinical trials.

Introduction

Escherichia coli, the type species of the *Escherichia* genus that includes mostly motile Gram negative bacilli, is the predominant facultative anaerobic constituent of normal colonic flora and usually colonizes the newborn infant within hours of birth. Thereafter and for the remainder of a human's life, *E. coli* performs important normal physiologic functions in the intestine.[1,2] Thus, under normal circumstances, *E. coli* usually remains confined within the intestinal lumen as a harmless (indeed, beneficial) saprophyte. *E. coli* are serotyped based on their lipopolysaccharide (LPS) O somatic, H flagellar and K capsular surface antigens. At present, more than 170 O serogroups are recognized based on the > 170 distinct O antigens. *E. coli* are often described by their O:H serotype. Many *E. coli* strains have capsular K antigens that overlie the O antigen.

In debilitated immunocompromised hosts, normal flora *E. coli* can act as opportunistic pathogens leading to sepsis and invasive infections. In immunologically competent hosts who suffer trauma that releases *E. coli* from the intestine into the peritoneum or into the bloodstream, or when critical anatomic barriers are disrupted (e.g., head trauma with tearing of the meninges), severe deep-seated infections may ensue caused by otherwise normal *E. coli.*

However, there also exist subsets of *E. coli* that possess arrays of specific virulence attributes that allow them to overcome host defense mechanisms and cause clinically important infections in healthy subjects who lack specific immunity. By virtue of these constellations of virulence attributes, these *E. coli* function as primary pathogens. The immunobiological characteristics of

New Bacterial Vaccines, edited by Ronald W. Ellis and Bernard R. Brodeur.

these subsets of pathogenic *E. coli*, the clinical syndromes they cause and strategies to develop vaccines against them are described in the ensuing paragraphs.

Clinical Syndromes and Causative Agents

Urinary Tract Infections

Urinary tract infections (UTI) are among the most common bacterial infections of humans. It is estimated that 11% of women 18 years of age and above suffer from symptomatic UTIs each year and that ~60% of women will experience a UTI during their lifetime.[3] Whereas UTIs may range clinically from asymptomatic bacteriuria to urosepsis, acute cystitis represents the most common symptomatic manifestation. Up to 44% of women who have cystitis will have a recurrence during the ensuing 12 months; most of these occur in individuals with a history of prior UTI.[4] The majority of women with recurrent episodes of symptomatic UTI have functionally and anatomically normal urinary tracts. However, individuals with abnormal urinary tracts, including those with spinal cord injuries, urethral catheters, renal calculi and partial urinary obstruction are at high risk of serious infection. The annual costs attributed to symptomatic UTI in the United States are estimated to exceed $1.6 billion.[3]

E. coli is by far the most common cause of UTI, accounting for at least 85% of episodes of cystitis, pyelonephritis and urosepsis in persons with normal urinary tracts. *E. coli* is also the commonest cause of UTI among males. In persons with urinary tract abnormalities, *E. coli* is also the dominant pathogen, although in such hosts with anatomical abnormalities or foreign bodies, a plethora of other less pathogenic bacteria can also cause symptomatic infection.[5]

Initiation of an *E. coli* UTI represents the culmination of a complex interaction between the bacteria and the human host defenses. Only in the first three months of life are UTIs more common in males. Thereafter, females are much more frequent victims of UTI. This remarkable gender difference has been attributed in part to the longer urethra in the male and the antibacterial properties of prostatic secretions. Physical manipulation of the female urethra can transfer bacteria from the urethra into the bladder.[6] "Milking" of the anterior urethra caused small numbers of bacteria to be recoverable from bladder urine collected by suprapubic puncture in 9 of 24 female subjects.[6] This observation helps to explain the increased incidence of cystitis in sexually active women ("honeymoon cystitis"), in comparison with age-matched sexually abstinent women.[7] Indeed, numerous studies have documented both a dose-dependent increase in the risk of symptomatic UTI with sexual intercourse and the presence of bacteriuria after sex.[8,9] These observations demonstrate that bacteria present in the vaginal introitus and periurethral area can play an important role in the steps leading to UTI. Indeed, studies have shown that women with recurrent UTI have a significantly higher prevalence (~50%) of *E. coli* colonization of their peri-urethral areas than normal women (~20%) ($p<0.001$). In women and girls with recurrent UTI who were followed in longitudinal studies, peri-urethral colonization with *E. coli* was found to precede and persist during UTI.[10-14] Finally, in the 1970s Swedish investigators showed that women suffering from UTI often exhibited a host risk factor. Using *E. coli* from UTI as the test organism, a quantitatively increased adherence was observed when the bacteria were reacted with uroepithelial cells from patients with recurrent UTI versus uroepithelial cells from normal individuals.[15,16]

While some women may be predisposed to developing UTI because of host factors, it is also clear that certain strains of *E. coli* are equipped with virulence properties for causing UTI. Indeed, outbreaks of UTI due to particular pathogenic clones have been observed, emphasizing the fact that certain strains are particularly pathogenic for the urinary tract.[16-18] Uropathogenic *E. coli* (UPEC) strains have been shown in epidemiological studies to be more likely than control strains to possess or express certain factors that are believed to play a role in virulence.[19] For example, despite the fact that the genes for type 1 somatic fimbriae are ubiquitous among *E. coli* strains and related organisms, UPEC are more likely to express these fimbriae than are strains from the fecal flora. Type 1 fimbriae have been demonstrated in animal models to be required for experimental UTI.[20] UPEC strains, especially those isolated from patients with pyelonephritis, are also more likely than control strains to express P fimbriae, which have been shown to enhance the pathogenesis of pyelonephritis in an animal model.[21] A variety of other fimbrial and afimbrial adhesins are more prevalent among UPEC strains and may play a role in pathogenesis.[19] One or more of these adhesins may be appropriate components to include in a UPEC vaccine to prevent UTI in susceptible women. Other factors associated with virulence based on animal models or epidemiologic studies and that may have relevance for vaccine development include hemolysin,[22] various iron acquisition systems,[23] and certain metabolic factors.[24,25]

Neonatal Meningitis

The incidence rate for meningitis is higher during the first month of life than during any other single month. Approximately one in every 3,000-4,000 infants develops *E. coli* meningitis, and ~80% of these *E. coli* strains express K1 capsular antigen. The K1 antigen is an acidic capsular polysaccharide (Ps), colominic acid, that is a 2→8 a-linked homopolymer of N-acetylneuraminic (sialic) acid. Notably, *E. coli* K1 is identical in chemical structure and antigenicity to the acidic capsular Ps of group B *Neisseria meningitidis.*[26-29]

At all ages, K1 *E. coli* are found in the colonic flora of 20-40% of individuals. Full term infants become colonized by transmission of *E. coli* K1 from their mothers. In ~1:4,000 neonates, the *E. coli* K1 invades the bloodstream and is carried to the meninges. It is not clear whether invasion occurs via the infant's nasopharynx or intestinal mucosa, or both.

Bacterial meningitis in the neonatal period is a devastating disease accompanied by high case-fatality, and survivors commonly suffer severe sequelae. Causative strains are commonly resistant to multiple antibiotics and, despite appropriate therapy with antibiotics to which the *E. coli* is sensitive in vitro, the clinical response to therapy is often unsatisfactory.

It was proposed that immunization of pregnant women with appropriate K1 vaccines might elicit high-titer IgG antibodies that would cross the placenta and provide passive protection to the human neonate during the first four weeks of life when risk of *E. coli* K1 meningitis is maximal. However, several factors mitigate against such a strategy. First, the incidence of *E. coli* K1 meningitis has diminished since the 1970s, becoming second in importance to group B streptococci. Second, safety concerns have been raised about vaccines that would stimulate anti-K1 antibodies, since such antibodies bind polysialosyl glycopeptides present in human fetal brain tissue.[30] Third, the clinical trials that would be required to generate data to document both the safety and efficacy of such a vaccine for licensure would be extremely complicated to perform.

Sepsis

Along with infections caused by *Klebsiella* and *Pseudomonas, E. coli* is one of the major pathogens associated with sepsis in immunocompromised hosts and in normal subjects who have interruptions of anatomical barriers from trauma. Because mortality from sepsis is high even when early therapy is initiated with antibiotics to which the *E. coli* is susceptible in vitro, a potential role has been identified for immunotherapy. Thus, *E. coli* vaccines have been considered as a way of eliciting antibodies in healthy subjects who could undergo plasmapheresis to provide a high-titer antibody source for preparation of immunoglobulin concentrates to be used in immunotherapy of sepsis. It has also been suggested that there may be a role for active immunization of highly targeted subjects such as trauma patients or even healthy soldiers, firemen and policemen to provide them with protection against sepsis should they experience trauma as an occupational hazard.[31]

One major challenge is to generate antibodies that would provide broad-spectrum protection against the majority of *E. coli* associated with sepsis. Three main targets have been investigated: lipid A antigens, core glycolipids such as J5, and an array of O Ps antigens representing the 12 most common O serogroups associated with sepsis (accounting for ~70% of *E. coli* sepsis isolates).

Diarrheal Disease

Within the species *E. coli*, there exist primary pathogens that cause various syndromes of diarrheal disease, including watery diarrhea, dysentery and hemorrhagic colitis, in different age groups under distinct epidemiologic settings. Collectively, these clinical gastrointestinal infections are referred to as *E. coli* diarrheal illness, even though the individual categories of diarrheagenic *E. coli* constitute quite discrete pathogens that can cause rather distinct clinical syndromes.

Strains of *E. coli* that cause diarrhea can be conveniently divided into six major categories: EPEC, ETEC, EIEC, EHEC, EAggEC and DAEC. Each category of diarrheagenic *E. coli* has a different pathogenesis, possesses distinct virulence attributes, and comprises a separate set of O:H serotypes. The individual categories can cause distinctive clinical syndromes and exhibit characteristic epidemiologic patterns. ETEC, EPEC, EIEC, EAggEC and DAEC are commonly isolated as agents of diarrheal disease among infants and young children in less-developed countries.[32] The different categories of diarrheagenic *E. coli* share certain pathogenesis motifs that include attachment to and interaction with intestinal mucosa, the elaboration of enterotoxins (all except DAEC), carriage of plasmids that encode virulence attributes and a set of O:H serotypes characteristic of each category.

EPEC

In the 1940s and 1950s, investigators in the United Kingdom, the USA and Europe found that *E. coli* strains of certain O:H serotypes, termed EPEC, were associated with sporadic cases of infant summer diarrhea and of epidemic gastroenteritis in hospital nurseries. Studies in adult volunteers in the 1950s in the USA and Japan confirmed the capacity of these strains to cause diarrheal illness, although at the time the virulence mechanisms remained unknown. EPEC used to be a common cause of diarrheal illness in Europe and North America but largely disappeared in the 1970s.[33] EPEC remains an important cause of diarrhea in young infants (less than 6 months of age) in many developing and newly industrializing countries where it is particularly associated with bottle feeding as a risk factor.[32-34]

EPEC carries a ~60 mega-Dalton (mD) plasmid that encodes Bundle Forming Pili (BFP) which foster the initial attachment of EPEC to intestinal epithelium.[35] This plasmid also regulates expression of a chromosomal gene encoding intimin, a 94-kD protein that mediates intimate attachment to enterocytes.[36] The gene encoding intimin is part of a large pathogenicity island, the Locus of Enterocyte Effacement (LEE),[37] that is also found in EHEC. The EspA and EspB proteins, also encoded within the LEE, form part of a translocation apparatus that delivers proteins directly to host epithelial cells.[38] One of these proteins is the translocated intimin receptor (Tir), which is inserted by the bacteria into the host cell membrane where it serves as a receptor for intimin.[39] The bacteria, once intimately attached to the host cell through this binding, induce actin condensation and other cytoskeletal changes in the enterocytes. The consequence of this interaction between EPEC and intestinal mucosa is a pathognomonic "attaching and effacing" intestinal lesion observed by electron microscopy.[40]

ETEC

In the late 1960s, largely based on investigations carried out in the Indian subcontinent, a new category of diarrheagenic *E. coli* was discovered that was associated with severe, cholera-like, watery diarrhea.[41] These ETEC strains elaborate enterotoxins, including a heat-labile enterotoxin (LT) that shares properties with cholera enterotoxin. In many developing countries, ETEC is the second most common cause (after rotavirus) of diarrheal dehydration in infants of a severity that requires rehydration at treatment centers.[42] ETEC is also the most common cause of travelers' diarrhea when adults from industrialized countries visit less-developed countries.

ETEC carry one or two ~60-mD plasmids that encode LT or heat-stable (ST) enterotoxins or both.[43] These plasmids usually also encode one or more fimbrial colonization factor antigens (CFAs) or genes encoding regulatory proteins necessary for the high-level expression of CFAs encoded by chromosomal genes.[43] LT closely resembles cholera enterotoxin (CT) in primary sequence, tertiary structure, antigenicity and mode of activity (ADP ribosylation). ST, which consists of peptides 18-19 amino acids in length, has a distinct mechanism of action (it activates guanylate cyclase, which results in an intracellular accumulation of GMP that leads to secretion) and is not immunogenic. Some ETEC strains capable of causing diarrhea express only LT or ST, whereas others elaborate both toxins.[44]

EIEC

Also in the late 1960s, another category of *E. coli* pathogen was identified that in many ways resembles *Shigella*, particularly in its ability to invade epithelial cells and in its capacity to cause dysenteric illness.[45] EIEC closely resembles *Shigella* in its pathogenesis, which involves both an early step of enterotoxin production leading to intestinal secretion and invasion of intestinal epithelium.[43] EIEC possesses virtually the identical 140-mD virulence plasmid as *S. flexneri*, which encodes an enterotoxin called *Shigella* enterotoxin 2 in *Shigella* and Enteroinvasive *E. coli* Toxin in EIEC.[46] Invasion plasmid antigens (IPAs) mediate the uptake of EIEC into enterocytes, which is followed by a process of intracellular and intercellular spread of EIEC, ultimately leading to death of the enterocyte. EIEC infection, like *Shigella*, is characterized by an influx of polymorphonuclear leukocytes into the lamina propria of affected intestinal mucosa.

EHEC

A multi-state outbreak of hemorrhagic colitis in the USA in the early 1980s caused by organisms of serotype O157:H7 led to the discovery of another distinct category of diarrheagenic *E. coli*[47,48] Milder forms of EHEC infection result in nonspecific diarrhea, while more severe forms can manifest as hemorrhagic colitis or HUS.[48] EHEC constitutes an emerging cause of diarrheal illness, hemorrhagic colitis and HUS (the most severe complication of EHEC infection) in industrialized countries (USA, Canada, UK, Japan, Germany, Italy, Australia). EHEC infections are mainly transmitted through the ingestion of contaminated (mainly ground) beef, other contaminated food and beverages (often cross-contaminated from beef), or through person-to-person contact (as in day-care centers and institutions for the elderly). EHEC carries a ~60-mD plasmid that appears to be involved in the expression of novel fimbriae.[43,49] Phages carried by EHEC encode powerful cytotoxins, Shiga toxin 1 or 2.[50] Finally, almost all EHEC harbor a Locus of Enterocyte Effacement (LEE) chromosomal pathogenicity island,[37] similar to that carried by EPEC and, like EPEC, they express a 94-kD protein that resembles intimin of EPEC (and shares considerable homology in the N-terminal region).[51] EHEC can cause attaching and effacing lesions of intestinal epithelial cells similar to those caused by EPEC.

EAggEC

In the 1980s it was found that *E. coli* strains that exhibit a unique pattern of adherence to HEp-2 cells in tissue culture, so-called aggregative adherence, were associated with diarrheal disease in infants in developing countries,[52,53] particularly the syndrome of persistent diarrhea.[54] Recent reports from Germany and the United Kingdom suggest that EAggEC diarrhea may also be common in some industrialized countries.[55] EAggEC is also being increasingly appreciated as a cause of travelers' diarrhea.[56]

EAggEC harbors a ~60-mD plasmid that encodes fimbrial attachment factors that mediate the pathognomonic aggregative adherence to HEp-2 cells.[57] EAggEC also expresses several enterotoxins that appear to contribute to pathogenesis of clinical illness, including two plasmid encoded toxins: the ~104-kD-plasmid-encoded enterotoxin (Pet) that exhibits a serine protease motif and acts as a autotransporter cytotoxin[58-61] and EAggEC heat-stable enterotoxin (EAST).[62,63] Whereas EAST was initially identified in association with EAggEC, more recent studies have also found this toxin in a proportion of ETEC, EPEC and EHEC strains.

DAEC

In some epidemiologic studies, *E. coli* strains that manifest a diffuse pattern of adherence to HEp-2 cells in tissue culture have also been associated with nonbloody diarrheal illness in young children in developing countries.[32,64,65] The geographic distribution of DAEC diarrhea is the least well mapped, with the most incriminating studies coming from Latin America (Mexico and Chile).[32,64] In some epidemiologic studies in developing countries, DAEC was more common in the preschool age group (3-5 years of age),[32] in contrast with EPEC, ETEC and EaggEC, which manifest the highest incidence in the first year of life.[32]

The pathogenesis of DAEC is the least understood of the different categories of diarrheagenic *E. coli*. The characteristic diffuse adherence to epithelial cells is mediated by fimbriae or afimbrial adhesins. Heretofore, no toxins specific for this category have been identified.

Vaccine Development Strategies and Experience with Vaccine Candidates

Vaccines Against UPEC

A variety of approaches might be used to create an effective UPEC vaccine. Among these strategies, two have produced some success in preclinical testing: a killed whole-organism vaccine administered intravaginally and a parenteral subunit vaccine composed of the type 1 fimbrial adhesin in complex with its chaperone.

Mucosal Whole-Cell Vaccine

A whole-cell vaccine composed of a mixture of heat-killed bacteria representing ten bacterial uropathogens (including six UPEC strains) has been formulated for vaginal administration. After testing in nonhuman primates, this vaccine has been administered in a Phase 1 and two Phase 2 trials to women suffering from recurrent UTI. The most recent trial consisted of a series of six vaginal suppository installations over a 14-week period.[66] The vaccine was well tolerated but only minimally efficacious, with a modest but statistically significant lengthening of the interval to first recurrence in the recipients of the vaccine compared to recipients of placebo. There was no significant difference between the recipients of vaccine and placebo in urine or vaginal levels of antibodies against *E. coli*.

Parenteral Fimbrial Tip Adhesin/Chaperone Protein Vaccine

The tip adhesin of type-1 fimbriae (FimH), which has been shown to be essential for the pathogenesis of UTI, has been used as an immunogen and tested in animals and humans. FimH is highly conserved among UPEC strains. It is thought that natural infection results in a poor antibody response to the adhesin because, in comparison to the protein that makes up the shaft of the pilus, FimH is present in small quantities. The adhesin is purified in complex with its chaperone and administered parenterally. Antibodies raised against this preparation block binding of a variety of UPEC strains to bladder cells *in vitro* and in mice administration of the vaccine resulted in a 100-fold reduction in bladder colonization.[67] The vaccine has also been tested in a small number of monkeys. Bacteriuria and pyuria developed after challenge in all four monkeys that received placebo and in one of four that received vaccine. Protection was correlated with vaginal IgG levels against the antigen.[68] These highly promising results have prompted the initiation of clinical trials[69] A Phase 1 clinical study has been completed, and the vaccine was well tolerated and immunogenic. Despite concerns, there was apparently no detectable effect of the vaccine on the normal bowel flora, however the results of this trial have not yet been published. Phase 2 studies are underway.

Vaccines Against Meningitis Caused by K1-Expressing E. coli

A variety of vaccine candidates have been prepared consisting either of the K1 or group B meningococcal Ps conjugated to an array of carrier proteins in attempts to make this polysaccharide immunogenic in rodent and primate animal models.[70-73] Despite promising preclinical results observed with some of these conjugates, there has not been a smooth progression to clinical trials because of the safety concerns outlined above.

Vaccines Against E. coli *Sepsis*

Phase 1 and 2 clinical trials have been carried out with multivalent vaccines consisting of *E. coli* O Ps conjugated to *P. aeruginosa* exotoxin A as the carrier protein.[31,74-76] These conjugates were well tolerated in clinical trials and moderately immunogenic. The O1, O2, O6-O8, and O15 conjugates elicited the strongest and the O4, O12, O16 and O25 conjugates evoked the weakest responses; O18 and O75 conjugates were intermediate in immunogenicity. ELISA antibody responses correlated with biological activity of the antibody including opsonophagocytic capacity and the ability of passively transferred antibody to protect mice against challenge.

Cross[31] has reviewed the generally disappointing results of passive protection immunotherapy clinical studies based on the administration of monoclonal antibodies to lipid A,[77,78] or of human antiserum from volunteers immunized with an *E. coli* J5 whole-cell vaccine.[79] Cross argues for active immunization of targeted persons in high-risk occupations (soldiers, firemen and policemen) who could benefit from having their immune status enhanced by supplemental administration of passive antibody at the time of trauma and risk of development of sepsis.

Vaccines Against ETEC Diarrhea

Target populations for ETEC vaccines include young infants in endemic areas and travelers who visit less-developed countries. Two critical virulence attributes dominate the pathogenesis of ETEC diarrhea: i) attachment of ETEC to the proximal small intestinal mucosa by means of fimbrial colonization factors, and; ii) the elaboration of LT or ST, leading to intestinal secretion.[43,80] ETEC strains are antigenically heterogeneous, exhibiting many different O:H serotypes, multiple antigenic types of fimbrial colonization factors, and three different toxin phenotypes (LT-only, ST-only or LT-ST).[43,44,80] To confer broad-spectrum protection, vaccines will have to immunize against this diverse assortment of ETEC pathogens. There is optimism that such broad protection will be achievable, because epidemiologic evidence and results of experimental challenge studies in volunteers convincingly show that strain-specific immunity follows ETEC infection.[81-83] Moreover, the cumulative immunologic stimulation from multiple infections with antigenically diverse ETEC strains results in broad-spectrum protection against ETEC diarrhea.[82,83] In developing countries, infants and young children often suffer 2-3 clinical ETEC diarrheal episodes yearly during the first three years of life; thereafter the incidence of ETEC diarrhea falls drastically.[84-86] The lower incidence observed in adults living in endemic areas is the result of acquired immunity rather than of other age-related host factors, since adults from industrialized countries who visit regions where pediatric ETEC diarrhea is endemic suffer high attack rates of ETEC travelers' diarrhea.[83,87] Similarly, travelers from industrialized countries who remain in less-developed countries for at least a year (and who therefore typically suffer multiple episodes of ETEC diarrhea) thereafter manifest significantly lower incidence rates of ETEC diarrhea than newly arrived travelers.[83]

Protective immunity to ETEC appears to be mediated by secretory IgA (sIgA) antibodies directed against fimbriae and LT; ST, a small peptide, does not elicit neutralizing antibodies following natural infection. A few prospective epidemiologic field studies suggest that acquired immunity is largely directed against ETEC fimbrial colonization factors.[88]

To provide broad-spectrum protection, a vaccine must contain fimbrial antigens expressed by the most prevalent ETEC pathogens.[89] The most common fimbrial colonization factor antigens (CFAs) of human ETEC are CFA/I and the fimbriae found within the CFA/II and CFA/IV families of antigens.[44,89] CFA/I is a single antigenic moiety, whereas coli surface antigens 1 (CS1), CS2 and CS3 constitute the CFA/II family of antigens.[43,89] All CFA/II strains express CS3, either alone or in conjunction with CS1 or CS2. CS4, CS5 and CS6 comprise the CFA/IV family of antigens and all CFA/IV strains express CS6, either alone or in conjunction with CS4 or CS5.[43,89] CS7, CS12, CS14, and CS17 are much less frequent. The expression of CFAs by ETEC closely correlates with the O:H serotype and toxin phenotype.[43,44,89,90]

CFA/I and CS1-6 have been found on the majority of ETEC isolates in various studies carried out worldwide.[43,44,89,90] Approximately 80-90% of isolates that elaborate both LT and ST express these CFAs, whereas they are found on ~50-60% of ST-only strains.[89,90] Generally, only a small proportion of LT-only strains bear these CFAs.[32,91] Thus, if a multivalent ETEC vaccine contained CFA/I and CS1-6, it could theoretically protect against the majority of ETEC strains in most geographic areas.[89] If an LT immunogen of some sort were included, even broader protection could derive. Finally, some of the less frequent fimbrial antigens (e.g., CS7 and CS17) may be incorporated into multivalent vaccines to further expand the coverage.

Killed Whole-Cell/Cholera Toxin B Subunit Combination Vaccine

The vaccine that is furthest along in development is one that consists of inactivated ETEC administered in combination with the B subunit BS of cholera toxin (CTB). The earliest inactivated whole-cell ETEC vaccine was developed by Evans et al who utilized ETEC inactivated with colicin E1, which did not damage the fimbrial protein antigens.[92] Oral immunization with such colicin E1-inactivated ETEC induced intestinal IgA antibody response against the homologous CFA (and against LT) and protected volunteers against experimental challenge with wild-type ETEC. However, further development of the colicin-inactivated vaccine was not pursued.

In the late 1980s a prototype oral ETEC vaccine was developed consisting of CTB in combination with formalin-killed ETEC strains expressing the most important CFAs. CTB was included because this antigen (as an oral killed whole-cell/CTB combination vaccine) had conferred significant protection for several months against LT-producing ETEC both among subjects in an endemic area and among vaccinated travelers.[93,94]

The initial prototype vaccine was subsequently replaced by an oral ETEC vaccine containing recombinant CTB (rCTB) in combination with five different formalin-inactivated *E. coli* strains expressing CFA/I and CS1-CS6.[95-99] Inactivation by formalin-treatment killed the ETEC without major loss in antigenicity of the different CFAs. Phase 1 and 2 trials of this ETEC-rCTB vaccine in Swedish, Bangladeshi, American and Egyptian volunteers showed that the vaccine was well tolerated and stimulated intestinal immune responses against the different CFAs of the vaccine in most subjects.[96,98-101] Safety/immunogenicity clinical trials were carried out with this inactivated ETEC vaccine in Egyptian preschool children, and the vaccine was shown to be well tolerated and immunogenic.[97,98,100] Two doses of vaccine or placebo (inactivated *E. coli* K-12) were administered 2 weeks apart to 97 children age 2-5 years. There was no significant difference in the occurrence of adverse responses in vaccinees versus controls. An antibody-secreting-cell response against CFA/I was recorded in 95% and against CS2 in 83% of these preschool age children.

Studies on the protective efficacy of the ETEC-rCTB vaccine are underway in European and American travelers, and a field trial of the efficacy of this vaccine is underway in Egypt in children 6-18 months of age.

Attenuated *E. coli* as Live Oral Vaccines Against ETEC

The feasibility of utilizing live bacteria expressing ETEC fimbriae as oral vaccines was demonstrated in clinical trials with prototype *E. coli* strain E1392-75-2A that expresses CS1 and CS3 fimbriae but lacks genes that encode LT and ST.[43,89,102] *E. coli* E1392-75-2A is a CFA/II-positive mutant that was derived in the Central Public Health Laboratory, Colindale, London wherein the genes encoding LT and ST spontaneously deleted from the CFA/II plasmid. Consequently, E1392-75-2A (which expresses CS1 and CS3 fimbrial antigens) is negative when tested with toxin assays and gene probes for LT and ST. Levine et al[43,89,102] utilized strain E1392-75-2A to explore fundamental questions of anti-colonization immunity in the absence of antitoxic immunity. All volunteers who were fed 10^{10} CFU doses of strain

E1392-75-2A developed significant rises in intestinal fluid SIgA antibody to CS1 and CS3 fimbriae. The geometric mean titer (GMT) of anti-fimbrial CS1 and CS3 SIgA antibody in these volunteers was 10-fold higher than the peak post-vaccination GMT of volunteers who received enteral immunization with multiple doses of purified CS1 and CS3 fimbriae.[103]

Vaccinees were challenged one month after immunization with a single 5×10^{10} CFU dose of E1392-75-2A or control with buffer. The pathogenic ETEC challenge strain used, E24377A, was of heterologous serotype O139:H28 but expressed CS1 and CS3 and elaborated LT and ST. The vaccinees were significantly protected ($p<0.005$, 75% vaccine efficacy) against ETEC diarrhea.[43] By means of bacteriological studies it was shown that anti-colonization immunity was responsible for the protection. In the challenge study, all participants, both vaccinees and un-immunized controls, excreted the ETEC challenge strain and there was no difference between the groups in the mean number of ETEC per gram of stool. In contrast, a striking difference was found in duodenal cultures that monitored colonization of the proximal small intestine, the critical site of ETEC-host interaction. The challenge strain was recovered from duodenal cultures of 5 of 6 controls (mean 7×10^3 CFU/mL) versus only 1 of 12 vaccinees (10^1 CFU/mL) ($p<0.004$). Levine et al interpreted these results to mean that sIgA anti-CS1 and anti-CS3 fimbrial antibody in the proximal intestine stimulated by live oral vaccine prevented challenge ETEC from colonizing the proximal small intestine. Since the immune response was not bactericidal, the ETEC organisms were carried by peristalsis to the large intestine where they could colonize without causing diarrheal illness.

Thus, one strategy to develop an ETEC vaccine involves assembling a collection of attenuated *E. coli* strains expressing the major fimbrial CFs and an LT antigen such as B subunit or mutant LT. Whereas strain E1392-75-2A provided invaluable information when used as a prototype live oral vaccine, it caused mild diarrhea in ~15% of the subjects who ingested it, an unacceptable rate of adverse reactions. Therefore, research is ongoing to prepare a live oral ETEC vaccine that will be acceptably immunogenic and efficacious without causing mild diarrhea or other adverse reactions. One approach being taken by British investigators is to introduce specific attenuating mutations into E1392-75-2A in an attempt to make it less reactogenic yet retain its immunogenicity.[104] Once an acceptable set of attenuating mutations is identified for E1392-75-2A, these mutations would be introduced into strains expressing other CFAs.

Attenuated *Salmonella* or *Shigella* Live Vectors Expressing ETEC Antigens

Attenuated *Shigella* and *Salmonella* can be used as live vector vaccines to express ETEC fimbrial antigens and LT antigens and deliver them to the immune system.[105-108]

Several investigators have constructed mutant LT molecules that have greatly diminished enterotoxic activity (they exhibit only minimal residual ADP-ribosyltransferase activity) yet in animal models elicit strong anti-LT responses and even serve as potent mucosal adjuvants for bystander antigens.[109,110] Two of the most promising mutant LTs, K63 and R72, were constructed by Rappuoli and coworkers from the wild-type LT of a porcine ETEC strain by substituting amino acids that contribute to the NAD binding site within the A subunit of LT.[111] The amino acid sequence of the LT found in human ETEC isolates (LTh) varies from the porcine LT (LTp) by only three amino acids in the A subunit and four in the B subunit.[112] Nevertheless, LTh and LTp each exhibits distinct epitopes and functions differently as an immunogen and as an antigen (in binding LT antibodies).[113,114] To develop a vaccine immunogen more appropriate for humans, Koprowski et al[106] constructed two nontoxic LTh derivatives with the mutations K63 or R72 and demonstrated expression of these mutant LTs by *E. coli* and attenuated *Shigella* live vectors.

The utility of attenuated *Shigella* as live vectors to coexpress CFA/I and CS3 fimbriae of ETEC and elicit SIgA mucosal antibody responses to those antigens has been clearly shown in a guinea pig model, clearing the way for proof-of-principle clinical trials[106,107,115] A multivalent live oral vaccine against both *Shigella* and ETEC is being developed based on the hypothesis that protection can be achieved if attenuated *Shigella* express ETEC fimbrial colonization factors and genetically detoxified LT from a human ETEC pathogen (LTh). In its final form, the multivalent *Shigella*/ETEC vaccine will contain five attenuated *Shigella* serotype strains (*S. dysenteriae* 1, *S. flexneri* 2a, *S. flexneri* 3a, and *S. sonnei*), each expressing two different ETEC CFAs and mutant LT.[106,116,117]. Notably, expression of the ETEC fimbriae and mutant LT does not diminish the capacity of the vector strain to protect against challenge with *Shigella* in a guinea pig model.[106]

Other ETEC Vaccines

Several other candidate ETEC vaccines have been tested in Phase 1 trials but were abandoned from further development because of modest immunogenicity or other drawbacks. These include purified CFA/II fimbriae administered orally,[103] CFA/II fimbriae in polylactide/polyglycolide microspheres,[118] and an LT/ST toxoid.[119]

Vaccines Against EPEC Diarrhea

It is during the first 12 months of life, and in the first six months in particular, that EPEC poses a notable disease risk.[32,33] Studies of molecular pathogenesis have identified several antigens that constitute potential immunogens. It is hypothesized that the stimulation of intestinal immune responses against these antigens could elicit protective immunity against EPEC disease. The antigens of interest include: 1) the bundle-forming pili (BFP) encoded by the EAF plasmid;[35] 2) intimin, the 94-kD protein encoded by *eae*, a chromosomal gene;[36,120] 3) the products of *espA* and *espB* (previously referred to as *eaeB*).[121-123] Each of these products has been demonstrated to be essential for virulence in experimental human or animal infections.[124-126]

SIgA intestinal antibody to BFP may interfere with bacterial binding or initial attachment of EPEC, whereas anti-intimin should prevent intimate attachment.[127] Finally, sIgA antibod ies against the gene product of *espB* may prevent signal transduction that ultimately culminates in secretion.[122] It is quite possible that these antibodies could work synergistically to enhance the protection that would be achieved by immunity to any single one of the antigens. Nevertheless, although EPEC vaccines are technically achievable, the epidemiologic need to immunize neonates or very young infants, in order to protect during the period of high risk, has impeded vaccine development efforts.

Vaccines Against EHEC

The public-health importance of HUS as a complication of EHEC diarrheal illness in human populations has led various authorities to consider immunologic means to prevent infection, disease or complications of disease. Immunization with antigens such as intimin (or its carboxyl terminus) that promote colonization would aim at preventing infection, whereas immunization with Shiga toxin B subunit, Stx toxoids or peptides representing toxin-neutralizing epitopes would be designed to prevent the pathologic effects of toxin-mediated clinically severe forms of disease.

Conjugate Vaccines

Parenteral conjugate vaccines consisting of a capsular Ps or O Ps of LPS covalently linked to a carrier protein have shown efficacy in the prevention of shigellosis and typhoid fever.[128,129] There is little pathogenetic or animal model basis for expecting anti-O antibodies to be protective against O157:H7.[130,131] Nevertheless, the excellent clinical results observed with typhoid Vi and *Shigella* O conjugate vaccines prompted investigators from the National Institute of Child Health and Human Development to explore the use of Ps conjugate vaccines to prevent HUS and other severe forms of EHEC disease.[132-134] Their early conjugates that utilized recombinant *P. aeruginosa* exotoxin were well tolerated by volunteers in a Phase 1 study, 81% of whom mounted significant rises in anti-O157 antibody.[134] Subsequent constructs that link the

O157 Ps to B subunit of Shiga toxin 1 and 2 would appear to be more promising, since such conjugates may induce neutralizing antitoxin that by itself may protect against severe forms of disease such as hemorrhagic colitis and hemolytic uremic syndrome.

Live Vector Vaccines

A popular approach in modern vaccine development is the use of attenuated strains of bacteria or viruses as carriers or live vectors in which to express foreign protective antigens and deliver them to the immune system. Attenuated *Vibrio cholerae* live vectors have been used to express B subunit of Stx 1 and demonstrate the capacity of various constructs to elicit neutralizing antitoxin in rabbits following oral immunization.[135,136] Calderwood and Butterton[136] also relate the expression of the *eae* gene product in *V. cholerae* from *eae* carried on a plasmid or integrated into the *V. cholerae* chromosome. Attenuated *Salmonella* has also been employed by other investigators to express Shiga toxin antigens.[137,138]

Toxoid Vaccines

Keusch et al[139] propose the use of a bivalent toxoid vaccine containing Stx1 and 2 antigens to stimulate neutralizing antitoxin. It is hypothesized that the elicitation of antitoxin would prevent the severe consequences of EHEC infection such as HUS and hemorrhagic colitis.

Passive Prophylaxis with Hyperimmune Globulin or Monoclonal Antibodies to Prevent Severe EHEC Disease

Another point at which to intervene against EHEC disease is to utilize specific antibodies or immune globulin in patients with uncomplicated EHEC illness with the aim of preventing further progression to life-threatening complications such as HUS and TTP. Such products might also be administered to individuals at high risk, e.g., as yet unaffected individuals who were involved in outbreaks or close contacts of HUS cases in day-care or nursing-home situations. The antibodies of greatest interest for passive administration are those that can neutralize Stx1 and 2. The practical success of this approach will require improved rapid diagnosis to identify EHEC infections sufficiently early to allow prompt administration of the antibodies before the onset of complications.

Immunoprophylaxis Viewed from the Public-Health Perspective

From the perspective of an epidemiologist charged with protecting the public health, Tauxe[140] points out that even if EHEC vaccines prove to be well tolerated and efficacious, there would be important obstacles to their licensure and implementation. In those parts of North America where the incidence of HUS is relatively high, e.g., the Pacific Northwest, the disease burden is distributed throughout childhood and adult ages, even though the incidence peaks in young children. This indicates that immunization would have to be universal to achieve control. If the US population were to be immunized against EHEC because of the "danger" posed by consumption of US ground beef and other foods, would it then be recommended that foreign travelers to the USA also be immunized? Could the USA continue to export beef to other countries if it deemed it prudent to protect its own population by immunization? What effect would this have on the US agricultural economy? Clearly, there are complexities to the economic and public policy issues that would be generated by the proposal to immunize human populations against EHEC disease.

Vaccines to Prevent EAggEC, EIEC and DAEC Diarrhea

There are no active programs to develop vaccines against EIEC or DAEC diarrheal disease. Some vaccines under development to prevent *Shigella* may provide a measure of protection against EIEC either by stimulating antibody to invasion plasmid antigens (IPAs) and *virG* (which are expressed by EIEC as well as *Shigella*) or by eliciting *Shigella* O antibodies that crossreact with EIEC O antigens.

Although there are no programs to develop EAggEC vaccines, there are several attractive antigens that could serve as the basis of rationale vaccine development strategies. These include the EAggEC fimbrial antigens such as AAFI and AAFII that mediate attachment and the pet enterotoxin.[57,58,62,141]

References

1. Simon GL, Gorbach SL. Intestinal flora in health and disease. Gastroenterol 1984; 86:174-93.
2. Drasar BS, Hill MJ. Human intestinal flora. London: Academic Press, 1974.
3. Foxman B, Barlow R, D'Arcy H et al. Urinary tract infection: self-reported incidence and associated costs. Ann Epidemiol 2000; 10:509-15.
4. Ikaheimo R, Siitonen A, Heiskanen T et al. Recurrence of urinary tract infection in a primary care setting: analysis of a 1-year follow-up of 179 women. Clin Infect Dis 1996; 22:91-9.
5. Warren JW. Clinical presentations and epidemiology of urinary tract infections. In: Mobley HL, Warren JW, eds. Urinary tract infections: molecular pathogenesis and clinical management. Washington, D.C.: ASM Press, 1996:3-27.
6. Bran JL, Levison ME, Kaye D. Entrance of bacteria into the female urinary bladder. N Engl J Med 1972; 286:626-9.
7. Kunin CM, McCormack RC. An epidemiologic study of bacteriuria and blood pressure among nuns and working women. N Engl J Med 1968; 278:635-42.
8. Hooton TM, Scholes D, Hughes JP et al. A prospective study of risk factors for symptomatic urinary tract infection in young women. N Engl J Med 1996; 335:468-74.
9. Hooton TM, Hillier S, Johnson C et al. Escherichia coli bacteriuria and contraceptive method. JAMA 1991; 265:64-9.
10. Stamey TA, Timothy M, Millar M et al. Recurrent urinary infections in adult women. The role of introital enterobacteria. Calif Med 1971; 115(1):1-19.
11. Stamey TA, Sexton CC. The role of vaginal colonization with enterobacteriaceae in recurrent urinary infections. J Urol 1975, 113:214-7.
12. Bailey RR, Gower PE, Roberts AP et al. Urinary-tract infection in nonpregnant women. Lancet 1973; 2:275-7.
13. Kraft JK, Stamey TA. The natural history of symptomatic recurrent bacteriuria in women. Medicine (Baltimore) 1977; 56:55-60.
14. Bollgren I, Winberg J. The periurethral aerobic flora in girls highly susceptible to urinary infections. Acta Paediatr Scand 1976; 65:81-7.
15. Svanborg-Eden C, Jodal U. Attachment of Escherichia coli to urinary sediment epithelial cells from urinary tract infection-prone and healthy children. Infect Immun 1979; 26:837-40.
16. Eden CS, Hanson LA, Jodal U et al. Variable adherence to normal human urinary-tract epithelial cells of Escherichia coli strains associated with various forms of urinary-tract infection. Lancet 1976; 1:490-2.
17. Manges AR, Johnson JR, Foxman B et al. Widespread distribution of urinary tract infections caused by a multidrug-resistant Escherichia coli clonal group. N Engl J Med 2001; 345:1007-13.
18. Phillips I, Eykyn S, King A et al. Epidemic multiresistant Escherichia coli infection in West Lambeth Health District. Lancet 1988; 1:1038-41.
19. Donnenberg MS, Welch RA. Virulence determinants of uropathogenic Escherichia coli. In: Mobley HL, Warren JW, eds. Urinary tract infectons: molecular pathogenesis and clinical management. Washington, D.C.: ASM Press; 1996:135-74.
20. Connell H, Poulsen LK, Klemm P. Expression of type 1 and P fimbriae in situ and localisation of a uropathogenic Escherichia coli strain in the murine bladder and kidney. Int J Med Microbiol 2000; 290:587-97.
21. Roberts JA, Marklund BI, Ilver D et al. The Gal(alpha 1-4)Gal-specific tip adhesin of Escherichia coli P-fimbriae is needed for pyelonephritis to occur in the normal urinary tract. Proc Natl Acad Sci USA 1994; 91:11889-93.
22. O'Hanley P, Lalonde G, Ji G. Alpha-Hemolysin contributes to the pathogenicity of piliated digalactoside-binding Escherichia coli in the kidney - efficacy of an alpha-hemolysin vaccine in preventing renal injury in the BALB/c mouse model of pyelonephritis. Infect Immun 1991; 59:1153-61.

23. Torres AG, Redford P, Welch RA et al. TonB-dependent systems of uropathogenic Escherichia coli: aerobactin and heme transport and TonB are required for virulence in the mouse. Infect Immun 2001; 69:6179-85.
24. Culham DE, Dalgado C, Gyles CL et al. Osmoregulatory transporter ProP influences colonization of the urinary tract by Escherichia coli. Microbiology 1998; 144(Pt 1):91-102.
25. Russo TA, Jodush ST, Brown JJ et al. Identification of two previously unrecognized genes (guaA and argC) important for uropathogenesis. Mol Microbiol 1996; 22:217-29.
26. Kasper DL, Winkelhake JL, Zollinger WD et al. Immunochemical similarity between polysaccharide antigens of Escherichia coli 07: K1(L):NM and group B Neisseria meningitidis. J Immunol 1973; 110:262-8.
27. Hurpin CM, Carosella ED, Cazenave PA. Bactericidal activity of two IgG2a murine monoclonal antibodies with distinct fine specificities for group B Neisseria meningitidis capsular polysaccharide. Hybridoma 1992; 11:677-87.
28. Kabat EA, Liao J, Osserman EF et al. The epitope associated with the binding of the capsular polysaccharide of the group B meningococcus and of Escherichia coli K1 to a human monoclonal macroglobulin, IgMNOV. J Exp Med 1988; 168:699-711.
29. Devi SJ, Schneerson R, Egan W et al. Identity between polysaccharide antigens of Moraxella nonliquefaciens, group B Neisseria meningitidis, and Escherichia coli K1 (nonO acetylated). Infect Immun 1991; 59:732-6.
30. Finne J, Leinonen M, Makela PH. Antigenic similarities between brain components and bacteria causing meningitis. Implications for vaccine development and pathogenesis. Lancet 1983; 2:355-7.
31. Cross AS, Opal SM, Bhattacharjee AK et al. Immunotherapy of sepsis: flawed concept or faulty implementation? Vaccine 1999; 17(Suppl 2):S13-S21.
32. Levine MM, Ferreccio C, Prado V et al. Epidemiologic studies of Escherichia coli infections in a low socioeconomic level periurban community in Santiago, Chile. Am J Epidemiol 1993; 138:849-69.
33. Levine MM, Edelman R. Enteropathogenic Escherichia coli of classic serotypes associated with infant diarrhea: epidemiology and pathogenesis. Epidemiol Rev 1984; 6:31-51.
34. Gomes TAT, Vieira MAM, Wachsmuth IK et al. Serotype-specific prevalence of Escherichia coli strains with EPEC adherence factor genes in infants with and withour diarrhea in Sao Paulo, Brazil. J Infect Dis 1989; 160:131-5.
35. Giron JA, Ho ASY, Schoolnik GK. An inducible bundle-forming pilus of enteropathogenic Escherichia coli. Science 1991; 254:710-3.
36. Jerse AE, Kaper JB. The eae gene of enteropathogenic Escherichia coli encodes a 94 kDa membrane protein, the expression of which is influenced by the EAF plasmid. Infect Immun 1991; 59:4302-9.
37. McDaniel TK, Jarvis KG, Donnenberg MS et al. A genetic locus of enterocyte effacement conserved among diverse enterobacterial pathogens. Proc Natl Acad Sci USA 1995; 92:1664-8.
38. Knutton S, Rosenshine I, Pallen MJ et al. A novel EspA-associated surface organelle of enteropathogenic Escherichia coli involved in protein translocation into epithelial cells. EMBO J 1998; 17:2166-76.
39. Kenny B, DeVinney R, Stein M et al. Enteropathogenic E. coli (EPEC) transfers its receptor for intimate adherence into mammalian cells. Cell 1997; 91:511-20.
40. Moon HW, Whipp SC, Argenzio RA et al. Attaching and effacing activities of rabbit and human enteropathogenic Escherichia coli in pig and rabbit intestines. Infect Immun 1983; 41:1340-51.
41. Sack RB, Gorbach SL, Banwell JG et al. Enterotoxigenic Escherichia coli isolated from patients with severe cholera-like disease. J Infect Dis 1971; 123:378-85.
42. Black RE, Merson MH, Huq I et al. Incidence and severity of rotavirus and Escherichia coli diarrhoea in rural Bangladesh. Lancet 1981; I:141-3.
43. Levine MM. Escherichia coli that cause diarrhea: enterotoxigenic, enteropathogenic, enteroinvasive, enterohemorrhagic, and enteroadherent. J Infect Dis 1987; 155:377-89.
44. Wolf MK. Occurrence, distribution, and associations of O and H serogroups, colonization factor antigens, and toxins of enterotoxigenic Escherichia coli. Clin Microbiol Rev 1997; 10:569-84.
45. DuPont HL, Formal SB, Hornick RB et al. Pathogenesis of Escherichia coli diarrhea. N Engl J Med 1971; 285:1-9.
46. Nataro JP, Seriwatana J, Fasano A et al. Identification and cloning of a novel plasmid-encoded enterotoxin of enteroinvasive Escherichia coli and Shigella strains. Infect Immun 1995; 63:4721-8.

47. Riley LW, Remis RS, Helgerson SD et al. Hemorrhagic colitis associated with a rare Escherichia coli serotype. N Engl J Med 1983; 308:681-5.
48. Griffin PM, Tauxe RV. The epidemiology of infections caused by Escherichia coli O157:H7, other enterohemorrhagic E. coli, and the associated hemolytic uremic syndrome. Epidemiol Rev 1991; 13:60-98.
49. Karch H, Heesemann J, Laufs R et al. A plasmid of Enterohemorrhagic Escherichia coli O157:H7 is required for expression of a new fimbrial antigen and for adhesion to epithelial cells. Infect Immun 1987; 55:455-61.
50. O'Brien AD, Newland JW, Miller SF et al. Shiga-like toxin-converting phages from Escherichia coli strains that cause hemorrhagic colitis or infantile diarrhea. Science 1984; 226:694-6.
51. Yu J, Kaper JB. Cloning and characterization of the eae gene of enterohaemorrhagic Escherichia coli O157:H7. Molec Microbiol 1992; 6:411-17.
52. Nataro JP, Kaper JB, Robins Browne R et al. Patterns of adherence of diarrheagenic Escherichia coli to HEp-2 cells. Pediatr Infect Dis J 1987; 6:829-31.
53. Vial PA, Robins Browne R, Lior H et al. Characterization of enteroadherent-aggregative Escherichia coli, a putative agent of diarrheal disease. J Infect Dis 1988; 158:70-9.
54. Bhan MK, Raj P, Levine MM et al. Enteroaggregative Escherichia coli associated with persistent diarrhea in a cohort of rural children in India. J Infect Dis 1989; 159:1061-4.
55. Huppertz HI, Rutkowski S, Aleksic S et al. Acute and chronic diarrhoea and abdominal colic associated with enteroaggregative Escherichia coli in young children living in western Europe. Lancet 1997; 349:1660-2.
56. Adachi JA, Jiang ZD, Mathewson JJ et al. Enteroaggregative Escherichia coli as a Major Etiologic Agent in Traveler's Diarrhea in 3 Regions of the World. Clin Infect Dis 2001; 32:1706-9.
57. Nataro JP, Deng Y, Maneval DR et al. Aggregative adherence fimbriae I of enteroaggregative Escherichia coli mediate adherence to HEp-2 cells and hemagglutination of human erythrocytes. Infect Immun 1992; 60:2297-304.
58. Eslava C, Navarro-Garcia F, Czeczulin JR et al. Pet, an autotransporter enterotoxin from enteroaggregative Escherichia coli. Infect Immun 1998; 66:3155-63.
59. Villaseca JM, Navarro-Garcia F, Mendoza-Hernandez G et al. Pet toxin from enteroaggregative Escherichia coli produces cellular damage associated with fodrin disruption. Infect Immun 2000; 68:5920-7.
60. Navarro-Garcia F, Sears C, Eslava C et al. Cytoskeletal effects induced by pet, the serine protease enterotoxin of enteroaggregative Escherichia coli. Infect Immun 1999, 67:2184-92.
61. Navarro-Garcia F, Canizalez-Roman A, Luna J et al. Plasmid-encoded toxin of enteroaggregative Escherichia coli is internalized by epithelial cells. Infect Immun 2001; 69:1053 60.
62. Navarro-Garcia F, Eslava C, Villaseca JM et al. In vitro effects of a high-molecular-weight heat-labile enterotoxin from enteroaggregative Escherichia coli. Infect Immun 1998; 66:3149-54.
63. Savarino SJ, Fasano A, Robertson DC et al. Enteroaggregative Escherichia coli elaborate a heat-stable enterotoxin demonstrable in an in vitro rabbit intestinal model. J Clin Invest 1991; 87:1450-5.
64. Giron JA, Jones T, Millanvelasco F et al. Diffuse-Adhering Escherichia coli (DAEC) As a Putative Cause of Diarrhea in Mayan Children in Mexico. J Infect Dis 1991; 163:507-13.
65. Baqui AH, Sack RB, Black RE et al. Enteropathogens associated with acute and persistent diarrhea in Bangladeshi children <5 years of age. J Infect Dis 1992; 166:792-6.
66. Uehling DT, Hopkins WJ, Beierle LM et al. Vaginal mucosal immunization for recurrent urinary tract infection: extended phase II clinical trial. J Infect Dis 2001; 183(Suppl 1):S81-S83.
67. Langermann S, Palaszynski S, Barnhart M et al. Prevention of mucosal Escherichia coli infection by FimH-adhesin-based systemic vaccination. Science 1997; 276:607-11.
68. Langermann S, Mollby R, Burlein JE et al. Vaccination with FimH adhesin protects cynomolgus monkeys from colonization and infection by uropathogenic Escherichia coli. J Infect Dis 2000; 181:774-8.
69. Langermann S, Ballou WR Jr. Vaccination utilizing the FimCH complex as a strategy to prevent Escherichia coli urinary tract infections. J Infect Dis 2001; 183(Suppl 1):S84-S86.
70. Fusco PC, Michon F, Tai JY et al. Preclinical evaluation of a novel group B meningococcal conjugate vaccine that elicits bactericidal activity in both mice and nonhuman primates. J Infect Dis 1997; 175:364-72.
71. Devi SJ, Robbins JB, Schneerson R. Antibodies to poly[(2——8)-alpha-N-acetylneuraminic acid] and poly[(2——9)-alpha-N-acetylneuraminic acid] are elicited by immunization of mice with Es-

cherichia coli K92 conjugates: potential vaccines for groups B and C meningococci and E. coli K1. Proc Natl Acad Sci USA 1991; 88:7175-9.

72. Zollinger WD, Moran EE, Devi SJ et al. Bactericidal antibody responses of juvenile rhesus monkeys immunized with group B Neisseria meningitidis capsular polysaccharide-protein conjugate vaccines. Infect Immun 1997; 65:1053-60.
73. Pavliakova D, Moncrief JS, Lyerly DM et al. Clostridium difficile recombinant toxin A repeating units as a carrier protein for conjugate vaccines: studies of pneumococcal type 14, Escherichia coli K1, and Shigella flexneri type 2a polysaccharides in mice. Infect Immun 2000; 68:2161-6.
74. Cryz SJ Jr, Cross AS, Sadoff JC et al. Safety and immunogenicity of Escherichia coli O18 O-specific polysaccharide (O-PS)-toxin A and O-PS-cholera toxin conjugate vaccines in humans. J Infect Dis 1991; 163:1040-5.
75. Cross A, Artenstein A, Que J et al. Safety and immunogenicity of a polyvalent Escherichia coli vaccine in human volunteers. J Infect Dis 1994; 170:834-40.
76. Cryz SJ Jr, Que JO, Cross AS et al. Synthesis and characterization of a polyvalent Escherichia coli O-polysaccharide-toxin A conjugate vaccine. Vaccine 1995; 13:449-53.
77. Ziegler EJ, Fisher CJ Jr., Sprung CL et al. Treatment of gram negative bacteremia and septic shock with HA-1A human monoclonal antibody against endotoxin. A randomized, double-blind, placebo-controlled trial. The HA-1A Sepsis Study Group. N Engl J Med 1991; 324:429-36.
78. Greenman RL, Schein RM, Martin MA et al. A controlled clinical trial of E5 murine monoclonal IgM antibody to endotoxin in the treatment of gram-negative sepsis. The XOMA Sepsis Study Group. JAMA 1991; 266:1097-102.
79. Ziegler EJ, McCutchan JA, Fierer J et al. Treatment of gram-negative bacteremia and shock with human antiserum to a mutant Escherichia coli. N Engl J Med 1982; 307:1225-30.
80. Levine M, Kaper J, Black RE et al. New knowledge on pathogenesis of bacterial enteric infections as applied to vaccine development. Microbiol Rev 1983; 47:510-50.
81. Levine MM, Nalin DR, Hoover DL et al. Immunity to enterotoxigenic Escherichia coli. Infect Immun 1979; 23:729-36.
82. Black RE, Merson MH, Rowe B et al. Enterotoxigenic Escherichia coli diarrhoea: acquired immunity and transmission in an endemic area. Bull WHO 1981; 59:263-8.
83. DuPont HL, Olarte J, Evans DG et al. Comparative susceptibility of Latin American and United States students to enteric pathogens. N Engl J Med 1976; 285:1520-1.
84. Black RE, Brown KH, Becker S et al. Longitudinal studies of infectious diseases and physical growth in rural Bangladesh. II. Incidence of diarrhea and association with known pathogens. Am J Epidemiol 1982; 115:315-24.
85. Black RE, Lopez de Romana G, Brown KH et al. Incidence and etiology of infantile diarrhea and major routes of transmission in Huascar, Peru. Am J Epidemiol 1989; 129:785-99.
86. Guerrant RL, Kirchhoff LV, Shields DS et al. Prospective study of diarrheal illness in Northeastern Brazil: Patterns of disease, nutritional impact, etiologies, and risk factors. J Infect Dis 1983; 148:986-97.
87. Merson MH, Morris GK, Sack DA et al. Travelers' diarrhea in Mexico. A prospective study of physicians and family members attending a congress. N Engl J Med 1976; 294:1299-305.
88. Cravioto A, Reyes RE, Ortega R et al. Prospective study of diarrhoeal disease in a cohort of rural Mexican children: incidence and isolated pathogens during the first two years of life. Epidemiol Infect 1988; 101:123-34.
89. Levine MM, Giron JA, Noriega F. Fimbrial vaccines. In: Klemm P, ed. Fimbriae: adhesion, biogenics, genetics and vaccines. Boca Raton: CRC Press, 1994.
90. Gaastra W, Svennerholm AM. Colonization factors of human enterotoxigenic Escherichia coli (ETEC). Trends Microbiol 1996; 4:444-52.
91. Qadri F, Das SK, Faruque ASG et al. Prevalence of toxin types and colonization factors in enterotoxigenic Escherichia coli isolated during a 2-year period from diarrheal patients in Bangladesh. J Clin Microbiol 2000; 38:27-31.
92. Evans DG, Evans DJ Jr, Opekun A et al. Nonreplicating whole cell vaccine protective against enterotoxigenic Escherichia coli (ETEC) diarrhea: stimulation of anti-CFA (CFA/I) and anti-enterotoxin (anti-LT) intestinal IgA and protection against challenge with ETEC belonging to heterologous serotypes. FEMS Microbiol Lett 1988; 47:117-25.

93. Clemens JD, Sack DA, Harris JR et al. Cross-protection by B subunit-whole cell cholera vaccine against diarrhea associated with heat-labile toxin-producing enterotoxigenic Escherichia coli: Results of a large-scale field trial. J Infect Dis 1988; 158:372-7.
94. Peltola H, Siitonen A, Kyrönseppä H et al. Prevention of travellers' diarrhoea by oral B-subunit/ whole-cell cholera vaccine. Lancet 1991; 338:1285-9.
95. Svennerholm A-M, Ahren C, Jertborn M. Oral inactivated vaccine against enterotoxigenic Escherichia coli. In: Levine MM, Woodrow GC, Kaper JB, Cobon GS, eds. New Generation Vaccines. 2nd ed. New York: Marcel Dekker,1997: 865-74.
96. Savarino SJ, Brown FM, Hall E et al. Safety and immunogenicity of an oral, killed enterotoxigenic Escherichia coli-cholera toxin B subunit vaccine in Egyptian adults. J Infect Dis 1998; 177:796-9.
97. Savarino SJ, Hall ER, Bassily S et al. Oral, inactivated, whole cell enterotoxigenic Escherichia coli plus cholera toxin B subunit vaccine: results of the initial evaluation in children. PRIDE Study Group. J Infect Dis 1999; 179:107-14.
98. Hall ER, Wierzba TF, Ahren C et al. Induction of systemic antifimbria and antitoxin antibody responses in Egyptian children and adults by an oral, killed enterotoxigenic Escherichia coli plus cholera toxin B subunit vaccine. Infect Immun 2001; 69:2853-7.
99. Ahren C, Jertborn M, Svennerholm AM. Intestinal immune responses to an inactivated oral enterotoxigenic Escherichia coli vaccine and associated immunoglobulin A responses in blood. Infect Immun 1998; 66:3311-6.
100. Qadri F, Wenneras C, Ahmed F et al. Safety and immunogenicity of an oral, inactivated enterotoxigenic Escherichia coli plus cholera toxin B subunit vaccine in Bangladeshi adults and children. Vaccine 2000; 18:2704-12.
101. Jertborn M, Ahren C, Holmgren J et al. Safety and immunogenicity of an oral inactivated enterotoxigenic Escherichia coli vaccine. Vaccine 1998; 16:255-60.
102. Levine MM. Travellers' diarrhoea: prospects for successful immunoprophylaxis. Scand J Gastroenterol Suppl 1983; 84:121-34.
103. Levine MM, Morris JG, Losonsky G et al. Fimbriae (pili) adhesins as vaccines. In: Lark DL, Normark S, Uhlin BE, Wolf-Watz H, eds. Protein-carbohydrate interactions in biological systems the molecular biology of microbial pathogenicity. London: Academic Press, 1986:143-5.
104. Turner AK, Terry TD, Sack DA et al. Construction and characterization of genetically defined aro omp mutants of enterotoxigenic Escherichia coli and preliminary studies of safety and immunogenicity in humans. Infect Immun 2001; 69:4969-79.
105. Giron JA, Xu J-G, Gonzalez CR et al. Simultaneous constitutive expression of CFA/I and CS3 colonization factors of enterotoxigenic Escherichia coli by aroC, aroD Salmonella typhi vaccine strain CVD 908. Vaccine 1995; 10:939-46.
106. Koprowski H2, Levine MM, Anderson RJ et al. Attenuated Shigella flexneri 2a vaccine strain CVD 1204 expressing colonization factor antigen I and mutant heat-labile enterotoxin of enterotoxigenic Escherichia coli. Infect Immun 2000; 68:4884-92.
107. Altboum Z, Barry EM, Losonsky G et al. Attenuated Shigella flexneri 2a ?guaBA strain CVD 1204 expressing enterotoxigenic Escherichia coli (ETEC) CS2 and CS3 fimbriae as a live mucosal vaccine against Shigella and ETEC infection. Infect Immun 2001; 69:3150-8.
108. Noriega FR, Losonsky G, Wang JY et al. Further characterization of ?aroA, ?virG Shigella flexneri 2a strain CVD 1203 as a mucosal Shigella vaccine and as a live vector vaccine for delivering antigens of enterotoxigenic Escherichia coli. Infect Immun 1996; 64:23-7.
109. Douce G, Giannelli V, Pizza M et al. Genetically detoxified mutants of heat-labile toxin from Escherichia coli are able to act as oral adjuvants. Infect Immun 1999; 67:4400-6.
110. Chong C, Friberg M, Clements JD. LT(R192G), a nontoxic mutant of the heat-labile enterotoxin of Escherichia coli, elicits enhanced humoral and cellular immune responses associated with protection against lethal oral challenge with Salmonella spp. Vaccine 1998; 16:732-40.
111. Rappuoli R, Pizza M, Douce G et al. Structure and mucosal adjuvanticity of cholera and Escherichia coli heat-labile enterotoxins. Immunol Today 1999; 20:493-500.
112. Yamamoto T, Gojobori T, Yokota T. Evolutionary origin of pathogenic determinants in enterotoxigenic Escherichia coli and Vibrio cholerae O1. J Bacteriol 1987; 169:1352-7.
113. Takeda Y, Honda T, Sima H et al. Analysis of antigenic determinants in cholera enterotoxin and heat- labile enterotoxins from human and porcine enterotoxigenic Escherichia coli. Infect Immun 1983; 41:50-3.

114. Levine MM, Young CR, Black RE et al. Enzyme-linked immunosorbent assay to measure antibodies to purified heat-labile enterotoxins from human and porcine strains of Escherichia coli and to cholera toxin: application in serodiagnosis and seroepidemiology. J Clin Microbiol 1985; 21:174-9.
115. Noriega FR, Losonsky G, Lauderbaugh C et al. Engineered ?guaB-A, ?virG Shigella flexneri 2a strain CVD 1205: construction, safety, immunogenicity and potential efficacy as a mucosal vaccine. Infect Immun 1996; 64:3055-61.
116. Noriega FR, Liao FM, Maneval DR et al. Strategy for cross-protection among Shigella flexneri serotypes. Infect Immun 1999; 67:782-8.
117. Levine MM, Galen J, Barry E et al. Attenuated Salmonella typhi and Shigella as live oral vaccines and as live vectors. Behring Inst Mitt 1997; 98:120-3.
118. Tacket CO, Reid RH, Boedeker EC et al. Enteral immunization and challenge of volunteers given enterotoxigenic E. coli CFA/II encapsulated in biodegradable microspheres. Vaccine 1994; 12:1270-4.
119. Klipstein FA, Engert RF, Houghten RA. Immunisation of volunteers with a synthetic peptide vaccine for enterotoxigenic Escherichia coli. Lancet 1986; I:471-3.
120. Levine MM, Nataro JP, Karch H et al. The diarrheal response of humans to some classic serotypes of enteropathogenic Escherichia coli is dependent on a plasmid encoding an enteroadhesiveness factor. J Infect Dis 1985; 152:550-9.
121. Kenny B, Lai LC, Finlay BB et al. EspA, a protein secreted by enteropathogenic Escherichia coli, is required to induce signals in epithelial cells. Mol Microbiol 1996; 20:313-23.
122. Tacket CO, Sztein MB, Losonsky G et al. Role of EspB in experimental human enteropathogenic Escherichia coli infection. Infect Immun 2000; 68:3689-95.
123. Parissi-Crivelli A, Parissi-Crivelli JM, Giron JA. Recognition of enteropathogenic Escherichia coli virulence determinants by human colostrum and serum antibodies. J Clin Microbiol 2000; 38:2696-700.
124. Bieber D, Ramer SW, Wu CY et al. Type IV pili, transient bacterial aggregates, and virulence of enteropathogenic Escherichia coli. Science 1998; 280:2114-8.
125. Donnenberg MS, Tacket CO, James SP et al. Role of the eaeA gene in experimental enteropathogenic Escherichia coli infection. J Clin Invest 1993; 92:1412-7.
126. Abe A, Heczko U, Hegele RG et al. Two enteropathogenic Escherichia coli type III secreted proteins, EspA and EspB, are virulence factors. J Exp Med 1998; 188:1907-16.
127. Loureiro I, Frankel G, Adu-Bobie J et al. Human colostrum contains IgA antibodies reactive to enteropathogenic Escherichia coli virulence-associated proteins: intimin, BfpA, EspA, and EspB. J Pediatr Gastroenterol Nutr 1998; 27:166-71.
128. Cohen D, Ashkenazi S, Green MS et al. Double-blind vaccine-controlled randomised efficacy trial of an investigational Shigella sonnei conjugate vaccine in young adults. Lancet 1997; 349:155-9.
129. Lin FYC, Ho VA, Khiem HB et al. The efficacy of a Salmonella Typhi Vi conjugate vaccine in two-to-five-year-old children. N Eng J Med 2001; 344:1263-8.
130. Conlan JW, Cox AD, KuoLee R et al. Parenteral immunization with a glycoconjugate vaccine containing the O157 antigen of Escherichia coli O157:H7 elicits a systemic humoral immune response in mice, but fails to prevent colonization by the pathogen. Can J Microbiol 1999; 45:279-86.
131. Conlan JW, KuoLee R, Webb A et al. Oral immunization of mice with a glycoconjugate vaccine containing the O157 antigen of Escherichia coli O157:H7 admixed with cholera toxin fails to elicit protection against subsequent colonization by the pathogen. Can J Microbiol 2000; 46:283-90.
132. Konadu E, Donohue-Rolfe A, Calderwood SB et al. Syntheses and immunologic properties of Escherichia coli O157 O-specific polysaccharide and Shiga toxin 1 B subunit conjugates in mice. Infect Immun 1999; 67:6191-3.
133. Konadu E, Robbins JB, Shiloach J et al. Preparation, characterization, and immunological properties in mice of Escherichia coli O157 O-specific polysaccharide-protein conjugate vaccines. Infect Immun 1994; 62:5048-54.
134. Konadu EY, Parke JCJ, Tran HT et al. Investigational vaccine for Escherichia coli O157: phase 1 study of O157 O-specificolysaccharide-Pseudomonas aeruginosa recombinant exoprotein A conjugates in adults. J Infect Dis 1998; 177:383-7.
135. Acheson DWK, Levine MM, Kaper JB et al. Protective immunity to Shiga-like toxin I following oral immunization with Shiga-like toxin I B-subunit-producing Vibrio cholerae CVD 103-HgR. Infect Immun 1996; 64:355-7.

136. Butterton JR, Ryan ET, Acheson DW et al. Coexpression of the B subunit of Shiga toxin 1 and EaeA from enterohemorrhagic Escherichia coli in Vibrio cholerae vaccine strains. Infect Immun 1997; 65:2127-35.
137. Su GF, Brahmbhatt HN, Wehland J et al. Extracellular export of Shiga toxin B-subunit/haemolysin A (C-terminus) fusion protein expressed in Salmonella typhimurium aroA-mutant and stimulation of B-subunit specific antibody responses in mice. Microb Pathog 1992; 13:465-76.
138. Conlan JW, KuoLee R, Webb A et al. Salmonella landau as a live vaccine against Escherichia coli O157:H7 investigated in a mouse model of intestinal colonization. Can J Microbiol 1999; 45:723-31.
139. Keusch GT, Acheson DW, Marchant C et al. Toxod-based active and passive immunization to prevent and/or modulate hemolytic uremic syndrome due to Shiga toxin-producing Escherichia coli. In: Kaper JB, O'Brien AD, eds. Escherichia coli O157:H7 and other Shiga toxin-producing E. coli strains. Washington,D.C.: ASM Press, 1998:409-18.
140. Tauxe RV. Public health perspective on immunoprophylactic strategies for Escherichia coli O157:H7: who or what would we immunize? In: Kaper JB, O'Brien AD, editors. Escherichia coli O157:H7and other Shiga toxin-producing E. coli strains. Washington, D.C.: ASM Press, 1998:445-52.
141. Czeczulin JR, Balepur S, Hicks S et al. Aggregative adherence fimbria II, a second fimbrial antigen mediating aggregative adherence in enteroaggregative Escherichia coli. Infect Immun 1997; 65:4135-45.

CHAPTER 9

A Vaccine for Gonorrhea

P. Frederick Sparling, Christopher E. Thomas and Weiyan Zhu

Summary

There is minimal evidence for naturally-acquired immunity to reinfection by the gonococcus. However, recent improvements in understanding the roles in pathogenesis played by a variety of cell surface molecules, availability of multiple models for infection including human volunteers, and development of techniques for delivering antigens for stimulating mucosal immune responses provide the means to determine whether a vaccine for gonorrhea is possible.

Introduction: Gonorrhea Is a Persistent Clinical Problem

Infection by *Neisseria gonorrhoeae* (the gonococcus) has been a problem for humans at least since the days of the Old Testament, being well described in Leviticus. The incidence of gonococcal infection has diminished substantially in the Western world in the past 15 years, but the infection is still common in certain populations (poor, African-American, inner city or rural SE) in the USA and is very common in many parts of Africa, Asia, Central and South America, and many aboriginal cultures. The decline of gonococci in the developed countries is due both to development of better diagnostic tests, better public and health professional awareness of the disease, and continued effective antibiotic treatment regimens. At present, ~300,000 cases of gonorrhea are diagnosed annually in the USA, which probably represents about one-half of the true incidence, based on estimates of unreported infection. Young persons are particularly likely to be infected, both because of behavioral risks associated with adolescence (multiple sex partners) and also increased susceptibility to infection in girls after the onset of sexual maturity.

The disease typically causes only mild urethritis in men but causes severe clinical illness in 10-20% of women, most usually in the form of salpingitis and resultant tubal scarring and infertility/ectopic pregnancy.[1-3] In the USA and Western Europe, only *Chlamydia trachomatis* infection is a more common cause of tubal scarring and infertility.[2] Bacteremia and arthritis occur in about 0.5% of infected persons, depending on the particular gonococcal strain and host factors.[3] Many genital infections are asymptomatic, in both males and females;[3] recent surveys of young USA military recruits by ligase chain reaction of urine showed that ~60% of infections were asymptomatic.[4] Pharyngeal or rectal infections are relatively common and are usually asymptomatic. The infected but asymptomatic person may carry the infection for months, and exposed partners may develop severe illness.[5] Neonates born to an infected asymptomatic mother may develop conjunctivitis and blindness as well as other complications.

In addition to the burden of disease caused by gonococci, especially in women, there is at least one other compelling reason to develop a vaccine, *viz.*, gonococcal infection is a cofactor in sexual transmission of HIV.[6] Gonococcal infection causes genital inflammation, which increases shedding of HIV in secretions of an HIV-infected person and increases the relative risk of transmission of HIV by ~3-fold in most studies.[6] A second reason to try to accelerate vaccine development is the worrisome increase in antibiotic resistance among gonococci in

New Bacterial Vaccines, edited by Ronald W. Ellis and Bernard R. Brodeur.

many parts of the world, including resistance to newer quinolones such as ciprofloxacin.[7,8] Ciprofloxacin is still useful in the USA and Europe but has lost its effectiveness in much of Asia, and resistance in Hawaii has climbed rapidly to 20% of isolates in the past year (personal communication, Susan Wang). If ciprofloxacin were to join penicillin G and tetracyclines on the list of antimicrobials no longer useful for gonococcal infection, public pressure for a vaccine certainly would increase.

Natural History of Infection

The first question regarding a possible vaccine is: does natural immunity exist? The answer unfortunately is that there is limited evidence for significant immunity after uncomplicated genital infection. In the modern antibiotic era, people commonly acquire gonorrhea, are treated, and reacquire a similar or identical infection within months.[3] Mild or asymptomatic infection may be carried for months without elimination of the organism if there is no antibiotic treatment.[3-5] Neither of these statements proves that there is not a limited amount of specific protective immunity after natural infection; they only state that if there is protective immunity, it is partial at best. Indeed, there are data that support the notion of antigen-specific (porin, or Por) partial immunity after natural infection, as discussed below. Early experimental studies in humans, shocking as they seem to the modern reader with a different ethical standard for using humans as volunteers, showed that symptoms and signs of untreated urethritis in men not infrequently resolved after several weeks.[9] There were many anecdotes in the pre-antibiotic era of spontaneous resolution of symptoms, including the famous case of James Boswell, who had more than two dozen discrete episodes of urethritis.[10] Before examining the immune response in detail, however, it will useful to review the surface structure of the gonococcus and the pathogenesis of infection both in vitro and in various in vivo model systems, including human experimental infections. In so doing, we will also examine most of the potential vaccine candidates.

Surface Structures: Variability in Expression and Antigenicity

The fundamental lesson of over two decades of intense study of cell surface antigens is that the gonococcal surface is remarkably variable. There is no capsule, a major point of difference from the meningococcus. The gonococcal surface is composed of lipooligosaccharides (LOS) and a variety of proteins. Many of these undergo high-frequency phase and antigenic variation, which presumably serves to provide specific structures for adherence to and invasion of different host cells as well as evasion of specific immune responses. There also are a variety of proteins that are expressed only under conditions of environmental stress, most of which were ignored until the relatively recent past, some of which may be vaccine candidates. There are some quite surprising surface-exposed proteins, such as ribosomal protein L 12 that appears to be involved in binding to and invasion of host cells,[11] and others that were only discovered by genomic sequencing.[12] Our knowledge of the outer membrane of the gonococcus is now extensive, although translation of this knowledge into prevention and vaccines has been very slow and frustrating.

Key Surface Antigens and Their Roles in Pathogenesis

If there is to be a vaccine for gonorrhea, it will be a subunit vaccine composed of one or more defined cell-surface antigens. Crude killed whole-cell vaccines have been tried in humans[13,14] and chimpanzees,[15] but they are likely to be more toxic than subunit vaccines, and a trial in humans showed no efficacy.[14] The questions include: which are the relevant immunogens, how will they be delivered, what tests can be used as surrogates for protection, and how will clinical trials be conducted? We will focus on the key surface molecules that play a critical role in pathogenesis of infection, some of which are or have been vaccine candidates, and others that are important because they interfere with what otherwise might be an effective host defense.

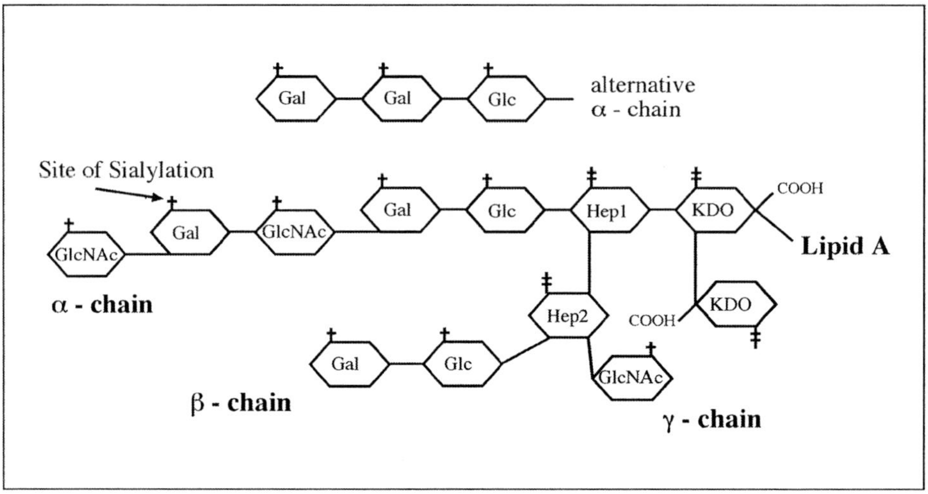

Figure 1. Apparent structure of gonococcal lipooligosaccharide (LOS) adapted from reference 17. The actual structure expressed by gonococci varies depending on phase variation in a number of glycosyltransferases and on sialylation, as described in the text.

LOS

Gonococci express an LOS that differs from many Gram negative LOS structures in that it lacks a repeating high-molecular-weight O antigen. It contains a typical lipid A, two 2-keto-3-deoxy-mannooctulosonic acid (KDO) molecules, and two heptoses; to these are attached three oligosaccharide chains designated α, β or γ.[16,17] The α-chain is attached to the first heptose, and the β- and γ-chains are attached to the second heptose (Fig. 1). Th oligosaccharide side-chains are variable, depending on the expression of several phase-variable glycosyltransferases that add carbohydrates to the LOS chain. The typical α-chain is the tetrasaccharide Glc-Gal-GlcNAc-Gal or lacto-N-neotetraose, which closely resembles host asialo-GM1 ganglioside.[18] Some species of LOS have a terminal GalNAc attached to the end of the lacto-N-neotetraose moiety; others express an alternative α-chain that consists only of Glc-Gal-Gal.[17] High-frequency variations in expression of many of the glycosyltransferases is due to slipped-strand mispairing, leading to insertion or deletion mutations in either a run of guanines or cytosines[17,19]within the structural genes, resulting in frame-shifting and an on-off phase variation.

These variations in LOS terminal sugars are highly important, because they dramatically affect the infectious phenotype of the organism. Gonococci that express the lacto-N-neotetraose moiety are capable of adding sialic acid to the terminal Gal, by virtue of a bacterial sialyltransferase and host-derived cytidine monophosphate N-acetyl neuraminic acid (CMP-NANA).[20-22] Loss of the terminal Gal results in inability to undergo sialylation of LOS (Fig. 2). Sialylated gonococci are resistant to the killing effects of complement (C'),[20-22] and resistant to neutrophilic leukocyte (PMN) uptake and killing, [23,24] but are less invasive for a variety of host cells.[25] Non-sialylated gonococci expressing full-length LOS containing the lacto-N-neotetraose moiety are sensitive to C' and opsonization, but are invasive for certain host cells even in the absence of Opa invasins (see below). Variants that express truncated LOS retain wild-type ability to attach to host cells, presumably by binding a host asialoglycoprotein receptor,[26] but are less invasive than those expressing full-length LOS.[27] The invasive phenotype of strain MS11 depends on expression of the first Glc on the α-chain.[17]

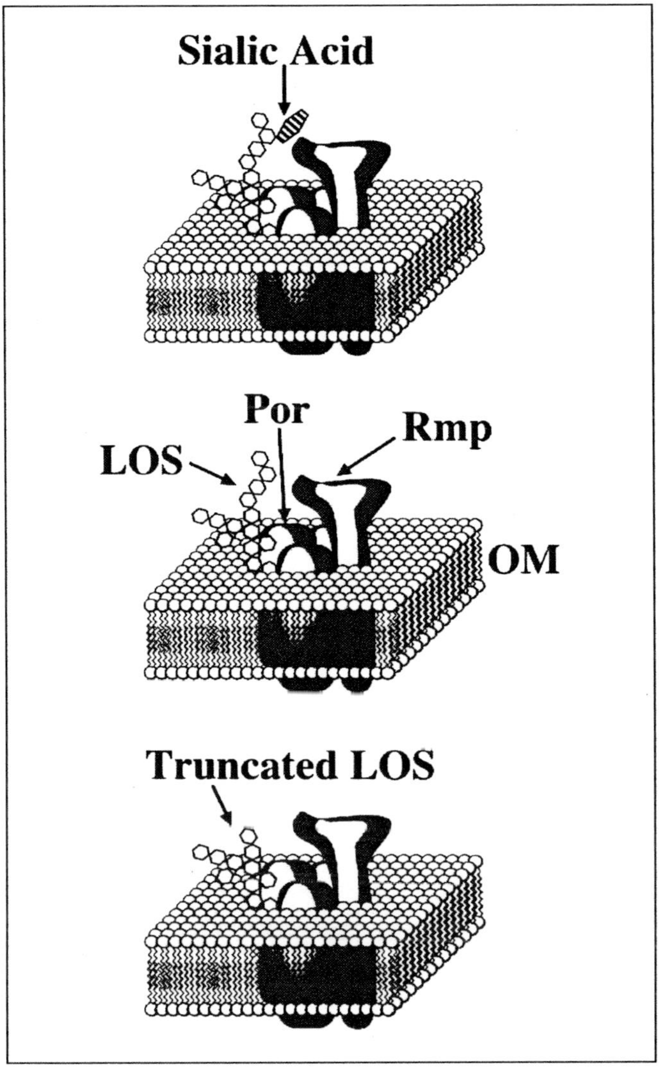

Figure 2. A cartoon of the relationship among LOS, Por and Rmp which are located in non-covalently attached clusters in the outer membrane. When LOS is sialylated, Por is partially masked. Rmp also protects Por by stimulating production of non-C'-fixing antibodies that block the activity of bactericidal antibodies.

Gonococcal LOS is a potential vaccine target. Rice and colleagues identified a monoclonal antibody (MAb) 2C7 that binds to ~94% of gonococcal clinical isolates but not to meningococci or host glycolipids.[28] Since the 2C7 MAb is both bactericidal and opsonic and since sialylation of LOS only partly interferes with bactericidal activity,[28] they suggested that the epitope defined by MAb 2C7 might be a potential vaccine candidate. The 2C7 epitope requires lactose as the β-chain,[29] and is immunogenic.[28] This same group developed an anti-idiotope MAb against MAb 2C7 that mimics the structure of the 2C7 target epitope, and the anti-idiotope MAb was immunogenic, resulting in bactericidal and opsonophagocytic antibodies against gonococci expressing the 2C7 epitope.[30] Thus, they suggested that such a strategy could be used to develop a vaccine.[30]

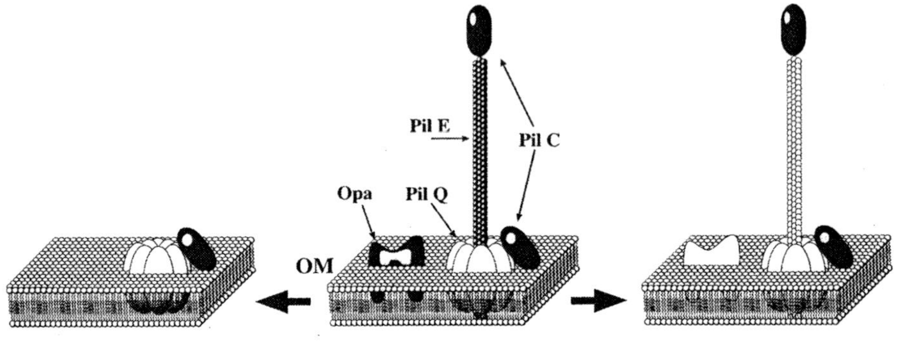

Figure 3. Variation in expression of the pilus and Opa adherence ligands. Individual cells express from none to up to five different Opa proteins, depending on translational frameshifts in *opa* genes. The pilus (assembled from the products of the *pilE* gene) is extruded through PilQ; pili also are subject to antigenic and phase variation. Adherence of the pilus to host receptors apparently is mediated by the tip adhesin PilC. Sizes are not to scale, and the cartoon is meant to illustrate concepts. See text for details.

Opacity (Opa) Proteins

Gonococci produce from none to up to at least five members at a time of a family of 10-12 surface-exposed outer membrane proteins (OMPs) collectively designated Opa, for their general property of increasing interbacterial adherence and therefore an opaque colony phenotype.[31] Not all Opa proteins cause opaque colonies, but all share a common structure and migrate in sodium dodecyl sulfate-polyacrylamide gel electrophoresis (SDS-PAGE) at differing apparent molecular weight (MW) depending on whether they are heat-denatured.[31] All are cationic, and all contain two hypervariable (HV-1 and HV-2) domains and one semivariable domain.[32] They are subject to high-frequency, RecA-independent phase variation due to slipped-strand mispairing in a CTCTT repeat located within the coding sequence for the signal peptide; the resultant frameshifting results in a high-frequency on-off variation for each of the 10-12 genes in the Opa family.[33] (Fig. 3) ecause the gene products are not identical, the on-off switch also results in antigenic variation. Recombination between genes in the Opa family also results in antigenic variation.[34]

Opa proteins are important to pathogenesis because they markedly affect adherence to and invasion of epithelial cells in vitro,[35-39] and there is strong selective pressure for their in vivo expression.[40,41] Likely pressures for in vivo expression include both the adherence and invasion phenotypes associated with Opa as well as the relative resistance to killing by C'.[42] Opa proteins also mediate non-opsonic uptake by neutrophils.[43-46] Adherence is mediated by binding to either one or both of two families of host cell receptors, the heparan sulfate proteoglycans (HSPG) or the CEACAM glycoproteins (previously known as the carcinoembryonic antigen (CEA) or the CD66 family).[47-50] One Opa protein binds strongly to HSPGs and leads to invasion of certain epithelial cells. HSPG-mediated binding and invasion are facilitated by the serum proteins vitronectin or fibronectin and their integrin receptors.[51-53] Syndecan 1 and 4 have been identified as key HSPGs in the internalization of gonococci into Chang epithelial cells.[54] Binding to HSPG receptors results in stimulation of intracellular signaling pathways and cytoskeletal rearrangements involving actin and microtubular polymerization.[55] The HV-1 domain of Opa is crucial to these interactions with the HSPG receptors, although other regions of the protein are also required for binding.[56]

Most Opa bind to one or several of the CEACAM family. The CEACAM (CD66) family includes multiple variants, which differ in their presence on various epithelial and phagocytic cells, thus accounting in part for tissue tropisms of different gonococci for different cell types. Interestingly, different Opa may bind the same CD66 variant equally well, despite differences in the structure of their HV regions. HV-2 appears most important to binding to CD66 receptors, but the binding site is complex and dependent on many regions of the protein coming together in particular conformations.[57] As in the case of binding to HSPG receptors, binding to CEACAM results in activation of intracellular signaling cascades (also involving acid sphingomyelinases)[58] and associated alterations in the cell surface and actin filaments.

It is unclear whether Opa are a vaccine target. There is some weak epidemiological evidence that an immune response to Opa is associated with reduced risk of salpingitis.[59] There are few data to support the notion that antibodies against Opa might block infection, and the variability in Opa expression and structure has stifled research in this area.

Porins (Por)

Unlike LOS and Opa, where there is at best modest interest in vaccine potential, Por has been a focus of intense interest as a vaccine candidate. Por has many potential virtues as a vaccine candidate: it is produced constitutively, is abundant and surface-exposed, and does not undergo phase or high-frequency antigenic variation. It is the target for MAbs that are bactericidal and opsonic and that protect cells in vitro.[60-63] An epidemiological study of female commercial sex workers in Nairobi, most of whom were HIV-infected and were exposed repeatedly to sexually-transmitted diseases (STDs) including gonorrhea, suggested that infection resulted in Por-serovar-specific partial immunity to reinfection.[64] An analogous study of repeat infections in rural North Carolina, among a population of principally males, failed to confirm this finding,[65] but the studies were different in several respects. Thus, interest in a Por-based vaccine continues.

Meningococci produce two porins: PorA, which is the basis of much current vaccine research,[66] and PorB, which does not appear to be as promising vaccine candidate. Gonococci do not produce a PorA, although they do have a silent *por A* pseudogene.[67] Because gonococcal porin is most closely related to meningococcal PorB, gonococcal porin also is designated PorB. It occurs in two antigenically distinct families, designated P.1A and P.1B, each of which is the product of the *porB* gene.[68] The P.1A and P.1B families can be divided into numerous minor antigenic variants (serovars) on the basis of their reactions with panels of Por-specific MAbs.[69] The differences in antigenicity of PorB results from variations in the eight surface-exposed loops.[62]

PorB provides a crucial pathway for entry of small molecules through the lipid-rich bacterial outer membrane and is essential for the bacterium, as evidenced by the inability to construct viable knockout mutations. Elegant work by several laboratories has shown that Por binds GTP[70,71] and serves as a voltage-gated ion channel.[72,73] Por translocates into mammalian membranes,[70,71] which may help gonococci to invade host cells. Interestingly, P.1A serovars translocate Por into lipid membranes more readily in vitro than P.1B serovars. Using isogenic strains varying only in their *porB* allele, van Putten and colleagues showed that invasion was enhanced specifically by the P.1A porin, as compared to P.1B.[70] This suggests that PorB plays a direct role in invasion of host cells. Moreover, PorB partially inactivates human neutrophils,[74] possibly helping to explain why gonococci are surprisingly resistant to neutrophil killing. Some evidence suggests that PorB also induces apoptosis in target cells.[75,76]

There is an epidemiological correlation between infection by strains of the P.1A serovar and disseminated (bacteremic) gonococcal infection.[3] Clearly, one reason might be the relatively greater ability of P.1A strains to invade host cells because of their greater ability to translocate porin into host cell membranes. Another reason is the resistance to normal human serum (NHS) and C' exhibited by almost all P.1A strains.[77,78] Many P.1B strains are sensitive to bactericidal effects of NHS.[77,78] These differences in susceptibility to killing by NHS are now known to be due to variations in loop structure, which directly affect C' sensitivity.[78] (Fig. 4)

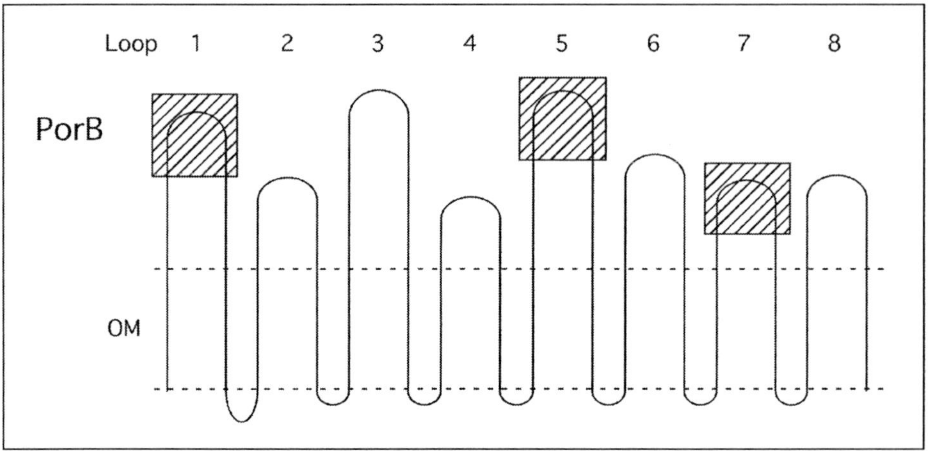

Figure 4. Noodle cartoon of the surface-exposed variable Por B loops. Shaded boxes indicate domains that either are crucial to pathogenesis because they are sites for binding C'-regulatory proteins C4bp and Factor H or are targets for protective antibodies, as discussed in the text.

Intrinscally serum-resistant P.1A strains bind the C' activation regulator Factor H to loop 5, and in many of these strains, the C' activation regulator C4bp also binds to loop 1. In those P.1B strains that are intrinsically resistant to killing by NHS, C4bp typically binds to a conformational epitope defined by the interactions between loops 5 and 7.[78] Strains that are intrinsically sensitive to NHS, and which fail to bind either C4bp or Factor H to PorB, may become phenotypically serum-resistant in vivo by binding Factor H to sialylated LOS.[77] Because most strains are sialylated significantly in vivo, all are phenotypically resistant to NHS on first isolation, although this is rapidly lost in vitro unless the bacteria are supplied with CMP-NANA.[79]

Evolution has provided PorB with other effective defenses against C'-mediated immune attack. In its native state, PorB exists as a trimer in the outer membrane.[80] Its immediate neighbors are LOS[81] and a protein designated reduction modifiable protein, or Rmp (Fig. 2). Proximity to LOS results not only in inactivation of C' when LOS is sialylated, but also in at least partial masking of PorB, limiting ability of anti-PorB antibodies to bind to the surface of intact organisms.[82] Since gonococci isolated directly from patients are usually sialylated,[77,81] this might limit efficacy of a PorB vaccine. Moreover, many epitopes of Rmp stimulate production of IgG non-C'-fixing antibodies that block the bactericidal effects of anti-PorB antibodies.[83-85] Antibodies to Rmp apparently enhance susceptibility to infection of persons sexually exposed to an infected partner.[86] Anti-Rmp antibodies also apparently interfered with the efficacy of an early human trial of a PorB vaccine that was contaminated by small amounts of Rmp.[87]

Despite all these difficulties, a PorB vaccine may still be possible. There is speculation that sufficiently high titers of anti-PorB antibodies will circumvent the effects of anti-Rmp antibodies.[87] Some of the MAbs against PorB described years ago by Heckels and colleagues were bactericidal against a broad range of either P.1A or P.1B serovars.[61-63] Antibodies against a loop 1 PorB peptide bound to the cell surface of many gonococci and were bactericidal.[82] Renatured recombinant PorB in liposomes stimulated production of antibodies that bound the cell surface of intact gonococci and were opsonic.[88] PorB also serves an adjuvant function by its effects on B cells.[89,90] Such considerations led to production by Wyeth-Lederle Vaccines of recombinant *E. coli*-derived renatured PorB from gonococcal strain FA1090,[91] which was tested recently in human volunteers for safety (Susan Hoiseth, personal communication). The hope is that such a vaccine might be tested in a human challenge model of gonorrhea (see below), which would allow relatively inexpensive and safe testing of proof of principle.

Pili

Another well-studied vaccine candidate is the pilus. Virtually all gonococci express pili on first isolation from patients,[92] although the ability to express pili is rapidly lost on in vitro subculture.[93] Early clinical research with human volunteers showed that only piliated gonococci were able to establish infection in the male urethra.[94] Pili are assembled from 15- to 20-kD pilin subunits, the products of the *pilE* gene, into large filamentous structures that are closely related to other pili in the type 4 family.[95] They are associated with ability to undergo DNA-mediated transformation[96] and with binding to a variety of human cells.[97,98] Pili thus represent a third class of adhesin, along with Opa and LOS. They undergo rapid phase and antigenic variation, reminiscent of variations in both Opa and LOS, but the mechanism is entirely different. Variations in pilin expression are due to recombination between *pilE* and other related incomplete (silent) *pilS* genes, containing variable amounts of slightly different versions of *pilE*, each of which lacks the 3' end of the gene. When the recombinational event produces a functional albeit different pilin product, the result is antigenic variation. When the product cannot be assembled into an intact pilus, the result is phase variation.[99]

Different pili show differences in their tropisms for particular epithelial cells,[98] although all pili seem able to promote binding to and agglutination of human red blood cells. Pili do not attach to non-human cells, providing part of the answer to why gonococci only infect humans. The receptor for pili is CD46,[95,100] which also serves as the receptor for binding the C' regulatory protein C3b and for many other microorganisms. Binding of pili to CD46 is associated with signaling events in the epithelial cell, analogous to but different in detail from the events that follow Opa-mediated binding.[101]

Antibodies to pili block attachment to human cells,[102-105] which led to a vigorous attempt to make a pilus-based vaccine. There was enthusiasm for a common (or at least not highly variable) peptide that seemed to be involved in attachment, especially since anti-peptide antibodies blocked attachment.[102,105] However, anti-pilus MAbs that blocked attachment were directed at variable epitopes,[103] showing that attachment was associated with the most variable domains on pili. Moreover, the common domains were not surface exposed on the intact pilus.[106] Little enthusiasm remains for a common pilus-peptide-based vaccine.

Other efforts focused on whole purified pili as the immunogen. Purified whole pili were relatively easily isolated, and anti-pilus antibodies also blocked attachment.[104,107] A vaccine composed of the Pgh3-2 pilus was given intramuscularly (in the deltoid), and human male volunteers were challenged intraurethrally with the homologous organism. The result was ~10- to 30-fold protection relative to no-vaccine controls,[108] This was very important if only because it provided proof of principle that a parenteral vaccine could block mucosal gonococcal infection. Mucosal IgG and IgA antibodies were produced that could block in vitro attachment to various cell types.[109] Unfortunately, the protection did not extend to a single other tested (heterologous) strain in human volunteers, and no protection was seen in a large field trial among US military in Korea.[110] Reasons for the failure of the pilus vaccine could be multiple, including use of a smaller dose in the field trial than in the preliminary experiments, although the vaccine did elicit an anti-pilus immune response.[110] The most likely explanation is that the pilus vaccine consisted only of a single antigenic type, and antigenic variation in clinical isolates allowed immune escape.

Although there is little known current effort to make a pilus vaccine, hope is not lost. The most exciting recent development is evidence that the minor pilus-related OMP PilC is an adhesin[111,112] and is associated with the pilus tip in immunoelectron microscopy.[113] (Fig. 3) PilC occurs in two versions, PilC1 and PilC2, which are somewhat different in their primary sequence. Both PilC1 and PilC2 are gonococcal adhesins.[114] PilC are the products of genes (*pilC*1 and *pilC*2), which undergo high-frequency phase variation fundamentally analogous in mechanism to that of *opa* (slipped-strand mispairing that results in translational frame shifting). When phase variation results in loss of expression of both PilC1 and PilC2, gonococci usually do not express pili.[115] This makes it difficult to unravel the relative roles of pili and PilC

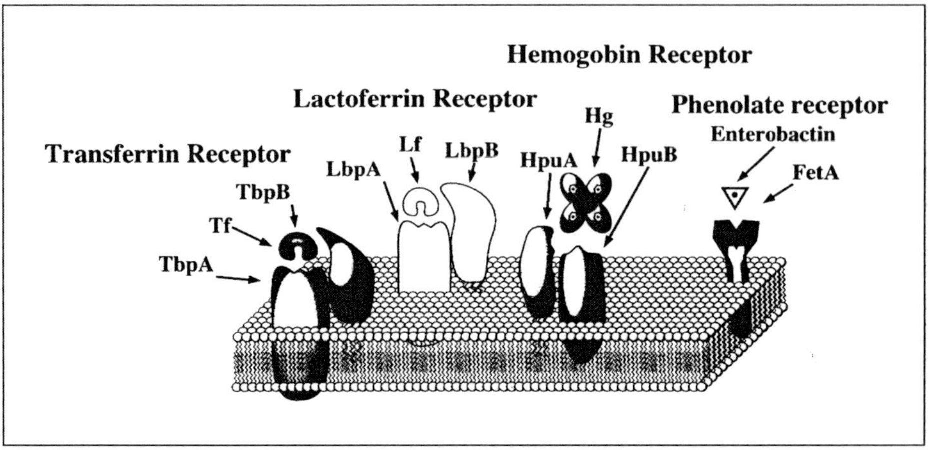

Figure 5. Conceptual view of iron-ligand receptors. Each is expressed by all gonococci except the lactoferrin receptor, which is found in only one-half of isolates.

in attachment. Mutants in *pilE* that do not express pili retain their ability to express PilC; PilC$^+$ PilE$^-$ strains do not attach well.[116] This could mean that pili are necessary to present the putative terminal tip (PilC) adhesin properly to its receptor on host cells. It is not known yet whether PilC binds directly to CD46. the N-terminus of PilC1 recently was shown to be involved in attachment.[114]

Other recent pertinent developments include demonstration that PilQ is the 75-kD subunit of the formerly identified high-MW common OMP antigen previously known as OMP-MC.[117,118] The PilQ product is one of many pilus-associated genes that are essential for pilus biogenesis and function.[118] PilQ is interesting because it is surface exposed, and much of the protein is common in different strains.[118] Its function is to make a multimeric channel in the outer membrane, through which the assembled pilus fiber is presented.[95] Since antibodies against OMP-MC are bactericidal,[119] vaccine development with PilQ may be possible.

Stress Proteins

Gonococci as well as most other bacteria produce a wide variety of other proteins when exposed to various conditions of stress. These include iron-regulated, oxygen-regulated, pH-regulated, and cell contact-induced proteins. Many or all of these are important to pathogenesis in some way, and some are potential vaccine components.

Iron-regulated Proteins

Gonococci produce a large and still relatively poorly characterized set of proteins that are repressed by iron, and others that are induced by iron.[120] The main focus has been on the surface proteins that serve as receptors for binding iron ligands and on the associated genes and gene products that activate these receptors and enable transit of iron released from the ligands into the cytoplasm. There are four quite well characterized receptors, including one for each of transferrin (Tf), lactoferrin (Lf), hemoglobin (Hb), and phenolate siderophores produced by other microorganisms.[121,122] These are designated respectively as the Tf, Lf, Hb, and Fet receptors (Fig. 5). The first three are organized along the same general lines, with a two- gene operon whose promoter is regulated by the iron-dependent transcriptional repressor Fur and tandem genes encoding first a lipoprotein and secondly an integral membrane protein.[121] These proteins are designated, respectively, TbpB and A, LbpB and A, HpuA and B, and FetA. The integral membrane protein is presumed by analogy to other systems to be a gated porin and is in each case essential to the function of the system. The lipoprotein is associated on the outer membrane with the integral membrane protein and facilitates the function of the receptor. In the case of the Hb receptor, the lipoprotein is essential.[123] The FetA receptor is composed only of an integral OMP, without an associated lipoprotein.

There is evidence for the role of iron-ligand receptors in infection. Using isogenic derivatives of the strain FA 1090, a strain that could produce neither the Tf nor the Lf receptor was shown to be non-infectious for male human volunteers.[124] Since strains expressing either the Tf[124] or Lf receptor are infectious in this model (J. E. Anderson et al, unpublished data), one of these receptors is crucial for infection. Of the two, the Tf receptor seems most important because at least half of gonococci in clinical isolates do not produce a functional Lf receptor, whereas all produce the Tf receptor.

One or more of these iron-ligand receptors might be useful in a vaccine. Using the meningococcus again as an example, the very closely related TF receptor lipoprotein TbpB may be a vaccine candidate, since it stimulates production of cross-reactive protective bactericidal antibodies in mice.[125,126] No comparable work has been done yet with gonococci. TbpA also may be a candidate, since a TbpA vaccine protected against experimental meningococcal infection.[127] Domains of TbpA that are directly involved in ligand binding offer a rational target for vaccine development.[128] Protection mediated by vaccination of animals with meningococcal TbpB is correlated with serum bactericidal activity,[125,126] whereas protection elicited by TbpA is not correlated with bactericidal serum titers.[127] This is relevant to considerations of what assays will be used in vitro as surrogates for potential vaccine efficacy. Of the other iron-ligand receptors, the FetA receptor may be the most promising because it is a major cell surface antigen during iron starvation and because antibodies against FetA are bactericidal for meningococci.[129] However, it undergoes rapid phase variation in levels of expression,[130] and bactericidal activity in meningococci is strain-specific.[129] The Hb receptor is not attractive because it apparently is expressed in vivo only in special circumstances.[131] The Lf receptor also is an unlikely vaccine candidate because the integral membrane protein LbpA is expressed in <50%, and the lipoprotein LbpB is expressed in only ~10% of isolates (G Biswas, J E Anderson and P F Sparling, unpublished data).

Other Stress Proteins

Gonococci respond to a relatively acidic environment by alterations in expression of many surface antigens, including down-regulation of Rmp,[132] up-regulation of novel OMPs and GroEL homologs,[132] and changes in LOS phenotype.[133] Sialylation of LOS may be enhanced under conditions of low pH.[134] Growth under anaerobic conditions also alters the organism in many important ways, including up-regulation of expression of a major OMP Pan1.[135] Antibodies are made against anaerobically-expressed proteins in natural infection,[136] which strongly suggests that anaerobic growth is a normal part of the infectious cycle. Exposure to sublethal concentrations of hydrogen peroxide results in up-regulation of catalase, by which gonococci defend themselves from neutrophil-mediated oxidative killing.[137]

Lessons Learned about Expression of Gonococcal Antigens from Studies of Infection in Patients and Human Volunteers

The first important observations were made in the 1960s by Kellogg and his colleagues at the CDC, who showed that gonococci isolated from patients have small-colony phenotypes; in vitro cultivation led to a large-colony phenotype. Only the small-colony phenotype isolates were infectious for male volunteers.[93,98] Small colonies were soon shown to be piliated, whereas the larger colonies were not piliated. Over the next several decades, a plethora of other important observations were made. Most colonies isolated directly from patients were opaque, suggesting that they expressed Opa.[31] Isolates from men almost always were opaque, but there was variability in expression of the opaque phenotype in women depending on the phase of the cycle.[138] LOS was shown to be substantially sialylated in vivo.[21] Recent evidence showed increased expression of the HpuAB Hb receptor early in the menstrual cycle,[131] suggesting that it along with the universally expressed Tf receptor is important in pathogenesis. Certain isolates are more likely to be found in patients with asymptomatic local infection, including those with the P.1A, serum-resistant, arginine-hypoxanthine-uracil (AHU)-requiring phenotype.[139] The same or similar isolates are associated with bacteremic disease.[140] Another clone with a P.1B, citrulline-uracil-requiring phenotype recently was associated with asymptomatic infection.[141] Intrinsic sensitivity to NHS, due to inability to bind C4bp or factor H to PorB, is associated with greater likelihood for producing both symptomatic mucosal disease and also salpingitis,[142] probably because such isolates generate more of the inflammatory and chemotaxis-promoting C' components.

In the past two decades, renewed use of human volunteers has allowed experimental insight into the pathogenesis of infection and of the potential efficacy of certain vaccine candidates. Great care has been taken to ensure the safety of the volunteers, and there have been no complications in studies of well over 400 volunteers. Because women might develop ascending infection of the fallopian tubes, only men have been used as experimental subjects. In order to prevent possible complications, infections usually have been terminated by antibiotic treatment immediately upon onset of earliest signs of infection, which has limited the ability to study the immune response or anything other than the very early stages of infection. Brinton et al [108] utilized male volunteers to show that a whole-pilus vaccine was safe and effective, at least against the homologous strain expressing the same antigenic type of pilus. Buchanan et al conducted studies of a PorB vaccine prepared from gonococcal membranes but were unable to show protection, possibly because the preparation was contaminated by small amounts of the blocking antigen Rmp.[87]

Investigators from the Walter Reed Army Institute of Research (WRAIR), the Rocky Mountain Laboratories of the NIH, and the University of North Carolina (UNC) in Chapel Hill have used male volunteers to explore the importance of particular antigens in infection. The WRAIR-NIH group utilized strain MS11, whereas the UNC group used strain FA1090 for most studies.[143] Both are P.1B strains, although they differ in several respects, including expression of the Lf receptor by MS11 but not FA1090. The estimated ID_{50} (infectious dose required to infect 50% of volunteers) was ~$1x10^5$ colony-forming units (CFU) of FA1090, which was at least 10-100 fold higher than that reported for MS11.[144] Challenge with a strain of MS11 isolated from volunteers was infectious at a very low inoculum as compared to the lab-passaged parent, which was correlated with in vivo selection of full-length LOS variants.[145] The apparent difference in infectivity of MS11 and FA1090 probably was not due to differences in the expressed LOS, since the in vivo-selected more-infectious derivative of MS11 expressed the same full-length lacto-N-neotetraose type of LOS that is expressed by all the FA1090 strains used by the UNC group. Challenge with non-Opa-expressing MS11 or FA1090 always resulted in rapid in vivo selection of Opa-expressing variants, although different Opa variants predominated in isolates recovered from different human subjects; it was common to isolate variants simultaneously expressing multiple Opa proteins.[40,41,146] Similarly, the particular type of expressed pilus changed rapidly, as soon as one day after inoculation, before any immune response could be generated.[147,148] One interpretation of these studies is that the Opa and Pilus variants were selected based on the particular types of receptors expressed in different volunteers, although recent work suggests that epithelial cells of the male urethra do not contain the usual CEACAM (CD66) receptors for most of the Opa proteins.[149]

Other studies utilized various deletion mutations to explore the importance of particular gene products. Loss of ability to express either Pili or Opa did not completely eliminate the ability of the strains to cause infection (Jane Cannon, personal communication). These results were surprising, given the strong evidence for in vivo selection of Pili and Opa. Likewise, loss of ability to make IgA protease had no effect on infection,[150] and mutation in sialyltransferase had minimal effects on the human male challenge results (Jane Cannon, personal communication). The only mutation that completely prevented infection was the loss of the Tf receptor, in a strain (FA1090) that was a natural Lf-receptor mutant.[124]

Unfortunately, it is not possible to study sufficient numbers of volunteers to answer all possible questions. Nevertheless, the human volunteer studies have paved the way for efficient testing of a vaccine, whenever one is ready.

Summary: Pathogenic Strategies Employed by Gonococci during Infection

On the basis of the details gleaned from the studies cited above as well as other in vitro studies, one may attempt a summary of how gonococci cause infection.

Transfer

There would be no gonorrhea without sexual transfer from one person to another. Male donors probably transmit infection by means of semen, which also may facilitate ascending infection of the female genital tract. Gonococci attach to spermatozoa by means of pili[151] and possibly other adhesins. While ~70% of female partners of infected males become infected, only ~25% of males are infected after a single sexual exposure to an infected woman.[152,153]

Adherence

Using a variety of adhesins, including pili, Opa and LOS, gonococci attach to specific receptors. Rapid antigenic variation may provide the "correct" ligand for binding the particular receptors found in the particular site (pharynx, cervix, urethra, rectum, conjunctiva, other) and person. There are many receptors as discussed above, including CD 46, CD66, HSPGs and the asialoglycoprotein receptor. The lutotropin receptor also apparently is a receptor for cell-surface-exposed ribosomal protein L12.[11]

Local Growth

For many gonococci, mucosal and neutrophil Lf is a source of usable Fe rather than an inhibitor of growth. When local inflammation occurs, Tf transudes onto the mucosal surface, which also provides many of the amino acids and other nutrients required for growth because the gonococcus has lost many of the relevant biosynthetic genes.

Escape from the Immune Response

Non-specific innate defenses are overcome. These include defensins, to which gonococci are relatively resistant due to an efflux pump for hydrophobic agents.[154] Both C' and IgG transude into the genital tract from serum and also are produced locally in the genital tract.[109,110,155,156] Semen inhibits the action of C',[157] which helps protect gonococci from attack by defenses that require C'. Specific acquired antibody and C' defenses are overcome by a variety of other methods, including down-regulation of C' activity by binding Factor H and C4bp to PorB and Factor H to sialylated LOS; masking of antigens by the effects of sialylation of LOS; antigenic and phase variation of targets of specific antibodies; possible destruction of IgA1 antibodies by the action of IgA protease;[158] shedding of membrane blebs that bind antibodies at a distance from the intact bacterium, thus subverting their effects;[159] binding of IgG non-C'-fixing blocking antibodies that interfere with the effects of bactericidal antibodies; escape from phagocytosis by neutrophils (in part) by means of rapid variation in expression of Opa protein and also by sialylation of LOS; relative resistance to killing by neutrophils after ingestion, possibly due to the effects of insertion of PorB into the neutrophil; and invasion of host cells, where antibody and C' cannot follow.

Local Inflammation and Issue Injury

Gonococcal whole cells and purified components (including Opa, IgA protease, and probably other gonococcal factors) trigger synthesis and release of inflammatory cytokines and chemokines in vitro, including IL-1, IL-6, IL-8, and TNF-α.[160-163] Tissues are damaged in cell or organ culture by the effects of TNF-α.[164,165] Tissue-damaging inflammation can be triggered in vitro by both LOS and peptidoglycan fragments.[166,167]

Given the evidence for stimulation of inflammatory cytokines in vitro, from either epithelial cells or macrophages, it is curious that there is only mixed evidence for production of cytokines in vivo. Analysis of urine from experimentally-infected men showed an inflammation-associated rise and fall in the levels of many of these cytokines, including IL-1, IL-6, IL-8 and TNF-α.[168] However, studies of serum and cervical mucous from women with naturally-acquired gonorrhea showed no or very minimal elevations in the same cytokines.[169] Conceivably, the relative lack of symptoms in many infected persons could be due to relative lack of production of inflammatory cytokines. Strain-specific differences in ability to generate the chemoattractant C5a probably also contributes to differences in the degree of inflammatory response.[77,78,142]

Invasion and Intracellular Growth

Binding by Opa and Pili to their receptors triggers signaling cascades and results in actin filament rearrangements and receptor-mediated invasion of epithelial cells. Invasion also occurs by macropinocytosis.[170] Transfer of PorB into the membranes of the host cell facilitates invasion. Invasion also is facilitated by expression of an HSPG-specific Opa protein and by phase variation of LOS to prevent its sialylation. Gonococci are able to grow in the cytoplasm of epithelial cells, in part due to the unexpected effect of IgA protease in cleaving the lysosomal protein LAMP1.[171] Interestingly, IgA protease may also inhibit TNF-mediated apoptosis by cleavage of a TNF receptor.[172] Ultimately, gonococci egress from the basal surface of epithelial cells into the interstitial spaces,[171] whence they may disseminate through the blood stream.

Dissemination

Bacteremic disease and seeding of joints and occasionally heart valves or meninges is facilitated by the Tf receptor and by the multiple mechanisms for evading the killing effects of C'.

The Immune Response

The immune response to naturally-acquired infection has been studied intermittently for decades. Most studies of the specificity of the immune response have used immunoblots or purified antigens as the methods of detection, with the result that conformation-dependent epitopes might be missed. Some studies did utilize whole cells, or a radioimmunoprecipitation assay that would allow recognition of conformational epitopes on the bacterial cell surface .[173] In many studies only a single strain was used, with the result that strain-variable epitopes would be missed. Almost all published studies did not attempt to use whole cells prepared so that stress proteins would be expressed, and thus less is known about the importance of stress proteins in the immune response to infection.

Humoral and mucosal IgG and IgA antibodies develop to a number of stable surface antigens after infection as well as antigenically-variable surface proteins and LOS.[173-176] Some studies also have noted an IgM response as well.[176,177] In many cases the identity of the respective antigens on immunoblots was not identified, but antibodies do certainly develop against PorB, Opa, Rmp, LOS, H.8, and pili.[173,175,176] Sera and genital secretions from normal persons denying infection by the gonococcus often have antibodies against OMPs and LOS, suggesting there are cross-reactive antibodies against common antigens from other bacteria.[178] Gonococcal infection may cause an increase in antibody titer to these antigens. The ability of sera to exert a bactericidal effect seems to reflect a stochastic balance between the amount of blocking IgG anti-Rmp and other C'-fixing antibodies against Por and other antigens.[87] Men with uncomplicated infection are be less likely to develop a demonstrable antibody response than women.[174-176] Absence of detectable antibody to certain gonococcal antigens has been correlated with development of salpingitis, suggesting antibodies or other aspects of the immune response may be protective.[179] Sera from patients often contain antibodies against the iron stress protein FbpA that mediates periplasmic iron transport,[179] and most patients with bacteremic disease contain antibodies against high molecular weight iron-stress proteins including TbpA and TbpB in a radioimmunoprecipitation assay (W. McKenna and P F Sparling, unpublished data). Antibodies also develop against anaerobic proteins.[136] The immune response to gonorrhea has been reviewed elsewhere.[180]

In genital secretions, the most abundant antibodies typically are of the IgG class, but there is also IgA, including secretory IgA.[176,177,181,182] Almost all studies have noted the brief persistence of serum and genital antibodies after treatment, with loss of most genital IgA within a few weeks and IgG within a few months.[176,177,181,182]

A TH1 response against IgA protease can be demonstrated in uncomplicated infections,[183] as can a TH2 response against PorB.[184] In general, relatively little is known about the relative importance of a TH1 or a TH2 response; the assumption has been that secretory (genital) antibodies are the essential components of a protective response. Now that we understand that gonococci are capable of invasion of and growth within epithelial cells, it would be helpful to better define the possible role of a cytotoxic TH1 response in protection and disease.

Two recent papers are worthy of more detailed discussion, regarding the relatively weak immune response and the apparent absence of protection after reinoculation of male volunteers, respectively. Hedges et al quantified the systemic and mucosal immune responses in men and women with uncomplicated infection and found a surprising paucity of antibodies in either serum or genital secretions.[185] Uninfected controls were included, and consideration was made for the confounding effects of other genital infections, which has rarely been done in other studies. Responses were followed over time, and the possibility was examined that rectal infection of women might promote a more vigorous response because of the presence of organized lymphatic tissues in the rectum. Assays used whole organisms (both a standard strain and the patient's own isolate) as the antigen in order to be able to detect conformational and/or variable epitopes. Results showed low levels of antibodies in >100 subjects, compared to other mucosal infections. Previous infection did not increase the levels of detected antibody, suggesting a lack of memory response, and rectal infection did not influence the results. Levels of cervical mucous antibodies were substantially higher than those of vaginal wash antibodies. There was a detectable IgA1 but almost no detectable IgA2 response. Women had a slightly higher response than men, who did not show any detectable increase in antibodies compared to uninfected controls. They hypothesized that gonococci might have means to suppress an immune response, which also was suggested by their earlier studies that showed a weak inflammatory cytokine response in vivo,[169] as compared to responses that can be elicited in vitro by gonococci or defined gonococcal antigens. Recent literature suggests mechanisms for suppression of the immune response by other mucosal bacteria,[186,187] but there is no evidence as to how gonococci might accomplish this. A very interesting recent paper by Boulton and Gray-Owen[188] showed that Opa-mediated in vitro binding to CEACAM1 on $CD4^+$ T lymphocytes suppressed their activation and proliferation. It also has been observed by Muenzner et al [189] that the same Opa is capable of upregulating CEACAM1 in epithelial cells. It remains to be determined whether CEACAM1 binding in vivo results in decreased immune responses, but further developments in this area of research are anticipated eagerly.

Schmidt et al of the WRAIR group rechallenged male volunteers with the same organism with which they had been infected about three weeks previously, to examine whether there was a protective response.[144] Overall, there was no evidence for protection against reinfection: 6 of 14 rechallenged volunteers exposed to an expected ID_{50} dose of MS11 became infected, compared to 5 of 10 uninfected controls. However, retrospective subgroup analysis suggested there might be some protection, since there was a trend for reduced infection rates in those volunteers with the most vigorous antibody responses to the first infection and the longest duration of untreated initial infection. They suggested that it might take at least 4-5 days of untreated gonorrhea to develop sufficient response to demonstrate protection. Numbers of subjects were too few to draw final conclusions, except that if there was protection, it was not great.

Animal Models for Studying Vaccines

Although gonorrhea is a natural infection only of humans, a variety of small animal models have been tried, with some success but no universal acceptance. These include infection of implanted subcutaneous chambers in several animals[190-195] and use of primates, especially chimpanzees. The small animal models were used to demonstrate protective immune responses.[192-195] The chimpanzee model was most interesting because it was possible to establish mucosal genital disease that closely mimicked human infection[196,197] and because a whole-cell vaccine elicited some protection.[198] Unfortunately, the unavailability as well as expense of chimpanzees makes this model impractical. The chimpanzee studies did demonstrate specific immune responses [199] but the data were insufficient to establish immunological correlates or surrogates for protection, which is one of the great needs in this field.

Recently there has been renewed interest in the use of mice as an infection model. Jerse and colleagues showed that controlled-release of estrogens as well as use of antibiotics to reduce the bacterial colonization of the vagina permitted gonococcal infection of the vagina, with a resultant neutrophilic leukocyte response .[200] There was in vivo selection for expression of Opa proteins,[200] and iron-stress proteins were produced as well (Ann Jerse, personal communication). Nasal vaccination with an outer membrane fraction reduced the duration of infection, validating the mouse model for vaccine development.[201] Of course, mice are not humans, and there are many differences in the genital tract of mice as compared to humans, including lack of a typical cervix. Mice also do not produce the important receptors (CD 46, CD66) for binding gonococcal adherence ligands, although it is entirely possible that this problem could be overcome by construction of transgenic mice. Because the immunology and genetics of mice are so well understood, there are many advantages to vigorous pursuit of the mouse model in hopes of future rational testing of vaccine candidates.

Possible Vaccine Candidates

There are many candidates, none of which stands out. Several have attractive features as potential vaccines. Each of the listed candidates either is known to be expressed by all gonococci or is expressed by the great majority. All are surface-exposed on the intact bacterium. Certainly all of these would need to be prepared from organisms that do not express Rmp, the blocking antigen, which can be done either in recombinant *E. coli* [91]or from *rmp*$^-$ gonococci. [202]

PorB

For reasons discussed above, porin is a candidate. Because the target epitopes probably occur on surface-exposed and somewhat variable loops, it might be necessary to use multiple serovars in a combination vaccine, as has been tried for meningococcal PorA-based vaccines.[203,204] Loops 1, 5 and 7 are critical to many pathogenically important properties and also contain some of the cross-protective epitopes identified by Heckels and colleagues,[205] and efforts might well focus on these peptides. Cyclic peptides might provide conformations critical to successful immunization with PorB peptides.[206]

Rmp

Although Rmp has a bad name because it contains common domains that stimulate blocking antibody production, there also are several common epitopes that are the targets of bactericidal antibodies,[207] and they should be further investigated for their vaccine potential.

PilC and PilQ

These surface-exposed proteins have received little attention in this regard but are found in all strains, and either are critical to host cell attachment (PilC) [111-114] or are already known to be targets for bactericidal antibodies (PilQ).[119] Although each is somewhat variable in its primary amino acid sequence from strain to strain, there are many parts of the proteins that are common.

TbpA and B

Both have been shown to be potential targets for meningococcal vaccines,[125-127] and their attractiveness is increased by evidence that they are critical for mucosal infection.[124] Each is somewhat variable, but there is a good chance that the transferrin-binding domains [128] will be found to be common.

The MAb 2C7 LOS Epitope

Although no published work on the anti-idiotope LOS vaccine[28-30] has appeared in recent years, the evidence that almost all gonococci make a common antigen on the b chain of LOS that is a target for opsonic and bactericidal antibodies warrants further research.

NspA

A common22-kD OMP, with no known function, is found in all meningococci and gonococci.[208] In the case of meningococci, it is the target of bactericidal and protective antibodies.[208] Further studies are warranted.

Genomic Neisseria Antigens (GNA)

Almost all vaccine work until now has focused on known OMPs. An exciting and awesome effort was undertaken coincident with the meningococcal MC58 genomic sequencing project to identify novel common antigens that could be vaccine targets.[12] A total of 570 putative surface-exposed or exported proteins were identified, and 350 of them were expressed as recombinant proteins in *E. coli*. Each was purified and used to immunize mice, and the sera were tested to verify surface-exposure of the antigen and bactericidal activity. Several were identified as possible vaccines by these criteria and by their presence in all tested meningococci and gonococci. One of these (GNA33) was predicted to be an enzyme involved in peptidoglycan metabolism, once again proving that our expectations about which proteins will be on the cell surface can be wrong. There is little evidence about their vaccine potential for gonococci, but one of the very promising aspects of this work is that a company has invested in its development. The potential market value of a vaccine for both meningococcal disease and gonorrhea could lead to commercial development, if further work justifies the initial hopes.

Other Antigens

Among several other possible candidates, IgA protease stand out because it is immunogenic, surface-exposed, and common to all strains.

Live Attenuated Vaccines

Mutation of the *aroA* gene resulted in attenuation of infection in a guinea pig subcutaneous chamber model.[209] Introduction into this strain of a second mutation in the *lpxLII* gene resulted in further reduction in the inflammatory response, as measured by ability to elicit inflammatory cytokines in vitro from either human macrophages or neutrophils.[210] The authors speculated that such an attenuated organism could be used as the foundation of a live vaccine[210]but clinical testing of a live vaccine would be very challenging, and public acceptance of a live attenuated vaccine for installation into the genital tract would be highly problematic.

Questions

There are many questions that need to be addressed if there is to be a gonococcal vaccine.

In What Model System(s) Will It Be Developed?

There are far too many variables and too little commercial interest at present to undertake development in humans; there will first need to be more convincing evidence of possible efficacy in a model system. This probably means that the mouse model will need to be expanded and improved. Tissue culture assays for attachment, invasion and toxicity also can help in development.

How Will Test Vaccines Be Administered?

The goal will be to generate protective antibodies on the genital mucosa; serum bactericidal or opsonic antibodies would be a bonus. Studies with the pilus vaccine showed that this could be accomplished with parenteral administration of a vaccine.[109,110] However, there have been major improvements in systems for mucosal vaccination, including delivery of antigens onto other mucosal surfaces, especially the nasal mucosa.[211] Use of adjuvants such as cholera toxin or its subunits may improve mucosal antibody responses substantially.[212,213] Activated vitamin D3 apparently also has the effect of increasing mucosal antibody levels after parenteral vaccination.[214-216] Novel vectors for delivering vaccines have been developed, including viral vectors that target dendritic cells directly.[217,218] DNA vaccines offer the possibility of rapid and inexpensive development of new antigens or mixtures of antigens, and they can de delivered so as to maximize mucosal responses.[219,220] If DNA or viral vector systems can be shown to be at least as efficacious as renatured recombinant proteins, work should proceed more rapidly because it is much easier to clone DNA than it is to purify and renature recombinant proteins. Many bacterial vectors also have been created in which foreign proteins can be expressed on the cell surface,[221-223] which might aid vaccine development.

What in Vitro Surrogates Can Be Used to Predict Efficacy?

Bactericidal activity of serum antibodies has been the usual in vitro assay for potential bacterial vaccines, but that might not be appropriate in this case. Gonorrhea is a mucosal infection, and the organism has many potentially effective means by which to evade bactericidal activity, especially on the mucosa where C' levels are less than those in serum and where there is little IgM antibody. Correlates for meningococcal vaccines may be irrelevant for gonorrhea. Since anti-pilus antibodies that block attachment are correlated with ability of a pilus vaccine to protect against homologous challenge, potential vaccines should be tested for their ability to block attachment to and invasion of relevant cells. Neutrophils are an apparently important genital mucosal defense, and therefore opsonic activity would be desirable in a vaccine. The minimum requirement for further development of any candidate or combinations of candidates should be the eliciting of antibodies that bind the cell surface of a diverse group of intact whole organisms. Since gonococci spend at least part of their life cycle within epithelial cells, it will be important to determine whether a cytotoxic TH1 response will help or hinder vaccine efficacy.

What Will Be the Goals for a Vaccine?

The primary goal probably should be to prevent infection, meaning growth on the mucosal surface. This has not been as easy to achieve for bacterial vaccines as prevention of the complications of infection, such as invasive meningococcal or *Haemophilus influenzae* type *b* or pneumococcal infections. Field testing for the prevention of the main clinical consequences of gonorrhea (salpingitis and increased transmission of HIV infection) would be very difficult, whereas trials to demonstrate decreased ability to initiate infection can be done easily in male volunteers, as a first step before testing populations of males and females in real-world situations. Even a modest decrease in transmission efficiency should have a great effect on incidence of the disease, and thus a vaccine would not have to be highly efficacious to be useful for public health. However, there are theoretical arguments that a partially effective vaccine might actually be worse than no vaccine, for the former might result in selective pressures for emergence of a more virulent variant.[224]

Who Will Support Development of a Vaccine?

Gonorrhea is not at the top of the world list for new vaccines, and countries that have health systems that can pay for such a vaccine have rapidly diminishing prevalence of infection. Commercial interest in a vaccine for gonorrhea that does not also prevent meningococcal infection is not high. It may be necessary for public bodies such as the NIH to support a more vigorous vaccine effort before pharmaceutical company support can be sustained.

Conclusions

Creation of a gonococcal vaccine will require a sustained effort, and persons involved in the effort will need to see the problem as a glass half-full rather than half-empty. Because the natural immune response to uncomplicated infection is not particularly vigorous, vaccines that generate a response that is much greater than that observed in nature should be possible. We know something about ways to avoid impediments to a vaccine, such as avoidance of blocking antigens in the formulation. The main question may be whether we in the developed world care enough about a disease that is much more prevalent in other distant and poorer societies to invest the time and resources that will be necessary before we will know whether such a vaccine can be created.

Acknowledgements

We thank J Cannon, M Cohen, C Elkins and A Jerse for helpful comments and discussions, and T Burnette for assistance in preparation of the manuscript. Author's unpublished studies were supported by the National Institutes of Health (grants AI31496 and AI26837) to P F Sparling.

References

1. Platt R, Rice PA, McCormack WM. Risk of acquiring gonorrhea and prevalence of abnormal adnexal findings among women recently exposed to gonorrhea. JAMA 1983; 250:3205-3209.
2. Westrom L, Eschenbach D. Pelvic inflammatory disease. In: Holmes KK, Mardh PA, Sparling PF et al. eds. Sexually Transmitted Diseases. 3rd ed. New York: McGraw-Hill Companies Inc., 1999:783-809.
3. Hook EW, Handsfield HH. Gonococcal infections in the adult. In: Holmes KK, Mardh PA, Sparling PF et al. eds. Sexually Transmitted Diseases. 3rd ed. New York: McGraw-Hill Companies, Inc., 1999:451-472.
4. Cecil JA, Howell MR, Tawes JJ et al. Features of Chlamydia trachomatis and Neisseria gonorrhoeae infection in male army recruits. J Infect Dis 2001; 184:1216-1219.
5. Handsfield HH, Lipman TO, Harnish JP et al. Asymptomatic gonorrhea in men. Diagnosis natural course, prevalence and significance. N Engl J Med 1974; 290:117-123.
6. Fleming DT, Wasserheit JN. From epidemiological synergy to public health policy and practice: the contribution of other sexually transmitted diseases to sexual transmission of HIV infection. Sex Transm Infect 1999; 75:3-17.
7. DeNeeling AJ, van Santen-Verheuvel M, Spaargaren J et al. Antimicrobial resistance of Neisseria gonorrhoeae and emerging ciprofloxacin resistance in the Netherlands, 1991 to 1998. Antimicrob Agents Chemother 2000; 44:3184-3185.
8. Tanaka M, Nakayama H, Haraoka M et al. Antimicrobial resistance of Neisseria gonorrhoeae and high prevalence of ciprofloxacin-resistant isolates in Japan, 1993-1998. J Clin Microbiol 2000; 38:521-525.
9. Hill J. Experimental infection with Neisseria gonorrhoeae. American Journal of Syphilis, Gonorrhea, and Venereal Diseases 1942; 27:733-771.
10. Ober WB. Boswell's gonorrhea. NY Academy of Medicine 1969; 45:587-636.
11. Spence JM, Clark VL. Role of ribosomal protein L12 in gonococcal invasion of Hec1B cells. Infect Immun 2000; 68:5002-5010.
12. Pizza M, Scarlato V, Masignani V et al. Identification of vaccine candidates against serogroup B meningococcus by whole-genome sequencing. Science 2000; 287:1816-1820.
13. Eyre J, Stewart B. The treatment of gonococcus infections by vaccines. Lancet 1909; 76-81.
14. Greenberg L, Diena B, Ashton F et al. Gonococcal vaccine studies in inuvik. Can J Pub Health 1974; 65:29-33.
15. Arko RJ, Duncan WP, Brown WJ et al. Immunity in infection with Neisseria gonorrhoeae: duration and serological response in the chimpanzee. J Infect Dis 1976; 133:441-447.
16. Yamasaki R, Kerwood D, Schneider H et al. The structure of lipooligosaccharide produced by Neisseria gonorrhoeae, strain 15253, isolated from a patient with disseminated infection. J Biol Chem 1994; 269:30345-30351.

17. Minor SY, Banerjee A, Gotschlich EC. Effect of α-oligosaccharide phenotype of Neisseria gonorrhoeae strain MS11 on invasion of chang conjunctival, Hec-1-b endometrial, and ME-180 cervical cells. Infect Immun 2000; 68:6526-6534.
18. Mandrell RE, Apicella MA. Lipo-oligosaccharides (LOS) mucosal pathogens: molecular mimicry and host-modification of LOS. Immunobiol 1993; 187:382-402.
19. Burch CL, Danaher RJ, Stein DC. Antigenic variation in Neisseria gonorrhoeae: production of multiple lipooligosaccharides. J Bacteriol 1997; 179:982-986.
20. Gill MJ, McQuillen DP, VanPutten JP et al. Functional characterization of a sialyltransferase-deficient mutant Neisseria gonorrhoeae. Infect Immun 1996; 64:3374-3378.
21. Parsons NJ, Cole J, Smith H. Resistance to human serum of gonococci in urethral exudates is reduced by neuraminidase. Proc R Soc Lond B Biol Sci 1990; 241:3-5.
22. Wetzler LM, Barry K, Blake M et al. Gonococcal lipooligosaccharide sialylation prevents complement-dependent killing by immune sera. Infect Immun 1992; 60:39-43.
23. Rest RF, Frangipane JV. Growth of Neisseria gonorrhoeae in CMP-N-acetylneuraminic acid inhibits nonopsonic (opacity-associated outer membrane protein-mediated) interactions with human neutrophils. Infect Immun 1992; 60:989-997.
24. Kim JJ, Zhou D, Mandrell RE et al. Effect of exogenous sialylation of lipooligosaccharide of Neisseria gonorrhoeae on opsonophagocytosis. Infect Immun 1992; 60:4439-4442.
25. van Putten JP. Phase variation of lipopolysaccharide directs interconversion of invasive and immuno-resistant phenotypes of Neisseria gonorrhoeae. EMBO J 1993; 12:4043-4051.
26. Porat N, Apicella MA, Blake M. Neisseria gonorrhoeae utilizes and enhances the biosynthesis of the asialoglycoprotein receptor expressed on the surface of the hepatic HepG2 cell line. Infect Immun 1995; 63:1498-1506.
27. Schwan E, Robertson BD, Brade H et al. Gonococcal rfaF mutants express Rd_2 chemotype LPS and do not enter epithelial host cells. Mol Microbiol 1995; 15:267-275.
28. Gulati S, McQuillan DP, Mandrell RE et al. Immunogenicity of Neisseria gonorrhoeae lipooligosaccharide epitope 2C7, widely expressed in vivo with no immunochemical similarity to human glycosphingolipids. J Infect Dis 1996; 174:1223-1237.
29. Yamasaki R, Koshino H, Kurono S et al. Structural and immunochemical characterization of a Neisseria gonorrhoeae epitope defined by a monoclonal antibody 2C7; the antibody recognizes a conserved epitope on specific lipooligosaccharides in spite of the presence of human carbohydrate epitopes. J Biol Chem 1999; 274:36550-8.
30. Gulati S, McQuillen DP, Sharon J et al. Experimental immunization with a monoclonal anti-idiotope antibody that mimics the Neisseria gonorrhoeae lipooligosaccharide epitope 2C7. J Infect Dis 1996; 174:1238-48.
31. Swanson J. Colony opacity and protein II compositions of gonococci. Infect Immun 1982; 37:359-368.
32. Connell TD, Shaffer D, Cannon JG. Characterization of the repertoire of hypervariable regions in the protein II (opa) gene family of Neisseria gonorrhoeae. Mol Microbiol 1990; 4:439-449.
33. Stern A, Brown M, Nickel P et al. Opacity genes in Neisseria gonorrhoeae: control of phase and antigenic variation. Cell 1986; 47:61-71.
34. Bhat KS, Gibbs CP, Barrera O et al. The opacity proteins of Neisseria gonorrhoeae strain MS11 are encoded by a family of 11 complete genes. Mol Microbiol 1991; 5:1889-1901.
35. Makino S, van Putten JP, Meyer TF. Phase variation of the opacity outer membrane protein controls invasion by Neisseria gonorrhoeae into human epithelial cells. EMBO J 1991; 10:1307-1315.
36. Sugasawara R, Cannon JG, Black WJ et al. Inhibition of Neisseria gonorrhoeae attachment to HeLa cells with monoclonal antibody directed against a protein II. Infect Immun 1983; 42:980-5.
37. Bessen D, Gotschlich EC. Interactions of gonococci with HeLa cells: attachment, detachment, replication, penetration, and the role of protein II. Infect Immun 1986; 54:154-60.
38. Dekker NP, Lammel C, Mandrell RE et al. Opa (protein II) influences gonococcal organization in colonies, surface appearance, size and attachment to human fallopian tube tissues. Microb Pathog 1990; 9:19-31.
39. Weel JF, Hopman CT, van Putten JP. In situ expression and localization of Neisseria gonorrhoeae opacity proteins in infected epithelial cells: apparent role of Opa proteins in cellular invasion. J Exp Med 1991; 173:1395-1405.
40. Swanson J, Barrera O, Sola J et al. Expression of outer membrane protein II by gonococci in experimental gonorrhea. J Exp Med 1988; 168:2121-2129.

41. Jerse AE, Cohen MS, Drown PM et al. Multiple gonococcal opacity proteins are expressed during experimental urethral infection in the male. J Exp Med 1994; 179:911-920.
42. Bos MP, Hogan D, Belland RJ. Selection of Opa+ Neisseria gonorrhoeae by limited availability of normal human serum. Infect Immun 1997; 65:645-650.
43. Belland RJ, Chen T, Swanson J et al. Human neutrophil response to recombinant neisserial Opa proteins. Mol Microbiol 1992; 6:1729-1737.
44. Fischer SH, Rest RF. Gonococci possessing only certain P.II outer membrane proteins interact with human neutrophils. Infect Immun 1988; 56:1574-1579.
45. Naids FL, Belisle B, Lee N et al. Interactions of Neisseria gonorrhoeae with human neutrophils: studies with purified PII (Opa) outer membrane proteins and synthetic Opa peptides. Infect Immun 1991; 59:4628-4635.
46. Kupsch E, Knepper B, Kuroki T et al. Variable opacity (Opa) outer membrane proteins account for the cell tropisms displayed by Neisseria gonorrhoeae for human leukocytes and epithelial cells. EMBO J 1993; 12:641-650.
47. Chen T, Belland RJ, Wilson J et al. Adherence of pilus- Opa+ gonococci to epithelial cells in vitro involves heparin sulfate. J Exp Med 1995; 182:511-517.
48. Virji M, Makepeace K, Ferguson DJ et al. Carcinoembryonic antigens (CD66) on epithelial cells and neutrophils are receptors for Opa proteins of pathogenic neisseriae. Mol Microbiol 1996; 22:941-950.
49. Bos MP, Grunert F, Belland RJ. Differential recognition of members of the carcinoembryonic antigen family by Opa variants of Neisseria gonorrhoeae. Infect Immun 1997; 65:2353-2361.
50. Gray-Owen SD, Lorenzen DR, Haude A et al. Differential Opa specificities for CD66 receptors influence tissue interactions and cellular response to Neisseria gonorrhoeae. Mol Microbiol 1997; 26:971-980.
51. Duensing TD, van Putten JP. Vitronectin mediates internalization of Neisseria gonorrhoeae by chinese hamster ovary cells. Infect Immun 1997; 65:964-970.
52. Gomez-Duarte OG, Dehio M, Guzman M et al. Binding of vitronectin to Opa-expressing Neisseria gonorrhoeae mediates invasion of HeLa cells. Infect Immun 1997; 65:3857-3866.
53. van Putten JP, Duensing TD, Cole RL. Entry of OpaA+ gonococci into HEp-2 cells requires concerted action of glycosaminoglycans, fibronectin and integrin receptors. Mol Microbiol 1998; 29:369-379.
54. Freissler E, auf der Heyde A, David G et al. Syndecan-1 and syndecan-4 can mediate the invasion of Opa$_{HSPG}$-expressing Neisseria gonorrhoeae into epithelial cells. Cell Microbiol 2000; 2:69-82.
55. Grassme HU, Gulbins E, Brenner B et al. Acidic sphingomyelinase mediates entry of Neisseria gonorrhoeae into nonphagocytic cells. Cell 1997; 91:605-615.
56. Grant CC, Bos MP, Belland RJ. Proteoglycan receptor binding by Neisseria gonorrhoeae MS11 is determined by the HV-1 region of OpaA. Mol Microbiol 1999; 32:233-42.
57. Virji M, Evans D, Hadfield A et al. Critical determinants of host receptor targeting by Neisseria meningitidis and Neisseria gonorrhoeae: identification of Opa adhesiotopes on the N-domain of CD66 molecules. Mol Microbiol 1999; 34:538-551.
58. Hauck CR, Grassme HU, Bock J et al. Acid sphingomyelinase is involved in CEACAM receptor-mediated phagocytosis of Neisseria gonorrhoeae. FEBS Lett 2000; 478:260-266.
59. Plummer F, Chubb H, Simonsen JN et al. Antibodies to opacity proteins (Opa) correlate with a reduced risk of gonococcal salpingitis. J Clin Invest 1994; 93:1748-1755.
60. Heckels JE, Fletcher JN, Virji M. The potential protective effect of immunization with outer-membrane protein I from Neisseria gonorrhoeae. J Gen Microbiol 1989; 135:2269-2276.
61. Virji M, Zak K, Heckels JE. Monoclonal antibodies to gonococcal membrane protein IB; use in investigation of the potential protective effect of antibodies directed against conserved and type-specific epitopes. J Gen Microbiol 1986; 132:1621-1629.
62. Mee BJ, Thomas H, Cooke SJ et al. Structural comparison and epitope analysis of outer-membrane PIA from strains of Neisseria gonorrhoeae with differing serovar specificities. J Gen Microbiol 1993; 139:2613-2620.
63. Butt NJ, Virji M, Vayreda F et al. Gonococcal outer-membrane protein PIB: comparative sequence analysis and localization of epitopes which are recognized by type-specific and cross-reacting monoclonal antibodies. J Gen Microbiol 1990; 136:2165-2172.
64. Plummer FA, Simonsen JN, Chubb H et al. Epidemiologic evidence for the development of serovar-specific immunity after gonococcal infection. J Clin Invest 1989; 83:1472-1476.

65. Fox KK, Thomas JC, Weiner DH et al. Longitudinal evaluation of serovar-specific immunity to Neisseria gonorrhoeae. Am J Epidemiol 1999; 149:353-358.
66. Morley SL, Pollard AJ. Vaccine prevention of meningococcal disease, coming soon? Vaccine 2002; 20:666-687.
67. Feavers IM, Maiden MC. A gonococcal porA pseudogene: implications for understanding the evolution and pathogenicity of Neisseria gonorrhoeae. Mol Microbiol 1998; 30:647-656.
68. Carbonetti N, Simnad V, Elkins C et al. Construction of isogenic gonococci with variable porin structure: effects on susceptibility to human serum and antibiotics. Mol Microbiol 1990; 4:1009-1018.
69. Knapp JS, Tam MR, Nowinski RC et al. Serological classification of Neisseria gonorrhoeae with use of monoclonal antibodies to gonococcal outer membrane protein I. J Infect Dis 1984; 150:44-48.
70. van Putten JP, Duensing TD, Carlson J. Gonococcal invasion of epithelial cells driven by P.IA, a bacterial ion channel with GTP binding properties. J Exp Med 1998; 188:941-952.
71. Rudel T, Schmid A, Benz R et al. Modulation of neisseria porin (PorB) by cytostolic ATP/GTP of target cells: parallels between pathogen accommodation and mitochondrial endosymbiosis. Cell 1996; 85:391-402.
72. Lynch EC, Blake MS, Gotschlich EC et al. Reconstitution of a voltage-dependent anion-preferring porin from Neisseria gonorrhoeae. Biophys J 1983; 41:62.
73. Lynch EC, Blake MS, Gotschlich EC et al. Studies of porins spontaneously transferred from whole cells and reconstituted from purified proteins of Neisseria gonorrhoeae and Neisseria meningitidis. Biophys J 1984; 45:104-7.
74. Haines KA, Yeh L, Blake M et al. Protein I, a translocatable ion channel form Neisseria gonorrhoeae, selectively inhibits exocytosis from human neutrophils without inhibiting O_2 - generation. J Biol Chem 1988; 263:945-951.
75. Muller A, Gunther D, Dux F et al. Neisserial porin (PorB) causes rapid calcium influx in target cells and induces apoptosis by the activation of cysteine proteases. EMBO J 1999; 18:339-52.
76. Muller A, Gunther D, Brinkmann V et al. Targeting of the pro-apoptotic VDAC-like porin (PorB) of Neisseria gonorrhoeae to mitochondria of infected cells. EMBO J 2000; 19:5332-5343.
77. Ram S, Mackinnon FG, Gulati S et al. The contrasting mechanisms of serum resistance of Neisseria gonorrhoeae and group B Neisseria meningitidis. Mol Immunol 1999; 36:915-928.
78. Ram S, Cullinane M, Blom A et al. C4bp binding to porin mediates stable serum resistance of Neisseria gonorrhoeae. Int Immunopharmacol 2001; 1:423-432.
79. Smith H, Parsons NJ, Cole JA. Sialylation of neisserial lipopolysaccharide: a major influence on pathogenicity. Microb Pathog 1995; 19:365-377.
80. Qi HL, Tai JY, Blake M. Expression of large amounts of neisserial porin proteins in Escherichia coli and refolding of the proteins into native trimers. Infect Immun 1994; 62:2432-2439.
81. Hitchcock PJ. Analyses of gonococcal lipopolysaccharide in whole-cell lysates by sodium dodecyl sulfate-polyacrylamide gel electrophoresis: stable association of lipopolysaccharide with the major outer membrane protein (Protein I) of Neisseria gonorrhoeae. Infect Immun 1984; 46:202-212.
82. Elkins C, Carbonetti NH, Varela VA et al. Antibodies to N-terminal peptides of gonococcal porin are bactericidal when gonococcal lipopolysaccharide is not sialylated. Mol Mirobiol 1992; 6:2617-2628.
83. Rice PA, Vayo HE, Tam MR et al. Immunoglobulin G antibodies directed against protein III block killing of serum-resistant Neisseria gonorrhoeae by immune serum. J Exp Med 1986; 164:1735-1748.
84. Joiner KA, Scales R, Warren KA et al. Mechanism of action of blocking immunoglobulin G for Neisseria gonorrhoeae. J Clin Invest 1985; 76:1765-1772.
85. Virji M, Heckels JE. Location of a blocking epitope on outer-membrane protein III of Neisseria gonorrhoeae by synthetic peptide analysis. J Gen Microbiol 1989; 135:1895-1899.
86. Plummer FA, Chubb H, Simonsen JN et al. Antibody to Rmp (outer membrane protein 3) increases susceptibility to gonococcal infection. J Clin Invest 1993; 91:339-343.
87. Blake M, Wetzler LM. Vaccines for gonorrhea: where are we on the curve? Trends Microbiol 1995; 3:469-474.
88. Elkins C, Barkley KB, Carbonetti NH et al. Immunobiology of purified recombinant outer membrane protein I of Neisseria gonorrhoeae. Mol Microbiol 1994; 14:1059-1075.
89. Ulmer JB, Burke CJ, Shi C et al. Pore formation and mitogenicity in blood cells by the class 2 protein of Neisseria meningitidis. J Biol Chem 1992; 267:19266-19271.

90. Mackinnon FG, Ho Y, Blake M et al. The role of B/T costimulatory signals in the immunopotentiating activity of Neisserial porin. J Infect Dis 1999; 180:755-61.
91. Matsuka YV, Dilts DA, Hoiseth S et al. Characterization of a subunit structure and stability of the recombinant porin from Neisseria gonorrhoeae. Protein Chem 1998; 17:719-728.
92. Sparling PF, Yobs AR. Colonial morphology of Neisseria gonorrhoeae isolated from males and females. J Bacteriol 1967; 93:513.
93. Kellogg DS Jr., Peacock WL Jr., Deacon WE et al. Neisseria gonorrhoeae. I. Virulence genetically linked to clonal variation. J Bacteriol 1963; 85:1274-1279.
94. Kellogg DS Jr., Cohen IR, Norins LC et al. Neisseria gonorrhoeae II. Colonial variation and pathogenicity during 35 months in vitro. J Bacteriol 1968; 96:596-605.
95. Tonjum T, Koomey M. The pilus colonization factor of pathogenic neisserial species: organelle biogenesis and structure/function relationships - a review. Gene 1997; 192:155-163.
96. Sparling PF. Genetic transformation of Neisseria gonorrhoeae to streptomycin resistance. J Bacteriol 1966; 92:1364-1371.
97. Swanson J. Studies on gonococcus infection. Pili: their role in attachment of gonococci to tissue culture cells. J Exp Med 1972; 137:571-589.
98. Jonsson A, Ilver D, Falk P et al. Sequence changes in the pilus subunit lead to tropism variation of Neisseria gonorrhoeae to human tissue. Mol Microbiol 1994; 13:403-416.
99. Swanson J, Koomey JM. Mechanisms for variation of pili and outer membrane protein II in Neisseria gonorrhoeae. In: Berg DE, Howe MM, eds. Mobile DNA. Washington, DC: 1989:743-761.
100. Kallstrom H, Blackmer-Gill D, Albiger B et al. Attachment of Neisseria gonorrhoeae to the cellular pilus receptor CD46: identification of domains important for bacterial adherence. Cell Microbiol 2001; 3:133-143.
101. Kallstrom H, Islam MS, Berggren PO et al. Cell signaling by the type IV pili of pathogenic neisseria. J Biol Chem 1998; 273:21777-82.
102. Rothbard J, Fernandez R, Wang L et al. Antibodies to peptides corresponding to a conserved sequence of gonococcal pilins block bacterial adhesion. Microbiology 1985; 82:915-919.
103. Virji M, Heckels JE. The role of common and type-specific pilus antigenic domains in adhesion and virulence of gonococci for human epithelial cells. J Gen Microbiol 1984; 130:1089-1095.
104. Tramont EC, Sadoff JC, Boslego JW et al. Gonococcal pilus vaccine: studies of antigenicity and inhibition of attachment. J Clin Invest 1981; 68:881-888.
105. Schoolnik GK, Tai JY, Gotschlich EC. The pilus peptide vaccine for the prevention of gonorrhea. Prog Allergy 1983; 33:314-331.
106. Parge HE, Forest K, Hickey MJ et al. Structure of the fibre-forming protein pilin at 2.6A resolution. Nature 1995; 378:32-38.
107. Siegel M, Olsen D, Critchow C et al. Gonococcal pili: safety and immunogenicity in humans and antibody function in vitro. J Infect Dis 1982; 145:300-310.
108. Brinton Jr CC, Wood SW, Brown A et al. The development of a neisserial pilus vaccine for gonorrhea and meningococcal meningitis. In: Robbins JB, Hill CM, Sadoff JC, eds. Bacterial Vaccines. New York: Thieme-Stratton Inc., 1982:140-159.
109. McChesney DG, Tramont EC, Boslego JW et al. Genital antibody response to a parenteral gonococcal pilus vaccine. Infect Immun 1982; 36:1006-1012.
110. Boslego JW, Tramont EC, Chung RC et al. Efficacy trial of a parenteral gonococcal pilus vaccine in men. Vaccine 1991; 9:154-162.
111. Rudel T, van Putten JPM, Gibbs CP et al. Interaction of two variable proteins (PilE and PilC) required for pilus-mediated adherence of Neisseria gonorrhoeae to human epithelial cells. Mol Microbiol 1992; 6:3439-3450.
112. Rudel T, Boxberger HJ, Meyer TF. Pilus biogenesis and epithelial cell adherence of Neisseria gonorrhoeae pilC double knock-out mutants. Mol Microbiol 1995; 17:1057-1071.
113. Rudel T, Scheuerpflug I, Meyer TF. Neisseria PilC protein identified as type-4 pilus tip-located adhesin. Nature 1995; 373:357-359.
114. Morand P, Tattevin P, Eugene E et al. The adhesive property of the type IV pilus-associated component PilC1 of pathogenic neisseria is supported by the conformational structure of the N-terminal part of the molecule. Mol Microbiol 2001; 40:846-856.
115. Jonsson AB, Nyberg G, Normark S. Phase variation of gonococcal pili by frameshift mutation in pilC, a novel gene for pilus assembly. EMBO J 1991; 10:477-488.

116. Rahman M, Kallstrom H, Normark S et al. PilC of pathogenic neisseria is associated with the bacterial cell surface. Mol Microbiol 1997; 25:11-25.
117. Tsai WM, Larsen SH, Wilde CE. Cloning and DNA sequence of the omc gene encoding the outer membrane protein-macromolecular complex from Neisseria gonorrhoeae. Infect Immun 1989; 57:2653-9.
118. Drake SL, Koomey M. The product of the pilQ gene is essential for the biogenesis of type IV pili in Neisseria gonorrhoeae. Mol Microbiol 1995; 18:975-986.
119. Corbett MJ, Black JR, Wilde CE. Antibodies to outer membrane protein - macromolecular complex (OMP-MC) are bactericidal for serum-resistant gonococci. In: Poolman J, Zanen HC, Meyer TF et al. eds. Gonococci and Meningococci. Dordrecht: Kluwer Academic Publishers, 1988:685-91.
120. Thomas CE, Sparling PF. Isolation and analysis of a fur mutant of Neisseria gonorrhoeae. J Bacteriol 1996; 178:4224-4232.
121. Schryvers AB, Stojiljkovic I. Iron acquisition systems in the pathogenic neisseria. Mol Microbiol 1999; 32:1117-1123.
122. Carson SD, Klebba PE, Newton SM et al. Ferric enterobactin binding and utilization by Neisseria gonorrhoeae. J Bacteriol 1999; 181:2895-901.
123. Chen C-J, Elkins C, Sparling PF. Phase variation of hemoglobin utilization in Neisseria gonorrhoeae. Infect Immun 1998; 66:987-993.
124. Cornelissen CN, Kelley M, Hobbs MM et al. The transferrin receptor expressed by gonococcal strain FA1090 is required for the experimental infection of human male volunteers. Mol Microbiol 1998; 27:611-16.
125. Danve B, Lissolo L, Mignon M et al. Transferrin-binding proteins isolated from Neisseria meningitidis elicit protective and bactericidal antibodies in laboratory animals. Vaccine 1993; 11:1214-1220.
126. Rockbi B, Mignon M, Maitre-Wilmotte G et al. Evaluation of recombinant transferrin-binding protein B variants from Neisseria meningitidis for their ability to induce cross-reactive and bactericidal antibodies against a genetically diverse collection of serogroup B strains. Infect Immun 1997; 65:55-63.
127. West D, Reddin K, Matheson M et al. Recombinant Neisseria meningitidis transferrin binding protein A protects against experimental meningococcal infection. Infect Immun 2001; 69:1561-1567.
128. Boulton IC, Yost M, Anderson J et al. Identification of discrete domains within gonococcal transferrin-binding protein A that are necessary for ligand binding and iron uptake functions. Infect Immun 2000; 68:6988-96.
129. Petterson A, Kuipers B, Pelzer M et al. Monoclonal antibodies against the 70-kilodalton iron-regulated protein of Neisseria meningitidis are bactericidal and strain specific. Infect Immun 1990; 58:3036-3041.
130. Carson SD, Stone BJ, Beucher M et al. Phase variation of the gonococcal siderophore receptor FetA. Mol Microbiol 2000; 36:585-593.
131. Anderson J, Leone P, Miller WC et al. Selection for expression of the gonococcal hemoglobin receptor during menses. J Infect Dis 2001; 184:1621-23.
132. Pettit RK, Martin ES, Filiatrault MJ. Alteration of gonococcal protein expression in acidic culture. Infect Immun 1996; 64:1039-1042.
133. Pettit RK, Martin ES, Wagner SM et al. Phenotypic modulation of gonococcal lipooligosaccharide in acidic and alkaline culture. Infect Immun 1995; 63:2773-2775.
134. Mandrell R, Smith H, Jarvis G et al. Detection and some properties of the sialyltransferase implicated in the sialylation of lipopolysaccharide of Neisseria gonorrhoeae. Microb Pathog 1993; 14:307-13.
135. Clark VL, Campbell LA, Palermo DA et al. Induction and repression of outer membrane proteins by anaerobic growith of Neisseria gonorrhoeae. Infect Immun 1987; 55:1359-1364.
136. Clark VL, Knapp JS, Thompson S et al. Presence of antibodies to the major anaerobically induced gonococcal outer membrane protein in sera from patients with gonococcal infections. Microb Pathog 1988; 5:381-390.
137. Zheng H, Hassett DJ, Bean K et al. Regulation of catalase in Neisseria gonorrhoeae. Effects of oxidant stress and exposure to human neutrophils. J Clin Investig 1992; 90:1000-1006.
138. James JF, Swanson J. Studies on gonococcus infection. XIII. Occurence of color/opacity colonial variants in clinical cultures. Infect Immun 1978; 19:332-340.
139. Crawford C, Knapp JS, Hale J et al. Asymptomatic gonorrhea in men caused by gonococci with unique nutritional requirements. Science 1977; 196:1352-1353.

140. Brunham RC, Plummer F, Slaney L et al. Correlation of auxotype and protein I type with expression of disease due to Neisseria gonorrhoeae. J Infect Dis 1985; 152:339-43.
141. Whittington WL, Holmes KK. Unique gonococcal phenotype associated with asymptomatic infection in men and with erroneous diagnosis of nongonococcal urethritis. J Infect Dis 2000; 181:1044-1048.
142. Ross SC, Densen P. Opsonophagocytosis of Neisseria gonorrhoeae: interaction of local and disseminated isolates with complement and neutrophils. J Infect Dis 1985; 151:33-41.
143. Cohen MS, Cannon JG. Human experimentation with Neisseria gonorrhoeae: progress and goals. J Infect Dis 1999; 179:S375-9.
144. Schmidt KA, Schneider H, Lindstrom JA et al. Experimental gonococcal urethritis and reinfection with homologous gonococci in male volunteers. Sex Transm Dis 2001; 28:555-564.
145. Schneider H, Griffiss JM, Boslego J et al. Expression of paragloboside-like lipooligosaccharides may be a necessary component of gonococcal pathogenesis in men. J Exp Med 1991; 174:1601-05.
146. Schmidt KA, Deal CD, Kwan M et al. Neisseria gonorrhoeae MS11mkC opacity protein expression in vitro and during human volunteer infectivity studies. Sex Transm Dis 1999; 27:278-83.
147. Swanson J, Robbins K, Barrera O et al. Gonococcal pilin variants in experimental gonorrhea. J Exp Med 1987; 165:1344-1357.
148. Seifert HS, Wright CJ, Jerse AE et al. Multiple gonococcal pilin antigenic variants are produced during experimental human infections. J Clin Invest 1994; 93:2744-2749.
149. Harvey HA, Jennings MP, Campbell CA et al. Receptor-mediated endocytosis of Neisseria gonorrhoeae into primary human urethral epithelial cells: the role of the asialoglycoprotein receptor. Mol Microbiol 2001; 42:659-672.
150. Johannsen DB, Johnston DM, Koymen HO et al. A Neisseria gonorrhoeae immunoglobulin A1 protease mutant is infectious in the human challenge model of urethral infection. Infect Immun 1999; 67:3009-13.
151. James-Holmquest AN, Swanson J, Buchanan TM et al. Differential attachment by piliated and nonpiliated Neisseria gonorrhoeae to human sperm. Infect Immun 1974; 9:897-902.
152. Holmes KK, Johnson DW, Trostle HJ. An estimate of the risk of men acquiring gonorrhea by sexual contact with infected females. Am J Epidemiol 1970; 91:170-74.
153. Lin JS, Donegan SP, Heeren TC et al. Transmission of Chlamydia trachomatis and Neisseria gonorrhoeae among men with urethritis and their female sex partners. J Infect Dis 1998; 178:1707-12.
154. Shafer WM, Qu X, Waring AJ et al. Modulation of Neisseria gonorrhoeae susceptibility to vertebrate antibacterial peptides due to a member of the resistance/nodulation/division efflux pump family. Proc Natl Acad Sci U S A 1998; 95:1829-1833.
155. Tramont EC. Inhibition of Neisseria gonorrhoeae by human genital secretions. J Clin Invest 1977; 59:117-123.
156. McMillan A, McNeillage G, Young H. Antibodies to Neisseria gonorrhoeae: a study of the urethral exudates of 232 men. J Infect Dis 1979; 140:89-95.
157. Brooks GF, Lammel CJ, Petersen BH et al. Human seminal plasma inhibition of antibody complement-mediated killing and opsonization of Neisseria gonorrhoeae and other gram-negative organisms. J Clin Invest 1981; 67:1523-1531.
158. Plaut AG, Gilbert JV, Artenstein MS et al. Neisseria gonorrhoeae and Neisseria meningitidis: extracellular enzyme cleaves human immunoglobulin A. Science 1975; 190:1103-05.
159. Dorward D, Garon CF, Judd RC. Export and intercellular transfer of DNA via membrane blebs of Neisseria gonorrhoeae. J Bacteriol 1989; 171:2499-2505.
160. Lorenzen DR, Dux F, Wolk U et al. Immunoglobulin A1 protease, an exoenzyme of pathogenic Neisseriae, is a potent inducer of proinflammatory cytokines. J Exp Med 1999; 190:1049-1058.
161. Makepeace BL, Watt PJ, Heckels JE et al. Interactions of Neisseria gonorrhoeae with mature human macrophage opacity proteins influence production of proinflammatory cytokines. Infect Immun 2001; 69:1909-1913.
162. Fichorova RN, Desai PJ, Gibson FC et al. Distinct proinflammatory host responses to Neisseria gonorrhoeae infection in immortalized human cervical and vaginal epithelial cells. Infect Immun 2001; 69:5840-5848.
163. Naumann M, Webler S, Bartsch C et al. Neisseria gonorrhoeae epithelial cell interaction leads to the activation of the transcription factors nuclear factor kB and activator protein 1 and the induction of inflammatory cytokines. J Exp Med 1997; 186:247-258.

164. McGee ZA, Clemens CM, Jensen RL et al. Local induction of tumor necrosis factor as a molecular mechanism of mucosal damage by gonococci. Microb Pathog 1992; 12:333-341.
165. McGee ZA, Jensen RL, Clemens CM et al. Gonococcal infection of human fallopian tube mucosa in organ culture: relationship of mucosal tissue TNF-α concentration to sloughing of ciliated cells. Sex Transm Dis 1999; 26:160-65.
166. Gregg CR, Melly MA, Hellerqvist CG et al. Toxic activity of purfied lipopolysaccharide of Neisseria gonorrhoeae for human fallopian tube mucosa. J Infect Dis 1981; 143:432-39.
167. Melly MA, McGee ZA, Rosenthal RS. Ability of monomeric peptidoglycan fragments from Neisseria gonorrhoeae to damage human fallopian-tube mucosa. J Infect Dis 1984; 149:378-85.
168. Ramsey KH, Schneider H, Cross AS et al. Inflammatory cytokines produced in response to experimental human gonorrhea. J Infect Dis 1995; 172:186-191.
169. Hedges SR, Sibley DA, Mayo MS et al. Cytokine and antibody responses in women infected with Neisseria gonorrhoeae: effects of concomitant infections. J Infect Dis 1998; 178:742-51.
170. Zenni MK, Giardina PC, Harvey HA et al. Macropinocytosis as a mechanism of entry into primary human urethral epithelial cells by Neisseria gonorrhoeae. Infect Immun 2000; 68:1696-1699.
171. Lin LP, Ayala J, Larson JA et al. The neisseria type 2 IgA1 protease cleaves LAMP1 and promotes survival of bacteria within epithelial cells. Mol Microbiol 1997; 24:1083-1084.
172. Beck SC, Meyer TF. IgA1 protease from Neisseria gonorrhoeae inhibits TNF alpha-mediated apoptosis of human monocytic cells. FEBS Lett 2000; 472:287-92.
173. Zak K, Diaz JL, Jackson D et al. Antigenic variation during infection with Neisseria gonorrhoeae: detection of antibodies to surface proteins in sera of patients with gonorrhea. J Infect Dis 1984; 149:166-174.
174. Ward ME, Glynn AA. Human antibody response to lipopolysaccharides from Neisseria gonorrhoeae. J Clin Path 1972; 25:56-59.
175. Lammel CJ, Sweet RL, Rice PA et al. Antibody-antigen specificity in the immune response to infection with Neisseria gonorrhoeae. J Infect Dis 1985; 152:990-1000.
176. Tapchaisri P, Sirisinha S. Serum and secretory antibody responses to Neisseria gonorrhoeae in patients with gonococcal infections. Br J Vener Dis 1976; 52:374-80.
177. McMillan A, McNeillage G, Young H et al. Secretory antibody response of the cervix to infection with Neisseria gonorrhoeae. Br J Vener Dis 1979; 55:265-270.
178. Hicks CB, Boslego JW, Brandt B. Evidence of serum antibodies to Neisseria gonorrhoeae before gonococcal infection. J Infect Dis 1987; 155:1276-1281.
179. Fohn MJ, Mietzner TA, Hubbard TW et al. Human immunoglobulin G antibody response to the major gonococcal iron-regulated protein. Infect Immun 1987; 55:3065-3069.
180. Elkins C, Sparling PF. Immunobiology of Neisseria gonorrhoeae. In: Quinn TC, ed. Sexually Transmitted Diseases. New York: Raven Press, 1992:113-39.
181. Kearns DH, O'Reilly RJ, Lee L et al. Secretory IgA antibodies in the urethral exudate of men with uncomplicated urethritis due to Neisseria gonorrhoeae. J Infect Dis 1973; 127:99-101.
182. O'Reilly RJ, Lee L, Welch BG. Secretory IgA antibody responses to Neisseria gonorrhoeae in the genital secretions for infected females. J Infect Dis 1976; 133:113-125.
183. Tsirpouchtsidis A, Hurwitz R, Brinkmann V et al. Neisserial immunoglobulin A1 protease induces specific T-cell responses in humans. Infect Immun 2002; 70:335-344.
184. Simpson SD, Ho Y, Rice PA et al. T lymphocyte response to Neisseria gonorrhoeae porin in individuals with mucosal gonococcal infections. J Infect Dis 1999; 180:762-73.
185. Hedges SR, Mayo MS, Mestecky J et al. Limited local and systemic antibody responses to Neisseria gonorrhoeae during uncomplicated genital infections. Infect Immun 1999; 67:3937-46.
186. Neish AS, Gewirtz AT, Zeng H et al. Prokaryotic regulation of epithelial responses by inhibition of IκB-α ubiquitination. Science 2000; 289:1560-1563.
187. Islam D, Bandholtz L, Nilsson J et al. Downregulation of bacterial peptides in enteric infections: A novel immune escape mechanism with bacterial DNA as a potential regulator. Nat Med 2001; 7:180-85.
188. Boulton IC, Gray-Owen SD. Neisserial binding to CEACAMI arrests the activation and proliferation of CD4+T lymphocytes. Nat Immunol 2002; 3(3):229-36.
189. Muenzner P, Billker O, Meyer TF et al. Nuclear factor-kappa B directs carcinoembryonic antigen-related cellular adhesion molecule 1 receptor expression in Neisseria gonorrhoeae-infected epithelial cells. J Biol Chem 2002; 277(9):7438-46.

190. Robertson JN. Protection by monospecific gonococcal antisera of the chicken embryo challenged with Neisseria gonorrhoeae. J Med Microbiol 1979; 12:283-89.
191. Arko Rj. Neisseria gonorrhoeae experimental infection of laboratory animals. Science 1972; 177:1200-1201.
192. Arko RJ. An imunologic model in laboratory animals for the study of Neisseria gonorrhoeae. J Infect Dis 1974; 129:451-55.
193. Scales RW, Kraus SJ. Development and passive transfer of immunity to gonococcal infection in guinea pigs. Infect Immun 1974; 10:1040-43.
194. Arko RJ, Smith S, Chen C. Neisseria gonorrhoeae: vaginal clearance and its correlation with resistance to infection in subcutaneous chambers in orally immunized estradiol-primed mice. Vaccine 1997; 15:1344-48.
195. Corbeil LB, Wunderlich AC, Lyons JM et al. Specific cross-protective antigonococcal immunity in the murine genital tract. Can J Microbiol 1984; 30:482-487.
196. Lucas CT, Chandler F, Martin JE et al. Transfer of gonococcal urethritis from man to chimpanzee. JAMA 1971; 216:1612-1614.
197. Brown WJ, Lucas CT, Kuhn US. Gonorrhoea in the chimpanzee: infection with laboratory-passed gonococci and by natural transmission. Br J Vener Dis 1972; 48:177-178.
198. Arko RJ, Kraus SJ, Brown WJ et al. Neisseria gonorrhoeae: effects of systemic immunization on resistance of chimpanzees to urethral infection. J Infect Dis 1974; 130:160-164.
199. Brown WJ, Lucas CT. Gonorrhoea in the chimpanzee: serological testing. Br J Vener Dis 1973; 49:441-445.
200. Jerse AE. Experimental gonococcal genital tract infection and opacity protein expression in estradiol-treated mice. Infect Immun 1999; 67:5699-5708.
201. Plante M, Jerse AE, Hamel J et al. Intranasal immunization with gonococcal outer membrane preparations reduces the duration of vaginal colonization of mice by Neisseria gonorrhoeae. J Infect Dis 2000; 182:848-55.
202. Wetzler LM, Blake M, Barry K et al. Gonococcal porin vaccine evaluation: comparison of Por proteosomes, liposomes, and blebs isolated from rmp deletion mutants. J Infect Dis 1992; 166:551-55.
203. van der Ley P, van der Biezen J, Poolman J. Construction of Neisseria meningitidis strains carrying multiple chromosomal copies of the porA gene for use in the production of a multivalent outer membrane vesicle vaccine. Vaccine 1995; 13:401-07.
204. Peeters M, Rumke HC, Sundermann LC et al. Phase 1 clinical trial with a hexavalent PorA containing meningococcal outer membrane vesicle vaccine. Vaccine 1996; 14:1009-1015.
205. Heckels JE, Virji M, Tinsley CR. Vaccination against gonorrhea: the potential protective effect of immunization with synthetic peptides containing epitopes of gonococcal outer-membrane protein IB. Vaccine 1990; 8:225-230.
206. Hoogerhout P, Donders EM, van Gaans van den Brink JA et al. Conjugates of synthetic cyclic peptides elicit bactericidal antibodies against a conformational epitope on a class 1 outer membrane protein of Neisseria meningitidis. Infect Immun 1995; 63:3473-3478.
207. Virji M, Zak K, Heckels JE. Outer membrane protein III of Neisseria gonorrhoeae: variations in biological properties of antibodies directed against different epitopes. J Gen Microbiol 1987; 133:3393-3401.
208. Martin D, Cadieux N, Hamel J et al. Highly conserved Neisseria meningitidis surface protein confers protection against experimental infection. J Exp Med 1997; 185:1173-1183.
209. Chamberlain LM, Strugnell R, Dougan G et al. Neisseria gonorrhoeae strain MS11 harbouring a mutation in gene aroA is attenuated and immunogenic. Microb Pathog 1993; 15:51-63.
210. Ellis C, Lindner B, Khan MA et al. The Neisseria gonorrhoeae lpxLII gene encodes for a late-functioning lauroyl acyl transferase, and a null mutation within the gene has a significant effect on the induction of acute inflammatory responses. Mol Microbiol 2001; 42:167-181.
211. Saunders NB, Shoemaker DR, Brandt BL et al. Immunogenicity of intranasally administered meningococcal native outer membrane vesicles in mice. Infect Immun 1999; 67:113-119.
212. Hajishengallis G, Hollingshead SK, Koga T et al. Mucosal immunization with a bacterial protein antigen genetically coupled to cholera toxin A2/B subunits. J Immunol 1995; 154:4322-4332.
213. George-Chandy A, Eriksson K, Lebens M et al. Cholera toxin B subunit as a carrier molecule promotes antigen presentation and increases CD40 and CD86 expression on antigen-presenting cells. Infect Immun 2001; 69:5716-5725.

214. Daynes R, Enioutina E, Butler S et al. Induction of common mucosal immunity by hormonally immunomodulated peripheral immunization. Infect Immun 1996; 64:1100-1109.
215. Enioutina E, Visic D, McGee ZA et al. The induction of systemic and mucosal immune responses following the subcutaneous immunization of mature adult mice: characterization of the antibodies in mucosal secretions of animals immunized with antigen formulations containing a vitamin D3 adjuvant. Vaccine 1999; 17:3050-3064.
216. Enioutina E, Visic D, Daynes R. The induction of systemic and mucosal immune response to antigen-adjuvant compositions administered into the skin: alterations in the migratory properties of dendritic cells appears to be important for stimulating mucosal immunity. Vaccine 2000; 18:2753-2767.
217. Davis N, Powell N, Greenwald GF et al. Attenuating mutations in the E2 glycoprotein gene of venezuelan equine encephalitis virus: construction of single and multiple mutants in a full-length cDNA clone. Virology 1991; 183:20-31.
218. Davis N, Brown K, Johnston R. A viral vaccine vector that expresses foreign gene in lymph nodes and protects against mucosal challenge. J Virol 1996; 70:3781-3787.
219. Amara RR, Villinger F, Altman J et al. Control of a mucosal challenge and prevention of AIDS by a multiprotein DNA/MVA vaccine. Science 2001; 292:69-74.
220. Bosarge JR, Watt JM, McDaniel DO et al. Genetic immunization with the region encoding the α-helical domain of PspA elicits protective immunity against Streptococcus pneumoniae. Infect Immun 2001; 69:5456-5463.
221. Huang Y, Hajishengallis G, Michalek SM. Induction of protective immunity against Streptococcus mutans colonization after mucosal immunization with attenuated Salmonella enterica serovar typhimurium expressing and S. mutans adhesin under the control of in vivo-inducible nirB promoter. Infect Immun 2001; 69:2154-2161.
222. Wang J, Michel V, Leclerc C et al. Immunogenicity of viral B-cell epitopes inserted into two surface loops of the Escherichia coli K12 LamB protein and expressed in an attenuated aroA strain of Salmonella typhimurium. Vaccine 1999; 17:1-12.
223. Klemm P, Schembri MA. Fimbrial surface display systems in bacteria: from vaccines to random libraries. Microbiology 2000; 146:3025-3032.
224. Gandon S, MacKinnon MJ, Nee S et al. Imperfect vaccines and the evolution of pathogen virulence. Nature 2001; 414:751-56.

Chapter 10

Group A *Streptococcus* Vaccine Research: Historical Synopsis and New Insights

Sean D. Reid, Kimmo Virtaneva and James M. Musser

Group A *Streptococcus* Distribution, Disease Complexity, Resurgence and Impact

Streptococcus pyogenes, commonly referenced to as Lancefield group A *Streptococcus* (GAS), is a gram positive human pathogen that causes a variety of diseases including pharyngitis, scarlet fever, necrotizing fasciitis, and streptococcal toxic shock syndrome (STSS). Post-infectious sequelae such as acute rheumatic fever (ARF), subsequent rheumatic heart disease (RHD), and acute glomerulonephritis can occur after GAS infection.[1] ARF and RHD are the most common causes of preventable pediatric heart disease globally. The only known reservoir of GAS is humans, and the organism is generally disseminated by individuals with symptomatic infection of the mucous membranes or skin, although asymptomatic carriers can also transmit the pathogen. GAS is the most common cause of bacterial upper respiratory tract infection in all age groups in the United States.[2] Prompt diagnosis and treatment of acute GAS pharyngitis is necessary to reduce the risk of transmission, and to prevent suppurative complications and post-streptococcal sequelae. The intent of this chapter is to provide a historical synopsis of GAS vaccine research, discuss recent advances in the field, and highlight prospects for the future. The reader is referred to refs. 1, and 3-8 for additional information about GAS pathogenesis and the history of GAS disease.

Disease in the United States and Other Western Countries

Approximately 15 million cases of streptococcal pharyngitis are estimated to occur annually in the United States, representing 15-30% of all childhood cases of acute pharyngitis and 5-10% of adult cases.[9] The annual direct health care costs associated with pharyngitis are approximately 2 billion dollars.[10]

Historically, GAS infections have been a major cause of morbidity and mortality in the United States. For example, nearly 25,000 patients were hospitalized with scarlet fever at Boston City Hospital between 1895-1905; the case-fatality rate was almost 15%. At the same time, scarlet fever was considered to be pandemic, and many cases were reported in Great Britain and in Europe.[3] Although many of the reports prior to the 1900's did not differentiate between scarlet fever and pharyngitis, the recorded numbers are striking.

The incidence of ARF in the United States was also high in the beginning of the 20th century with mortality rates due to rheumatic fever (RF) reaching 7 per 100,000 cases.[4] During World War II, a very large RF outbreak occurred among recruits at Great Lakes U.S. Naval training center, with 21,209 cases recorded. Moreover, examination of 13 million armed forces recruits in 1943 identified almost 100,000 individuals with clinical findings consistent with RF and RHD.[11]

New Bacterial Vaccines, edited by Ronald W. Ellis and Bernard R. Brodeur.

Morbidity and mortality rates due to GAS infections and post-streptococcal sequelae decreased after World War II.[3,6,11] By 1965 the number of reported RF cases in the U.S. had dropped to 4,998, and by 1984 the number had decreased to 117 cases. The RF mortality rate by 1981 was 0.5 cases per 100,000.[3,11] Widespread use of penicillin to treat GAS pharyngitis and improved access to medical care were responsible for some of this decline. Better nutrition and standards of hygiene also were thought to have played a role.

The decline in the case rate of ARF did not continue. Outbreaks of ARF occurred in the 1980's and early 1990's in Utah, Ohio, New York, Tennessee and Missouri,[4,6] but the reasons for the resurgence remains unknown. Similar increases in Europe have not been documented.

Resurgence of Invasive Disease

The late 1980's and early 1990's saw an increase in the incidence of invasive GAS infections including the number of cases of streptococcal toxic shock (Fig. 1). Increases were documented in many countries, including the United States, Canada, United Kingdom, Sweden, Norway, Finland, New Zealand, Australia, and Japan.[6] In the majority of cases, resurgent disease was associated with GAS strains belonging to two clonal lineages (ET1 and ET2) which expressed

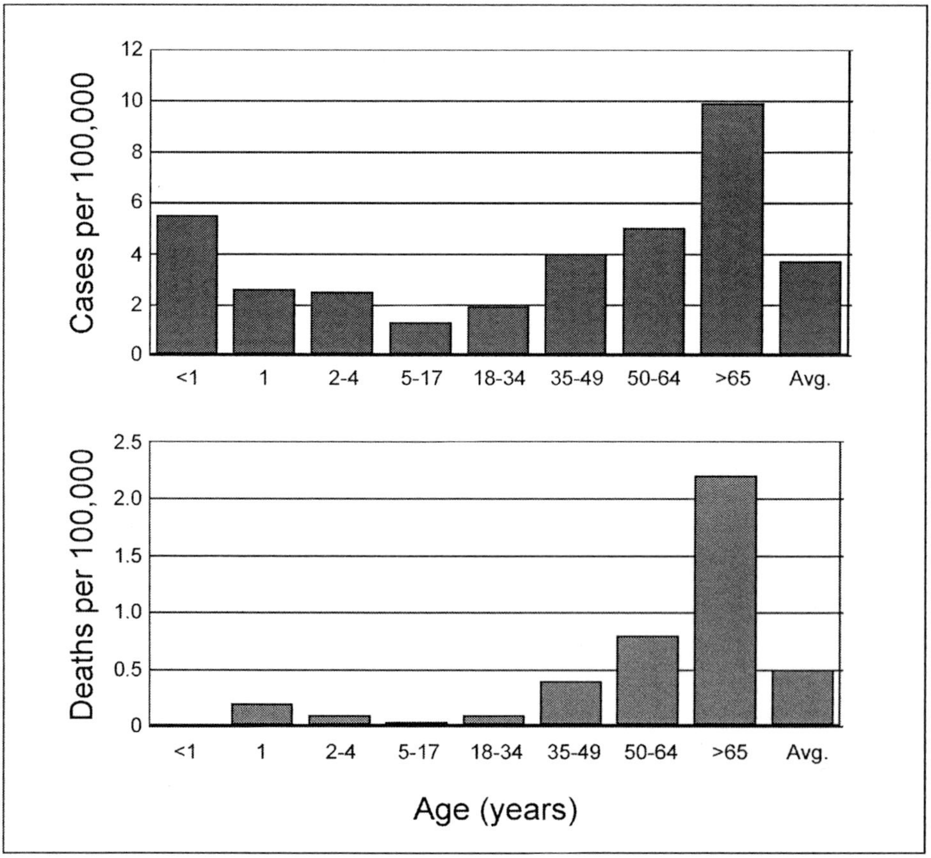

Figure 1. Morbidity and mortality associated with invasive group A streptococcal disease for the year 2001 based on the surveillance of 30,675,124 persons from 9 states. The data were collected as part of the Active Bacterial Core Surveillance (ABCs), Emerging Infections Program Network (http://www.cdc.gov/ncidod/dbmd/abcs/gas01.pdf).

M protein serotypes 1 and 3 respectively.[12] Furthermore, members of these clones were found to produce an exotoxin (streptococcal pyrogenic exotoxin A, SpeA) that is a superantigen.[6] The molecular basis of the reemergence of GAS disease is unknown, but a change in herd immunity (i.e., the immune status of a host population) is one possible contributing factor. For example, a series of studies demonstrated that patients with mild GAS infections had high serum antibody levels to streptococcal pyrogenic exotoxin B (SpeB). Conversely, patients with severe GAS infections had low SpeB antibody levels, and those with fatal infections had the lowest measured levels of antibody directed against SpeB.[13-16]

Strains of GAS can vary considerably from one another at the genetic level and this variation can affect disease severity.[17] Therefore, it is possible that an additional factor leading to the resurgence of severe GAS disease was the emergence of a new genetic variant of GAS with increased fitness. Hoe et al[18] have studied a hypervariable gene (*sic*) that inhibits human complement function. Comparative sequencing of *sic* from >1100 strains of GAS isolated from a population-based surveillance of disease in three countries indicated that *sic* undergoes rapid diversification on human mucosal surfaces.[18-20] Interestingly, the *sic* gene is limited to serotype M1 GAS. Recent evidence suggests that Sic inhibits binding of GAS to human epithelial cells thereby preventing internalization and killing, and promoting long-term survival and dissemination.[21]

Replacement of GAS M Protein Serotype in Host Populations

Several studies have reported shifts in the predominant M protein serotype infecting civilian populations over a period of months to years.[22-26] Moreover, a recent epidemiological study of GAS pharyngitis in a semi-closed population of 500 children and adults documented a rapid change in the most abundant M protein serotype.[27] In a 6-month period (July 1, 1999 – Dec. 31, 1999), 92% of isolates obtained from 111 throat cultures positive for GAS were serotype M1.[27] In the following three months (Jan. 1, 2000 – Mar. 31, 2000), M6 was the most predominate serotype (84%), isolated from 126 throat cultures positive for GAS.[27] It is unclear if this observation represents a common but seldom documented epidemiological event among GAS populations, or if serotype replacement is limited to a subset of abundant serotypes.

GAS Disease in Developing Countries

GAS is responsible for considerable global morbidity and mortality.[6] Thus, it is clear that the disease burden in the developing world should be taken into account in any consideration of a GAS vaccine. Globally, an estimated 12 million people are currently affected by RF/RHD; 2 million patients need repeated hospitalization and one million will require heart surgery within five to twenty years (http://www.who.int/inf-pr-1999/en/pr99-73.html). Developing countries face an annual incidence of RF/RHD that is 100-200 times higher than in developed countries,[28] resulting in 0.4 million deaths per year (http://www.who.int/inf-pr-1999/en/pr99-73.html). RHD is the most common cause of preventable heart disease in children in many developing countries.[29] In 1986, the World Health Organization (WHO) conducted a five year comprehensive study of RF/RHD in sixteen developing countries located in five regions around the world.[30] A total of 1.4 million school children were screened, and an average of 2.2 per 1,000 were diagnosed with RF/RHD. The prevalence was higher in Africa (4.7 cases per 1,000) and in the Eastern Mediterranean countries (4.4 cases per 1,000). Smaller studies have identified additional areas where the prevalence of RF/RHD is unusually high. For example, the prevalence of RF/RHD was reported to be 6.9 cases per 1,000 children in poor areas of Johannesburg, South Africa,[31] and a remarkably high prevalence of 24 cases per 1,000 was found in an Aboriginal community in Northern Australia.[32]

Streptococcal pyoderma is also common in developing countries where poor hygiene and crowding predominate. However, only limited data bearing on molecular pathogenesis, epidemiology, and health care burden are available.[33-36]

Historical Account of Early GAS Vaccine Efforts

In general, early vaccine studies focused on two approaches to stimulate an immune response to protect against GAS infection. One strategy sought to stimulate local mucosal immunity and the other to induce circulating type-specific immunity. In 1906, Gabritschewsky developed a whole-cell vaccine from streptococci isolated from a case of scarlet fever.[37] Administration of this vaccine to thousands of children in Europe appeared to reduce the number of cases of scarlet fever, however, complications associated with GAS disease were not significantly reduced.[37] In 1924, Dick and Dick reported that a vaccine consisting of streptococcal erythrogenic toxin (scarlet fever toxin) provided protection against scarlet fever.[38] Coburn and Pauli later demonstrated that antibodies to erythrogenic toxin inhibited the formation of the scarletinal rash, but did not prevent streptococcal infection.[39] Nonetheless, these efforts stimulated additional investigations, and in 1946 Watson, Rothbard and Swift presented evidence that M type-specific immunity could be achieved in nonhuman primates by intranasal inoculation of GAS.[40]

Protective Immunity by Type-Specific IgG

Rebecca Lancefield is responsible for the early work that elucidated the basis of type-specific immunity against GAS. Her extensive characterization of the M protein established it as an important determinant of virulence, and demonstrated that it elicited protective anti-M antibody in the serum of immunized animals and the serum of humans following GAS pharyngitis.[41-43] These studies also indicated that anti-M antibody was type-specific.[41-43] Later work by Hirst and Lancefield demonstrated that active immunization of mice with M protein also conferred type-specific protection.[44] These studies stimulated investigations in which heat-killed GAS strains of specific M types were used to vaccinate human subjects. However, bactericidal antibodies were produced only in some vaccines. For example, Rantz and colleagues demonstrated that subcutaneous vaccination of human volunteers with varying concentrations of heat killed type 3 or type 17 organisms elicited type-specific antibodies only in those individuals who received higher doses of M protein over an extended period.[45] Similarly, only a subset of human volunteers vaccinated with partially purified M19 protein generated type-specific antibodies.[46]

Beachey, Dale, and colleagues have contributed extensively to efforts designed to formulate a multivalent M protein vaccine.[47-49] One such multivalent vaccine has been developed from the NH_2-terminal portion of M protein peptides from types 1, 3, 5, 6, 19, and 24 GAS.[50] This hexavalent vaccine was immunogenic in rabbits and mice, and evoked bactericidal antibodies against each of the serotypes represented in the formulation. Evidence also has been presented that the vaccine does not evoke an autoimmune response in mice or rabbits.[10,50] Currently, the hexavalent vaccine formulation is being tested in a phase I human clinical trial conducted at the Center for Vaccine Development at the University of Maryland. The trial is a dose-escalating study consisting of three groups of human volunteers. Initial results from the trial indicate that the majority of individuals in the first two groups developed serum antibodies against the hexavalent vaccine (J. Dale, personal communication). In addition, many individuals developed either primary or secondary opsonic antibodies (J. Dale, personal communication). The results from the immunization of the third group of volunteers is forthcoming. Importantly, the phase I trial demonstrated that the vaccine was safe, well-tolerated, and immunogenic.

The results from study of the hexavalent M protein vaccine have prompted Dale and colleagues to develop a 26-valent formulation.[51] This vaccine is composed of four different recombinant fusion proteins, each containing six or seven M protein fragments chosen because they are representative of serotypes frequently recovered from cases of GAS disease, or because they are historically "rheumatogenic."[51] In rabbit models, the vaccine was immunogenic, and the sera was broadly opsonic against many of the 26 different GAS serotypes.[51] Importantly, the 26-valent rabbit antisera showed bactericidal activity against some strains of serotype M4 streptococci suggesting that protection may be conferred against serotypes not represented in the 26-valent formulation.[51] Indirect immunofluorescence assays indicated that immune sera did not cross-react with tissue samples of human heart, brain, kidney, or cartilage.[51] A phase I human trial to test the safety of the 26-valent formulation (under the direction of Dr. Scott Halperin) has been completed. The vaccine was safe, well-tolerated, and highly immunogenic (J. Dale, personal communication). The vaccine has now entered phase II clinical trials, in which 70 additional adult volunteers have been enrolled. The phase II trials will be expanded to include preschool age children, pending initial results and appropriate regulatory approvals (J. Dale, personal communication).

Recently, a similar multi-determinant strategy was used to construct a septavalent vaccine from NH_2-terminal regions representing M types common among Australian Aboriginal populations. The vaccine produced a specific T cell-dependent immune response in mice.[52]

Nontype-Specific Protection and Mucosal Immunity

The mechanism by which natural mucosal immunity is attained has remained unclear. Evidence suggests that IgA present on the host mucosal surface inhibits GAS colonization in the nasopharynx. Fox and associates[53-56] demonstrated that intranasal delivery of purified M protein provided more effective protection of human subjects from homologous challenge than subcutaneous delivery. Evidence to support the development of mucosal immunity to multiple GAS strains is shown by the general decrease in incidence of streptococcal pharyngitis in adults, presumably due to naturally acquired immunity.[9,57]

Fischetti and colleagues have explored the possibility of a mucosal vaccine for nonserotype-specific protection against GAS based on the M protein. The structure of M protein consists of two N-terminal repeat regions (designated A and B) which are antigenically variable. Antibodies directed against these regions are able to confer M type-specific protection. Adjacent to the variable A and B regions is a set of amino acid repeats which are conserved in the species (designated C-repeats). Fischetti et al[58] demonstrated that human patient sera contained antibodies to the C-repeat region of several different M protein serotypes, but the sera did not necessarily possess antibodies to the N-terminal epitopes of the same serotypes. Furthermore, passive immunization of mice with pooled human and rabbit anti-M protein sIgA resulted in protection of mice from GAS colonization after intranasal challenge.[58] Subsequent investigation determined that active immunization of mice with the conserved region of the M6 protein (delivered as a cholera toxin B subunit conjugate) was able to protect against homologous and heterologous colonization.[59,60]

Good and colleagues have constructed a peptide consisting of amino acids 344-355 of the M protein C region which contains a conformational B-cell epitope.[61] The peptide, referred to as J8, was synthesized directly onto the amino groups of a polylysine core resulting in a lipid core peptide construct with a lipidic anchor moiety and self-adjuvanting properties (LCP-J8).[61] Parenteral immunization of mice with LCP-J8 in the absence of additional adjuvant led to the development of high titers of specific J8 antibodies.[61] J8 antisera was opsonic for 4 heterologous GAS strains and was not cross-reactive with human heart tissue.[61] The results suggest that it may be possible to generate an efficacious GAS vaccine without the need for potentially toxic adjuvants.

Several immunization methods have resulted in protecting mice from GAS colonization after intranasal challenge including attenuated *Salmonella typhimurium* expressing M6 protein,[62] live *Salmonella dublin* expressing the N-terminal epitope of M5 protein,[63] and vaccinia virus expressing recombinant M6 protein.[64] In addition, the gram positive human oral commensal *Streptococcus gordonii* has been used as a live vector to immunize mice. *S. gordonii* expressing the NH_2 terminal region of M6 protein fused with either allergen Ag5.2 from white face hornet venom, or E7 papillomavirus type 16, elicited mucosal IgA and a specific IgG response.[65,66]

Table 1. Group A streptococcal vaccine candidates I

Antigen	Mass[a]	Putative Function / Homolog
M protein (Emm)	21.7-kDa	Antiphagocytic
Group A carbohydrate (GRA)	36% of cell wall weight	Serologic classification
C5a peptidase (SCPA)	128.2-kDa	Inhibits complement-derived chemotactic activity
Streptococcal pyrogenic exotoxin A (SpeA)	25.8-kDa	Superantigen
Streptococcal pyrogenic exotoxin B (SpeB)	40.3-kDa / 27.6-kDa[b]	Cysteine protease
Streptococcal pyrogenic exotoxin C (SpeC)	24.4-kDa	Superantigen
Streptococcal protective antigen (Spa)	58.9-kDa	Antiphagocytic
Streptococcus pyogenes fibronectin-binding protein I (Sfbl)	71-kDa	Fibronectin binding
Fibronectin binding protein 54 (FBP54)	54-kDa	Fibronectin binding
R28 protein (R28)	126.9-kDa	Adhesin
Streptococcal heme-associated protein (Shp).	29.2-kDa	Associates with heme in a 1:1 ratio

a. Approximate molecular weight
b. Made as a zymogen that undergoes proteolytic processing to a mature, enzymatically active form.

Additional GAS Vaccine Candidates

The search for an efficacious GAS vaccine has not been limited to M protein (Tables 1 and 2). GAS carbohydrate (GRA), C5a peptidase (SCPA), streptococcal pyrogenic exotoxin A (SpeA), streptococcal pyrogenic exotoxin B (SpeB), streptococcal pyrogenic exotoxin C (SpeC), streptococcal protective antigen (Spa), fibronectin-binding proteins (Sfb1 and FBP54), and R28 protein have been investigated as vaccine candidates in model systems.

GAS carbohydrate. The majority of GAS associated diseases occur during childhood, and adults older than 18 rarely get disease. Antibodies to multiple M protein serotypes are rarely found in human sera suggesting that antibodies to other GAS components contribute to natural immunity. Antibodies to GAS carbohydrate (GRA) are present in human sera,[67,68] and antibody titers to GRA peak around the age of 17.[69] These observations led Zabriskie and colleagues to pursue the idea that antibodies to GRA contribute to adult protection against GAS. Their work has shown that antibodies to GRA are opsonic,[70] promote phagocytosis of multiple GAS M serotypes,[70] and passively protect mice against heterologous intraperitonal challenge.[71]

C5a peptidase. SCPA is an endopeptidase that cleaves and inactivates human complement-derived chemotaxin C5a. It is believed that SCPA inhibits normal complement-derived chemotactic activity during the host inflammatory response, resulting in delayed recruitment of phagocytes and aiding GAS colonization.[72] Mice infected with GAS with an inactivated *scpA* gene clear GAS more efficiently from the nasopharynx than control animals infected with wild-type GAS.[73] Antibodies generated against a purified, enzymatically inactive form of SCPA made from a serotype M49 strain were able to neutralize C5a peptidase activity of M1, M6, M12, and M49 GAS in vitro.[74] These results led Ji et al[73] to investigate a possible protective role for SCPA. Mice immunized intranasally with inactive SCPA made from a serotype M49 strain had high levels of specific secretary IgA and serum IgG antibodies, and reduced levels of colonization of GAS serotypes M1, M2, M6, M11, and M49.[73] Limited sequence data indicate that *scpA* alleles are greater than 98% similar, suggesting that SCPA antibodies may confer protection against many GAS serotypes.[74,75]

Table 2. Group A streptococcal vaccine candidates II

GAS Antigen	Immunogen/ Treatment	Delivery Mechanism[a]	Vaccination Study	Protection[b]	Ref.
Emm	6-valent and 26-valent type-specific multimeric peptide	s.c.	Human Phase I	SS, ND	10, 49a, personal communication
Emm	39 type-specific heteropeptides	s.c.	Mouse	SS	50
Emm	non-type specific peptide	commensal vector	Mouse	ND	159
Emm	lipid core peptide construct	s.c.	Mouse	ND	58a
GRA	rabbit anti-GRA antibodies	s.c.	Mouse	SS	72
SCPA	purified SCPA protein	nasal	Mouse	NS	70
SpeA	purified SpeA	s.c.	Rabbit	SS	73
SpeB	purified SpeB, rabbit anti-SpeB antibodies	i.p., air sac	Mouse	SS	81-83
SpeC	SpeC mutant proteins	s.c.	Rabbit	SS	76
Spa	rabbit anti-Spa antibodies	i.p.	Mouse	ND	91, personal communication
Sfbl	Sfbl polypeptides	intranasal	Mouse	SS	89, 90
FBP54	purified FBP54 protein	s.c., oral	Mouse	SS	88
R28	rabbit anti-R28 antibodies	i.p.	Mouse	SS	96, 97

a. s.c subcutaneous, i.p. intraperitoneal
b. ND no data available, SS statistically significant, NS not statistically significant

Streptococcal pyrogenic exotoxin A. SpeA has been identified as the pyrogenic exotoxin most commonly associated with streptococcal toxic shock syndrome.[6] Rabbits immunized with purified SpeA do not develop STSS and are resistant to lethal challenge with serotype M1 and M3 organisms.[76] Due to the pyrogenic and toxic nature of the SpeA protein, Schlievert and colleagues have focused on producing nontoxic derivatives that elicit the production of protective antibodies. Single-, double-, triple-, and hexa-amino acid mutants were constructed and tested.[77,78] Each of the mutants lacked superantigenicity, elicited production of SpeA-specific antibodies in rabbits, and provided protection against lethal challenge with native SpeA in rabbit models.[77,78]

Streptococcal pyrogenic exotoxin C. Similar to their studies involving SpeA, Schlievert and colleagues have used the three dimensional structure of SpeC to predict residues important for interaction with host molecules or proper structural formation.[79] Site-specific mutagenesis has been used to generate a nontoxic form of the protein. Double- and triple-site SpeC mutants elicited antibodies that protected against STSS in rabbit models.[79]

Streptococcal pyrogenic exotoxin B. SpeB was first discovered and characterized by Elliot while investigating the inability to type certain strains of GAS with antisera directed against M protein.[80] SpeB has been studied extensively and the reader is directed to refs 15 and 78 for additional information. Briefly, SpeB is an extracellular cysteine protease capable of cleaving human fibronectin, vitronectin, human interleukin 1β precursor, kininogen, urokinase receptor, and human matrix metalloproteinase in vitro.[78-80] SpeB is expressed by virtually all GAS strains and sequence analysis of *speB* in 200 strains from global sources indicates that the protein is very highly conserved.[75,82] Initial evidence suggestive of an immunoprophylaxis role for SpeB was based on observations that patients with mild GAS infections have higher acute antibody levels to SpeB than patients with fatal streptococcal diseases.[16] Kapur et al[84] demonstrated that mice passively immunized with rabbit anti-SpeB antibodies and mice actively immunized with purified SpeB had significantly increased survival against intraperitoneal challenge with GAS.[81] Lukomski et al[85] showed that inactivation of SpeB results in decreased colonization, and reduced skin pathology and lethality in mice. Further support of these findings was provided by Kuo et al[86] who showed that a *speB* mutant strain caused less mortality and tissue damage than protease-positive strains when inoculated into BALB/c mice. Subsequent immunization with SpeB provided protection against challenge with GAS.[83]

Recently, Ashbaugh et al[87] reported that inactivation of *speB* did not result in decreased virulence in mice. These results are inconsistent with the observation that immunization with SpeB protects mice against invasive disease, suggesting that extensive in vitro passage or genetic manipulation of strains constructed by the investigators produced an experimental artifact.

Fibronectin binding proteins. Numerous GAS proteins bind fibronectin, including SfbI, SfbII, protein F2, PFBP, and FBP54.[88-92] In general, the structure of these proteins consists of a variable N-terminus and a conserved C-terminus containing a 37-48 amino acid repeat responsible for fibronectin-binding.[90] Recently, two of these proteins, Sfb1 and FBP54, have been shown to elicit protective immunity in murine models of GAS infection. Intranasal immunization of mice with Sfb1 afforded 80% and 90% protection versus homologous and heterologous challenge respectively.[92] However, intraperitoneal immunization was only 30% protective.[92] A subsequent study demonstrated that vaccination of mice with polypeptides spanning the fibronectin binding domain of SfbI provided protection against heterologous GAS challenge.[93]

Mice immunized subcutaneously, orally, or nasally with FBP54 develop FPB54 specific antibodies.[91] Mucosal levels of IgA antibody were also increased. The majority of immunized mice challenged intraperitoneally with M1, M3, or M12 GAS strains survived the challenge.[91] The deduced amino acid sequence of FBP54 was 98% conserved among 9 clinical isolates representing 7 M types (including M1 and M3). Given the variable distribution of other fibronectin-binding proteins in the natural population of GAS, a more extensive study on the distribution of FBP54 will need to be conducted.

Streptococcal protective antigen. Spa was discovered after Dale et al[94] demonstrated that an M protein-negative mutant of type 18 GAS was opsonized by antisera raised against a crude pepsin extract of the mutant. Passive immunization with anti-Spa and anti-M18 antiserum was required to provide protection against the M18 parent strain.[94] Spa antisera opsonized serotype M3 and M28 strains, but was ineffective against strains expressing serotype M1, M2, M5, M6, M13, M14, M19, or M24 protein. ARF patients also demonstrated measurable levels of antibody against Spa.[95]

R28 protein. The R28 protein was originally described by Lancefield, and was shown later to be associated with cases of puerperal sepsis ("childbed fever") in Britain.[96-98] Passive and active immunization of mice with antibodies to R28 or its Group B streptococcal homolog (Rib) provided protection against challenge with two R28+, serotype M28 strains.[99,100] Evidence suggests that the R28 protein is limited to M28 strains and some M2 and M48 strains,[101] suggesting that the immunoprophylaxis utility will be limited.

Streptococcal heme-associated protein (Shp). Analysis of a serotype M1 genome identified Shp among a number of previously uncharacterized extracellular proteins. Shp was found to associate with heme in a 1:1 ratio and flow cytometric analysis indicated Shp was located on the GAS cell surface.[102] ELISA analysis showed that 24 of 28 patients with invasive GAS disease had significantly higher levels of anti-Shp antibodies in convalescent-phase sera compared to acute-phase sera.[102] Analysis of serum samples obtained from patients with pharyngitis yielded similar results. Mice immunized with recombinant Shp and adjuvant had elevated anti-Shp titers, and a direct bactericidal assay indicated that mouse anti-Shp antibody significantly inhibited the growth of an M1 strain in vitro.[102] Given that iron is essential for GAS growth and regulates virulence factor expression, inhibition of Shp activity may be therapeutically advantageous.[1,102]

GAS Mediated Autoimmunity in Human Infection

Primary GAS infections can be followed by nonsuppurative post streptococcal sequelae that are autoimmune in nature. The more common of these diseases are ARF and RHD, but they also include acute glomerulonephritis, guttate psoriasis, and neuropsychological disorders.[4,103,104] The exact relationship between GAS infection and guttate psoriasis and neuropsychological disorders is not clear at this time. The association of antecedent GAS pharyngitis with ARF was described in two reports, one by Coburn and the other by Collis.[105,106] The researchers observed that in cases of pharyngitis followed by ARF, hemolytic streptococci (GAS) could be cultured from patients' throats during throat symptoms, but could not be recovered from the throat during rheumatic symptoms. However, GAS could be cultured from tonsils excised from patients during rheumatic symptoms.[105,106] Collis, based on the observation that patients with a history of recurring ARF experience repeated cases of tonsillitis, noted "the possibility of an altered body reaction being produced in persons who have had previous streptococcal infections."[106] Cavelti later associated auto antibodies against the heart with ARF.[107]

There is continued concern that a GAS vaccine would stimulate the autoimmune sequelae it was designed to protect against. For example, two of twenty-one healthy siblings of rheumatic patients who were immunized with partially purified type 3 M-protein developed rheumatic fever during a vaccine trial at the House of the Good Samaritan in Boston.[108] However, it remains unclear if vaccination with M-protein caused ARF in these individuals. Studies in the 1960's and 1970's identified many candidate cross-reactive antigens including, M protein, M-associated protein, group A polysaccharide, and hyaluronic acid capsule.[1,109-113] Subsequent studies using monoclonal antibodies (MAbs) against GAS and human heart tissue identified myosin as the cross-reactive antigen in the heart and localized the cross reactive antigens of GAS to the cell wall and cell membrane. These experiments identified M protein and N-acetylglucosamine, a component of GRA, as cross-reactive antigens, but suggested there may be others.[114-122] Additional work has shown that the α-helical M protein is cross reactive with α-helical coiled-coil proteins including, cardiac and skeletal tropomyosin, vimentin, laminin and keratin.[1,123-125] Experiments using affinity purified human antimyosin antibodies isolated from ARF patient sera have confirmed that the cross-reactive antigens identified with MAbs (M protein, *N*-acetylglucosamine) are present in ARF patient sera.[126-128] For additional information on GAS mediated autoimmunity, the reader is directed to ref. 1 for a recent scholarly review.

The mechanism for the cross-reactivity of M protein has been suggested to be T-cell mediated since heart muscle proteins are intracellular and are not able to bind antibodies. The presence of CD4+ T cells in the heart of RHD patients has been demonstrated, which suggests T cells play a role in the molecular mimicry of the M protein (M5 in this study).[129] Recently, three out of six Lewis rats immunized with recombinant type 6 streptococcal protein were reported to develop valvulitis and localized myocarditis.[130] Rheumatic valve sections showed infiltration of CD4+ lymphocytes in the rat hearts with valvulitis.[130] However, no direct evidence exists to demonstrate that the cross-reactive human antibodies are a direct consequence of GAS infection or are due to a secondary response to the damage of the host tissue.

Newly Described Extracellular Proteins and Antigens of GAS

Abundant chromosomal, allelic, and serologic diversity in GAS has hindered vaccine development, understanding of pathogen-host interactions, and differences in strain behavior.[17] For more than 40 years it has been known that patients with GAS infections produce antibodies to a large number of extracellular proteins,[131-135] but most of these antigens have not been identified. Availability of genome sequences has permitted virulence factors and therapeutics candidates to be identified very rapidly by comparative genomics and other post-genomic methods.[136-142]

Table 3. Chromosomal location and putative function of 5 GAS genes encoding novel extracellular proteins

Gene (*spy* No.)[a]	Chromosomal Location[b]	Putative Function of Encoded Protein[c]	LPXTG[d]
spy0747	607,542-610,274	Extracellular nuclease	LPKTG
spy0843	694,643-697,669	Cell surface protein	LPRTG
spy0872	718,489-720,501	2',3'-cyclic-nucleotide 2'-phosphodiesterase	LPITG
spy1361	1,127,063-1,129,441	Internalin homolog	No
spy1972	1,639,165-1,642,662	Pullulanase	LPKTG

a. *spy* No. refers to the corresponding numerical identifier of each ORF as listed in GenBank.
b. The chromosomal location of each gene in the sequenced GAS M1 strain ATCC 700294.[154]
c. Putative function as determined by BLAST analysis.
d. Amino acid motif used to anchor proteins to the cell wall in gram positive organisms. Single letter amino acid abbreviations are used (L, leucine; P, proline; K, lysine; R, arginine; I, isoleucine; T, threonine; G, glycine)

Many new extracellular and cell wall anchored proteins of GAS have recently been described,[140,141] and accumulating evidence suggests that further analysis of the suitability of these proteins as candidate antigens for conferring protective immunity is warranted.

A recent analysis[143] of the genomes of 4 GAS strains (serotypes M1, M3, M5, and M18) led to the discovery of five genes (*spy0747*, *spy0843*, *spy0872*, *spy1361*, and *spy1972*) that encode novel extracellular proteins (Table 3). The five proteins have conventional gram positive amino terminal secretion signal sequences, and 4 of the 5 proteins (Spy0747, Spy0843, Spy0872, and Spy1972) have a carboxyterminal LPXTG motif that covalently links gram positive virulence factors to the bacterial cell surface.[144-146] Sequencing and population genetic analysis of these genes in 37 strains representing 12 M serotypes revealed restricted allelic variation, indicating that the proteins are very well conserved in the species. Western immunoblot analysis of convalescent sera obtained from 80 patients with invasive infections, noninvasive soft tissue infections, pharyngitis, and rheumatic fever confirmed that all 5 proteins are made during the course of host-pathogen interactions in multiple GAS infection types (Table 4).[143]

To address questions concerning the regulation and differential expression of these 5 genes, gene transcript levels were analyzed by real-time reverse transcriptase PCR (TaqMan) assays.[140,143] TaqMan analysis of isogenic mutant strains implicated the GAS virulence gene regulators *covR* (negative regulator of several GAS virulence factors, including cysteine protease and capsule)[147,148] and *mga* (positive regulator of M protein, C5a peptidase, streptococcal inhibitor of complement, and streptococcal collagen-like protein 1)[149-151] in the control of expression of several of the genes. Transcription of *spy0747* and *spy0843* was up regulated in the absence of the CovR repressor, whereas expression of *spy1972* was down regulated in the absence of the positive regulator encoded by *mga*.[140]

Inasmuch as considerable allelic and chromosomal variation exists in natural populations of GAS, strain variation in the level of transcription of each gene was studied with TaqMan analysis of representative serotype M1, M3, and M18 strains.[143] Analysis was conducted with total RNA isolated at 6 time points throughout the growth curve (A_{600} = 0.05, 0.1, 0.2, 0.4, 0.6, 0.8). The results indicated that the maximum transcript level and the time of maximal expression differed among the 5 genes for each of the 3 strains.[143] This observation implies that although a protein may be genetically conserved and capable of interacting with the host during infection, variation in the level and timing of gene expression and subsequent protein synthesis among strains may alter the role of the protein in host-pathogen interactions.

Table 4. Percent immunoreactivity of recombinant GAS proteins with human sera obtained from patients with GAS infections

Protein (Spy No.)[a]	Pharyngitis (n=9)[b]	ARF (n=40)[c]	Invasive (n=27)[d]
Spy0747	89	85	81
Spy0843	78	90	74
Spy0872	22	15	37
Spy1361	56	70	67
Spy1972	78	88	85

a. Spy No. refers to the corresponding numerical identifier of each ORF as listed in GenBank.
b. Convalescent-phase sera isolated from 9 individuals with recent episodes of GAS pharyngitis.
c. Convalescent-phase sera isolated from 40 individuals with a history of ARF.
d. Convalescent-phase sera isolated from 27 individuals with invasive GAS disease.

More than 50 extracellular proteins with the LPXTG motif have been described in gram positive bacteria, and many of them are virulence factors.[152] It was recently confirmed that the LPXTG containing proteins Spy0843 and Spy1972 are displayed on the GAS cell surface and accessible to antibody.[143] Importantly, all GAS cell-surface proteins with an LPXTG anchor motif or closely related amino acid sequence that have been extensively studied (M protein, C5a peptidase, serum opacity factor, a fibronectin-binding protein, and streptococcal protective antigen) are virulence factors and most contribute to protective immunity in mouse models.[74,94,153-155] Hence, it will be important to determine if immunization with these newly-identified extracellular proteins can stimulate a protective immune response.

Post Genomic Strategies to Study Host-Pathogen Interactions

The ever increasing number of completed genome sequences has opened the door to the study of the complex interactions between a pathogen and its host. The availability of the 3,200 Mb human genome sequence[156,157] and the 1.8-1.9 Mb genome sequence of serotype M1, M3, and M18,[158,159,160] provide a resource to assist discovery of new vaccine candidates and aid our understanding of the pathogenic mechanisms of streptococcal disease and post-streptococcal sequelae. The first genome-wide expression profiling of GAS was published recently by Smoot et al[161] In this study, genome wide changes in gene expression in response to three physiologically relevant temperatures (29°, 37°, and 40°C) were investigated by DNA microarray analysis. The results demonstrated that GAS has the ability to alter gene transcription extensively on the basis of temperature.[161] In addition, 28 genes encoding putative extracellular proteins were differentially expressed in response to temperature.[161] This suggests that the type of GAS infection may influence the number of possible protective antigens expressed.

Combining DNA microarray and quantitative RT-PCR analysis, Graham et al[162] used a genome wide approach to study the two component GAS regulatory system, *covRS* (*cov*, control of virulence). Comparison of a wildtype M1 strain and its nonpolar isogenic derivative (inactive *covR*) indicated that CovR influences transcription of 15% (n=271) of all chromosomal genes in vitro, including many that encode extracellular proteins and those involved in stress and adaptation responses.[162] Altered CovR mediated gene expression was also seen in vivo in a mouse model of soft-tissue infection.[162] Of note, CovR was involved in multiple gene regulatory networks, influencing the expression of other genes encoding transcriptional regulators.[162] Similar results were seen in an earlier study which investigated the role of Rgg in GAS gene regulation.[163] Genome wide transcript profiles of a serotype M49 strain and its isogenic derivative (inactive *rgg*) generated by microarray analysis revealed that Rgg influences transcription of >10 genes encoding putative or proven virulence factors.[163] In addition, Rgg

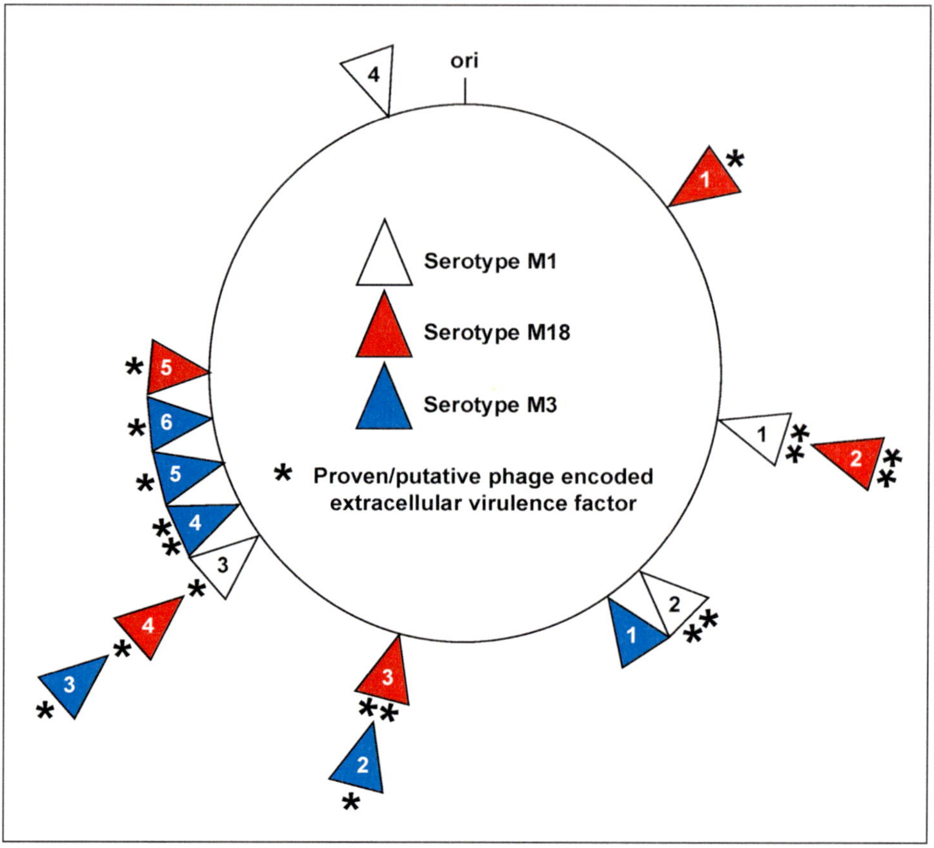

Figure 2. Variation in the number, integration site, and virulence complement of GAS prophage. The core GAS genome is shown (~1.7 Mbp) and phage integration sites are indicated by triangles color-coded to match the GAS strain. The prophage of each strain are numbered clockwise from the origin of replication (Ori). Stacked triangles indicate the phage share the same chromosomal integration site. Each asterisk represents a phage encoded proven/putative extracellular virulence factor. Strain-to-strain variation in phage content and phage encoded virulence factors may substantially alter strain virulence, resistance to the host innate immune response, and the landscape of the GAS cell surface. This variation may complicate development of novel therapeutics and vaccination strategies. (Modified from Beres SB, et al. Proc Natl Acad Sci 2002; 99:10078-83, with permission.)

influences the expression of *covRS*, *mga* (another known regulator of GAS virulence genes), and several putative regulators.[163] Elucidation of the complex regulatory circuits in GAS will undoubtedly provide insight into GAS pathogenesis and identify new therapeutic targets overlooked by other methods of investigation.

Perhaps the most important discovery to derive from the comparison of the available GAS genomes is the extent to which prophage contribute to variation in gene content between strains, including genes likely to contribute to GAS pathogenesis (Fig. 2). The 3 sequenced GAS genomes differ in the number of prophage, the composition (assortment) of prophage, and the position of chromosomal integration.[160] Importantly, 13 of the 15 prophage present in the 3 sequenced GAS genomes encode at least one proven or putative virulence factor, the majority of which were unknown prior to the determination of the genome sequences.[158,159,160] These factors can be separated into two functional groups, the first composed of PTSags SpeA,

SpeC, SpeH, SpeI, SpeK, SpeL, SpeM, and SSA, and the second composed of degradative enzymes, including DNAses and a phospholipase A_2. Antibodies against many of these proteins are present in convalescent sera from human patients indicating that these prophage-encoded molecules are produced during the course of human infection. These genes are located adjacent to the phage chromosomal integration site, and some have a G +C content that is not characteristic of the GAS genome or resident prophage. This suggests that some of these putative or proven virulence factor genes were acquired from another organism by lateral gene transfer. To summarize, bacteriophages are a major source of variation in GAS virulence determinant content, and they encode novel proteins capable of eliciting an immune response, perhaps contributing to host protection.

Final Comments

In this chapter we have reviewed the current status of GAS vaccine research. The technology of the post-genomic era has facilitated the discovery of several new GAS vaccine candidates, providing new promise for a field that was previously limited to the investigation of the immunological protection stimulated by M protein and a few other molecules. However, the pathogenesis of GAS infections is complicated, and it is likely that a vaccine made from a single antigen will not protect against all forms of GAS infection and post-infectious sequelae. Although severe episodes of GAS disease are relatively rare, ARF and RHD account for a substantial proportion of the disease burden of developing countries with millions more at risk. Moreover, GAS pharyngitis is a major cause of childhood morbidity and economic loss in developed countries. Thus, continued focus on the development of new strategies for vaccine discovery is warranted. Future research must investigate GAS in the context of its natural host as the best insights into the molecular basis of pathogenesis and the immunological protection against disease will come from in vivo studies in relevant animal models (nonhuman primates) or infected humans.[164-167]

References

1. Cunningham MW. Pathogenesis of group A streptococcal infections. Clin Microbiol Rev 2000; 13:470-511.
2. Pichichero ME. Group A beta-hemolytic streptococcal infections. Pediatr Rev 1998; 19:291-302.
3. Katz AR, Morens DM. Severe streptococcal infections in historical perspective. Clin Infect Dis 1992; 14:298-307.
4. Bisno AL. Group A streptococcal infections and acute rheumatic fever. N Engl J Med 1991; 325:783-793.
5. Lennon DR. Acute rheumatic fever. In: Feigin RD, Cherry JD, eds. Textbook of pediatric infectious diseases. Philadelphia: WB Saunders, 1996:371-383.
6. Musser JM, Krause RM. The revival of group A streptococcal diseases, with a commentary on staphylococcal toxic shock syndrome. In: Krause RM, ed. Emerging infections. Academic Press, 1998:185-218.
7. Streptococci and the Host. In: Horaud T, Bouvet A, Leclercq R, et al. eds. Advances in Experimental Medicine and Biology. New York: Plenum Press, 1997:418.
8. Gram-Positive Pathogens. Fischetti VA, Novick RP, Ferretti JJ et al. eds. Washington, D.C.: ASM Press, 2000.
9. Bisno AL. Primary care: acute pharyngitis. N Engl J Med 2001; 344:205-211.
10. Dale JB. Group A streptococcal vaccines. Infect Dis Clin North Am 1999; 13:227-243.
11. Quinn RW. Comprehensive review of morbidity and mortality trends for rheumatic fever, streptococcal disease, and scarlet fever: the decline of rheumatic fever. Rev Infect Dis 1989; 11:928-953.
12. Musser JM, Hauser AR, Kim MH et al. Streptococcus pyogenes causing toxic-shock-like syndrome and other invasive diseases: clonal diversity and pyrogenic exotoxin expression. Proc Natl Acad Sci USA 1991; 88:2668-2672.
13. Norrby-Teglund A, Pauksens K, Holm SE et al. Relation between low capacity of human sera to inhibit streptococcal mitogens and serious manifestation of disease. J Infect Dis 1994; 170:585-591.
14. Norrby-Teglund A, Kaul R, Low DE et al. Plasma from patients with severe invasive group A streptococcal infections treated with normal polyspecific IgG inhibits streptococcal superantigen-induced T cell proliferation and cytokine production. J Immunol 1996; 156:3057-3064.

15. Musser JM. Streptococcal superantigen, mitogenic factor, and pyrogenic exotoxin B expressed by Streptococcus pyogenes. Structure and function. Prep Biochem Biotechnol 1997; 27:143-172.
16. Holm SE, Norrby A, Bergholm AM et al. Aspects of pathogenesis of serious group A streptococcal infections in Sweden, 1988-1989. J Infect Dis 1992; 166:31-37.
17. Reid SD, Hoe NP, Smoot LM et al. Group A Streptococcus: allelic variation, population genetics, and host-pathogen interactions. J Clin Invest 2001; 107:393-399.
18. Hoe NP, Nakashima K, Lukomski S et al. Rapid selection of complement-inhibiting protein variants in group A Streptococcus epidemic waves. Nat Med 1999; 5:924-929.
19. Hoe NP, Kordari P, Cole R et al. Human immune response to streptococcal inhibitor of complement, a serotype M1 group A Streptococcus extracellular protein involved in epidemics. J Infect Dis 2000; 182:1425-1436.
20. Hoe NP, Vuopio-Varkila J, Vaara M et al. Distribution of streptococcal inhibitor of complement variants in pharyngitis and invasive isolates in an epidemic of serotype M1 group A Streptococcus infection. J Infect Dis 2001; 183:633-639.
21. Hoe NP, Ireland RM, DeLeo FR et al. Insight into the molecular basis of pathogen abundance: group A Streptocuccus inhibitor of complement inhibits bacterial adherence and internalization into human cells. Proc Natl Acad Sci USA 2002; 99:7646-7651.
22. Wannamaker L. The epidemiology of streptococcal infections. In: McCarty M, ed. Streptococcal infections. Columbia University Press, 1954.
23. Cornfeld D, Hubbard J. A four-year study of the occurrence of beta-hemolytic streptococci in 64 school children. N Eng J Med 1961; 264:211-215.
24. Anthony B, Kaplan E, Wannamaker L et al. The dynamics of streptococcal infections in a defined population of children: serotypes associated with skin and respiratory infections. Am J Epidemiol 1976; 104:652-666.
25. Gaworzewska E, Colman G. Changes in the pattern of infection caused by Streptococcus pyogenes. Epidemiol Infect 1988; 100:257-269.
26. Martin P, Hoiby E. Streptococcal serogroup A epidemic in Norway 1987-1988. Scand J Infect Dis Suppl 1990; 22:421-429.
27. Kaplan E, Wotton J, Johnson D. Dynamic epidemiology of group A streptococcal serotypes associated with pharyngitis. Lancet North Am Ed 2001; 358:1334-1337.
28. Olivier C. Rheumatic fever—is it still a problem? J Antimicrob Chemother 2000; 45 Suppl:13-21.
29. Stollerman GH. Changing streptococci and prospects for the global eradication of rheumatic fever. Perspect Biol Med 1997; 40:165-189.
30. Nordet P. WHO programme for the prevention of rheumatic fever/rheumatic heart disease in 16 developing countries: report from Phase I (1986-90). WHO Cardiovascular Diseases Unit and principal investigators. Bull World Health Organ 1992; 70:213-218.
31. McLaren MJ, Markowitz M, Gerber MA. Rheumatic heart disease in developing countries: the consequence of inadequate prevention. Ann Intern Med 1994; 120:243-245.
32. Carapetis JR, Wolff DR, Currie BJ. Acute rheumatic fever and rheumatic heart disease in the top end of Australia's Northern Territory. Med J Aust 1996; 164:146-149.
33. Lawrence DN, Facklam RR, Sottnek FO et al. Epidemiologic studies among Amerindian populations of Amazonia. I. Pyoderma: prevalence and associated pathogens. Am J Trop Med Hyg 1979; 28:548-558.
34. Taplin D, Lansdell L, Allen AM et al. Prevalence of streptococcal pyoderma in relation to climate and hygiene. Lancet 1973; 1:501-503.
35. Brahmadathan KN, Koshi G. Epidemiology of streptococcal pyoderma in an orphanage community of a tropical country. J Trop Med Hyg 1988; 91:306-314.
36. Bessen DE, Carapetis JR, Beall B et al. Contrasting molecular epidemiology of group A streptococci causing tropical and nontropical infections of the skin and throat. J Infect Dis 2000; 182:1109-1116.
37. Thompson D, Thompson R. The role of the streptococci in scarlet fever. Annals of the Pickett-Thompson research laboratory 1930; 4:244-252.
38. Dick GF, Dick G. Scarlet fever toxin in preventive immunization. JAMA 1924; 82:544-545.
39. Massell BF. Rheumatic Fever and Streptococcal Infection. Boston: Harvard University Press, 1997.
40. Watson RF, Rothbard S, Swift HF. Type-specific protection and immunity following intranasal inoculation of monkeys with group A hemolytic streptococci. J Exp Med 1946; 84:127-142.
41. Lancefield RC. The antigenic complex of Streptococcus haemolyticus. I. Demonstration of a type specific substance in extracts of Streptococcus haemolyticus. J Exp Med 1928; 47:91 103.
42. Lancefield RC, Todd EW. Antigenic differences between matt hemolytic streptococci and their glossy variants. J Exp Med 1928; 48:769-790.

43. Dochez AR, Avery OT, Lancefield RC. Studies on the biology of Streptococcus. I. Antigenic relationships between strains of Streptococcus haemolyticus. J Exp Med 1919; 30:179-213.
44. Hirst GK, Lancefield RC. Antigenic properties of the type-specific substances derived from group A hemolytic streptococci. J Exp Med 1939; 69:425-445.
45. Rantz LA, Randall E, Rantz HH et al. Immunization of human beings with group A hemolytic streptococci. Am J Med 1949; 6:424-432.
46. Schmidt WC. Type-specific antibody formation in man following injection of streptococcal M protein. J Infect Dis 1960; 106:250-255.
47. Beachey EH, Seyer JM, Dale JB et al. Type-specific protective immunity evoked by synthetic peptide of Streptococcus pyogenes M protein. Nature 1981; 292:457-459.
48. Beachey EH, Seyer JM, Dale JB. Protective immunogenicity and T lymphocyte specificity of a trivalent hybrid peptide containing NH2-terminal sequences of types 5, 6, and 24 M proteins synthesized in tandem. J Exp Med 1987; 166:647-656.
49. Dale JB, Chiang EY, Lederer JW. Recombinant tetravalent group A streptococcal M protein vaccine. J Immunol 1993; 151:2188-2194.
50. Dale JB. Multivalent group A streptococcal vaccine designed to optimize the immunogenicity of six tandem M protein fragments. Vaccine 1999; 17:193-200.
51. Hu MC, Walls MA, Stroop SD et al. Immunogenicity of a 26-valent group A streptococcal vaccine. Infect Immun 2002; 70:2171-2177.
52. Brandt ER, Sriprakash KS, Hobb RI et al. New multi-determinant strategy for a group A streptococcal vaccine designed for the Australian Aboriginal population. Nat Med 2000; 6:455-459.
53. Fox EN, Waldman RH, Wittner MK et al. Protective study with a group A streptococcal M protein vaccine. Infectivity challenge of human volunteers. J Clin Invest 1973; 52:1885-1892.
54. Waldman RH, Lee JD, Polly SM et al. Group A streptococcal M protein vaccine: protection following immunization via the respiratory tract. Dev Biol Stand 1975; 28:429-434.
55. Polly SM, Waldman RH, High P et al. Protective studies with a group A streptococcal M protein vaccine. II. Challenge of volunteers after local immunization in the upper respiratory tract. J Infect Dis 1975; 131:217-224.
56. D'Alessandri R, Plotkin G, Kluge RM et al. Protective studies with group A streptococcal M protein vaccine. III. Challenge of volunteers after systemic or intranasal immunization with Type 3 or Type 12 group A Streptococcus. J Infect Dis 1978; 138:712-718.
57. Breese BB. Beta-hemolytic streptococcal diseases. Boston: Houghton Mifflin Professional Publishers, Medical Divison, 1978:1-287.
58. Bessen D, Fischetti VA. Passive acquired mucosal immunity to group A streptococci by secretary - immunoglobulin A. J Exp Med 1988; 167:1945 1950.
59. Bessen D, Fischetti VA. Influence of intranasal immunization with synthetic peptides corresponding to conserved epitopes of M protein on mucosal colonization by group A streptococci. Infect Immun 1988; 56:2666-2672.
60. Bessen D, Fischetti VA. Synthetic peptide vaccine against mucosal colonization by group A streptococci: I. Protection against a heterologous M serotype with shared C repeat region epitopes. J Immuno 1990; 145:1251-1256.
61. Olive C, Batzloff MR, Horváth A et al. A lipid core peptide construct containing a conserved region determinant of the group A streptococcal M protein elicits heterologous opsonic antibodies. Infect Immun 2002; 70:2734-2738.
62. Poirier TP, Kehoe MA, Beachey EH. Protective immunity evoked by oral administration of attenuated aroA Salmonella Typhimurium expressing cloned streptococcal M protein. J Exp Med 1988; 168:25-32.
63. Newton SM, Kotb M, Poirier TP et al. Expression and immunogenicity of a streptococcal M protein epitope inserted in Salmonella flagellin. Infect Immun 1991; 59:2158-2165.
64. Fischetti VA, Hodges WM, Hruby DE. Protection against streptococcal pharyngeal colonization with a vaccinia:M protein recombinant. Science 1989; 244:1487-1490.
65. Medaglini D, Pozzi G, King TP et al. Mucosal and systemic immune responses to a recombinant protein expressed on the surface of the oral commensal bacterium Streptococcus gordonii after oral colonization. Proc Natl Acad Sci USA 1995; 92:6868-6872.
66. Oggioni MR, Manganelli R, Contorni M et al. Immunization of mice by oral colonization with live recombinant commensal streptococci. Vaccine 1995; 13:775-779.
67. Schmidt WC, Moore DJ. The determination of antibody to group A streptococcal polysaccharide in human sera by agglutination. J Exp Med 1965; 121:793-806.
68. Karakawa WW, Osterland CK, Krause RM. Detection of group specific antibodies in human sera. J Exp Med 1965; 122:195-210.

69. Zimmerman RA, Auernheimer AH, Taranta A. Precipitating antibody to group A streptococcal polysaccharide in humans. J Immunol 1971; 107:832-841.
70. Salvadori LG, Blake MS, McCarty M et al. Group A Streptococcus-liposome ELISA antibody titers to group A polysaccharide and opsonophagocytic capabilities of the antibodies. J Infect Dis 1995; 171:593-600.
71. Zabriskie JB, Poon-King T, Blake MS et al. Phagocytic, serological, and protective properties of streptococcal group A carbohydrate antibodies. Adv Exp Med Biol 1997; 418:917-919.
72. Wexler DE, Chenoweth DE, Cleary PP. Mechanism of action of the group A streptococcal C5a inactivator. Proc Natl Acad Sci USA 1985; 82:8144-8148.
73. Ji Y, Carlson B, Kondagunta A et al. Intranasal immunization with C5a peptidase prevents nasopharyngeal colonization of mice by the group A Streptococcus. Infect Immun 1997; 65:2080-2087.
74. Chen CC, Cleary PP. Complete nucleotide sequence of the streptococcal C5a peptidase gene of Streptococcus pyogenes. J Biol Chem 1990; 265:3161-3167.
75. Dale JB, Cleary PP, Fischetti VA et al. Group A and group B streptococcal vaccine development. A round table presentation. Adv Exp Med Biol 1997; 418:863-868.
76. Schlievert PM, Assimacopoulos AP, Cleary PP. Severe invasive group A streptococcal disease: clinical description and mechanisms of pathogenesis. J Lab Clin Med 1996; 127:13-22.
77. Roggiani M, Stoehr JA, Leonard BA et al. Analysis of toxicity of Streptococcal pyrogenic exotoxin A mutants. Infect Immun 1997; 65:2868-2875.
78. Roggiani M, Assimacopoulos AP, Schlievert PM. Exotoxins of Streptococcus pyogenes. In: Stevens DL, Kaplan EL, eds. Streptococcal Infections. New York: Oxford University Press, 2000:57-75.
79. McCormick JK, Tripp TJ, Olmsted SB et al. Development of streptococcal pyrogenic exotoxin C vaccine toxoids that are protective in the rabbit model of toxic shock syndrome. J Immunol 2000; 165:2306-2312.
80. Elliot SD. A proteolytic enzyme produced by group A streptococci with special reference to its effect on the type-specific M antigen. J Exp Med 1945; 81:573-592.
81. Burns Jr EH, Marciel AM et al. Activation of a 66-kilodalton human endothelial cell matrix metalloprotease by Streptococcus pyogenes extracellular cysteine protease. Infect Immun 1996; 64:4744-4750.
82. Kapur V, Topouzis S, Majesky MW et al. A conserved Streptococcus pyogenes extracellular cysteine protease cleaves human fibronectin and degrades vitronectin. Microb Pathog 1993; 15:327-346.
83. Kapur V, Majesky MW, Li LL et al. Cleavage of interleukin 1 ß (IL-1 ß) precursor to produce active IL-1 ß by a conserved extracellular cysteine protease from Streptococcus pyogenes. Proc Natl Acad Sci USA 1993; 90:7676-7680.
84. Kapur V, Maffei JT, Greer RS et al. Vaccination with streptococcal extracellular cysteine protease (interleukin-1 ß convertase) protects mice against challenge with heterologous group A streptococci. Microb Pathog 1994; 16:443-450.
85. Lukomski S, Sreevatsan S, Amberg C et al. Inactivation of Streptococcus pyogenes extracellular cysteine protease significantly decreases mouse lethality of serotype M3 and M49 strains. J Clin Invest 1997; 99:2574-2580.
86. Kuo CF, Wu JJ, Lin KY et al. Role of streptococcal pyrogenic exotoxin B in the mouse model of group A streptococcal infection. Infect Immun 1998; 66:3931-3935.
87. Ashbaugh CD, Wessels MR. Absence of a cysteine protease effect on bacterial virulence in two murine models of human invasive group a streptococcal infection. Infect Immun 2001; 69:6683-6688.
88. Kreikemeyer B, Talay SR, Chhatwal GS. Characterization of a novel fibronectin-binding surface protein in group A streptococci. Mol Microbiol 1995; 17:137-145.
89. Jaffe J, Natanson-Yaron S, Caparon MG et al. Protein F2, a novel fibronectin-binding protein from Streptococcus pyogenes, possesses two binding domains. Mol Microbiol 1996; 21:373-384.
90. Rocha CL, Fischetti VA. Identification and characterization of a novel fibronectin-binding protein on the surface of group A streptococci. Infect Immun 1999; 67:2720-2728.
91. Kawabata S, Kunitomo E, Terao Y et al. Systemic and mucosal immunization with fibronectin-binding protein FBP54 induce protective immune responses against Streptococcus pyogenes challenge in mice. Infect Immun 2001; 69:924-930.
92. Guzman CA, Talay SR, Molinari G et al. Protective immune response against Streptococcus pyogenes in mice after intranasal vaccination with the fibronectin-binding protein SfbI. J Infect Dis 1999; 179:901-906.
93. Schulze K, Medina E, Talay SR et al. Characterization of the domain of fibronectin binding protein I of Streptococcus pyogenes responsible for elicitation of a protective immune response. Infect Immun 2001; 69:622-625.
94. Dale JB, Chiang EY, Liu S et al. New protective antigen of group A streptococci. J Clin Invest 1999; 103:1261-1268.

95. McLellan DG, Chiang EY, Courtney HS et al. Spa contributes to the virulence of type 18 group A streptococci. Infect Immun 2001; 69:2943-2949.
96. Lancefield RC, Perlmann GE. Preparation and properties of a protein (R antigen) occurring in streptococci of group A, type 28 and in certain streptococci of other serological groups. J Exp Med 1952; 96:83-97.
97. Gaworzewska E, Colman G. Changes in the pattern of infection caused by Streptococcus pyogenes. Epidemiol Infect 1988; 100:257-269.
98. Colman G, Tanna A, Efstratiou A et al. The serotypes of Streptococcus pyogenes present in Britain during 1980-1990 and their association with disease. J Med Microbiol 1993; 39:165-178.
99. Stalhammar-Carlemalm M, Areschoug T, Larsson C et al. The R28 protein of Streptococcus pyogenes is related to several group B streptococcal surface proteins, confers protective immunity and promotes binding to human epithelial cells. Mol Microbiol 1999; 33:208-219.
100. Stalhammar-Carlemalm M, Areschoug T, Larsson C et al. Cross-protection between group A and group B streptococci due to cross-reacting surface proteins. J Infect Dis 2000; 182:142-149.
101. Lancefield RC. Differentiation of group A streptococci with a common R antigen into three serological types, with special reference to the bactericidal test. J Exp Med 1957; 106:525-544.
102. Lei B, Smoot LM, Menning HM et al. Identification and characterization of a novel heme-associated cell surface protein made by group A Streptococcus. Infect Immun 2002; 70:4494-4500.
103. Allen AJ, Leonard HL, Swedo SE. Case study: a new infection-triggered, autoimmune subtype of pediatric OCD and Tourette's syndrome. J Am Acad Child Adolesc Psychiatry 1995; 34:307-311.
104. Valdimarsson H, Baker BS, Jonsdottir I et al. Psoriasis: a T-cell-mediated autoimmune disease induced by streptococcal superantigens? Immunol Today 1995; 16:145-149.
105. Coburn AF. The factor of infection in the rheumatic states. Baltimore: The Williams and Wilkins Company, 1931.
106. Collis WRF. Acute rheumatism and haemolytic streptococci. Lancet 1931; 1:1341-1345.
107. Cavelti PA. Auto antibodies in rheumatic fever. Proc Soc Exp Biol Med 1945; 60:379-381.
108. Massell BF, Honikman LH, Amezcua J. Rheumatic fever following streptococcal vaccination. Report of three cases. JAMA 1969; 207:1115-1119.
109. Widdowson JP, Maxted WR, Pinney AM. An M-associated protein antigen (MAP) of group A streptococci. J Hyg (Lond) 1971; 69:553-564.
110. Widdowson JP. The M-associated proteins of group A streptococci. In: Read SE, Zabriskie JB, eds. Streptococcal disease and the immune response. New York: Academic Press, 1980:125-147.
111. Sandson J, Hamerman D, Janis R. Immunologic and chemical similarities between the Streptococcus and human connective tissue. Trans Assoc Am Physicians 1968; 81:249-257.
112. Goldstein I, Halpern B, Robert L. Immunological relationship between Streptococcus A polysaccharide and the structural glycoproteins of heart valve. Nature 1967; 213:44-47.
113. Beachey EH, Stollerman GH. Mediation of cytotoxic effects of streptococcal M protein by nontype-specific antibody in human sera. J Clin Invest 1973; 52:2563-2570.
114. Barnett LA, Cunningham MW. A new heart-cross-reactive antigen in Streptococcus pyogenes is not M protein. J Infect Dis 1990; 162:875-882.
115. Cunningham MW, Russell SM. Study of heart-reactive antibody in antisera and hybridoma culture fluids against group A streptococci. Infect Immun 1983; 42:531-538.
116. Cunningham MW, Krisher K, Graves DC. Murine monoclonal antibodies reactive with human heart and group A streptococcal membrane antigens. Infect Immun 1984; 46:34-41.
117. Cunningham MW, Hall NK, Krisher KK et al. A study of anti-group A streptococcal monoclonal antibodies cross-reactive with myosin. J Immunol 1986; 136:293-298.
118. Dale JB, Beachey EH. Epitopes of streptococcal M proteins shared with cardiac myosin. J Exp Med 1985; 162:583-591.
119. Dale JB, Beachey EH. Multiple, heart-cross-reactive epitopes of streptococcal M proteins. J Exp Med 1985; 161:113-122.
120. Dale JB, Beachey EH. Human cytotoxic T lymphocytes evoked by group A streptococcal M proteins. J Exp Med 1987; 166:1825-1835.
121. Shikhman AR, Cunningham MW. Immunological mimicry between N-acetyl-ß-D-glucosamine and cytokeratin peptides. Evidence for a microbially driven anti-keratin antibody response. J Immunol 1994; 152:4375-4387.
122. Adderson EE, Shikhman AR, Ward KE et al. Molecular analysis of polyreactive monoclonal antibodies from rheumatic carditis: human anti-N-acetylglucosamine/anti-myosin antibody V region genes. J Immunol 1998; 161:2020-2031.
123. Fenderson PG, Fischetti VA, Cunningham MW. Tropomyosin shares immunologic epitopes with group A streptococcal M proteins. J Immunol 1989; 142:2475-2481.

124. Cunningham MW, Antone SM, Gulizia JM et al. Cytotoxic and viral neutralizing antibodies crossreact with streptococcal M protein, enteroviruses, and human cardiac myosin. Proc Natl Acad Sci USA 1992; 89:1320-1324.
125. Cunningham MW, Antone SM, Gulizia JM et al. Alpha-helical coiled-coil molecules: a role in autoimmunity against the heart. Clin Immunol Immunopathol 1993; 68:118-123.
126. Dale JB, Beachey EH. Sequence of myosin-crossreactive epitopes of streptococcal M protein. J Exp Med 1986; 164:1785-1790.
127. Cunningham MW, McCormack JM, Talaber LR et al. Human monoclonal antibodies reactive with antigens of the group A Streptococcus and human heart. J Immunol 1988; 141:2760-2766.
128. Cunningham MW, McCormack JM, Fenderson PG et al. Human and murine antibodies cross-reative with streptococcal M protein and myosin recognize the sequence GLN-LYS-SER-LYS-GLN in M protein. J Immunol 1989; 143:2677-2683.
129. Guilherme L, Cunha-Neto E, Coelho V et al. Human heart-infiltrating T-cell clones from rheumatic heart disease patients recognize both streptococcal and cardiac proteins. Circulation 1995; 92:415-420.
130. Quinn A, Kosanke S, Fischetti VA et al. Induction of autoimmune valvular heart disease by recombinant streptococcal M protein. Infect Immun 2001; 69:4072-4078.
131. Halbert SP, Swick L, Sonn C. The use of precipitin analysis in agar for the study of human streptococcal infections. II. Ouchterlony and Oakley techniques. J Exp Med 1955; 101:557-575.
132. Halbert SP, Swick L, Sonn C. The use of precipitin analysis in agar for the study of human streptococcal infections. I. Oudin technic. J Exp Med 1955; 101:539-556.
133. Halbert SP. The use of precipitin analysis in agar for the study of human streptococcal infections. III. The purification of some of the antigens detected by these methods. J Exp Med 1958; 108:385-410.
134. Halbert SP, Auerbach T. The use of precipitin analysis in agar for the study of human streptococcal infections. IV. Further observations on the purification of group A extracellular antigens. J Exp Med 1960; 113:131-157.
135. Halbert SP, Keatinge SL. The analysis of streptococcal infections. VI. Immunoelectrophoretic observations on extracellular antigens detectable with human antibodies. J Exp Med 1961; 113:1013-1028.
136. Grandi G. Antibacterial vaccine design using genomics and proteomics. Trends Biotechnol 2001; 19:181-188.
137. Janulczyk R, Rasmussen M. Improved pattern for genome-based screening identifies novel cell wall-attached proteins in gram-positive bacteria. Infect Immun 2001; 69:4019-4026.
138. Musser JM, Kaplan SL. Pneumococcus research transformed. N Engl J Med 2001; 345:1206-1207.
139. Pizza M, Scarlato V, Masignani V et al. Identification of vaccine candidates against serogroup B Meningococcus by whole-genome sequencing. Science 2000; 287:1816-1820.
140. Reid SD, Green NM, Buss JK et al. Multilocus analysis of extracellular putative virulence proteins made by group A Streptococcus: population genetics, human serologic response, and gene transcription. Proc Natl Acad Sci USA 2001; 98:7552-7557.
141. Lei B, Mackie S, Lukomski S et al. Identification and immunogenicity of group A Streptococcus culture supernatant proteins. Infect Immun 2000; 68:6807-6818.
142. Chakravarti DN, Fiske MJ, Fletcher LD et al. Application of genomics and proteomics for identification of bacterial gene products as potential vaccine candidates. Vaccine 2000; 19:601-612.
143. Reid SD, Green NM, Sylva GL et al. Post genomic analysis of four novel antigens of group A Streptococcus: Growth-phase-dependent gene transcription and human serologic response. J Bact 2002 in press.
144. Fischetti VA, Pancholi V, Schneewind O. Conservation of a hexapeptide sequence in the anchor region of surface proteins from gram-positive cocci. Mol Microbiol 1990; 4:1603-1605.
145. Navarre WW, Schneewind O. Surface proteins of gram-positive bacteria and mechanisms of their targeting to the cell wall envelope. Microbiol Mol Biol Rev 1999; 63:174-229.
146. Schneewind O, Model P, Fischetti VA. Sorting of protein A to the staphylococcal cell wall. Cell 1992; 70:267-281.
147. Levin JC, Wessels MR. Identification of csrR/csrS, a genetic locus that regulates hyaluronic acid capsule synthesis in group A Streptococcus. Mol Microbiol 1998; 30:209-219.
148. McIver KS, Thurman AS, Scott JR. Regulation of mga transcription in the group A Streptococcus: specific binding of mga within its own promoter and evidence for a negative regulator. J Bacteriol 1999; 181:5373-5383.
149. McIver KS, Subbarao S, Kellner EM et al. Identification of isp, a locus encoding an immunogenic secreted protein conserved among group A streptococci. Infect Immun 1996; 64:2548-2555.

150. McIver KS, Scott JR. Role of mga in growth phase regulation of virulence genes of the group A Streptococcus. J Bacteriol 1997; 179:5178-5187.
151. Lukomski S, Nakashima K, Abdi I et al. Identification and characterization of the scl gene encoding a group A Streptococcus extracellular protein virulence factor with similarity to human collagen. Infect Immun 2000; 68:6542-6553.
152. Fischetti VA. Surface proteins on gram-positive bacteria. In: Fischetti VA, Novick RP, Ferretti JJ, Portnoy DA, Rood JI, eds. Gram-Positive Pathogens. Washington, D. C.: ASM Press, 2000:11-24.
153. Courtney HS, Hasty DL, Li Y et al. Serum opacity factor is a major fibronectin-binding protein and a virulence determinant of M type 2 Streptococcus pyogenes. Mol Microbiol 1999; 32:89-98.
154. Rasmussen M, Muller HP, Bjorck L. Protein GRAB of Streptococcus pyogenes regulates proteolysis at the bacterial surface by binding α2-macroglobulin. J Biol Chem 1999; 274:15336-5344.
155. Lukomski S, Nakashima K, Abdi I et al. Identification and characterization of a second extra cellular collagen-like protein made by group A Streptococcus: control of production at the level of translation. Infect Immun 2001; 69:1729-1738.
156. Lander ES, Linton LM, Birren B et al. Initial sequencing and analysis of the human genome. Nature 2001; 409:860-921.
157. Venter JC, Adams MD, Myers EW et al. The sequence of the human genome. Science 2001; 291:1304-1351.
158. Ferretti JJ, McShan WM, Ajdic D et al. Complete genome sequence of an M1 strain of Streptococcus pyogenes. Proc Natl Acad Sci USA 2001; 98:4658-4663.
159. Smoot JC, Barbian KD, Van Gompel JJ et al. Genome sequence and comparative microarray analysis of serotype M18 group A Streptococcus strains associated with acute rheumatic fever outbreaks. Proc Natl Acad Sci USA 2002; 99:4668-4673.
160. Beres SB, Sylva GL, Barbian KD et al. Genome sequence of a serotype M3 strain of group A Streptococcus: phage-encoded toxins, the high-virulence phenotype, and clone emergence. Proc Natl Acad Sci USA 2002; 99:10078-10083.
161. Smoot LM, Smoot JC, Graham MR et al. Global differential gene expression in response to growth temperature alteration in group A Streptococcus. Proc Natl Acad Sci USA 2001; 98:10416-10421.
162. Graham MR, Smoot LM, Migliaccio CA et al. Virulence control in group A Streptococcus by a two-component gene regulatory system: global expression profiling and in vivo infection modeling. Proc Natl Acad Sci USA 2002; 99:13855-13860.
163. Chaussee MS, Sylva GL, Sturdevant DE et al. Rgg influences the expression of multiple regulatory loci to coregulate virulence factor expression in Streptococcus pyogenes. Infect Immun 2002; 70:762-770.
164. Ashbaugh CD, Moser TJ, Shearer MH et al. Bacterial determinants of persistent throat colonization and the associated immune response in a primate model of human group A streptococcal pharyngeal infection. Cell Microbiol 2000, 2:283-292.
165. Lengeling A, Pfeffer K, Balling R. The battle of two genomes: genetics of bacterial host/pathogen interactions in mice. Mamm Genome 2001; 12:261-271.
166. Bessen DE, Fischetti VA. Vaccines against Streptococcus pyogenes infections. In: Levine MM, Woodrow GC, Kaper JB, Cobon GS, eds. New generation vaccines: Dekker M, 1997:783-802.
167. Virtaneva K, Graham Mr., Porcella SF et al. Group A Streptococcus gene expression in human and cynomologus macaques with acute pharygitis. Infect Immun 2003; In Press.

Chapter 11

Academic Pursuits of Vaccines against Group B *Streptococcus*

Lawrence C. Paoletti

Introduction

Today's welcome declines in the prevalence of early-onset group B *Streptococcus* (GBS) neonatal disease—due to active surveillance and use of intrapartum antibiotic prophylaxis [1]—may become tomorrow's problematic emergence of GBS strains bearing antibiotic resistance.[2,3] Vaccines against GBS offer the best hope for lasting protection against this opportunistic pathogen. This chapter will review research that has led to the development of promising vaccines against GBS disease. The progress towards effective GBS vaccines has been made through the unwavering determination of scientists with expertise in medicine, pediatrics, carbohydrate chemistry, immunology, microbiology, genetics, and epidemiology. Indeed, the GBS vaccinologist has gained a working knowledge of these independent fields of study that we hope will soon culminate in effective prevention of diseases caused by GBS.

Ecological Niches of GBS

Before it was recognized as a human pathogen, *Streptococcus agalactiae* (group B *Streptococcus* [GBS]) was well known as a primary cause of bovine mastitis and thus was mainly a health concern of the dairy industry.[4] Contaminated milk is not the source of human disease, but milk-borne outbreaks of streptococcal disease may have been associated with acute udder infection of dairy cattle.[5] *Streptococcus* colonize intestines of the human newborn in the first two weeks of life, but their numbers drop quickly to the low numbers present in the gastrointestinal tract of adults.[6] GBS, although considered a common member of the healthy adult colonic microflora, are present in low numbers relative to other streptococcal species and especially to other intestinal bacteria such as those belonging to the genus *Bacteroides*.[7]

Epidemiology of GBS Disease

Strategies for vaccine design and implementation are based on active surveillance of the population to determine who is most at risk of contracting disease. Schrag and coworkers, who studied invasive GBS disease in selected counties in the United States from 1993 to 1998,[1] showed (Table 1) that invasive GBS disease is most common in newborns less than 3 months of age and in adults. Both early-onset (<7 days of age) and late-onset (>7 days to 3 months of age) neonatal disease accounted for 2,196 (28%) of 7,834 total invasive GBS cases, while childhood (3 months to 14 years of age) cases accounted for only 2%.[1] Nonpregnant adults aged 15 to 64 years and the elderly (>65 years) each accounted for 33% of the total invasive cases. Pregnant women accounted for 4% in this study. The case fatality rates for neonatal, childhood, and adult GBS disease were 7.5%, 9.0%, and 23%, respectively. Most of the adults with invasive GBS disease had one of several underlying conditions, including diabetes mellitus, cardiovascular

New Bacterial Vaccines, edited by Ronald W. Ellis and Bernard R. Brodeur.

Table 1. Cases and fatality rates of invasive GBS disease in selected counties in the United States, 1993-1998 [1]

Population	No. of Cases (% of Total)	Case Fatality Rate (%)*
Newborn		
Early onset (<7 days of age)	1,584 (20)	4.7
Late onset (7-89 days of age)	612 (8)	2.8
Childhood		
(90 days – 14 years)	175 (2)	9
Adult		
15 – 64 years	2,559 (33)	8
≥65 years	2,559 (33)	15
Pregnant girls and women	345 (4)	0.003

A total of 7,834 cases from counties in Maryland, California, Georgia, Atlanta, Tennessee, Minnesota, Oregon, and New York. Population ranged from 12 million in 1993 to over 20 million in 1998.
*Disease outcome was available for 7,636 (97%) of the 7,834 cases.

disease, or cancer.[1] On the basis of this and other reports,[8-10] GBS no longer can be considered solely a neonatal pathogen but one that can cause disease in all age groups, particularly in immunocompromised adults and the elderly. Although the mode of transmission is unclear, elderly adults residing in nursing homes had a higher incidence of invasive GBS disease than did those living in the community,[11] a particular concern as the number of elderly adults in the United States population increases.

Two independent studies showed associations between GBS isolated from stool and rectal cultures and vaginal colonization, implicating the intestinal tract as the primary reservoir for vaginal or urogenital colonization among pregnant women.[12,13] GBS infection is not considered a sexually transmitted disease, although vaginal GBS colonization and acquisition have been associated with sexual activity.[14] Multiple sexual partners and frequent sexual intercourse (three or more times per week) were associated with increased risk of acquiring vaginal GBS. Colonization of the vagina during pregnancy is a known risk-factor for neonatal GBS disease. GBS is passed from mother to newborn during birth.[15,16] The newborn can aspirate GBS during birth, which can manifest as pneumonia and a subsequent bacteremia. In some cases, GBS bacteremia can lead to meningitis, which often results in neurological deficiencies.[17]

Association between GBS Disease and the Absence of Polysaccharide Specific Antibody

In the mid 1970s, Baker and colleagues investigated whether there were associations between maternal antibody to GBS capsular polysaccharide (CPS), vaginal colonization, and neonatal outcome in pregnant women.[18] They found an unambiguous association between low levels of maternal antibody to type III CPS and susceptibility of the newborn to GBS disease. In contrast, 22 (76%) of 29 pregnant women vaginally colonized with GBS whose babies were healthy possessed serum antibody specific to type III CPS.[18] This study also showed that women with GBS-specific capsular antibody transplacentally transfer these antibodies to the newborn, providing the essential rationale for developing a vaccine based on GBS CPS. A recent study by Campbell and coworkers[19] of pregnant women at time of delivery described an association between vaginal/rectal colonization with types Ia, II, III, and V and the presence of type-specific serum IgG, extending the above described studies that were limited only to serotype

III. No such correlation existed for serotype Ib, which was the least prevalent serotype among the colonized cohort. Interestingly, the lowest median level of type-specific IgG to GBS serotypes Ia, Ib, II, III and V was in sera from women <20 years of age and the highest among women 30 years and older.[19] These lower levels of antibody among teenagers may account for the increased risk of GBS disease in neonates born to this age group.

GBS Targets of Protective Immunity

The first step in vaccine development is identification of antigens on the pathogen that are either a central cause of disease or involved with persistence of illness.[20] The careful work of Rebecca Lancefield in describing GBS antigens thought to provide protection against infections in animals gave researchers a first clue to viable vaccine targets.

Carbohydrates

Group B Carbohydrate

GBS expresses two distinct surface-associated carbohydrates: the group B carbohydrate and the capsular polysaccharide (CPS) antigens. The group B carbohydrate is a highly branched structure of rhamnose, galactose, *N*-acetylglucosamine, and glucitol as the main sugar constituents.[21] Antibody to this surface structure is not protective against encapsulated GBS strains,[22] hence this polysaccharide has not been considered a candidate for development as a human vaccine. In direct contrast, antibody to the CPS antigens has been shown to protect against GBS infection and therefore has been the primary focus of vaccine development. Indeed, Rebecca Lancefield not only began to delineate serotypes based on cross-adsorption of polyclonal rabbit serum raised against whole encapsulated GBS, but also established the principle of polysaccharide-specific protection in mice using polyclonal rabbit serum to whole GBS.[23,24]

Type-Specific Carbohydrates

With an understanding that the CPS antigens were critical for immune protection against GBS disease, investigators began to determine the fine chemical composition and structure of these surface antigens. In the mid-1970s a collaborative effort was initiated to isolate, purify, and perform structural analyses of CPSs of clinically important GBS serotypes including types Ia,[25] Ib,[26] II,[27] and III.[27,28] Striking among the findings was the structural and antigenic heterogeneity among these four structures, despite the fact that they are composed of only four sugars: glucose, galactose, *N*-acetylglucosamine, and sialic acid. Structural analyses are now complete for all GBS serotypes including types IV,[29] V,[30] VI,[31] VII,[32] and VIII.[33] Although some of these structures are unique in that they lack *N*-acetylglucosamine (types VI and VII) or have rhamnose (found abundantly in the structure of the group B antigen) as a component sugar (type VIII), all nine possess a side chain composed of or terminating with the 9-carbon sugar sialic acid.[34]

Of the nine GBS CPSs, type III CPS has been the most thoroughly studied. It is composed of 100 to 150 pentasaccharide repeating unit polymers of glucose, galactose, *N*-acetyl glucosamine, and sialic acid.[27] Using immune rabbit serum to whole GBS type III bacteria or to chemically depolymerized type III CPSs, Jennings and coworkers demonstrated the presence of two distinct pools of antibody-binding epitopes: the major epitope was dependent on the presence of the side chain sialic acid sugar, and another was specific for a region on the backbone.[35] They showed that sialic acid can ionically interact with the backbone *N*-acetylglucosamine residue, thus imparting a conformational structure to the polymer. These results were expanded by Wessels and coworkers, who demonstrated a clear association between type III oligosaccharide chain length and high-affinity antibody binding. These results provided solid evidence of the recognition by specific antibodies of an epitope created by the conformation of the polymer as it increased in length from 2.6 to 92 repeating units.[28,36] With purified type III oligosaccharides,[37] Brisson and colleagues applied nuclear magnetic resonance and molecular dynamic techniques to show that the fully sialylated structure formed an extended helix within a random coil formation.[38,39] NMR measurements on sialylated as well as desialylated type III oligosaccharides confirmed previous observations of the importance of the sialic acid residue in creating the conformational epitope of native GBS type III CPS.

Immune rabbit sera to conjugate vaccines prepared with varying lengths of GBS type III oligosaccharides end-linked to tetanus toxoid (TT) also were used to study the effects of conformational epitopes on antibody affinity and function.[40] Higher binding affinity to native type III polysaccharide, elicited by conjugate vaccines prepared with oligosaccharides of 14 and 25 repeating units, corresponded to higher functional activity compared with the conjugate vaccine prepared with oligosaccharides of 6 repeating units. The relatively weak immunogenicity and functional activity of the oligosaccharide conjugate vaccine prepared with 6 repeating units was attributed to a loss of conformational epitopes.[40]

A potential shortcoming of the conformational studies with GBS type III CPS was that they were all performed with antibody raised in rabbits or mice. Would antibody from humans who received a type III conjugate vaccine also recognize a conformation-dependent epitope? The answer to this question awaited clinical trials with a GBS type III conjugate vaccine and will be discussed later in this chapter.

Protein Antigens

Several GBS surface proteins have been shown to be important for GBS pathogenesis, and some have been tested as vaccine candidates or as carrier proteins for the CPSs.[34] Although promising results have been obtained in animal protection studies with GBS proteins as vaccine candidates, none thus far have entered clinical trials in humans.

Alpha C Protein

The alpha C protein, which exhibits a laddering profile on sodium dodecyl sulfate-polyacrylamide gels, is an attractive target as a vaccine candidate as it is found on the surface of about 50% of all GBS clinical isolates and on 70% of nontype III GBS.[41] A conjugate vaccine comprising type III CPS coupled to a two-repeating unit alpha C protein conferred 95% protection against GBS type III challenge to neonatal mice born to actively vaccinated dams and 60% survival among pups challenged with GBS type Ia strain A909 bearing the alpha C protein.[41] In addition, 73% of mouse pups born to dams vaccinated with uncoupled two-repeat alpha C protein alone survived challenge with GBS type Ia, thus demonstrating the utility of this protein as both an effective carrier for GBS CPS and an immunogen against alpha C protein-bearing GBS.

Beta C protein

The beta C protein is found on 10% to 25% of all GBS isolates mainly of those bearing type Ib CPS, and unlike the alpha C protein, it is sensitive to digestion with trypsin.[34] GBS beta C protein, which induces protective antibodies in animals,[42-44] also has been a good carrier protein for GBS type III CPS. A type III CPS-beta C protein conjugate elicited in mice protective antibodies against strains of GBS bearing either the type III antigen or the beta C protein.[45]

Rib

Rib protein, present on GBS type III strains, is structurally similar to, but antigenically distinct from, the alpha C protein. Both are laddering proteins that are resistant to trypsin digestion.[46] Antiserum to Rib protected mice against challenge against Rib-containing GBS but not against those strains containing the alpha C protein.[47] A vaccine mixture composed of both Rib and alpha C proteins resulted in complete protection against GBS type III strains in mice.[47]

C5a Peptidase

A conserved surface protein, C5a peptidase, found on all strains of GBS has recently been shown to induce opsonically active antibody in experimental animals.[48] Although much work remains to be done on the application of C5a peptidase as either a carrier protein or an immunogen, promising results were obtained with antibody raised in animals to a GBS type III-C5a peptidase conjugate vaccine.[48] Cheng and colleagues demonstrated the ability of antibodies to III-C5a peptidase antibody to opsonize GBS serotypes Ib, III, and V for in vitro phagocytic killing, implying that C5a peptidase may induce antibody with serotype-independent activity.[48] The ability of C5a peptidase alone or as a carrier protein for CPS antigens to induce cross-serotype protection awaits experimentation in an animal model such as the maternal vaccination-neonatal mouse model of GBS disease used extensively with other GBS vaccines.[49]

Sip

A GBS protein called surface immunogenic protein (Sip) with an apparent molecular mass of 53 kDa has been detected on strains of all nine GBS serotypes.[50] Antibody to Sip bound mainly to polar and septal surface regions of GBS, suggesting localization to areas of new wall growth.[51] Active vaccination of adult mice with 20 μg of recombinant Sip protein mixed with Quil A adjuvant induced antibody that reacted with whole GBS of serotypes Ia, Ib, III, and V. These mice were partially (70%) to completely (100%) protected against challenge with strains of GBS types Ia, Ib, II, III, V, and VI.[50] This vaccine was also ≥78% effective against GBS challenge in neonatal mice born to actively vaccinated dams.[52] Sip represents yet another protein that induces protective and cross-serotype immunity to GBS in mice. This protein may be developed as a stand-alone vaccine or perhaps as a useful carrier protein for carbohydrate antigens from other encapsulated pathogens. The role of the Sip antigen in GBS virulence and pathogenesis remains to be elucidated.

Clinical Trials with GBS Vaccines

Native CPSs

The type III CPS was the first to be tested as a vaccine because this serotype was responsible for about two-thirds of invasive GBS disease.[53] No preclinical testing of purified GBS CPSs could have substantiated their use in clinical trials because, like many bacterial polysaccharides, they are poorly immunogenic in rabbits and mice. However, the strong correlation between low maternal CPS-specific antibody and neonatal GBS disease[18] prompted testing of purified type III CPS vaccines in several phase 1 trials. By the mid-1980s approximately 300 healthy adults had received a GBS CPS vaccine at doses ranging from 10 to 150 μg.[54-58] The high level of safety with GBS CPS vaccine allowed for a phase 1 trial with type III CPS in pregnant women.[59] This trial would become one of the most important clinical studies with the "first-generation" GBS (native, uncoupled type III CPS) vaccine. At least three important principles were established with this landmark study: a) the CPS vaccine was safe and well tolerated; b) the immunogenicity of the vaccine depended on the preexisting immune status of the individual; and c) a direct correlation existed between maternal and cord blood levels of CPS-specific IgG.[59] Clearly, the approach of maternal vaccination to provide the neonate with circulating specific antibody and possibly to prevent neonatal GBS disease was feasible. However, it was necessary to improve the immunogenicity of the CPS, since only ~60% of the recipients of the type III CPS vaccine mounted an immune response. Subsequent research focused on methods to improve the immunogenicity of GBS CPS antigens. Conjugation technology had been applied to improve the immunogenicity of *Haemophilus influenzae* type b polysaccharide, which eventually became the first polysaccharide-protein conjugate licensed for use in humans. Now, glycoconjugate vaccines against several other pathogens are licensed or have advanced to phase 3 clinical trials.[60]

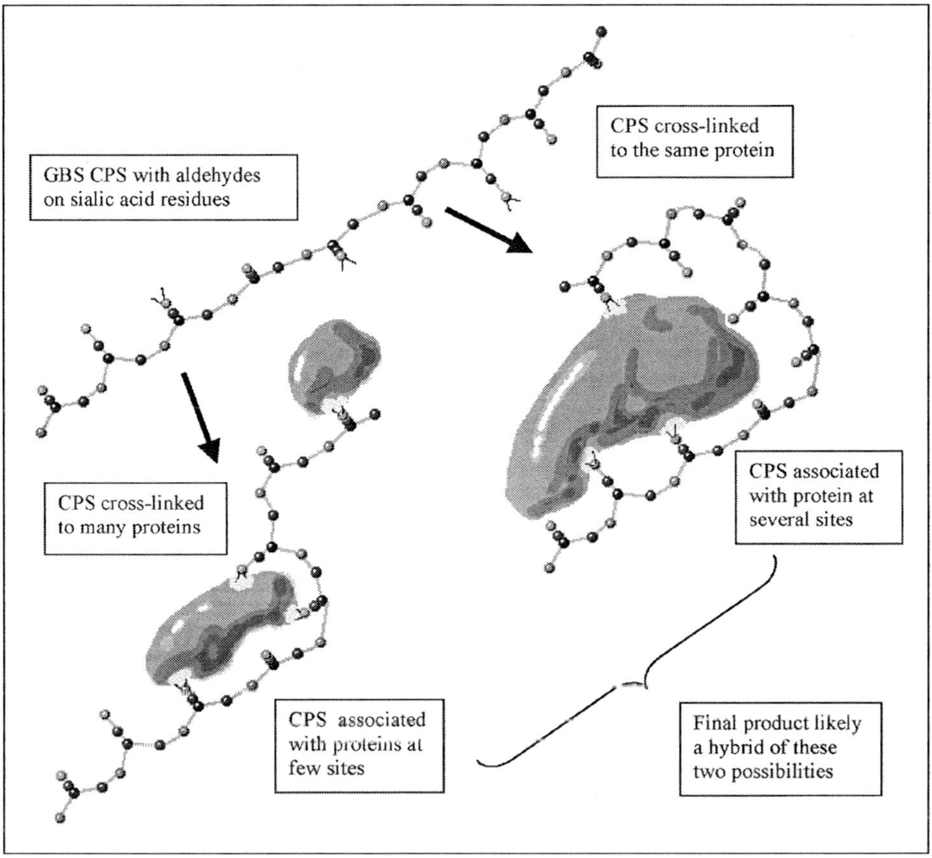

Figure 1. Schematic representation of potential molecular interactions between GBS capsular polysaccharides (CPS) and proteins. Chains of group B streptococcal CPS with aldehyde groups created on a targeted number of sialic acid sugars can cross-link several proteins (left arrow) or can associate with the same protein at several sites (right arrow). Because protein elution profiles from conjugation reactions are often broad indicating a wide range of molecular masses,[41,63,107] the final product is most likely a composite of these two possibilities. Illustration by Tom Dicesare.

Conjugated GBS CPSs

The results of studies by Wessels and colleagues revealed that sialic acid was an important virulence factor for type III CPS.[61] Oxidation of this CPS with sodium periodate, which creates aldehydes on a portion of the sialic acid residues, does not destroy epitopes critical for the maintenance of antigenicity.[35] The importance of this finding cannot be overstated, as it delineated a way for targeted, direct coupling of GBS CPS to proteins by a well-known chemical reaction called reductive amination.[62] This reaction was used to improve the immunogenicity of GBS CPS antigens by coupling them individually to immunogenic proteins carriers (Fig. 1).

Taking advantage of the chemical structures of the CPS antigens, the "second generation" of GBS vaccines consisted of the CPS-protein conjugates linked covalently without the use of a spacer molecule. Selection of GBS serotypes to target for vaccine development was based on epidemiological findings of those associated with neonatal GBS disease. Isolates from GBS-colonized newborns consisted mostly of serotype Ia (31.6%) followed by types II (25%), III (22.4%), V (11.8%), and Ib (7.9%); 1.3% were nontypable.[16] These serotypes are also

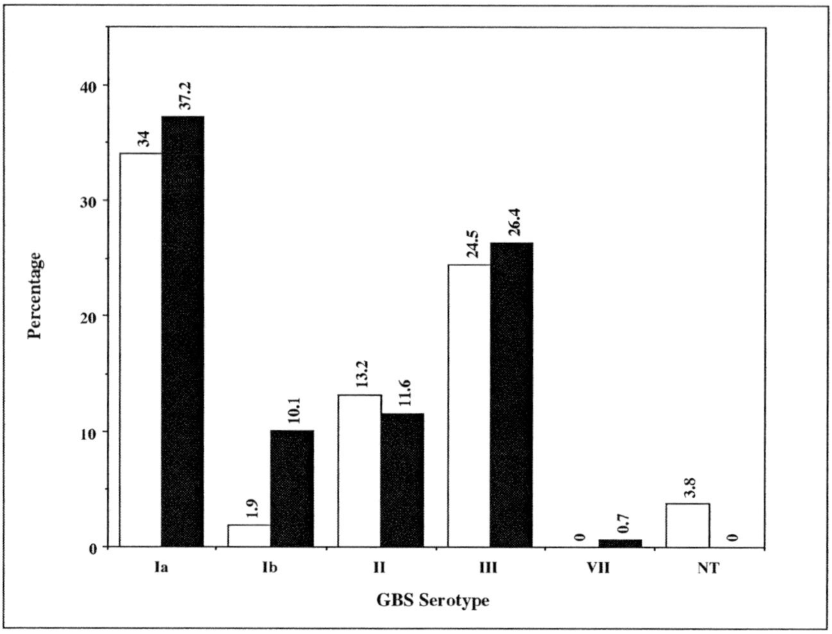

Figure 2. Distribution of invasive group B streptococcal serotypes among pregnant women (white bars, n = 53) and neonates <7 days of age (black bars, n = 129). Data from Zaleznik et al.[108]

responsible for invasive GBS disease among both pregnant women and neonates (Fig. 2). As with the CPS vaccines, the first GBS conjugate vaccines were prepared with serotype III, because this serotype was responsible for the majority of invasive GBS disease.[53]

Two conjugate vaccines were prepared with full-length type III CPS, and a third was prepared with type III oligosaccharides. Native type III CPS was coupled to TT either by reductive amination via aldehydes created by periodate oxidation on a selected number of sialic acid residues[63] or by carbodiimide reduction using adipic acid dihydrazide as a spacer.[64] GBS type III CPS conjugate vaccines elicited in animals high-titered, opsonically active IgG to the GBS CPS at levels that dramatically eclipsed those elicited by uncoupled type III CPS. To date, only GBS CPS conjugate vaccines prepared with the former coupling method have entered human clinical trials.

In addition to these vaccines, a GBS type III oligosaccharide—prepared by digesting native CPS with endo-β-galactosidase—was covalently linked to TT via its reducing end using an 8-carbon spacer molecule.[65] Like the full-length CPS, the oligosaccharide-TT conjugate vaccine also raised in animals high-titered, opsonically active IgG. Type III oligosaccharide conjugates, although useful tools to study the immune-system recognition of carbohydrate polymers of varying chain lengths,[40] were not practical to develop for even small clinical studies because of the labor-intensive methods needed to create the oligosaccharides. In addition, selecting an oligosaccharide with the optimal chain length is clearly not as efficient as using native CPS, and the need for a spacer molecule added another step to the conjugation reaction, reasons that prompted the abandonment of oligosaccharide conjugate vaccines for a more focused effort on the development of conjugates using full-length CPS. It is worth noting that ozonolysis[66] and a chemoenzymatic method[67] are two new ways of efficiently creating oligosaccharides from GBS CPSs. These advances may prompt a manufacturer to reexamine the feasibility of generating GBS oligosaccharide conjugate vaccines.

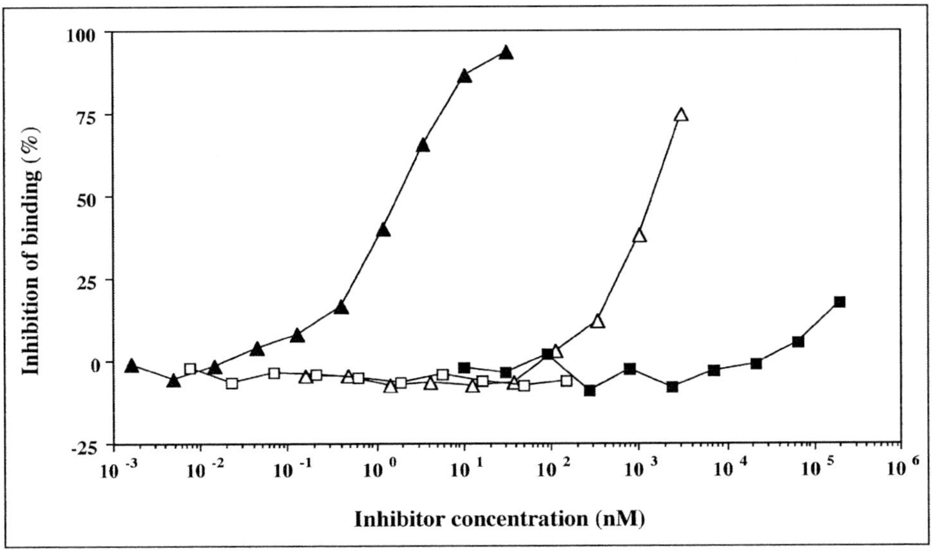

Figure 3. Human antibody to group B streptococcal type III-tetanus toxoid conjugate vaccine recognizes a conformational epitope. Inhibition of binding of antibody to type III CPS as the target antigen on an ELISA plate by native type III polysaccharide (closed triangles), 25-repeating unit type III polysaccharide (open triangles), 1-repeating unit type III oligosaccharides (closed squares), and human serum albumin (open squares).[70] Copyright 1996 by Journal of Clinical Investigation. Reproduced with permission of Journal of Clinical Investigation in the format Trade Book via Copyright Clearance Center.

All nine currently identified GBS CPSs possess side chains composed of or terminating with sialic acid, which allows this nine-carbon sugar to be used on each type CPS as a site for the formation of aldehydes that can in turn be used to couple to amino groups on proteins. Indeed, conjugate vaccines with Ia, Ib, II, III, and V—those most prevalent in the United States—have been tested preclinically and clinically.

Clinical Trials of GBS Type III Conjugate *Vaccine*

Several preclinical trials with conjugate vaccines prepared with GBS type III CPS[63,64,68,69] led to the first testing of a type III CPS-TT (III-TT) vaccine in healthy nonpregnant women. One hundred women of childbearing age were randomized in phase 1 and phase 2 trials to receive a single dose at one of three concentrations of III-TT vaccine, of uncoupled type III CPS, or of saline placebo. Overall, the conjugated and unconjugated type III CPS vaccines were well tolerated, with little reactogenicity noted.[70] Serum levels of type III CPS-specific IgG rose sharply in a dose-dependent fashion only two weeks after vaccination with the conjugate vaccine. Elevated levels of specific antibody persisted for 26 weeks. Type III CPS-specific IgG concentrations correlated closely (r = 0.71) with functional activity as measured with an in vitro opsonophagocytic killing assay. The relative affinities for native type III CPS of GBS type III CPS-specific antibody were nearly identical, whether the antibodies were elicited by the III-TT vaccine or the native type III CPS vaccine. This finding indicated that periodate oxidation of the CPS followed by reductive amination coupling to a protein did not destroy critical binding epitopes.[70] Indeed, antibody from healthy adults vaccinated with a GBS III-TT vaccine recognized a conformation-dependent epitope as had been shown previously with vaccine-induced antibody from animals. The conformation-dependent epitope (Fig. 3) was evident by the higher affinity binding of the III-TT antibody to native type III CPS (~150 repeating units) than to shorter saccharides of 25 repeating units in length and no binding to one-repeating unit oligosaccharides.[70] Human antibody to III-TT vaccine was functionally active in vitro and therapeutically active against GBS infection in a neonatal mouse model.[71] These first successful trials with the second-generation GBS vaccine led the way for additional trials with conjugate vaccines of GBS CPS antigens of other clinically relevant serotypes.

Clinical Trials of GBS Types Ia and Ib Conjugate Vaccines

Although some scientists may consider type Ia and type Ib CPSs to be identical, the results of several investigators[23,26,68] showed that these closely related structures indeed are both antigenically and immunologically distinct. Whereas cross-protective antibody can be raised in rabbits immunized with Ia-TT,[72] complete protection in mouse pups required active vaccination of dams with conjugate vaccines prepared with both type Ia and type Ib CPSs.[68]

Preclinical studies in rabbits and mice provided the necessary evidence of efficacy to progress to phase 1 and 2 testing of both Ia-TT and Ib-TT vaccines in healthy nonpregnant women of childbearing age.[73] These vaccines were individually administered at Ia CPS doses of 60, 15 and 3.75 μg and Ib CPS doses of 63, 15.75, and 3.94 μg in the absence of an adjuvant. As with the III-TT vaccine, the Ia-TT and the Ib-TT vaccines were generally well tolerated. Brisk rises in type-specific serum IgG levels were measured two weeks after a single intramuscular vaccination for both conjugate vaccines. Type-specific antibodies evoked by the conjugate vaccines persisted at ~50% of peak values through 1 year. Type-specific IgG levels to both types Ia and Ib CPS correlated strongly with opsonic titers in phagocytosis assays.[73] These two clinical trials expanded the repertoire of GBS conjugate vaccines tested safely in humans and demonstrated the utility of the reductive amination coupling procedure as a method useful to augment the immunogenicity of CPSs other than type III in humans.

Clinical Trials of GBS Type II Conjugate Vaccine

Unlike type Ia, Ib, and III CPSs, type II possesses two monosaccharide side chains, one of galactose and the other of sialic acid.[74] In the generation of conjugate vaccines, relatively higher amounts of sodium periodate were required to oxidize the sialic acid residues, perhaps due to the proximal positions of the side chain saccharides to the backbone of the polymer. This technical hurdle was overcome by increasing the ratio of periodate to sialic acid residues, and type II conjugate vaccines were prepared again using TT as the carrier protein and were tested for efficacy in mice.[75] It was determined that efficacious type II conjugates could be prepared using type II CPS with 30 - 60% of its sialic acid residues oxidized. A clinical grade GBS type II-TT was prepared with 35% sialic acid oxidation and evaluated in phase 1 and 2 trials. It was the first GBS conjugate vaccine vialed as a lyophilized preparation using sucrose as the excipient. The conjugate vaccine was reconstituted with phosphate-buffered saline containing 0.01% thimerosal and was randomly administered at a CPS concentration of 57, 14.3, or 3.6 μg to nonpregnant healthy women of childbearing age; another group received a 45-μg dose of uncoupled type II CPS. One subject who received the 14.3-μg dose developed fever (37.8^{0}C) chills, malaise, and headache 17 hours later. These reactions resolved after 36 hours, and no other serious adverse events were reported.[75] Two weeks after vaccination, the II-TT elicited a sharp rise in type-specific IgG response that was dose dependent and durable at levels above baseline after 2 years. Immune serum obtained from recipients of the conjugate vaccines was opsonically active in vitro against GBS type II. In addition to a strong IgG response, this conjugate vaccine also elicited type II CPS-specific serum antibody of the IgM and IgA isotype.[75] Why this conjugate vaccine, and to a lesser extent uncoupled type II CPS, evoked these three antibody isotypes is currently unknown.

Clinical Trial of GBS type V Conjugate Vaccines

While preclinical studies with GBS types Ia, Ib, II, and III were underway, a new GBS serotype—type V—emerged among both infants and adults.[76-80] An international effort resulted in the rapid isolation, purification, and structural analysis of the new type V CPS.[30] Because the type V CPS contained a side chain that terminated with sialic acid, the reductive amination coupling procedure used successfully with other GBS serotypes was also used with this CPS to create conjugate vaccines. GBS type V-TT vaccines elicited type-specific IgG in rabbits that was functionally active against GBS type V in vitro.[81] Moreover, these vaccines were efficacious in newborn pups against type V challenge in the maternal vaccination-neonatal mouse model of GBS disease.[81] Two lots of clinical GBS type V vaccines were prepared with TT and cross-reactive material (CRM_{197}), a mutant diphtheria protein, as the carrier proteins. Preliminary results showed that both of these conjugate vaccines were safe and immunogenic in healthy adults.[82]

Preclinical Trials of Conjugate Vaccines of Other GBS Serotypes

Preclinical and clinical GBS vaccine development has focused on those serotypes most prevalent in the United States. In addition, conjugate vaccines with serotypes VI and VIII—serotypes prevalent thus far only in Japan[83]—have also been generated and shown to be more immunogenic in animals than homologous uncoupled CPS.[84] GBS CPS conjugate vaccines have also been useful in generating high-titered, polyclonal rabbit antisera that are monospecific with respect to the CPS and useful in many studies including serotyping. Towards that end, high-titered types IV and VII CPS-specific rabbit sera have been made with use of conjugate vaccines prepared with these two CPSs.[84b]

Advanced Clinical Trials

All of the GBS clinical trials discussed thus far were designed to establish the safety and immunogenicity in healthy nonpregnant adults of a single dose of a single serotype conjugate in the absence of an adjuvant. Attention has now focused on ways of improving the immunogenicity of the already improved CPS conjugate vaccines by use of an adjuvant and by administration of two doses. We also sought to determine whether immune interference would occur by combining two different conjugates and administering them simultaneously. Most recently, a III-TT vaccine was administered to women early in the third trimester of their pregnancy.

Bivalent Vaccine Trial

An effective GBS vaccine will protect against multiple GBS serotypes, namely types Ia, Ib, II, III, and V, which are currently the most prevalent in the United States. To establish the safety of each new vaccine, clinical trials with GBS conjugate vaccines were performed with a single serotype conjugate vaccine. With the safety of each conjugate vaccine established, a trial was initiated to study the safety of and immune response to two GBS CPS conjugate vaccines administered simultaneously. GBS type II-TT and type III-TT were combined and administered as a single intramuscular injection to healthy adults, while control groups received each monovalent vaccine at the same dose as in the bivalent preparation. All vaccines were well tolerated. Following vaccination, ≥4-fold rises in type II CPS-specific IgG were measured in serum from ≥80% of subjects who received the monovalent or bivalent preparation of II-TT; and a 4-fold rise in type III CPS-specific IgG was measured in serum from >90% of recipients of the monovalent or bivalent preparation of III-TT.[85] These results indicate that no apparent immune interference existed between the two serotypes. Whether immune interference will exist when more than two GBS CPS conjugate vaccines are simultaneously administered can only be determined by further experimentation.

Adjuvant and Two-Dose Studies

A GBS III-TT vaccine adsorbed to aluminum hydroxide was administered to healthy adults at suboptimal concentrations, and type III CPS-specific IgG responses were compared with those who received unadsorbed III-TT.[86] Alum did not improve the immune response to either the III CPS or the TT component of the vaccine, an unexpected result given previous studies in baboons in which the presence of alum was essential to induce an immune response.[69] Unlike humans, the baboons vaccinated with III-TT vaccine had not been exposed previously to the carrier protein TT. Whether carrier priming influenced the ability of alum to augment the immune response is not known. Indeed, little is known regarding the augmentative role of alum with glycoconjugate vaccines.

The effects of a booster dose on the immune response were determined by giving healthy adults two doses 21 months apart of III-TT vaccine without alum.[69] The second dose of III-TT restored type III CPS-specific IgG levels to those achieved 1 month after administration of the first dose. However, the most pronounced effect was seen not in those with preexisting levels of type III CPS-specific IgG >0.05 μg/mL but in the minority of subjects who had preexisting levels <0.05 μg/mL, who had a 300% increase in geometric mean IgG levels.[69] This study may be useful in determining a vaccination schedule necessary to achieve high levels of specific antibody for an adult population.

Maternal Vaccination

A milestone in GBS vaccine development was recently achieved with the administration of a type III-TT conjugate to third-trimester pregnant women. In a double-blind, placebo-controlled trial, 30 women at a mean gestation of 31.2 weeks were randomized to receive either a single dose of III-TT (12.5 μg CPS) or saline placebo.[87] All subjects delivered at >37 weeks gestation, and all had normal healthy babies. Maternal geometric mean serum concentration of type III CPS-specific IgG at delivery was 9.8 μg/mL and correlated closely ($r^2 = 0.96$) with infant cord blood values. Antiserum from infants of vaccinated mothers was opsonically active in vitro against type III GBS.[87] These results indicate that a GBS conjugate vaccine can be safely administered to pregnant women during the early third trimester, that maternally derived specific IgG can cross the placenta, and that antibody from infants is opsonically active against viable GBS.

Target Populations to Receive GBS Vaccines

Pregnant Women

The first clinical report of neonatal sepsis due to GBS was published in 1964,[88] 25 years after the first report of GBS disease in an adult.[89] Clinical reports published in the 1960s[88,90,91] showed a steady increase in the prevalence of GBS among neonates. Vaccine efforts galvanized around preventing neonatal GBS disease, by means of maternal vaccination. Although maternal vaccination is the best strategy for the prevention of neonatal GBS disease, there are several obstacles to its being universally accepted.[92] Foremost among them is the concern of vaccine safety. Clearly, any vaccine ought to be safe, and well tolerated and have a little or no risk of causing harm. Liability concerns are interwoven with any medical intervention, but perhaps at a higher level of sensitivity when the patient is pregnant.[93] The interested reader is referred to a discussion on delivery of vaccines to pregnant women in a report on vaccines issued recently by the Institutes of Medicine.[94]

GBS conjugate vaccines have been developed with the goal of generating a safe and effective vaccine that can be administered to pregnant women. Tetanus toxoid has been chosen as the carrier protein for almost all clinical GBS vaccine trials because of its long record of safe global use in women during pregnancy to prevent neonatal tetanus.[95] Several animal models, including baboons, have demonstrated placental transport of GBS conjugate vaccine-induced IgG to provide protection against infection to the offspring.[45,96] And as described above, the first clinical trial of a GBS conjugate vaccine in pregnant women demonstrated its safety and immunogenicity.[87]

Women of Childbearing Age

Vaccination of women of childbearing age with a GBS conjugate vaccine may be a viable alternative to maternal vaccination as a means of protecting newborns. Indeed, a higher proportion of neonates born to women given *H. influenzae* type b (Hib) conjugate vaccine before pregnancy had protective antibody than did offspring of those who did not receive an Hib conjugate vaccine.[97] Although the long-term functional activity of GBS conjugate vaccine-induced antibody remains to be determined, CPS-specific IgG at ~50% of peak levels was measured in recipients of a GBS type Ia-TT and Ib-TT vaccine 1 year after vaccination, suggesting a sustained and durable response to a single dose of vaccine.[73]

Elderly and/or Immunocompromised Adults

The percentage of cases and case fatality rates of invasive GBS disease among those 65 years and older were among the highest of all age groups,[1] making this population the most at need for an effective vaccine. Because of the increased prevalence in GBS disease among the elderly, particularly, those in nursing homes and with underlying illnesses, future testing of GBS CPS conjugate vaccines in the elderly is warranted.

Future of GBS Vaccine Research and Implementation

Antigen Discovery

On the basis of epidemiological data, extensive preclinical and clinical testing, and record of safety and immunogenicity, the first effective GBS vaccine for use in the United States will most likely be multivalent in design, incorporating types Ia, Ib, II, III, and V CPSs. These CPSs will most likely be individually coupled to two or more protein carriers similar to the formulation of the 7-valent pneumococcal conjugate vaccine.[98]

However, the future of GBS vaccine research will likely progress along two separate paths. The CPS-based path will focus on improving existing technology for coupling oligosaccharides from each serotype of interest to a single protein carrier. Procedures for efficiently generating oligosaccharides from GBS exist[66,67] as does end link coupling technology, as demonstrated by Laferriere et al with pneumococcal type 14 oligosaccharides.[99] Challenges with this technology include binding oligosaccharides from each major serotype to a single carrier protein in a reproducible fashion to satisfy manufacturing quality-control standards.

The second path will focus on GBS proteins involved with colonization and/or invasion. With the exception of the alpha C protein[100] and C5a peptidase,[48] the function of GBS proteins developed as vaccine candidates has yet to be determined. Perhaps one of the several GBS protein antigens described earlier is involved with colonization and/or invasion of host tissue. The whole genome of *S. pneumoniae* sequences, was used to identify surface proteins that may serve as important targets of immunity.[101,102] Sequencing the whole genome of GBS may expedite identification of yet unrevealed antigens involved in pathogenicity and complement genetic approaches such as signature-tagged mutagenesis, which has already identified many genes thought to play a role in in vivo survival of GBS.[103]

Indeed, our understanding of GBS lags behind that of many other bacterial pathogens. We have yet to determine 1) which surface proteins act as adhesins; 2) which proteins are involved with invasion; 3) the tissue ligands for these receptors; and 4) whether any putative adhesins or invasins are potential vaccine candidates.[104] New directions in GBS vaccine development may arise from studies of attachment and invasion, particularly through the use of the newly described technology: the dynamic in vitro attachment and invasion system (DIVAS). DIVAS was developed to study GBS attachment and invasion with GBS cells held at specific and controlled conditions of growth, metabolism, and nutrient levels.[105] Experiments performed in DIVAS with GBS type III strains substantiated earlier findings that CPS is not critical to the invasion of A549 respiratory epithelial cells.[106] However, GBS type III strain M781 invaded A549 cells only when held at a fast growth rate as opposed to a relatively slow rate of growth.[105] In addition, GBS expressed several proteins solely under growth conditions conducive for effective invasion of respiratory epithelial cells. These proteins may be important targets of protective immunity, especially at mucosal sites where GBS colonization can be retarded or ablated.

Table 2. Milestones in GBS vaccine development

Year	Finding
1938	Rebecca Lancefield demonstrates passive protection against GBS disease in mice using rabbit serum to whole GBS[23]
1976	Correlation demonstrated between low CPS-specific antibody and neonatal susceptibility to disease.[18]
1980	Structure of GBS type III CPS revealed the presence of side chains with terminal sialic acid residues.[27]
1981	Antigenicity of the type III CPS retained after periodate oxidation and borohydride reduction, indicating that direct, covalent coupling of this CPS to a protein can be achieved without use of a spacer molecule.[35]
1988	Type III CPS vaccine administered safely to third trimester pregnant women. Correlation shown between maternal and cord blood serum type III CPS-specific IgG.[59]
1990	Improved immunogenicity in animals to CPS antigens by covalent coupling to immunogenic nonGBS protein carriers.[63,64]
1991	First GBS type III CPS coupled to tetanus toxoid conjugate vaccine prepared for use in humans.[49]
1994	Multivalent protection in mice with a tetravalent conjugate vaccine.[68]
1994	First vaccine prepared and evaluated preclinically using type III CPS conjugated to GBS beta C-protein, demonstrating the use of the protein as both a carrier and an immunogen.[45]
1995	First lot of type III-tetanus toxoid conjugate prepared under good manufacturing practices (GMP).[49]
1996	First clinical study in nonpregnant women of GBS CPS conjugate vaccine performed with a type III CPS coupled to tetanus toxoid.[70]
1998	First clinical trial in healthy adults of type III-tetanus toxoid conjugate prepared under GMP.[82]
1999	Administration in healthy adults of a GBS bivalent conjugate vaccine.[85]
2001	Phase I testing in pregnant women of a GMP lot of type III-tetanus toxoid conjugate vaccine.[87]

Induction of Mucosal Immunity

Induction of systemic humoral responses - mainly IgG responses - has been the goal in the development of GBS vaccines to prevent neonatal disease because this is the only isotype of antibodies that crosses the placenta. Relatively little attention has been given to the induction of mucosal immune responses to GBS conjugate vaccines. Would induction of secretory IgA in the vagina abrogate GBS colonization? How would a GBS conjugate vaccine be designed to induce a mucosal immune response? And how would such a vaccine be delivered? A key to addressing these questions awaits the development of an animal model to study GBS colonization and mucosal immunity.

Summary

An effective vaccine for GBS has recently been given a high priority by the National Academy of Sciences, Institute of Medicine. It was one of seven vaccines in the Level I (most favorable) category, as it is anticipated to save both health care costs and quality-adjusted life years if administered to "women during first pregnancy and to high-risk adults (at age 65 years and to people less than 65 years with serious, chronic health conditions)".[94] Because of the over 30 years of NIH-funded research on GBS pathogenesis, virulence properties, epidemiological surveillance and vaccine development (Table 2), a safe and immunogenic vaccine has now been developed against the five major serotypes prevalent in the United States. Academic pursuits have provided the blueprints necessary for the vaccine industry to now develop and manufacture a safe, effective multivalent vaccine against invasive GBS disease.

Acknowledgments and Dedication

I thank Angel Rosas and Jean C. Lee for critical review of this manuscript, and Jaylyn Olivo for editorial assistance. This article is dedicated to the myriad of scientists particularly Dennis L. Kasper, Michael L. Wessels, Lawrence C. Madoff, Carol J. Baker, Morven S. Edwards, Marcia Rench and Harold J. Jennings who, along with their colleagues, have been instrumental the GBS vaccine effort. Research described in this article was funded primarily by grants and contracts (AI-25152 and AI-75326) from the NIH-NIAID. The author is a recipient of the William Randolph Hearst Award from Harvard Medical School.

References

1. Schrag SJ, Zywicki S, Farley MM et al. Group B streptococcal disease in the era of intrapartum antibiotic prophylaxis. N Engl J Med 2000; 342(1):15-20.
2. Pearlman MD, Pierson CL, Faix RG. Frequent resistance of clinical group B streptococci isolates to clindamycin and erythromycin. Obstet Gyneco 1998; 92(2):258-261.
3. Fernandez M, Hickman ME, Baker CJ. Antimicrobial susceptibilities of group B streptococci isolated between 1992 and 1996 from patients with bacteremia or meningitis. Antimicrob Agents Chemother1998; 42(6):1517-1519.
4. Baker C, Edwards M. Group B streptococcal infections. In: Remington J, Klein J, eds. Infectious diseases of the fetus and newborn infant. Philadelphia: WB Saunders, 1990:742-811.
5. Freeman BA. Burrows Textbook of microbiology. Philadelphia: WB Saunders Co., 1979.
6. Cooperstock MS, Zedd AJ. Intestinal flora or infants. In: Hentges DJ, ed. Human intestinal microflora in health and disease. New York: Academic Press, 1983:79-99.
7. Finegold SM, Sutter VL, Mathisen GE. Normal indigenous intestinal flora. In: Hentges DJ, ed. Human intestinal microflora in health and disease. New York: Academic Press, 1983:3-31.
8. Harrison LH, Ali A, Dwyer DM et al. Relapsing invasive group B streptococcal infection in adults [see comments]. Ann Intern Med 1995; 123(6):421-427.
9. Jackson LA, Hilsdon R, Farley MM et al. Risk factors for group B streptococcal disease in adults. Ann. Intern. Med. 1995; 123:415-420.
10. Harrison LH, Elliott JA, Dwyer DM et al. Serotype distribution of invasive group B streptococcal isolates in Maryland: implications for vaccine formulation. J Infect Dis. 1998; 177(4):998-1002.
11. Henning KJ, Hall EL, Dwyer DM et al. Invasive group B streptococcal disease in Maryland nursing home residents. J Infect Dis 2001; 183(7):1138-1142.
12. Dillon HJ, Gray E, Pass MA et al. Anorectal and vaginal carriage of group B streptococci during pregnancy. J Infect Dis 1982; 145(6):794-799.
13. Anthony BF, Eisenstadt R, Carter J et al. Genital and intestinal carriage of group B streptococci during pregnancy. J Infect Dis 1981; 143(6):761-766.
14. Meyn LAD, Moore DM, Hillier SL et al. Association of sexual activity with colonization of vaginal acquisition of group B Streptococcus in nonpregnant women. Am J Epidemiol 2002; 155:949-957.
15. Baker CJ, Barrett FF. Transmission of group B streptococci among parturient women and their neonates. J Pediat 1973; 83(6):919-925.
16. Hickman ME, Rench MA, Ferrieri P et al. Changing epidemiology of group B streptococcal colonization. Pediatrics 1999; 104(2 Pt 1):203-209.
17. Baker CJ. Group B streptococcal infections. Clin Perinatol 1997; 24(1):59-70.
18. Baker CJ, Kasper DL. Correlation of maternal antibody deficiency with susceptibility to neonatal group B streptococcal infection. N Engl J Med 1976; 294:753-756.
19. Campbell JR, Hillier SL, Krohn MA et al. Group B streptococcal colonization and serotype-specific immunity in pregnant women at delivery. Obset Gyneco 2000; 96:498-503.
20. Rappuoli R, Del Giudice G. Identification of vaccine targets. In: Paoletti LC, McInnes PM, eds. Vaccines. From concept to clinic. A guide to the development and clinical testing of vaccines for human use. Boca Raton: CRC Press, 1999:1-17.
21. Michon F, Brisson JR, Dell A et al, Multiantennary group-specific polysaccharide of group B Streptococcus. Biochemistry 1988; 27(14):5341-5351.

22. Marques MB, Kasper DL, Shroff A et al. Functional activity of antibodies to the group B polysaccharide of group B streptococci elicited by a polysaccharide-protein conjugate vaccine. Infect Immun 1994; 62(5):1593-1599.
23. Lancefield RC. Two serological types of group B hemolytic streptococci with related, but not identical, type-specific substances. J Exp Med 1938; 67:25-40.
24. Lancefield RC. A serological differentiation of specific types of bovine hemolytic streptococci (group B). J Exp Med 1934; 59:441-458.
25. Jennings HJ, Rosell KG, Kasper DL. Structure and serology of the native polysaccharide antigen of type Ia group B Streptococcus. Proc Natl Acad Sci U S A 1980;77(5):2931-2935.
26. Jennings HJ, Katzenellenbogen E, Lugowski C et al. Structure of native polysaccharide antigens of type Ia and type Ib group B Streptococcus. Biochemistry 1983; 22(5):1258-1264.
27. Jennings HJ, Rosell KG, Kasper DL. Structural determination and serology of the native polysaccharide antigen of type-III group B Streptococcus. Can J Biochem 1980; 58(2):112-120.
28. Wessels MR, Pozsgay V, Kasper DL et al. Structure and immunochemistry of an oligosaccharide repeating unit of the capsular polysaccharide of type III group B Streptococcus. A revised structure for the type III group B streptococcal polysaccharide antigen J Biol Chem 19; 262(17):8262-8267.
29. Wessels MR, Benedi WJ, Jennings HJ et al. Isolation and characterization of type IV group B Streptococcus capsular polysaccharide. Infect Immun 1989; 57(4):1089-1094.
30. Wessels MR, DiFabio JL, Benedi VJ et al. Structural determination and immunochemical characterization of the type V group B Streptococcus capsular polysaccharide. J Biol Chem 1991; 266(11):6714-6719.
31. Kogan G, Uhrin D, Brisson J-R et al. Structure of the type VI group B Streptococcus capsular polysaccharide determined by high resolution NMR spectroscopy. J Carbohy Chem 1994; 13:1071-1078.
32. Kogan G, Brisson JR, Kasper DL et al. Structural elucidation of the novel type VII group B Streptococcus capsular polysaccharide by high resolution NMR spectroscopy. Carbohydr Res 1995; 277(1):1-9.
33. Kogan G, Uhrin D, Brisson JR et al. Structural and immunochemical characterization of the type VIII group B Streptococcus capsular polysaccharide. J Biol Chem 1996; 271(15):8786-8790.
34. Paoletti LC, Madoff LC, Kasper DL. Surface structures of group B Streptococcus important in human immunity. In: Fischetti VA, Novick, RP Ferretti, JJ, Portnoy, DA, Rood, J.I., eds. Grampostive pathogens Washington DC: ASM Press, 2000:137-153.
35. Jennings HJ, Lugowski C, Kasper DL. Conformational aspects critical to the immunospecificity of the type III group B streptococcal polysaccharide. Biochem 1981; 20:4511-4518.
36. Wessels MR, Munoz A, Kasper DL. A model of high-affinity antibody binding to type III group B Streptococcus capsular polysaccharide. Proc Natl Acad Sci USA 1987; 84:9170-9174.
37. Paoletti LC, Johnson KD. Purification of preparative quantities of group B Streptococcus type III oligosaccharides. J Chromatogr A 1995; 705(2):363-368.
38. Zou W, Mackenzie R, Therien L et al. Conformational epitope of the type III group B Streptococcus capsular polysaccharide. J Immunol 1999; 163(2):820-825.
39. Brisson JR, Uhrinova S, Woods RJ et al. NMR and molecular dynamics studies of the conformational epitope of the type III group B Streptococcus capsular polysaccharide and derivatives. Biochemistry 1997; 36(11):3278-3292.
40. Paoletti LC, Kasper DL, Michon F et al. Effects of chain length on the immunogenicity in rabbits of group B Streptococcus type III oligosaccharide-tetanus toxoid conjugates. J Clin Invest 1992; 89(1):203-209.
41. Gravekamp C, Kasper DL, Paoletti LC et al. Alpha C protein as a carrier for type III capsular polysaccharide and as a protective protein in group B streptococcal vaccines. Infect Immun 1999; 67(5):2491-2496.
42. Fusco PC, Perry JW, Liang SM et al.Bactericidal activity elicited by the beta C protein of group B streptococci contrasted with capsular polysaccharides. XIIIth Lancefield International Symposium on Streptococci and Streptococcal Diseases 1996; P201.
43. Madoff LC, Michel JL, Gong EW et al. Protection of neonatal mice from group B streptococcal infection by maternal immunization with beta C protein. Infect Immun 1992; 60(12):4989-4994.
44. Michel JL, Madoff LC, Kling DE et al. Cloned alpha and beta C-protein antigens of group B streptococci elicit protective immunity. Infect Immun 1991; 59(6):2023-2028.

45. Madoff LC, Paoletti LC, Tai JY et al. Maternal immunization of mice with group B streptococcal type III polysaccharide-beta C protein conjugate elicits protective antibody to multiple serotypes. J Clin Invest 1994; 94(1):286-292.
46. Stalhammar-Carlemalm M, Stenberg L, Lindahl G. Protein rib: a novel group B streptococcal cell surface protein that confers protective immunity and is expressed by most strains causing invasive infections. J Exp Med 1993; 177(6):1593-1603.
47. Larsson C, Stalhammar-Carlemalm M, Lindahl G. Protection against experimental infection with group B Streptococcus by immunization with a bivalent protein vaccine. Vaccine 1999; 17(5):454-458.
48. Cheng Q, Carlson B, Pillai S et al. Antibody against surface-bound C5a peptidase is opsonic and initiates macrophage killing of group B streptococci. Infect Immun 2001; 69(4):2302-2308.
49. Paoletti LC. Potency of clinical group B streptococcal conjugate vaccines. Vaccine 2001; 19(15-16):2118-2126.
50. Brodeur BR, Boyer M, Charlebois I et al. Identification of group B streptococcal Sip protein, which elicits cross-protective immunity. Infect Immun 2000; 68(10):5610-5618.
51. Rioux S, Martin D, Ackermann HW et al. Localization of surface immunogenic protein on group b Streptococcus. Infect Immun 2001; 69(8):5162-5165.
52. Martin D, Rioux S, Gagnon E et al. Maternal Sip-specific antibodies confer protection to mouse neonates challenged with serologically distinct group B streptococcal isolates. Paper presented at: American Society for Microbiology. Orlando, Florida: 2001.
53. Baker CJ. Group B streptococcal infections. Adv Intern Med 1980; 25(475):475-501.
54. Baker CJ, Edwards MS, Kasper DL. Immunogenicity of polysaccharides from type III, group B Streptococcus. J Clin Invest 1978; 61(4):1107-1110.
55. Baker CJ, Kasper DL. Group B streptococcal vaccines. Rev Infect Dis 1985; 7(4):458-467.
56. Eisenstein TK, De CB, Resavy D et al. Quantitative determination in human sera of vaccine-induced antibody to type-specific polysaccharides of group B streptococci using an enzyme-linked immunosorbent assay. J Infect Dis 1983; 147(5):847-856.
57 Kasper DL, Baker CJ, Galdes B et al. Immunochemical analysis and immunogenicity of the type II group B streptococcal capsular polysaccharide. J Clin Invest 1983; 72:260-269
58. Fischer G, Horton RE, Edelman R. From the National Institute of Allergy and Infectious Diseases. Summary of the National Institutes of Health workshop on group B streptococcal infection J Infect Dis 1983; 148(1):163-166.
59. Baker CJ, Rench MA, Edwards MS et al. Immunization of pregnant women with a polysaccharide vaccine of group B Streptococcus. N Engl J Med 1988; 319(18):1180-1220.
60. Ada G. Vaccines and Vaccination. N Engl J Med October 4, 2001 2001; 345(14):1042-1053.
61. Wessels MR, Rubens CE, Benedi VJ et al. Definition of a bacterial virulence factor: sialylation of the group B streptococcal capsule. Proc Natl Acad Sci U S A 1989; 86(22):8983-8987.
62. Paoletti LC, Wessels MR, Kasper DL. Optimization of group B streptococcal glycoconjugate vaccines. In: R. M. Chanock FB, H.S. Ginsberg, and E. Norrby, eds. Vaccines 95 Molecular approaches to the control of infectious diseases Cold Spring Harbor: Cold Spring Harbor Laboratory Press, 1995:213-217.
63. Wessels MR, Paoletti LC, Kasper DL et al. Immunogenicity in animals of a polysaccharide-protein conjugate vaccine against type III group B Streptococcus. J Clin Invest 1990; 86(5):1428-1433.
64. Lagergard T, Shiloach J, Robbins JB et al.Synthesis and immunological properties of conjugates composed of group B Streptococcus type III capsular polysaccharide covalently bound to tetanus toxoid. Infect Immun 1990; 58(3):687-694.
65. Paoletti LC, Kasper DL, Michon F et al. An oligosaccharide-tetanus toxoid conjugate vaccine against type III group B Streptococcus J Biol Chem 1990; 265(30):18278-18283.
66. Wang Y, Hollingsworth RI, Kasper DL. Ozonolysis for selectively depolymerizing polysaccharides containing beta-D-aldosidic linkages. Proc Natl Acad Sci U S A 1998; 95(12):6584-6589.
67. Zou W, Laferriere CA, Jennings HJ. Oligosaccharide fragments of the type III group B streptococcal polysaccharide derived from S. pneumoniae type 14 capsular polysaccharide by a chemoenzymatic method Carbohydr Res 1998; 309(3):297-301.
68. Paoletti LC, Wessels MR, Rodewald AK et al. Neonatal mouse protection against infection with multiple group B streptococcal (GBS) serotypes by maternal immunization with a tetravalent GBS polysaccharide-tetanus toxoid conjugate vaccine. Infect Immun 1994; 62(8):3236-3243.

69. Paoletti LC, Kennedy RC, Chanh TC et al. Immunogenicity of group B Streptococcus type III polysaccharide- tetanus toxoid vaccine in baboons. Infect Immun 1996; 64(2):677-679.
70. Kasper DL, Paoletti LC, Wessels MR et al. Immune response to type III group B streptococcal polysaccharide- tetanus toxoid conjugate vaccine. J Clin Invest 1996; 98(10):2308-2314.
71. Paoletti LC, Pinel J, Rodewald AK et al. Therapeutic potential of human antisera to group B streptococcal glycoconjugate vaccines in neonatal mice. J Infect Dis 1997; 175(5):1237-1239.
72. Wessels MR, Paoletti LC, Rodewald AK et al. Stimulation of protective antibodies against type Ia and Ib group B streptococci by a type Ia polysaccharide-tetanus toxoid conjugate vaccine. Infect Immun 1993; 61(11):4760-4766.
73. Baker CJ, Paoletti LC, Wessels MR et al. Safety and immunogenicity of capsular polysaccharide-tetanus toxoid conjugate vaccines for group B streptococcal types Ia and Ib. J Infect Dis 1999; 179:142-150.
74. Jennings HJ, Rosell KG, Katzenellenbogen E et al. Structural determination of the capsular polysaccharide antigen of type II group B Streptococcus. J Biol Chem 1983; 258(3):1793-1798.
75. Baker CJ, Paoletti LC, Rench MA et al. Use of capsular polysaccharide-tetanus toxoid conjugate vaccine for type II group B Streptococcus in healthy women. J Infect Dis 2000; 182(4):1129-1138.
76. Jelinkova J, Motlova J. Worldwide distribution of two new serotypes of group B streptococci: type IV and provisional type V. J Clin Microbiol 1985; 21(3):361-362.
77. Galloway A, Deighton CM, Deady J et al. Type V group B streptococcal septicaemia with bilateral endophthalmitis and septic arthritis [letter]. Lancet193; 341(8850):960-961.
78. Rench MA, Baker CJ. Neonatal sepsis caused by a new group B streptococcal serotype. J Pediatr 1993; 122(4):638-640.
79. Greenberg DN, Ascher DP, Yoder BA et al. Group B Streptococcus serotype V [letter]. J Pediatr 1993; 123:494-495.
80. Harrison LH, Dwyer DM, Johnson JA. Emergence of serotype V group B streptococcal infection among infants and adults [letter]. J Infect Dis 1995; 171(2):513.
81. Wessels MR, Paoletti LC, Pinel J et al. Immunogenicity and protective activity in animals of a type V group B streptococcal polysaccharide-tetanus toxoid conjugate vaccine. J Infect Dis 1995; 171(4):879-884.
82. Paoletti LC, Baker CJ, Kasper DL. Neonatal group B streptococcal disease: progress towards a multivalent maternal vaccine. Paper presented at: The First Annual Conference on Vaccine Research. Washington DC: 1998.
83. Lachenauer CS, Kasper DL, Shimada J et al. Serotypes VI and VIII predominates among group B streptococci from pregnant Japanese women. ICAAC abstract no K-80 1997.
84. Paoletti LC, Pinel J, Johnson KD et al. Synthesis and preclinical evaluation of glycoconjugate vaccines against group B Streptococcus types VI and VIII. J Infect Dis 1999; 180(3):892-895.
84b. Paoletti LC, Kasper DL. Conjugate vaccines against group B Streptococcus types IV and VII. J Infect Dis 2002; 186:123-126.
85. Fernandez M, Paoletti LC, Kasper DL et al. Evaluation of a bivalent group B streptococcal polysaccharide-tetanus toxoid conjugate vaccine. Paper presented at: 37th Annual Meeting of the Infectious Diseases Society of America. Philadelphia, PA:1999.
86. Paoletti LC, Rench MA, Kasper DL et al. Effects of alum adjuvant or a booster dose on immunogenicity during clinical trials of group B streptococcal type III conjugate vaccines. Infect Immun 2001; 69:6696-6701.
87. Baker CJ, Rench MA, McInnes PM. Safety and immunogenicity of group B streptococcal (GBS) type III capsular polysaccharide (CPS)-tetanus toxoid (III-TT) conjugate vaccine in pregnant women. San Francisco, California: Paper presented at: Infectious Diseases Society of America 39th Annual Meeting, 2001.
88. Eickhoff TC, Klein JO, Daly AK et al. Neonatal sepsis and other infections due to group B beta-hemolytic streptococci. New Engl J Med 1964; 271:1221-1228.
89. Fry RM. Fatal infections by haemolytic streptococcus group B. Lancet 1938;1:199-201.
90. Butter MNW, de Moor CE. Streptococcus agalactiae as a cause of meningitis in the newborn, and of bacteraemia in adults. Differentiation of human and animal varieties J Microbiol Serol 1967; 33:439-450.
91. Hood M, Janney A, Dameron G. Beta hemolytic streptococcus group B associated with problems of the perinatal period. Amer Obstet Gynecol 1961; 2:809-818.

92. Erramouspe J. Challenges on the prevention of perinatal group B streptococcal infection. Infections in Medicine 2000;17:49-56.
93. Trannoy E. Will ethical and liability issues and public acceptance allow maternal immunization? Vaccine 1998; 6(14-15):1482-1485.
94. Stratton KR, Durch JS, Lawrence RS, eds. Vaccines for the 21st Century. A tool for decisionmaking Washington DC: National Academy Press, 2000.
95. Englund J, Mbawuike I, Hammill H et al.al immunization with influenza or tetanus toxoid vaccine for passive antibody production in young infants. J Infect Dis 1993; 68(3):647-656.
96. Paoletti LC, Pinel J, Kennedy RC et al. antibody transfer in baboons and mice vaccinated with a group B streptococcal polysaccharide conjugate. J Infect Dis 2000;181(2):653-658.
97. Santosham M, Englund JA, McInnes P et al. Safety and antibody persistence following Haemophilus influenzae type b conjugate or pneumococcal polysaccharide vaccines given before pregnancy in women of childbearing age and their infants. Pediatr Infect Dis J 2001; 20(10):931-940.
98. Rennels MB, Edwards KM, Keyserling HL et al. Safety and immunogenicity of heptavalent pneumococcal vaccine conjugated to CRM197 in United States infants. Pediatrics 1998; 101(4 Pt 1):604-611.
99. Laferriere CA, Sood RK, de Muys JM et al. Streptococcus pneumoniae type 14 polysaccharide-conjugate vaccines: length stabilization of opsonophagocytic conformational polysaccharide epitopes. Infect Immun 1998; 66(6);2441-2446.
100. Madoff LC, Michel JL, Gong EW et al. Group B streptococci escape host immunity by deletion of tandem repeat elements of the alpha C protein. Proc Natl Acad Sci U S A 1996; 93(9):4131-4136.
101. Wizemann TM, Heinrichs JH, Adamou JE et al. Use of a whole genome approach to identify vaccine molecules affording protection against Streptococcus pneumoniae infection. Infect Immun 2001; 69(3):1593-1598.
102. Musser JM, Kaplan SL. Pneumococcal Research Transformed. N Engl J Med October 18, 2001 2001; 345(16):1206-1207.
103. Jones AL, Knoll KM, Rubens CE. Identification of Streptococcus agalactiae virulence genes in the neonatal rat sepsis model using signature tagged mutagenesis. Mol Microbiol 2000; 37(6):1444-1455.
104. Wizemann TM, Adamou JE, Langermann S. Adhesins as targets for vaccine development. Emerg Infect Dis 1999; 5(3):395-403.
105. Malin G, Paoletti LC. Use of a dynamic in vitro attachment and invasion system (DIVAS) to determine influence of growth rate on invasion of respiratory epithelial cells by group B Streptococcus. Proc Natl Acad Sci 2001; 98(23):13335-13340.
106. Hulse ML, Smith S, Chi EY et al. Effect of type III group B streptococcal capsular polysaccharide on invasion of respiratory epithelial cells. Infect Immun 1993; 61:4835-4841
107. Wessels MR, Paoletti LC, Guttormsen HK et al. Structural properties of group B streptococcal type III polysaccharide conjugate vaccines that influence immunogenicity and efficacy. Infect Immun 1998; 66(5):2186-2192.
108. Zaleznik DF, Rench MA, Hillier S et al. Invasive disease due to group B Streptococcus in pregnant women and neonates from diverse population groups. Clin Infect Dis 2000;30(2):276-281.

Chapter 12

Helicobacter pylori Vaccines

Gabriela Garcia and Jacques Pappo

Summary

Helicobacter pylori is a motile, Gram negative spiral organism with gastric trophism. Approximately half of the world's population is infected with *H. pylori*, and the infection persists for life unless treated with antimicrobials and a proton-pump inhibitor. Commonly acquired during childhood, the infection stimulates the immune system to commit a relatively high frequency of immune effector cells throughout the course of the infection, but the natural immune response against this organism does not effect clearance nor does it confer protective immunity against reinfection after antimicrobial therapy.[1] Cases of spontaneous clearance in animal and human populations remain largely unexplained, but mathematical and animal models have strongly suggested an important role for the host response in regulating the severity of *H. pylori* disease.[2,3] Colonization of the gastric mucosa results in gastritis, mucosal atrophy and metaplasia.[4] These damaging infection outcomes are linked to the genesis of Th1 cells and persistent proinflammatory signaling. Gastroduodenal ulcer disease develops in ~10% of infected subjects, and a small subset (~1%) can progress to develop adenocarcinoma and mucosal B cell lymphoma.[5,6] Based on evidence from animal infection models, as well as from human clinical trials, the concept of immunization against *H. pylori* has evolved from the strict notion of vaccine-mediated "sterilizing immunity" to the ability to greatly attenuate the severity of the infection and to protect from the chronic inflammatory sequelae secondary to infection.

Host Immune Program and Disease Pathogenesis

Considerable evidence has established that *H. pylori* reshapes the immunologic machinery of the stomach. Binding of *H. pylori* to epithelial cells signals for activation of NF-κB transcription factor[7] and production of RANTES, GROα, MIP-1α, MCP-I, IL-1β, IL-6, IL-8, IL-12, and TNFα (reviewed in ref. 8). Recent evidence has shown that IL-1 gene polymorphisms controlling the magnitude of host inflammatory responses are associated with gastric disease.[9] *H. pylori* infection upregulates expression of CD11b/CD18 integrin and its receptor, intercellular-adhesion molecule-1 (CD54) mediating leukocyte transmigration,[10,11,12] and stimulates gastric epithelial cell expression of the T cell costimulatory molecules CD80 and CD86.[13] The *H. pylori*-driven restructuring of the gastric microenvironment results in continuous leukocyte recruitment and activation. Thus, *H. pylori*-infected gastric tissue harbors substantially greater frequencies of leukocytes than the uninfected stomach. Gastric T-cell populations are dominated by the $CD4^+$ phenotype[14] and constitute an enriched source (1-10%) of *H. pylori*-specific T cells compared with peripheral T cells.[15,16] There is clear evidence that *H. pylori* polarizes T helper (Th) cell responses and that skewing of the host response during natural infection results in failed immune protection and contributes to disease pathogenesis. Gastric T cells isolated from biopsies of *H. pylori*-infected subjects exhibit a predominant proinflammatory Th1 phenotype characterized by a high frequency of IFN-γ-secreting cells

New Bacterial Vaccines, edited by Ronald W. Ellis and Bernard R. Brodeur.

relative to IL-4$^+$ cells.[14,17] The finding that live *H. pylori* preferentially stimulates production of IL-12,[18] a cytokine selective for Th1 cell development, may explain why the majority of Th cell clones derived from *H. pylori*-infected patients are comprised of Th1 effector cells.[15,19] Because *H. pylori* augments expression of epithelial class II MHC,[20,21] T cells homing to gastric inflammatory sites may be further engaged by *H. pylori* antigens, leading to redundant cycles of Th1 cell activation, expansion and mucosal damage. Interestingly, the class II MHC heterodimer itself can function as an *H. pylori* receptor.[22] On the other hand, recent evidence points to the ability of *H. pylori* to induce Th cell apoptosis and thus to control the size of the gastric T cell pool as a strategy for immune evasion,[23] raising the possibility of preferential retention of Th1 cells via negative selection of Th2 cells.

Raison D'être for Vaccination

Because *H. pylori* delivers powerful stimuli that bias the host Th phenotype, vaccination could be envisaged as a strategy to re-program a dominant Th1 response consistent with infection and gastric inflammation into a host immune response capable of attenuating the bacterial load and gastric disease.

The global *H. pylori* burden is in the order of 10^{16} organisms.[24] Successful clinical treatment of the infection with triple therapy and a proton-pump inhibitor[25] is threatened by the specter of antibiotic and multidrug-resistant *H. pylori* [26,27,28] and by treatment failures due to adverse events and poor patient compliance.[29] Vaccination should protect from drug resistant *H. pylori*, curb the rising rate of resistant strains, and should prevent reinfection, especially in at-risk populations.[1] A recent mathematical model describing the impact of a vaccine on the cost of *H. pylori*-associated disease supports vaccine development on the basis of cost and health benefits.[30] However, a central argument in favor of vaccination resides in the potential to deviate the host-bacterial equilibrium established in natural infection and, by extension, to interfere with the evolution of *H. pylori*-mediated gastritis and mucosal damage. Thus, vaccination would be expected to reduce the risk of ulcer disease and gastric cancer.

Surrogate Models of Human Vaccine Efficacy

The development of a surrogate *H. pylori* infection based on the murine *H. felis* infection model[31] greatly stimulated the field of vaccination against Helicobacter infection (Table 1). Studies showing protection from challenge upon oral immunization emerged in short order.[32,33] The principle of vaccination in the control of Helicobacter infection was widely confirmed in the prevention of infection[34,35] and as a strategy for the treatment or cure of an ongoing infection.[36,37] While oral immunization in this model was judged to be completely protective, these findings require careful interpretation, as the histologic and urea hydrolysis assays employed to describe efficacy are unable to detect relatively low infection levels in the order of 10^4-10^5 organisms/gm of gastric biopsy. The successful adaptation of *H. pylori cagA*$^+$ and *cagA* mutant strains to murine hosts of varied genetic backgrounds led to the establishment of infection models displaying a wide range of infection density.[38,39] Observations of vaccine-mediated prophylactic and therapeutic protection largely supported those in the *H. felis* model (Fig. 1), but immune protection, when assessed by quantitative bacterial culture, was found to range from clearance in models with low colonization density[38] to attenuation of the infection by $\geq 10^1$ CFU/gm when the *H. pylori* burden more closely resembled that of human populations.[40-42] The recent development of models of progressive atrophy, metaplasia and gastric adenocarcinoma in *H. felis*-infected hypergastrinemic transgenic mice[43] and in *H. pylori*-infected Mongolian gerbils[44] provides the opportunity to directly examine the ability of vaccination on protection not only from infection but also from the evolution of *H. pylori* disease. In ferrets, oral immunization cleared *H. mustelae* infection in ~30% of ferrets. [45] Mucosal vaccination likewise diminished the infection density in the gnotobiotic piglet[46] and feline[47] *H. pylori* infection models. In rhesus monkeys, vaccination was ineffective[48] or modestly effective[49] in preventing infection from experimental challenge. Whereas oral immunization may have

Table 1. Experimental models of Helicobacter infection and vaccine efficacy

Animal Model	Organism	Salient Features	Vaccination Outcome
Mouse	*H. felis*	Gastritis, metaplasia, atrophy and carcinoma in mutant (IL-10 $^{-/-}$) and transgenic (INS-GAS) strains	Mucosal immunization generates long-term protection from challenge and "cures" established infection. Immune protection associated with gastric infiltration of $CD4^+$ and $CD8^+$ cells of unknown Th function → post-immunization gastritis. Protection assayed by histology and/or urea hydrolysis
Mouse	Adapted *H. pylori* $cagA^+$ or $cagA^-$ strains	Varying degrees of gastritis and infection density specified by host genetic background. Ulcerative lesions. Mucosal atrophy after long-term infections	Mucosal immunization protects from challenge. Therapeutic immunization diminishes *H. pylori* burden. Vaccination prevents reinfection. Parenteral immunization protective in some models. Protection is Ab-independent but requires gastric $CD4^+$ T-cell effectors. Efficacy assessed by quantitative bacterial culture
Gerbil	Adapted *H. pylori*	Gastritis, ulcer, metaplasia, adenocarcinoma	Unknown
Ferret	*H. mustelae*. Natural infection, reinfection post-antimicrobial eradication	Multifocal atrophic gastritis, ulcer	Mucosal immunization with MDP adjuvant is not protective and promotes mucosal damage. Therapeutic vaccine efficacious in ca. 30% of naturally infected ferrets
Cat	*H. pylori*. Natural infection. Experimental infection variable	Lymphofollicular gastritis	Prophylactic immunization protects against challenge
Germ-free piglet	*H. pylori*	Gastritis, ulcer	Mucosal and parenteral immunizations protect. Parenteral vaccination exacerbates gastritis
Rhesus monkey	*H. pylori*. Enzootic. Long-term infection with some strains	Gastritis, atrophy	Immune protection highly variable by oral, parenteral, or combined vaccination routes. Therapeutic protection not established

interfered with the natural transmission,[3] therapeutic protection in chronically infected rhesus monkeys remains to be demonstrated conclusively.[50] While the differences in host susceptibility to infection, genetic strain adaptation, immunization schemes, and efficacy readouts do not

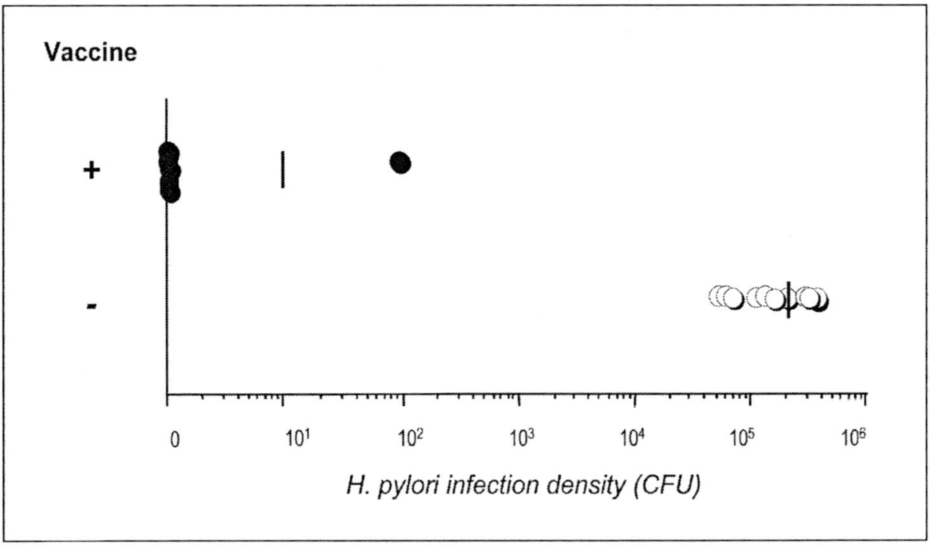

Figure 1. Effect of mucosal vaccination on *H. pylori* infection. Groups of 10 C57BL/6 mice were immunized intranasally with 100 μg *H. pylori* lysate antigen and 10 μg cholera toxin (CT) adjuvant (●), or with 10 μg CT adjuvant alone (○) 4 times weekly. The mice were subsequently challenged with 10^6 CFU *H. pylori* SS1, and the effect of immunization assessed 2 weeks later by quantitative bacterial culture. The points represent the infection level (colony forming units; CFU) in gastric biopsies excised from each mouse, and the solid lines indicate the group means. Immunization protected from infection relative to treatment with CT alone ($p<0.0001$; Wilcoxon rank sum analysis).

enable a clear finding of an animal model predictive of human vaccine efficacy, the advent of an acute human challenge model[51] now permits the direct study of outcomes of prophylactic immunization in humans.

Vaccine Effector Pathways and Post-Immunization Gastritis

The observation that protective oral immunization is temporally associated with IgA antibody induction[35] led to the equivocal assumption that IgA must effect protection.[52] Indeed, oral immunization yields a high frequency of IgA$^+$ cells in the gastric mucosa[40] and passive administration of IgA antibody may interfere with the acquisition of infection in mice[53] and humans.[54] However, the magnitude of the anti-*H. pylori* IgA response post-vaccination does not predict the extent of immune protection.[40] Recent studies in B cell-deficient μMT mice now indicate that prophylactic [55] and therapeutic protection[56] are B cell and antibody-independent and that B-cell deficiency has no demonstrable effect on the severity of the infection, but instead may lead to spontaneous clearance.[57] While a putative role for the involvement of T cells in vaccine immunity likewise could be made from observations that oral immunization greatly expands the resident gastric Th population, only recently has it been shown directly that immune protection is dependent on the emergence of activated CD4$^+$ T cells and that vaccine efficacy is strictly dependent on intact class II MHC function.[42] Furthermore, adoptive transfer of αβ$^+$ CD4$^+$ T cells is both necessary and sufficient for control of the *H. pylori* burden in unimmunized recipients.[58] The precise mechanism whereby Th cell effectors mediate clearance has not been defined. However, we hypothesize that gastric mucosal T cells engaged during immunization, particularly those which home to gastric epithelium (the so-called αβ$^+$CD4$^+$ CD11a^{hi} CD103$^+$ gastric intraepithelial lymphocytes),[59] perturb the host-bacterial balance by regulating epithelial cell receptors mediating adhesive interactions with their *H. pylori* cognate ligands. The finding that T-cell-related cytokines profoundly alter epithelial cell function is consistent with this notion. [60]

The available evidence points to vaccination as an approach to redirect a Th1-dominant response committed during infection to a Th2 phenotype associated with protection. Vaccination downregulates IFN-γ responses and gives rise to the expression of IL-4 and IL-5, consistent with a Th2 profile. [61,62] Whereas vaccine protection can be generated in Th1-deficient mice,[63] the absence of IL-4 compromises the protective effect of vaccination. [64] There is direct evidence that adoptive transfer of a Th2 cell line limits the severity of the infection resulting from *H. felis* challenge. [65] Activation of a vaccine-specific Th2 program is of great consequence to the host, since Th2 responses attenuate the severity of chronic inflammation and gastric atrophy, [66,67] while a Th1-background promotes mucosal injury. [68] Importantly, the proinflammatory cytokine migration inhibitory factor, secreted by T cells during chronic inflammatory reactions, can inactivate transcription of p53 tumor suppressor. [69]

A downstream effect of vaccination has been the development of gastritis of greater severity than that observed in unimmunized hosts. In murine vaccination models, this "post-immunization gastritis" is characterized by the accumulation in the gastric corpus of $CD4^+$ and $CD8^+$ cells of unknown Th lineage and function. [70] It has become clear from long-term protection studies that the coordinate development of gastritis in immunized mice is an evanescent event, especially driven by challenge with *H. felis*. [71,72] Thus, the gastritis associated with vaccination may simply reflect influx and amplification of Th cell effectors in the target end organ. The frequency of *H. pylori*-specific Th cells that must infiltrate gastric tissue to effect protection, their precise temporal and spatial phenotypic balance, and factors that regulate their differentiation during vaccination are unknown.

H. pylori Vaccine Targeting and Antigen Discovery

Because *H. pylori* is a noninvasive mucosal pathogen, a widespread strategy for immunization has been the stimulation of mucose-associated lymphoid tissues. Accordingly, antigen targeted to oral, nasal, small intestinal, and rectal tissues has been used successfully to protect against infection.[32,33,35,40] Efficacy has shown a strict adjuvant requirement, as multiple immunizations in the absence of adjuvant, while able to generate relatively high levels of serum IgG and mucosal IgA, failed to confer protective efficacy.[73] The mucosal adjuvants cholera toxin (CT) and the closely related *E. coli* heat-labile toxin (LT) are AB_5 toxin molecules employed as prototypical adjuvants for Helicobacter immunization, but their toxicity in humans has buttressed the search for detoxified mutant adjuvants. One such example is a genetically detoxified mutant LTK63 molecule with a serine to lysine substitution at position 63, capable of mediating immune protection upon oral immunization.[41] Immunization with the orally active muramyl dipeptide adjuvant has not proven efficacious, but instead, appeared to lead to mucosal damage.[74] Parenteral immunization with alum, Freund's adjuvant, and with DNA-based vaccines elicited varying degrees of efficacy, [75,76,77] but repeated alum immunizations in rhesus monkeys were largely ineffective.[49] While additional evidence from murine models shows a glycolipid adjuvant and the saponin adjuvant QS21 to be highly efficacious, especially when delivered to the infra-diaphragmatic region to target the draining gastric lymph nodes,[78,79] parenteral immunization in other *H. pylori* vaccination models using similar adjuvants has resulted in the exacerbation of gastritis.[80,49] Lastly, suppression of experimental infections also has been achieved using adenovirus-[81] and *Salmonella typhimurium*-vectored vaccines.[82]

A substantial number of vaccine antigens have been identified by proteomic analyses using sera from infected subjects.[83,84] The antigens urease, catalase, heat-shock proteins HspA and HspB, and the neutrophil-activating protein NapA have demonstrable efficacy in infection models [35,85,86,87] while the protective function of flagellar proteins, elongations factors and other *H. pylori* enzymes identified by this method remains undefined. On the other hand, selection of the virulence factors CagA and VacA as protective *H. pylori* vaccine antigens[38] has been supported by in vitro assays of Th cell usage.[88] Genomic analyses have further identified five paralogous gene families in both sequenced *H. pylori* strains containing either a type-I or type-II leader peptide and a C-terminal hydrophobic motif. The largest outer membrane family is comprised of 21 proteins and is represented by the Hop vaccine candidates with porin function and adhesive activity to gastric epithelial cells.[89] The genomics approach has also proven to be a valuable tool for antigen selection, since it has revealed that candidate vaccine antigens may be susceptible to antigenic diversification. While the intrinsic properties of antigen-adjuvant pairs in concert with immunization routes have not been studied systematically for their ability to bias gastric Th cell differentiation, such studies are paramount for precisely dissecting an outcome of immune protection from the potential to magnify the underlying Th1-mediated gastric disease.

Clinical Trials

The safety and immunogenicity of recombinant *H. pylori* urease and LT adjuvant was examined in a double-blind placebo-controlled control vaccine trial in *H. pylori* infected subjects.[90] An oral immunization schedule similar to that developed in murine models (4 weekly doses) effected only a modest reduction of bacterial load (~10^1 CFU/biopsy) in 6/14 subjects. While oral vaccination generated IgG and IgA antibody-secreting cells, 66% of the volunteers experienced a significant diarrheal illness attributable to LT. In a second trial, the safety and immunogenicity of an *H. pylori* whole cell vaccine administered with the mutant LT_{R192G} adjuvant was tested in *H. pylori*-infected adults.[91] Subjects were orally immunized 3 times every 2 weeks. Vaccination resulted in mild to moderate adverse events consisting of diarrhea, vomiting and fever. Whereas vaccination gave rise to serum IgG and mucosal IgA antibody responses, there was no measurable effect on *H. pylori* infection at trial completion. Two additional clinical studies have been conducted in uninfected human volunteers using recombinant Salmonella-vectored urease. Single dose immunizations with a *phoP/phoQ* attenuated *S. enterica* serovar Typhimurium resulted in a modest IgA response,[92] but immunization with *S. enterica* serovar Typhi did not.[93] The clinical experience accrued from these early trials, coupled to the active search for mucosal adjuvants and surrogate markers of protection, provides the scaffolding for clinical management in the not-so-distant future of *H. pylori* gastroduodenal disease by vaccination.

References

1. Ramirez-Ramos A, Gilman RH, Leon-Barua R et al. Rapid recurrence of Helicobacter pylori infection in Peruvian patients after successful eradication. Clin Infect Dis 1997; 25:1027-1031.
2. Blaser MJ, Kirschner D. Dynamics of Helicobacter pylori colonization in relation to the host response. Proc Natl Acad Sci USA 1999; 96:8359-8364.
3. Dubois AC, Lee K, Fiala N et al. Immunization against natural Helicobacter pylori infection in nonhuman primates. Infect Immun 1998; 66:4340-4346.
4. Sipponen P, Hyvarinen H, Seppala K et al. Pathogenesis of the transformation from gastritis to malignancy. Alim Pharmacol Thera 1998; 12:61-71.
5. Correa P, Miller M. Helicobacter pylori and gastric atrophy – cancer paradoxes. J Nat Cancer Inst 1995; 87:1731-1732.
6. Wotherspoon AC, Doglioni C, Diss TC et al. Regression of primary low-grade B-cell gastric lymphoma of mucosa-associated lymphoid tissue type after eradication of Helicobacter pylori. Lancet 1993; 342:575-577.
7. Keates S, Hitti Y, Upton M et al. Helicobacter pylori infection activates NF-κB in gastric epithelial cells. Gastroenterology 1997; 113:1099-1109.
8. Ibraghimov A, Pappo J. The immune response against Helicobacter pylori - a direct linkage to the development of gastroduodenal disease. Microbes Infect 2000; 2:1073-1077.
9. El-Omar EM, Carrington M, Chow WH et al. Interleukin-1 polymorphisms associated with increased risk of gastric cancer. Nature 2000; 404:398-402.
10. Crowe SE, Alvarez L, Dytoc M et al. Expression of interleukin 8 and CD54 by human gastric epithelium after Helicobacter pylori infection in vitro. Gastroenterology 1995; 108:65-74.

11. Hansen PS, Go MF, Varming K et al. Proinflammatory activation of neutrophils and monocytes by Helicobacter pylori in patients with different clinical presentations. Infect Immun 1999; 67:3171-3174.
12. Hatz RA, Rieder G, Stolte M et al. Pattern of adhesion molecule expression on vascular endothelium in Helicobacter pylori-associated antral gastritis. Gastroenterology 1997; 112:1908-1919.
13. Ye G, Barrera C, Fan X et al. Expression of B7-1 and B7-2 costimulatory molecules by gastric epithelial cells. Potential role in $CD4^+$ T cell activation during Helicobacter pylori infection. J Clin Invest 1997; 99:1628-1636.
14. Bamford KB, Fan X, Crowe SE et al. Lymphocytes in the human gastric mucosa during Helicobacter pylori have a T helper cell 1 phenotype. Gastroenterology 1998; 114:482-492.
15. D'Elios MM, Manghetti M, De Carli M et al. T helper 1 effector cells specific for Helicobacter pylori in the gastric antrum of patients with peptic ulcer disease. J Immunol 1997; 158:962-967.
16. Di Tommaso A, Xiang Z, Bugnoli M et al. Helicobacter pylori-specific $CD4^+$ T-cell clones from peripheral blood and gastric biopsies. Infect Immun 1995; 63:1102-1106.
17. Lindholm C, Quiding-Jarbrink M, Lonroth H et al. Local cytokine response in Helicobacter pylori-infected subjects. Infect Immun 1998; 66:5964-5971.
18. Haeberle HA, Kubin M, Bamford KB et al. Differential stimulation of interleukin-12 (IL-12) and IL-10 by live and killed Helicobacter pylori in vitro and association of IL-12 production with gamma interferon-producing T cell sinthehumangastric mucosa. Infect Immun 1997; 65(10):4229-35.
19. Sommer F, Faller G, Konturek P et al. Antrum- and corpus mucosa-infiltrating $CD4^+$ lymphocytes in Helicobacter pylori gastritis display a Th1 phenotype. Infect Immun 1998; 66:5543-5546.
20. Engstrand L, Scheynius A, Pathlso C et al. Association of Campylobacter pylori with induced expression of class II transplantation antigens on gastric epithelial cells. Infect Immun 1989; 57:827-832.
21. Wee A, The M, Kang JY. Association of Helicobacter pylori with HLA-DR antigen expression in gastritis. J Clin Pathol 1992; 45:30-33.
22. Fan X, Crowe SE, Behar S et al. The effect of class II major histocompatibility complex expression on adherence of Helicobacter pylori and induction of apoptosis in gastric epithelial cells: a mechanism for T helper cell type-1 mediated damage. J Exp Med 1998; 187:1659-1669.
23. Wang J, Brooks EG, Bamford KB et al. Negative selection of T cells by Helicobacter pylori as a model for bacterial strain selection by immune evasion. J Immunol 2001; 167:926-934.
24. Cover TL. Commentary: Helicobacter pylori transmission, host factors, and bacterial factors. Gastroenterology 1997; 113:S29-S30.
25. Lind T, Megrau F, Unge P et al. The MACH2 study: Role of omeprazole in eradication of Helicobacter pylori with 1-week triple therapies. Gastroenterology 1999; 116:248-253.
26. Megraud F. Resistance of Helicobacter pylori to antibiotics. Aliment Pharmacol Ther 1997; 11:43-53.
27. Graham DY. Antibiotic resistance in Helicobacter pylori: implications for therapy. Gastroenterology 1998; 115:1272-1277.
28. Debets-Ossenkopp YJ, Herscheid AJ, Pot RGJ et al. Prevalence of Helicobacter pylori resistance to metronidazole, claritromycin, amoxycillin, tetracycline and trovafloxicin in The Netherlands. J Antimicrob Chemother 1999; 43:511-515.
29. Chiba N, Rao BV, Rademaker JW et al. Meta-analysis of the efficacy of antibiotic therapy in eradicating Helicobacter pylori. Amer J Gastroenterol 1992; 87:1716-1727.
30. Rupnow MF, Owens DK, Shachter R et al. Helicobacter pylori vaccine development and use: a cost-effectiveness analysis using the Institute of Medicine Methodology. Helicobacter 1999; 4:272-280.
31. Lee A, Fox JG, Otto G et al. A small animal model of human Helicobacter pylori active chronic gastritis. Gastroenterology 1990; 99:1315-1323.
32. Czinn SJ, Nedrud JG. Oral immunization against Helicobacter pylori. Infect Immun 1991; 59:2359-2363.
33. Chen M, Lee A, Hazell SL. Immunisation against Helicobacter infection in a mouse Helicobacter felis model. Lancet 1992; i:1120-1121.
34. Michetti P, Corthesy-Thelaz I, Davin C et al. Immunization of Balb/c mice against Helicobacter felis infection with Helicobacter pylori urease. Gastroenterology 1994; 107:1002-1011.
35. Pappo J, Thomas WD, Kabok Z et al. Effect of oral immunization with recombinant urease on murine Helicobacter felis gastritis. Infect Immun 1995; 63:1246-1252.

36. Doidge C, Gus I, Lee A et al. Therapeutic immunization against Helicobacter infection. Lancet 1994; 343:913-914.
37. Corthesy-Theulaz I, Porta N, Glauser M et al. Oral immunization with Helicobacter pylori urease B subunit as a treatment against Helicobacter infection in mice. Gastroenterology 1995; 109:115-121.
38. Marchetti M, Arico B, Burroni D et al. Development of a mouse model of Helicobacter pylori infection that mimics human disease. Science 1995; 267:1655-1658.
39. Lee A, O'Rourke J, De Ungria MC et al. A standardised mouse model of Helicobacter pylori infection: introducing the Sydney strain. Gastroenterology 1997; 112:1386-1397.
40. Kleanthous H, Myers GA, Georgakopoulo KM et al. Rectal and intranasal immunizations with recombinant urease induce distinct local and serum immune responses in mice and protect against Helicobacter pylori infection. Infect Immun 1998; 66:2879-2886.
41. Marchetti M, Rossi M, Giannelli V et al. Protection against Helicobacter pylori infection in mice by intragastric vaccination with H. pylori antigens is achieved using a nontoxic mutant of E. coli heat-labile enterotoxin (LT) as adjuvant. Vaccine 1998; 16:33-37.
42. Pappo J, Torrey D, Castriotta L et al. Helicobacter pylori infection in immunized mice lacking Major Histocompatability Complex class I and class II functions. Infect Immun 1999; 67:337-341.
43. Wang TC, Dangler CA, Chen D et al. Synergistic interaction between hypergastrinemia and Helicobacter infection in a mouse model of gastric cancer. Gastroenterology 2000; 118:36-47.
44. Watanabe T, Tada M, Naga H et al. Helicobacter pylori infection induces gastric cancer in mongolian gerbils. Gastroenterology 1998; 115:642-648.
45. Cuenca R, Blanchard TG, Czinn SG et al. Therapeutic immunization against Helicobacter mustelae infection in naturally infected ferrets. Gastroenterology 1996; 110:1770-1775.
46. Eaton KA, Ringler SR, Krakowka S. Vaccination of gnotobiotic piglets against Helicobacter pylori. J Infect Dis 1998; 178:1399-1405.
47. Batchelder M, Fox JG, Monath T et al. Oral vaccination with recombinant urease reduces gastric Helicobacter pylori colonization in the cat. Gastroenterology 1996; 110:A58.
48. Solnick JV, Canfield DR, Hansen LM et al. Immunization with recombinant Helicobacter pylori urease in specific-pathogen-free rhesus monkeys (Macaca mulatta). Infect Immun 2000; 68:2560-2565.
49. Lee CK, Soike K, Giannasca P. Immunization of rhesus monkeys with a mucosal prime, parenteral boost strategy protects against infection with Helicobacter pylori. Vaccine 1999; 17:3072-3082.
50. Lee CK, Soike K, Hil J et al. Immunization with recombinant Helicobacter pylori urease decreases colonization levels following experimental infection of rhesus monkeys. Vaccine 1999; 17:1493-1505.
51. Graham DY, Opekun AR, Osato MS et al. Challenge model for H. pylori infection in human volunteers. Gut 1999; 45:A57.
52. Lee CK, Weltzin R, Thomas WDJ et al. Oral Immunization with recombinant Helicobacter pylori urease induces secretory IgA antibodies and protects mice from challenge with Helicobacter felis. J Infect Dis 1995; 172:161-172.
53. Czinn SJ, Cai A, Nedrud JG. Protection of germ-free mice from infection by Helicobacter felis after active oral or passive IgA immunization. Vaccine 1993; 11:637-642.
54. Thomas JE, Austin S, Dale A et al. Protection by human milk IgA against Helicobacter pylori infection in infancy. Lancet 1993; 342:121.
55. Blanchard TG, Czinn SJ, Redline RW et al. Antibody-independent protective mucosal immunity to gastric helicobacter infection in mice. Cell Immunol 1999; 191:74-80.
56. Sutton P, Wilson J, Kosaka T et al. Therapeutic immunization against Helicobacter pylori infection in the absence of antibodies. Immunol Cell Biol 2000; 78:28-30.
57. Roth K, Kapadia S, Martin S et al. Cellular immune responses are essential for the development of Helicobacter felis-associated gastric pathology. J Immunol 1999; 163:1490-1497.
58. Kabok Z, Gao W, Pappo J. Function of murine Helicobacter-specific $CD4^+$ T cells in protection against Helicobacter pylori in C57BL/6 and MHC class $II^{-/-}$ knockout mice. Gut 1999; 45:A58.
59. Ibraghimov A, Kabok Z, Garcia G et al. Gastric $CD4^+$ intraepithelial lymphocytes: a novel mucosa-associated lymphoid compartment induced in mice by Helicobacter pylori infection. Mucosal Immunol 2000; 8:9-12.
60. Panja A, Goldberg S, Eckmann L et al. The regulation and functional consequence of proinflammatory cytokine binding on human intestinal epithelial cells. J Immunol 1998; 161:3675-3684.

61. Saldinger PF, Porta N, Launois P et al. Immunization of BALB/c mice with Helicobacter urease B induces a T helper 2 response absent in Helicobacter infection. Gastroenterology 1998; 115:891-897.
62. Goto T, Nishizono A, Fujioka T et al. Local secretory immunoglobulin A and postimmunization gastritis correlate with protection against Helicobacter pylori infection after oral vaccination of mice. Infect Immun 1999; 67:2531-2539.
63. Sawai N, Kita M, Kodama T et al. Role of gamma interferon in Helicobacter pylori-induced gastric inflammatory responses in a mouse model. Infect Immun 1999; 67:279-285.
64. Kabok Z, Gao W, Castriotta L et al. Administration of anti-interleukin 4 monoclonal antibody exacerbates murine Helicobacter pylori infection. Gut 1998; 43:A30.
65. Mohammadi M, Nedrud J, Redline R et al. Murine CD4 T cell responses to Helicobacter infection: TH1 cells enhance gastritis and TH2 cells reduce bacterial load. Gastroenterology 1997; 113:1848-1857.
66. Berg DJ, Lynch NA, Lynch RG et al. Rapid development of severe hyperplastic gastritis with gastric epithelial dedifferentiation in Helicobacter felis-infected IL-$10^{-/-}$ mice. Am J Pathol 1998; 152:1377-1386.
67. Fox JG, Beck P, Dangler CA et al. Concurrent enteric helminth infection modulates inflammation and gastric immune responses and reduces helicobacter-induced gastric atrophy. Nature Med 2000; 6:536-542.
68. Monteleone G, McDonald TT, Wathen NC et al. Enhancing lamina propria Th1 cell responses with interleukin 12 produces severe tissue injury. Gastroenterology 1999; 117:1069-1077.
69. Hudson JD, Shoaibi MA, Maestro R et al. A proinflammatory cytokine inhibits p53 tumor suppressor activity. J Exp Med 1999; 190:1375-1382.
70. Ermak TH, Ding R, Ekstein B et al. Gastritis in urease-immunized mice after Helicobacter felis challenge may be due to residual bacteria. Gastroenterology 1997; 113(4):1118-28.
71. Sutton P, Danon SJ, Walker M et al. Post-immunisation gastritis and Helicobacter infection in the mouse: a long term study. Gut 2001; 49:467-473.
72. Garhart CA, Redline RW, Nedrud JG et al. Clearance of Helicobacter pylori infection and resolution of postimmunization gastritis in a kinetic study of prophylactically immunized mice. Infect Immun 2002; 70:3529-3538.
73. Weltzin R, Kleanthous H, Guirakhoo F et al. Novel intranasal immunization techniques for antibody induction and protection of mice against gastric Helicobacter felis infection. Vaccine 1997; 15:370-376.
74. Whary MT, Palley LS, Batchelder M et al. Promotion of ulcerative duodenitis in young ferrets by oral immunization with Helicobacter mustelae and muramyl dipeptide. Helicobacter 1997; 2:65-77.
75. Yamaguchi H, Osaki T, Kai M et al. Immune response against a cross-reactive epitope on the Heat Shock Protein 60 homologue of Helicobacter pylori. Infect Immun 2000; 68:3448-3454.
76. Todoroki I, Takashi J, Watanabe K et al. Suppressive effects of DNA Vaccines encoding Heat Shock Protein on Helicobacter pylori-induced gastritis in mice. Biochem Biophys Res Commun 2000; 277:159-163.
77. Gottwein JM, Blanchard TG, Targoni OS et al. Protective anti-Helicobacter immunity is induced with aluminum hydroxide or complete Freund's adjuvant by systemic immunization. J Infect Dis 2001; 184:308-314.
78. Guy B, Hessler C, Fourage S et al. Systemic immunizaton with urease protects mice against Heliocbacter pylori infection. Vaccine 1998; 16:850-856.
79. Guy B, Hessler C, Fourage S et al. Comparison between targeted and untargeted systemic immunizations with adjuvanted urease to cure Helicobacter pylori infection in mice. Vaccine 1999; 17:1130-1135.
80. Eaton KA, Krakowka S. Chronic active gastritis due to Helicobacter pylori in immunized gnotobiotic piglets. Gastroenterology 1992; 103:1580-1586.
81. Jiang B, Jordana M, Xing Z et al. Replication-defective adenovirus infection reduces Helicobacter felis colonization in the mouse in a gamma interferon- and Interleukin-12-dependent manner. Infect Immun 1999; 67:4539-4544
82. Corthesy-Theulaz IE, Hopkins S, Bachmann D et al. Mice are protected from Helicobacter pylori infection by nasal immunization with attenuated Salmonella typhimurium phoPc expressing urease A and B subunits. Infect Immun 1998; 66:581-586.
83. McAtee CP, Fry KE, Berg DE. Identification of potential diagnostic and vaccine candidates of Helicobacter pylori by proteome technologies. Helicobacter 1998; 3:163-169.

84. Kimmel B, Bosserhoff A, Frank, R. et al. Identification of immunodominant antigens from Helicobacter pylori and evaluation of their reactivities with sera from patients with different gastroduodenal pathologies. Infect Immun 2000; 68:915-920.
85. Ferrero RL, Thiberge JM, Kansau I et al. The groES homolog of Helicobacter pylori confers protective immunity against mucosal infection in mice. Proc Natl Acad Sci USA 1995; 92:6499-6503.
86. Radcliff FJ, Hazell SL, Kolesnikow T et al. Catalase, a novel antigen for Helicobacter pylori vaccination. Infect Immun 1997; 65:4668-4674.
87. Satin B, Giudice GD, Bianca VD et al. The neutrophil-activating protein (HP-NAP) of Helicobacter pylori is a protective antigen and a major virulence factor. J Exp Med 2000; 191:1467-1476.
88. D'Elios MM, Manghetti M, Almerigogna F et al. Different cytokine profile and antigen-specificity repertoire in Helicobacter pylori-specific T cell clones from the antrum of chronic gastritis patients with or without peptic ulcer. Eur J Immunol 1997; 27:1751-1755.
89. Alm RA, Ling LSL, Moir DT et al. Genomic-sequence comparison of two unrelated isolates of the human gastric pathogen Helicobacter pylori. Nature 1999; 397:176-180.
90. Michetti P, Kreiss C, Kotloff KL et al. Oral immunization with urease and Escherichia coli heat-labile enterotoxin is safe and immunogenic in Helicobacter pylori-infected adults. Gastroenterology 1999; 116:804-812.
91. Kotloff KL, Sztein MB, Wasserman SW et al. Safety and immunogenicity of oral inactivated whole-cell Helicobacter pylori vaccine with adjuvant among volunteers with or without subclinical infection. Infect Immun 2001; 69:3581-3590
92. Angelakopoulos H, Hohmann EL. Pilot study of phoP/phoQ-deleted Salmonella enterica serovar typhimurium expressing Helicobacter pylori urease in adult volunteers. Infect Immun 2000; 68:2135-2141.
93. DiPetrillo MD, Tibbetts T, Kleanthous H et al. Safety and immunogenicity of phoP/phoQ-deleted Salmonella typhi expressing Helicobacter pylori urease in adult volunteers. Vaccine 1999; 18:449-459.

Chapter 13

Lyme Disease Vaccine

Janine Evans and Erol Fikrig

Epidemiology and Ecology

Lyme disease occurs throughout the world. Most cases of Lyme borreliosis are reported from temperate regions and coincide with the distribution of the principal vector, ticks of the *Ixodes ricinus* complex, including *I. ricinus*, which is found in most of Europe; *Ixodes persulcatus*, which is found in eastern Europe and Asia; *Ixodes pacificus*, found in the northwestern United States; and *Ixodes scapularis* is found in the eastern and central United States.[1] (Fig. 1)

In the United States, Lyme disease is the most common tick-borne illness. This is likely to be true for Europe as well. Between 1992 and 1998, the number of cases of Lyme disease reported to the United States Centers for Disease Control and Prevention by 49 states was 88,967.[2] The true number of cases of Lyme disease is likely to be much higher. It is estimated that there are 7 to 12 unreported cases for each reported case. The majority (88% of nationally reported cases) were geographically restricted to the northeast, the upper Midwest, and northern California, areas of established enzootic cycles of *Borrelia burgdorferi*, the etiologic agent of Lyme disease. Sporadic cases in states without established enzootic transmission of *B. burgdorferi* may have occurred in limited, unrecognized foci or during visits to endemic areas outside the state of residence, or may have been due to misclassification or misdiagnosis.

Lyme has been reported from almost all countries in Europe. It is particularly prevalent in European countries located in the temperate zones including Sweden, Germany, Austria, and the central portion of the former Soviet Union extending from the Baltic Sea to the Pacific Ocean.[1] Results from a carefully designed, prospective, population-based study of Lyme disease in southern Sweden reported an annual incidence of 69 cases per 100,000 inhabitants (range 26-160 per 100,000).[3] Similar findings have been reported from Germany and Slovenia.[4,5]

Foci of *B. burgdorferi* are highly localized and dependent on environmental factors that are favorable to vector ticks, their maintenance hosts (especially deer), and to animal reservoirs (especially rodents).[1,6] Many mammalian and avian species are reservoir competent and are capable of infecting larval ticks with *B. burgdorferi*. All *Ixodes* ticks have four developmental states: egg, larva, nymph, and adult. Each of the three motile stages feed only once before molting into the next stage. In the northeastern United States, where the epizootiology of Lyme disease has been most extensively studied, the white-footed mouse, *Peromyscus leuopus*, is the principal reservoir species, and the white-tailed deer is the preferred maintenance host of adult *I. scapularis*. In this region, infection rates in nymphal ticks range from 10% to more than 50%. In the southern United States, immature *I. scapularis* feed primarily on lizards, which are reservoir incompetent, resulting in infection rates of less than 1% in nymphal and adult ticks. In northern (*I. ricinus*) and Eastern Europe (*I. persulcatus*), feeding cycles are similar to those in the northern United States, which accounts for the high infection rates in these tick species. The pattern of spread of Lyme disease and its vectors in the northeastern U.S. and Europe derives from the recent proliferation of deer, and the abundance of deer has resulted from the

New Bacterial Vaccines, edited by Ronald W. Ellis and Bernard R. Brodeur.

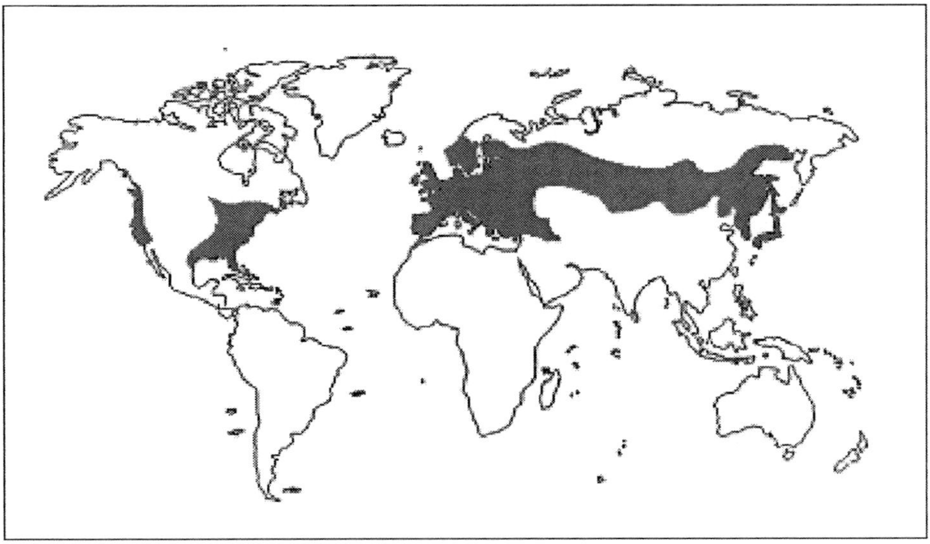

Figure 1. Map showing geographic distribution of Lyme disease worldwide. The distribution of Lyme disease occurs predominantly in temperate zones and coincides with the distribution of the tick vector, *Ixodes ricinus*. The highlighted regions indicate areas endemic for Lyme disease. Reprinted with permission from Eucalb website "http://www.dis.strath.ac.uk/vie/LymeEU/."

process of reforestation. Environmental and socioeconomic factors, such as the growth of suburban communities into farmland and wooded regions and increasing exposure of humans to deer and deer ticks, contribute to the emergence of Lyme disease.

Lyme disease affects all age groups, although the greatest number of cases occur in children under the age of 10 and middle aged adults.[2,7] The incidence of early clinical manifestations peaks from June to August and tapers off in the early fall, coinciding with periods when nymphal ticks are feeding. Adult ticks, abundant during the early and late fall, are less likely to transmit the disease because they prefer deer as hosts and are more readily detected. Late manifestations of disease may occur at any time.

Bacteriology

Borrelia species, along with the leptospira and treponema, belong to the eubacterial phylum of spirochetes. (Fig. 2) As a group, Borrelia species are fastidious, microaerophilic bacteria that grow best at 33°C in a complex, liquid medium called Barbour-Stoenner-Kelly medium. *B. burgdorferi* can be cultured fairly easily from tick and skin biopsy specimens. In people, it is rarely cultured from other sites of infection. *B. burgdorferi* grow slowly, elongating for 12 to 24 hours prior to dividing. After 10 to 15 passages in culture, many isolates of *B. burgdorferi* lose pathogenicity and are no longer infectious.[8,9]

Structurally, Borrelia have a protoplasmic cylinder that is surrounded first by a cell membrane, then by flagella, and finally by an outer membrane.[10] The genome of *B. burgdorferi* B31 has been sequenced and contains a linear chromosome and twenty-one extrachromosomal elements, including 12 linear and 9 circular plasmids.[11,12] The chromosome contains 853 genes encoding a basic set of proteins for DNA replications, transcription, translation, solute transport and energy metabolism. There are no genes for cellular biosynthetic reactions. The biologic function of most of the products of plasmid genes is not known. Many components of the outer membrane are encoded by genes located on extrachromosomal plasmids; theoretically, allowing the organism to make antigenic changes more readily. Plasmids are also thought

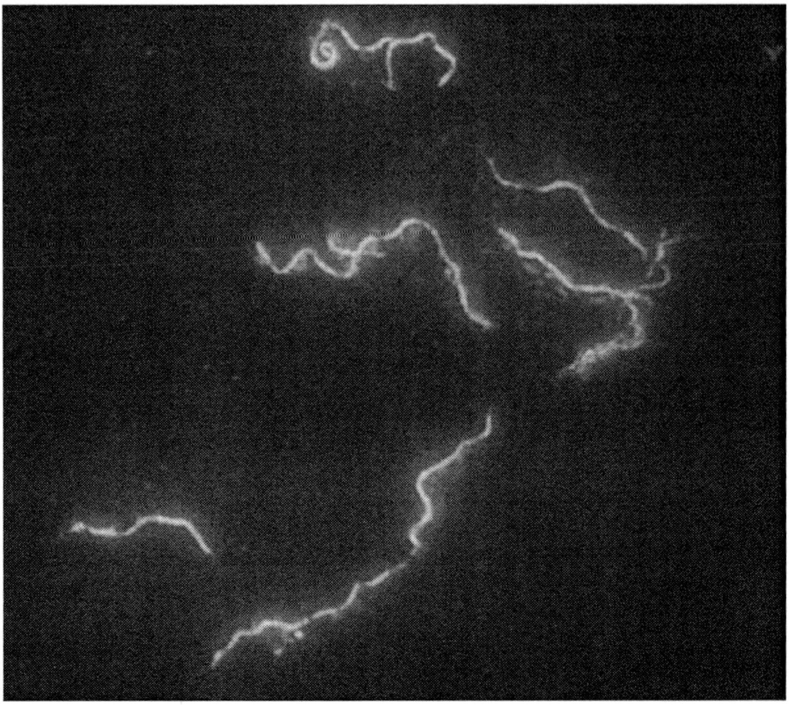

Figure 2. Immunoflourescent photograph of the spirochete, *Borrelia burgdorferi*, the causative agent of Lyme disease. Note the coiled appearance of the organism. Many strains of *B. burgdorferi* have been isolated to date. Photo courtesy of Ruth R. Montgomery, Yale University.

to code for proteins that are important in pathogenicity, antigenic variation or immune evasion, since the loss of infectivity of isolates after passage has been correlated with the loss of particular plasmids in culture.

Some of the genes of *B. burgdorferi* have been isolated and cloned. The protein products of some of the cloned genes have been characterized, including outer surface proteins (Osps) termed OspA , OspB , OspC , OspD, numerous paralogues of OspE and OspF, and *p*G.[13-17] Many of the Osps are lipoproteins and their expression by *B. burgdorferi* varies during the course of infection. A 41 kD antigen, FlaB, is located on the flagellum, and is similar to flagellar antigens of other spirochetes.[18] Two heat shock proteins from the Hsp60 and Hsp70 families have been identified and are cross-reactive with equivalent antigens in other bacteria.[9] Additional antigens include the 22 kD, 39 kD, 55 kD (P55), 83 kD, 93, 100 kD proteins, decorin-binding protein (Dbp)A, and a fibronectin-binding protein (BBK32).[19-23]

B. burgorferi expresses a surface lipoprotein, VlsE (Vmp-like sequence, expressed) that undergoes antigenic variation.[24] Antigenic variation is a method used by certain microbes to avoid or suppress the host immune response. Variable antigens contain both invariable and variable domains. Invariable short regions are interspersed within the variable domains. Antigenic variation affects only the variable domain. Invariable domains and short regions are thought to be important in maintaining the functional structure of the molecule. VlsE contains six invariable short regions (IR1-6) and these IRs are conserved among strains and genospecies of *B. burgdorferi*. The vls genetic locus has the potential to produce millions of antigenic variants during infection of a mammalian host. Unlike the invariable regions of other organisms that are not antigenic during natural infections, the most conserved of the IRs, IR6 is immunodominant in LD patients.

Genetic analysis of Borrelia isolated from North America, Europe, and Asia has led to the identification of distinct genospecies. To date, at least 10 different Borrelia species have been described within the *B. burgdorferi sensu lato* complex: *B. burgdorferi sensu stricto, B. garinii, B. afzelii, B. japonica, B. andersonii, B. valaisiana, B. lusitaniae, B. tanukii, B. turdi*, and *B. bissettii* sp.nov. Only *B. burgdorferi sensu strico, B. garinii*, and *B. afzelii* have been associated with significant human disease.[25] *B. burgdorferi sensu stricto* has been reported to be the most prevalent species in ticks from North America whereas *B. afzelii, B. sensu stricto*, and *B. garinii* are all commonly found in Europe. In some parts of Europe, all three species have been found in the same region and mixed infections have been reported.

Each of the 3 major pathogenic species can be divided into subspecies, each demonstrating differences in genetic, phenotypic, and immunological heterogeneity.[26] More than 100 different isolates from the United States have been identified. The outer surface proteins of *B. burgdorferi sensu strico* are heterogeneous, and multiple isolates are often in a single tick. The results of some studies suggest that specific genetic subtypes of *B. burgdorferi sensu strico* influence disease pathogenesis.[27] *B. burgdorferi* may use surface antigen modulation as a mechanism for evading the immune response. A variant form of OspA has been identified from one of four synovial fluid samples obtained from an individual with chronic Lyme arthritis, and later from two additional serum specimens from people who resided in the vicinity of the index case.[28] It may be that distinct *B. burgdorferi* variant proteins present themselves serially to the immune system and thus serve as a mechanism for disease persistence.[29]

Animal Models

Experimental models of Lyme disease partially mimic human infection and have contributed to our understanding of the pathogenesis of Lyme disease and the development of effective strategies for prevention. Several laboratory animal species have been investigated as potential models of infection, including rabbits, hamsters, dogs, and mice.[30,31] However, disease expression varies between animal species. Rabbits and guinea pigs develop cutaneous lesions of erythema migrans but do not display other signs of disease. Hamsters develop arthritis, but only when inoculated in the footpad and irradiated. Infection in dogs produces fever, anorexia, fatigue, and most commonly limb and joint disorders. Monkeys infected with *B. burgdorferi* develop erythema migrans and neurologic disease.[32] Inoculation of *B. burgdorferi* into laboratory mice produces a disseminated infection, with acute inflammatory polyarthritis, and carditis. In general, disease regresses in immunocompetent mice over several months, but the animals remain persistently infected. The study of disease in mice is preferred because there is better characterization of immunologic and genetic data. Studies using different inbred strains of mice (C3H/He, SWR, C57BL, SJL, and Balb/c mice) have shown that mouse genotype and age significantly influence disease severity.[31] For example, immunocompetent C3H mice developed severe joint and heart disease while C57BL/6 mice displayed only mild disease. Severe combined immunodeficient (SCID) mice develop an overwhelming disseminated infection, not seen in their immunocompetent counterparts.[33]

Pathogenesis

Spirochetes are present in low copy number in the midgut of unfed nymphal ticks. Studies have shown that on attachment of ticks to a host, the bacteria multiplied quickly, with a doubling time close to 4 hours, and reached a maximum number after 72 hours of attachment, likely in response to the blood meal and changes in temperature.[34,35] During an initial 15-hour period, the spirochetes appeared restricted to the tick gut, but after 48 hours they had disseminated to the salivary glands, supporting previous data that indicated the risk of infection prior to 36 hours of tick attachment is low.[36]

B. burgdorferi undergoes alterations in antigenic structure during its life cycle. In the tick midgut and in culture, spirochetes express OspA and OspB in abundance while they produce little or no OspC. In response to the blood meal and prior to entry into the mammalian host,

Osp A/B are cleared from the spirochete surface and OspC is expressed. The rapid upregulation of OspC during tick feeding suggests that this protein is involved in transmission and early colonization of the spirochetes in mammals.[37] BBK32 and BBK50 are also induced during tick engorgement. During mammalian infection, several genes are induced, including OspE/F paralogues, Mlps, vls, eppa, and *p*G.[38,39] It is likely that spirochetes alter the expression of outer surface proteins as a means of adapting to differences in its environment and as a mechanism to evade the mammalian host's immune defenses.

From its point of entry in the skin, *B. burgdorferi* spreads locally in 60 to 80 percent of patients and produces the characteristic early skin lesion, erythema migrans. *B. burgdorferi* later disseminates through the blood and lymphatic system to invade distant organs after a period of spirochetemia. Although spread of an organism is the result of complex interactions between many bacterial and host factors, specific binding of host cells or extracellular matrix by the organism may play an important role in colonization. Movement of spirochetes through the skin or through the basement membranes of endothelium is likely to require the elaboration of proteases. It has been determined that *B. burgdorferi* does not produce collagenase, elastase, hyaluronidase, or other enzymes that digest extracellular matrix components.[40] *B. burgdorferi* may take advantage of host enzymes to spread through the skin. Host derived plasmin, a trypsin-like serine proteinase was found to be important for tissue invasion by spirochetes as demonstrated in cell cultures and in mice genetically deficient in plasminogen.[41]

Glycoaminoglycan (GAG) binding may also contribute to the attachment of the Lyme disease spirochete to host cells and matrix.[42] Mammalian cells ubiquitously express GAGs, and this binding could explain the adherance of *B. burgdorferi* to a variety of cell types in vitro.[43] *B. burgdorferi* have been shown to bind to fibronectin, decorins, and integrins, all of which may contribute to their localization in connective tissue and joints.[44,45]

Immunologic Response to the Spirochete

The presence of *B. burgdorferi* elicits strong host immune responses with the subsequent release of inflammatory mediators. *B. burgdorferi* induces a host inflammatory response, at least in part, through activation of vascular endothelium.[41] Endothelial cell adhesion molecules mediate the attachment of circulating leukocytes to the blood vessel wall and direct inflammatory leukocytes to the site of spirochetal infection.

Histopathologic studies have indicated that mixed, predominantly mononuclear cellular infiltrates with monocytes/macrophages, but also T and B lymphocytes are present in infected tissues.[46] It is believed that a combined effect of local spirochetal infection with an intense immunologic reaction to the organism is responsible for disease expression.

The macrophages and neutrophils of the innate immune system provide the first line of defense against infection.[47,48] The innate immune system, including the Toll-like receptors (TLR) is ancient and serves as an important defense mechanism against bacterial antigens such as endotoxin or lipoproteins that act as the major inflammatory stimulus associated with infection. Lipoproteins, including *B. burgdorferi* OspA, are recognized by TLR2, thereby providing insight into initial pathogen recognition by the host.

The theoretical possibility that *B. burgdroferi* OspA may contribute to the pathogenesis of Lyme arthritis had been examined by Steere and his colleagues. In 1990, Steere et al reported that chronic Lyme arthritis was associated with the presence of major histocompatability complex (MHC) class II antigen, human leukocyte antigen DR2 and DR4 haplotype.[49] Antibody reactivity to two outer surface proteins of *B. burgdorferi* (OspA and OspB) and T cell responses to OspA that may cross react with human lymphocyte antigen-1 (hLFA-1) have been associated with chronic antibiotic-resistant Lyme arthritis.[50,51] A mechanism of molecular mimicry in the pathogenesis of chronic antibiotic-resistant Lyme arthritis has been proposed but alternatives have also been suggested.[29,52,53]

Immunization

Antibody is essential for the killing of *B. burgdorferi*, suggesting that humoral immunity is an important host defense mechanism.[54,55] The protective effect of antibody has been demonstrated in animals. Passive immunization with *B. burgdorferi* antiserum protected hamsters from challenge with an intraperitoneal inoculation of spirochetes.[56] Passive immunization using polyclonal antiserum to *B. burgdorferi* in immunocompetent C3H and in severe combined immunodeficient mice was also protective against intradermal or intraperitoneal inoculation with *B. burgdorferi* sensu stricto if given prior to or at the time of spirochetal challenge.[57,58] No protection occurred when antibodies were given after the infection suggesting that protection from humoral immunity occurs primarily because of spirochete destruction within the tick and not within the mammalian host.[58] The full spectrum of antigens capable of eliciting the production of protective antibodies is not known. Monoclonal antibodies to OspA and OspB, but not those to nonsurface structures of *B. burgdorferi* have also been shown to be protective.

Following infection, borreliacidal activity was present at 7 days, peaked at weeks 3 to 5, and thereafter decreased.[59] It was demonstrated that *B. burgdorferi* activated the classical and alternative complement pathways but was resistant to the nonspecific bactericidal property of human serum. Subsequent studies have shown both complement-dependent and complement-independent antibody mechanisms are capable of conferring protection from infection.[60]

In 1986, Russell Johnson performed the first active immunization study.[61] Hamsters actively immunized with spirochetal lysates were effectively protected from infection from challenge using a homologous strain of *B. burgdorferi*. However, hosts challenged with a heterologous isolate were poorly protected.

Using the C3H/He mouse model, Fikrig and his colleagues evaluated the capacity of recombinant *B. burgdorferi* OspA to induce protection. Mice were immunized with *Escherichia coli* expressing OspA, or with 20 ug of purified recombinant OspA transferase fusion proteins in complete Freund's adjuvant and boosted twice at bimonthly intervals.[57,62] Mice immunized with either recombinant protein, but not controls, developed strong IgG reactivity to these antigens at 14 days after the last boost. OspA-vaccinated mice challenged with an intradermal inoculum of either 10^7 or 10^4 low passage virulent *B. burgdorferi* N40 were fully protected from infection and disease, as determined by culture from internal tissues or by examination of histopathologic specimens. OspB-immunized mice were protected against low (10^2) but not high (10^4) dosage of *B. burgdorferi* N40. Other laboratories confirmed and extended these studies.[63,64]

It was uncertain whether immunization with OspA would induce long-lasting protective immunity. It is known that *B. burgdorferi* can persist in its hosts for long periods of time. In human disease, spirochetes have been cultured from, or have been demonstrated in tissue specimens years following initial infection.[65-67] Similar results have been observed in animal models. Studies addressing longevity of protection from Lyme disease using OspA vaccination were performed in C3H mice. Mice challenged with *B. burgdorferi* N40 up to 4 months after vaccination retained their immune status. Furthermore, mice sacrificed at time points up to 180 days were shown to be free of infection.[68]

The cross-protection afforded by vaccination with monovalent OspA and OspB proteins is unknown. Antigenic differences in OspA and OspB have been demonstrated between and within *B. burgdorferi* genospecies, including *B. burgdorferi* sensu stricto, *B. afzelii*, and B. garinii.[14,69,70] Moreover, spirochetes with mutations, frame shifts or recombination between OspA and OspB have been isolated.[71,72] These observations suggest that a single OspA or B antigen, cloned from a single isolate, may not be sufficient to provide broad cross-protective immunity.[73]

Studies have tried to address the degree of cross-protection conferred following vaccination with a single isolate protein. When mutations are created in the Osp genes of *B. burgdorferi*, subsequent infection using the altered spirochetes can produce disease in vaccinated hosts, especially if the mutations result in variability with the C-terminus of OspA or OspB.[74-77] Moreover, spirochete diversity can influence protective immunity in syringe-inoculation studies.[78-80] However, vaccination with OspA from a single isolate (*B. burgdorferi* N40) has been shown to protect mice against infection by ticks, even when those ticks carried *B. burgdorferi* that were antigenically heterogeneous.[81,82]

Mode of Action

The mode of action of OspA vaccines appears to be vector-specific.[83] Evidence from animal studies indicated that the expression of OspA by *B. burgdorferi* varies during the course of infection. During the initiation of tick feeding, spirochetes residing in the tick gut primarily express OspA. OspA expression then decreases as the spirochetes multiply, and migrate to the tick salivary gland.[84] OspA vaccines appear to exert their principal protective effect by eliciting antibodies that kill Lyme disease spirochetes within the tick gut. Established infection is not affected due to loss of OspA expression in mammalian hosts.[85] Because of this unusual mode of action, a critical level of anti-OspA circulating antibody, at the time of a tick bite, is important in the development of protective immunity.

Human Trials

Two vaccine preparations of lipidated recombinant OspA (rOspA) developed by SmithKline Beecham Pharmaceuticals and Pasteur Merieux Connaught were found to be safe and immunogenic in Phase I and Phase II clinical trials.[86-88]

The results of two large safety and efficacy trials using rOspA preparations have been reported.[89,90] Both studies enrolled approximately 10,000 volunteers each in double-blind, placebo-controlled trials conducted in endemic areas for Lyme disease. Recipients were given three injections of either 30ug of OspA lipoprotein or saline; the first two injections were given 1 month apart in the spring, and a booster dose followed 12 months later. Steere and The Lyme Disease Vaccine Study Group reported that in the first year, after two injections, vaccine efficacy with the LYMErix[tm] rOspA preparation was 49% and increased to 76% in the second year, after the third injection.[89] The age range of the volunteers was between 15 and 70 years. Serologic testing to detect asymptomatic infections with *B. burgdorferi* was performed on study subjects at entry and 12 and 20 months later. The efficacy of the vaccine in preventing asymptomatic infection was 83% in the first year and 100% after the third innoculation. Overall, vaccine efficacy against definite LD and asymptomatic seroconversion was 80% after three doses. (Table 1)

The Pasteur Merieux Connaught rOspA preparation, Imulyme[tm], was given to volunteers between 18 and 92 years of age.[90] In the first year, following two injections, the vaccine efficacy in preventing clinical Lyme disease was 68% and increased to 92% after the third injection. Vaccinees older than 60 years were less protected than younger vaccinees, suggesting that the vaccine may not be as efficacious in older recipients. (Table 1)

rOspA vaccination elicited an antibody response in most individuals. Antibodies reactive with a protective, conformational epitope of OspA, termed LA-2 equivalent antibody, were measured by Steere and his colleagues in a subset of individuals enrolled in the Phase III safety and efficacy trial.[89] A geometric mean antibody titer (GMT) of greater than 1400 ELISA units/ml (EL.U/ml) correlated with protection from Lyme disease during one tick season (spring and summer). Antibody GMT levels of 6,006 EL.U/ml occurred after the third injection and declined over the next 10 months to levels below 1400 EL.U/ml. Most of the antibody loss occurred in the first 7 months after which the rate of decline leveled off (Fig. 3).

Adverse effects were more common in the subjects who received the rOspA vaccine than in individuals that received placebo. Soreness, redness, and swelling at the injection site were the

Table 1. Efficacy of OspA-containing vaccines against* Borrelia burgdorferi *infection

Percent Vaccine Efficacy (95% CI)

	SmithKline Beecham	**Pasteur Merieux Connaught**
First year, after two injections		
Definite Cases	49 (15-69)	68 (36-85)
Asymptomatic	83 (32-97)	NA
Second year, after three injections		
Definite Cases	76 (56-86)	92 (69-97)
Asymptomatic	100 (26-100)	NA
No booster dose given	NA	0 (0-60)

CI, confidence interval; NA, not available
Reprinted with permission from Evans J, Fikrig E Vaccines, Third Edition edited by Stanley A Plotkin and Walter Orenstein Philadelphia, W.B. Saunders Co. 1999.

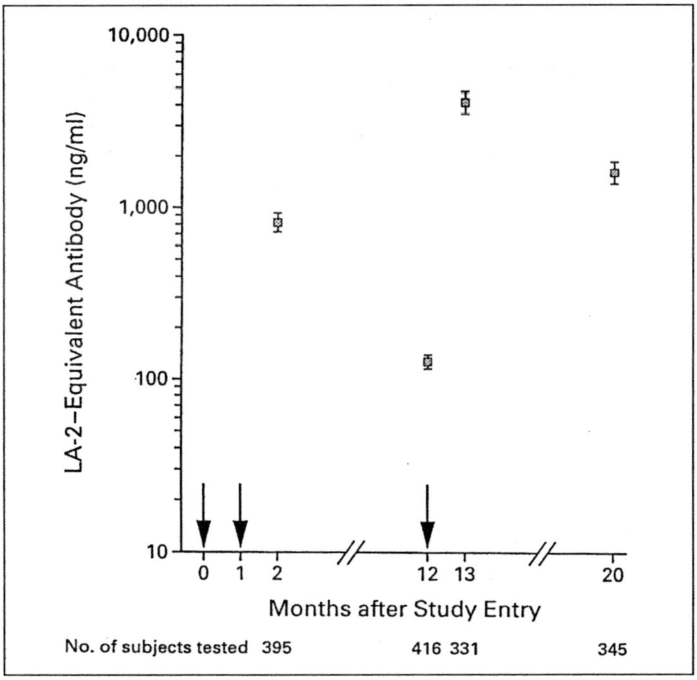

Figure 3. Levels of antibody to the protective epitope of OspA (LA-2-equivalent antibody). After the second injection, the geometric mean antibody titer increased to 816 ng per milliliter after the second injection and declined during the subsequent 10 months. A marked anamnestic response was seen after the third injection, at month 13. The I bars indicated 95 percent confidence intervals. Arrows indicate injections. Reprinted with permission from Steere AC, Sikand VK, Meurice F, et al NEJM 1998;339:209-215.

most frequently reported events. Typically, these symptoms were mild or moderate in severity and self-limited, lasting a median of three days. No hypersensitivity reactions occurred. Thirty days or more after the injections, there were no significant differences between vaccine and placebo recipients in the type or frequency of symptoms. The vaccine also appears to be safe in individuals with a prior history of Lyme disease.[88] Recently, an uncontrolled case report examined 4 individuals who developed transient arthritis following vaccination with OspA.[91] In all four cases the arthritis was of limited duration without subsequent sequelae.

LYMErix™ was approved by the Food and Drug Administration (FDA) in 1999 for use in individuals aged 15 and older. The sales of Lymerix brand vaccine were halted in spring of 2002 by GlaxoSmithKline reportedly due to poor sales. The vaccine remains approved by the FDA.

Additional Considerations

The large safety and efficacy trials administered the rOspA vaccines on a 0,1,and 12 month dosing schedule. Alternative vaccination schedules of 0,1, 6 months and 0,1,2 months have also been studied.[92,93] Adequate GMT of OspA antibodies were achieved using the shorter dosing schedules. Such accelerated schedules can provide protection against Lyme disease prior to the onset of the first tick season after vaccination.

It is unknown how long protective immunity lasts after the third dose of vaccine. Based upon the results of the immunogenicity studies it is likely that additional booster injections will be necessary. There are currently no publications on the immunogenicity of a booster dose upon which to base further recommendations regarding subsequent vaccine doses.

Serologic testing of individuals vaccinated with rOspA frequently produced false-positive results in ELISA assays using whole *B. burgdorferi* specimens. Western blot analysis can assist in discriminating between *B. burgdorferi* infection and previous immunization with rOspA.[94] Anti-OspA antibodies typically do not develop after natural infection.[95]

The Centers for Disease Control Advisory Committee on Immunization Practices has published recommendations for the use of the Lyme disease vaccine.[96] (Table 2) The decision to vaccinate against Lyme disease should be determined on an individual basis, taking into account the risk of exposure to infected tick vectors. Vaccination for Lyme disease should be considered for persons aged 15-70 years who engage in activities (e.g., recreational, property maintenance, occupations, or leisure) that results in frequent or prolonged exposure to tick-infested habitats. Vaccination for Lyme disease may be considered for individuals who are exposed to tick-infested habitats, but whose exposure is neither frequent nor prolonged and travelers to endemic areas, depending upon their risk of exposure. The rOspA vaccine is not recommended for persons with no or minimal exposure to infected ticks. It is also not recommended for pregnant women, children, and persons with treatment resistant Lyme disease. There is no available data regarding vaccination of individuals with immunodeficencies or patients with chronic joint or neurologic illnesses. Vaccination may be considered for persons with a prior history of successfully treated Lyme disease.

The results of a randomized, placebo-controlled safety and immunogenicity trial performed in children and adolescents has recently been published. [97] A total of 4090 healthy children and adolescents (age range: 4-18) participated at seventeen investigational sites in Lyme endemic areas. Children were randomized to receive either 30 mug of OspA vaccine (N=3063) or placebo ((N=1024) on a 1,2,12 month dosing schedule. The majority of adverse events were self-limited local reactions, similar to those experienced by adults. Eight volunteers experienced more generalized symptoms with chills, total body aching, urticaria (seven vaccine, 1 placebo). One recipient developed transient ankle swelling after dose 2. The results of the immunogenicity analysis reported 100% seroconversion with all recipients producing GMT >1400 EL.U/ml after the third injection. The use of LYMErix™ in children has not received FDA appoval.

Table 2. ***Recommendations for use of recombinant outer-surface Protein A vaccine for the prevention of Lyme disease. Advisory Committee on Immunization Practices, 1999.***

	Vaccination Recommendation
Persons who reside, work, or recreate in areas of high or moderate risk	
Persons aged 15–70 years whose exposure to tick-infested habitat is frequent or prolonged	Should be considered
Persons aged 15–70 years who are exposed to tick-infested habitat, but whose exposure is not frequent or prolonged	May be considered
Persons whose exposure to tick-infested habitat is minimal or none	Not recommended
Persons who reside, work, or recreate in areas of low or no risk	Not recommended
Travelers to areas of high or moderate risk	
Travelers aged 15–70 years whose exposure to tick-infested habitat is frequent or prolonged	Should be considered
Children aged <15 years	Not recommended
Pregnant women	
Health-care providers are encouraged to register vaccinations of pregnant women by calling SmithKline Beecham, toll free, at (800) 366-8900, ext. 5231	Not recommended
Persons with immunodeficiency	No available data
Persons with musculoskeletal disease	Limited data available
Persons with previous history of Lyme disease	
Persons aged 15–70 years with previous uncomplicated Lyme disease who are at continued high risk	Should be considered
Persons with treatment-resistant Lyme arthritis	Not recommended
Persons with chronic joint or neurologic illness related to Lyme disease and persons with second- or third-degree atrioventricular block	No available data
Other Recommendations	
Vaccine schedule	
Three doses administered by intramuscular injection as follows: Initial dose, followed by a second dose 1 month later, followed by a third dose 12 months after the first dose	
Second dose (year 1) and third dose (year 2) administered several weeks before the beginning of the disease-transmission season, which is usually April	
Boosters	
Existing data indicate that boosters might be needed, but additonal data are required before recommendations can be made regarding booster schedules	
Simultaneous administration with other vaccines	
Additional data needed	
If simultaneous administration is necessary, use separate syringes and separate injection sites	

Reprinted with permission from MMWR 1999 48:1-26.

Future Vaccines

Potential limitations with use of a single protein recombinant OspA vaccine preparation include a lack of cross-protection for diverse *B. burgdorferi* strains and evasion of the immune system by spirochetes that have truncated outer surface proteins and do not bind protective antibodies.[71,77,98] Multiple antigen vaccines may prove to be more effective.

Recent work has identified other Borrelia proteins that are immunogenic, although they display strain heterogeneity that is similar to OspA. One such protein, outer surface protein C (OspC) has been identified as another possible vaccine candidate. [99] OspC is expressed in abundant amounts by *B. burgdorferi* and, in natural infections, induces a strong early immune response. [100,101] OspC expression appears to correlate negatively with OspA as it increases in response to ticks feeding and contact with human tissues. [102] Animal studies have indicated that vaccination with recombinant OspC is also effective against challenge with limited strains of *B. burgdorferi*. [103,104] Strain heterogeneity is likely to limit the usefulness of OspC as a vaccine candidate. [105] Human trials have not been performed using OspC.

Vaccinations using other Borrelia proteins have been explored. Potential candidates include OspB, OspF, DbpA, and a 110 kD fusion protein containing a portion of a *B. burgdorferi* heat shock protein (HSP70)[106-108] Moreover, immunization with BBK32 (P35) and BBK50 (P37), two Borrelia proteins that are selectively induced in vivo, provide protective immunity as well. [109] Vaccination experiments using OspD, OspE, or Borrelia proteins 30 kD, 83 kD, or P55 kD did not appear to protect animals from infection. [110,111]

Experience with vaccines against Lyme disease, both in animals is increasing yearly. Important advances in understanding immunity against *B. burgdorferi*, including the antigens that elicit protective responses, and the mode of action of OspA in the vector, contribute to our knowledge of the spirochete.

Note

Yale University has a licensing agreement with GlaxoSmithKline for the OspA-based Lyme disease vaccine, and Dr. Fikrig receives a portion of the royalties paid to the University under this agreement.

References

1. Steere AC. Lyme disease: A growing threat to urban populations. Proc Nathl Acad Sci 1994; 91:2378-2383.
2. Orloski KA, Hayes EB, Campbell GL. Surveillance for Lyme disease- United States, 1992-1998. MMWR 2000; 49:1-11.
3. Berglund J, Eitrem R, Ornstein K et al. An epidemiologic study of Lyme disease in southern Sweden. NEJM 1995; 333:1319-1324.
4. Spielman A. The emergence of Lyme disease and human Babesiosis in a changing environment. J N Y Acad Sci 1995; 146-156.
5. Strle F, Stantic-Pavlinic M. Lyme disease in Europe. NEJM 1996; 334:803.
6. Barbour AG ,Fish D. The biological and social phenomenon of Lyme Disease. Science 1993; 260:1610-1616.
7. Shapiro ED. Lyme disease in children, In: Rahn DW, Evans J, eds. Lyme Disease. Philadelphia: American College of Physicians, 1998:123-136.
8. Barbour AG. Isolation and Cultivation of Lyme Disease Spirochetes. Yale J Biol Med 1984; 57:521-525.
9. Pfister H, Wilske B, Weber K. Lyme borreliosis: basic science and clinical aspects. Lancet 1994; 343:1013-1016.
10. Hayes SF, Burgdorfer W. Ultrastructure of Borrelia burgdorferi. In: Weber K, Burgdorfer W, eds. Aspects of Lyme borreliosi., Berlin: 1993:29-43.
11. Fraser CM, Casjens S, Huang WM et al. Genomic sequence of a Lyme disease spirochaete, Borrelia burgdorferi. Nature 1997; 390:580-586.
12. Porcella SF, Schwan TG. Borrelia burgdorferi and Treponema pallidum: a comparison of functional genomics, environmental adaptations and pathogenic mechanisms. J Clin Invest 2001; 107:651-656.
13. Barbour AG , Hayes SF. Biology of Borrelia Species. Microbiol Rev 1986; 50:381-400.
14. Wilske B, Barbour AG, Bergstrom S et al. Antigenic variation and strain heterogeneity in Borrelia spp. Res Microbiol 1992; 143:583-596.

15. Ramamoorthy R, Povinelli L, Phillip MT. Molecular characterization, genomic arrangement, and expression of bmpD, a new member of the bmpD class of genes encoding membrane proteins of Borrelia burgdorferi. Infect Immun 1996; 64:1259-1264.
16. Lam TT, Nguyen TP, Montgomery RR et al. Outer surface proteins E and F of Borrelia burgdorferi, the agent of Lyme disease. Infect. Immun 1994; 62(1):290-298.
17. Wallich R, Brenner C, Kramer MD et al. Molecular cloning and immunological characterization of a novel linear-plasmid-encoded gene, pG, of Borrelia burgdorferi expressed only in vivo. Infect Immun 1995; 63(9):3327-3335.
18. Wallich R, Schaible UE, Simon MM et al. Nucleotide sequence of the Borrelia burgdorferi flagellin. Nuc Acid Res 1989; 17:8869.
19. Scriba M, Ebrahim S, Schlott T et al. The 39-kilodalton protein of Borrelia burgdorferi: a target for bactericidal human monoclonal antibodies. Infect Immun 1993; 61:4523-4526.
20. Feng S, Das S, Lam T et al. A 55-kilodalton antigen encoded by a gene on a Borrelia burgdorferi 49-kilobase plasmid is recognized by antibodies in sera from patients with Lyme disease. Infect Immun 1995; 63(9):3459-66.
21. LeFebvre RB, Perng GC, Johnson RC. The 83-kilodalton antigen of Borrelia burgdorferi which stimulates immunoglobulin M (IgM) and IgG responses in infected hosts is expressed by a chromosomal gene. Infect Immun 1990; 63:1673-1675.
22. Caputa AC, Murtaugh MP, Bey RF et al. 110-kilodalton recombinant protein which is immunoreactive with sera from humans, dogs, and horses with Lyme borreliosis. J Clin Micro 1992; 29:2418-2423.
23. Hagman KE, Lahdenne P, Popova TG et al. Decorin-binding protein of Borrelia burgdorferi is encoded within a two-gene operon and is protective in the murine model of Lyme borreliosis. Infect Immum 1998; 66:5379-5387.
24. Liang FT, Alvarez AL, Gu Y et al. An immunodominant conserved region within the variable domain of VlsE, the variable surface antigen of Borrelia burgdorferi. J Immunol 1999; 163(10):5566-73.
25. Wang G, van Dam AP, Schwartz I et al. Molecular typing of Borrelia burgdorferi sensu lato: taxonomic, epidemiological, and clinical implications. Clin Microbiol Rev 1999; 12(4):633-53.
26. Liveris D, Varde S, Iyer R et al. Genetic diversity of Borrelia burgdorferi in Lyme disease patients as determined by culture versus direct PCR with clinical specimens. J Clin Microbiol 1999; 37(3):565-9.
27. Wormser GP, Liveris D, Nowakowski J et al. Association of specific subtypes of Borrelia burgdorferi with hematogenous dissemination in early Lyme disease. J Infect Dis 1999; 180(3):720-5.
28. Malawista SE, Montgomery RR, Wang XM et al. Geographic clustering of a outer surface protein A mutant of Borrelia burgdorferi. Possible implications of multiple variants for Lyme disease persistence. Rheumatology 2000; 39:537-541.
29. Malawista SE. Resolution of Lyme arthritis, acute or prolonged: a new look. Inflammation 2000, 24:493-504.
30. Philipp MT, Johnson BJ. Animal models of Lyme disease: pathogenesis and immunoprophylaxis. Trends in Microbiol 1994; 2:431-437.
31. Barthold SW. Animal models for Lyme disease. Lab Invest 1995; 72:127-128.
32. Pachner AR, Delaney E, O'Neill T et al. Inoculation of nonhuman primates with the N40 strain of Borrelia burgdorferi leads to a model of Lyme neuroborreliosis faithful to the human disease. Neurol 1995; 45(1):165-72.
33. Schaible U, Kramer M, Museteanu C. et al. The severe combine immunodeficient mouse: a laboratory model of Lyme arthritis and carditis. J Exp Med 1989; 170:240-247.
34. de Silva AM, Fikrig E. Growth and migration of Borrelia burgdorferi in Ixodes ticks during blood feeding. Am J Trop Med Hyg 1995; 53(4):397-404.
35. Ribeiro J, Mather T, Piesman J et al. Dissemination and salivary delivery of Lyme disease spirochetes in vector ticks (Acari: Ixodidae). J Med Entomol 1987; 24:201-205.
36. Piesman J. Dynamics of Borrelia burgdorferi transmission by nymphal Ixodes dammini ticks. J Inf Dis 1993; 167:1082-1085.
37. de Silva AM, Fikrig E. Borrelia burgdorferi genes selectively expressed in ticks and mammals. Parasitology Today 1997; 13:267-270.
38. Anguita J, Samanta S, Revilla B et al. Borrelia burgdorferi gene expression in vivo and spirochete pathogenicity. Infect Immun 2000; 68:1222-1230.

39. de Silva AM, Fikrig E, Hodzic E et al. Immune evasion by tickborne and host-adapted Borrelia burgdorferi. J Inf Dis 1998; 177: 395-400.
40. Klempner MS, Noring R, Epstein MP et al. Binding of human plasminogen and urokinase-type plasminogen activator to the Lyme disease spirochete, Borrelia burgdorferi. JID 1995; 171:1258-1265.
41. Fuchs H, Wallich R, Simon MM et al. The outer surface protein A of the spirochete Borrelia burgdorferi is a plasmin(ogen) receptor. Proc Natl Acad Sci USA 1994; 91:12594-12598.
42. Issacs RD. Borrelia burgdorferi bind to epithelial cell proteoglycans. J Clin Invest 1994; 93:809-819.
43. Leong JM, Wang H, Magoun L et al. Different classes of proteoglycans contribute to the attachment of Borrelia burgdorferi to cultured endothelial and brain cells. Infect Immun 1998; 66:6045-6048.
44. Guo BP, Brown EL, Dorward DW et al. Decorin-binding adhesins from Borrelia burgdorferi. Mol Microbiol 1998; 30:711-723.
45. Coburn J, Magoun L, Bodary SC et al. Integrins alpha(v)beta3 and alpha5beta1 mediate attachment of Lyme disease spirochetes to human cells. Infect Immun 1998; 66:1946-1952.
46. Duray P, Steere AC. Clinical pathologic correlations of Lyme disease by stage. Ann NY Acad Sci 1988; 539:65-79.
47. Brightbill HD, Libraty DH, Krutzik SR et al. Host defense mechanisms triggered by microbial lipoproteins through toll-like receptors. Science 1999; 285(5428):732-6.
48. Yang RB, Mark MR, Gurney AL et al. Signaling events induced by lipopolysaccharide-activated toll-like receptor 2. J Immunol 1999; 163:639-643.
49. Steere AC, Dwyer E, Winchester R. Association of chronic Lyme arthritis with HLA-DR4 and HLA-DR2 alleles. New Engl J Med 1990; 323:219-223.
50. Kalish R, Leong JM, Steere AC. Association of treatment-resistant chronic Lyme arthritis with antibody reactivity to OspA and OspB of Borrelia burgdorferi. Infect Immun 1993; 61:2774-2779.
51. Gross DM, Forsthuber T, Tary-Ledmann M et al. Identification of LFA-1 as a candidate autoantigen in treatment-resistant Lyme arthritis. Science 1998; 281:703-706.
52. Maier b, Molinger M, Cope AP et al. Multiple cross-reactive self-ligands for Borrelia burgdorferi -specific HLA-DR4-restricted T Cells. Eur J Immunol 2000; 30:448-457.
53. Benoist C , Mathis D. Autoimmunity provoked by infection: how good is the case for T cell epitope mimicry? Nat Immunol 2001; Sep 2:797-801.
54. Kochi SK, Johnson RC. Role of Immunoglobulin G in killing of Borrelia burgdorferi by the classical complement pathway. Inf Imm 1988; 56:314-321.
55. Johnson RC, Kodner C, Russell M. Passive immunization of hamsters against experimental infection with Borrelia burgdorferi. Infect Immun 1986; 53:713-716.
56. Schmitz JL, Schell RF, Hejka AG et al. Passive immunizaion prevents induction of Lyme arthritis in LSH hamster. Infect Immun 1990; 58:144-148.
57. Fikrig E, Barthold SW, Kantor FS et al. Protection of mice against the Lyme disease agent by immunizing with recombinant OspA. Science 1990; 250:553-556.
58. Schaible UE, Wallich R, Kramer MD et al. Protection against Borrelia burgdorferi infection in SCID mice is conferred by presensitized spleen cells and partically by B. but not T cells alone. Int Immunol 1994; 6:671-681.
59. Schmitz JL, Schell RF, Lovrich SD et al. Characterization of the protective antibody response to Borrelia burgdorferi in experimentally infected LSH hamsters. Infect Immun 1991; 59:1916-1921.
60. Bockenstedt LK, Barthold S, Deponte K et al. Borrelia burgdorferi infection and immunity in mice deficient in the fifth component of complement. Infect Immun 1993; 61:2104-2107.
61. Johnson RC, Kodner C, Russell M et al. Active immunization of hamsters against experimental infection with Borrelia burgdorferi. Infect Immun 1986; 54:897.
62. Fikrig E, Barthold SW, Marcantonio N et al. Roles of OspA, OspB and flagellin in protective immunity to Lyme borreliosis in laboratory mice. Infect Immun 1992; 59:553-559.
63. Erdile LF, Brandt M, Warakomski DJ et al. Role of attached lipid in immunogenicity of Borrelia burgdorferi OspA. Infect Immun 1993; 61:81-90.
64. Chang Y, Appel MJG, Jacobson RH et al. Recombinant OspA protects dogs against infection and disease caused by Borrelia burgdorferi. Infect Immun 1995; 63:3543-3549.
65. Asbrink E , Hovmark A. Successful cultivation of spirochetes from the skin lesions of patients with erythema chronica migrans afzelius and acrodermatitis chronica atrophicans. Acta Pathol Microbiol Immunol Scand 1985; 93:161-163.

66. Hoffmann JC, Stichtenoth DO, Zeidler H et al. Lyme disease in a 74-year old forest owner with symptoms of dermatomyositis. Arth Rheum 1995; 38:1157-1160.
67. Stanek G, Klein J, Bittner R et al. Isolation of Borrelia burgdorferi from the myocardium of a patient with longstanding cardiomyopathy. N Eng J Med. 1990; 322:249-252.
68. Fikrig E, Barthold SW, Kantor FS et al. Long term protection of mice from Lyme disease by immunizing with recombinant OspA. Infect Immun 1992; 60:773-778.
69. Zumstein G, Fuchs R, Hofmann A et al. Genetic polymorphism of the gene encoding the outer surface protein A (OspA) of Borrelia burgdorferi. Med Microbiol Immunol 1992; 181:57-70.
70. Jonsson M, Noppa L, Barbour AG et al. Heterogeneity of outer membrane proteins in Borrelia burgdorferi: comparison of osp operons of three isolates of different geographic origins. Infect Immun 1992; 60:1845-1853.
71. Sadziene A, Rosa PA, Thompson PA et al. Antibody-resistant mutants of Borrelia burgdorferi: in vitro selection and characterization. J Exp Med 1992; 176:799-809.
72. Fikrig E, Liu B, Fu LL et al. An OspA frame shift, identified from DNA in Lyme arthritis synovial fluid, results in an outer surface protein A that does not bind protective antibodies. 1995.
73. Lovrich SD, Callister SM, DuChateau BK et al. Abilities of OspA proteins from different seroprotective groups of Borrelia burgdorferi to protect hamsters from infection. Infect Immun 1995; 63:2113-2119.
74. Sears J, Fikrig E, Nakagawa T et al. Molecular mapping of OspA-mediated protection against Borrelia burgdorferi, the Lyme disease agent. J Immunol 1991; 147:1995-2001.
75. McGrath BC, Dunn JJ, Gorgone G et al. Idenfication of an immunologically important hypervariable domain of major outer surface protein A of Borrelia burgdorferi. Infect Immun 1995; 63:1356-1361.
76. Fikrig E, Tao H, Kantor FS et al. Borrelia burgdorferi lacking the carboxyl terminus of OspB evade immune destruction. Proc Natl Acad Sci USA 1993; 90:4092-4096.
77. Bockenstedt LK, Fikrig E, Barthold SW et al. Inability of truncated recombinant OspA proteins to elicit protective immunity to Borrelia burgdorferi in mice. J Immun 1993; 151:900-906.
78. Lovrich SD, Callister SM, Lim LCL et al. Seroprotective groups among isolates of Borrelia burgdorferi. Infect Immun 1993; 61:4367-4374.
79. Gern L, Schaible UE, Simon MM. Mode of inoculation of the Lyme disease agent Borrelia burgdorferi influences infection and immune responses in inbred strains of mice. J Inf Dis 1993; 167:971-975.
80. Roehrig JT, Peisman J, Hunt AR et al. The hamster immune response to tick-transmitted Borrelia burgdorferi differs from the response to needle-inoculated, cultured organisms. J Immunol 1992; 149:3648-3653.
81. Telford SR, Kantor FS, Lobet Y et al. Efficacy of human Lyme disease vaccine formulations in a mouse model. JID 1995; 171:1368-1370.
82. Fikrig E, Telford SR, Wallich R et al. Vaccination against Lyme disease caused by diverse Borrelia burgdorferi. J Exp Med 1995; 181:215-221.
83. Shih C, Spielman A, Telford SR. Short report: mode of action of protective immunity to Lyme disease spirochetes. Am J Trop Med Hyg 1995; 52:72-74.
84. de Silva AM, Fikrig E. Arthropod- and host-specific gene expression by Borrelia burgdorferi. J Clin Invest 1997; 99:377-379.
85. Fikrig EF, Telford SR, Barthold SW et al. Elimination of Borrelia burgdorferi from vector ticks feeding on OspA-immunized mice. Proc Natl Acad Sci USA 1992; 89:5418-5421.
86. Keller D, Koster FT, Marks DH. et al. Safety and immunogenicity of a recombinant outer surface protein A Lyme vaccine. JAMA 1994; 271:1764-1768.
87. Van Hoecke CV, Comberbach M, De Grave D et al. Evaluation of the safety, reactogenicity, and immunogenicity of three reccombinant outer surface protein (OspA) Lyme vaccines in healthy adults. Vaccine 1997; 14:1620-1626.
88. Schoen RT, Meurice F, Brunet CM et al. Safety and immunogenicity of an outer surface protein A vaccine in subjects with previous Lyme disease. J Infect Dis 1995; 1324-1329.
89. Steere AC, Sikand VK, Meurice F et al. Vaccination against Lyme disease with recombinant Borrelia burgdorferi outer-surface lipoprotein A with adjuvant. NEJM 1998; 339:209-215.
90. Sigal LH, Adler-Klein D, Bryant G et al. A vaccine consisting of recombinant Borrelia burgdorferi outer-surface protein A to prevent Lyme disease. NEJM 1998; 339: 216-222.
91. Rose CD, Fawcett PT, Gibney KM. Arthritis following recombinant outer surface protein A vaccination for Lyme disease. J Rheum 2001; 28:2555-2557.

92. Van Hoecke C, Lebacq E, Beran J et al. Alternative vaccination schedules (0, 1, and 6 months versus 0, 1, and 12 months) for a recombinant OspA Lyme disease vaccine. Clin Infect Dis 1999; 28(6):1260-4.
93. Schoen RT, Sikand VK, Caldwell MC et al. Safety and immunogenicity profile of a recombinant outer-surface protein A Lyme disease vaccine: clinical trial of a 3-dose schedule at 0,1 and 2 months. Clin Therapeutics 2000; 22:315-325.
94. Aguero-Rosenfeld ME, Roberge J, Carbonaro CA et al. Effects of OspA vaccination on Lyme disease serologic testing. J Clin Microbiol 1999; 37(11):3718-21.
95. Steere AC. Lyme disease. N Engl J Med 1989; 321:586-594.
96. Advisory Committee on Immunization Practices: Recommendations for the use of Lyme disease vaccine. MMWR 1999; 48(RR-7):1-25.
97. Sikand VK, Halsey N, Krause PJ et al. Safety and immunogenicity of a recombinant Borrelia burgdorferi outer surface protein A vaccine against Lyme disase in healthy children and adolescents: a randomized controlled trial. Pediatrics 2001; 108:123-128.
98. Fikrig ET, H., Kantor FS, Barthold SW et al. Evasion of protective immunity by Borrelia burgdorferi by truncation of outer surface protein B. Proc Natl Acad Sci 1993; 90:4092-4096.
99. MBow ML, Gilmore RD, Titus RG. An OspC-specific monoclonal antibody passively protects mice from tick-transmitted iinfection by Borrelia burgdorferi B31. Infect Immun 1999; 67:5470-5472.
100. Padula SJ, Sampieri A, Dias F et al. Molecular characterization and expression of p23 (OspC) from a North American strain of Borrelia burgdorferi. Infection & Immunity 1993; 61(12):5097-105.
101. Padula SJ, Dias F, Sampieri A et al. Use of recombinant OspC from Borrelia burgdorferi for serodiagnosis of early Lyme disease. J Clin Micro 1994; 32:1733-1738.
102. Ohnishi J, Piesman J, de Silva AM. Antigenic and genetic heterogeneity of Borrelia burgdorferi populations transmitted by ticks. Proc Natl Acad Sci USA 2001; 98:670-675.
103. Bockenstedt LK, Hodzic E, Feng S et al. Borrelia burgdorferi strain-specific ospC-mediated immunity in mice. Infect Immun 1997; 65:4661-4667.
104. Probert WS, Crawford M, Cadiz RB et al. Immunization with outer surface protein (Osp)A, but not OspC, provides cross-protection of mice challenged with North American isolates of Borrelia burgdorferi. J Inf Dis 1997; 400-404.
105. Wang I, Dykhuizen DE, Qiu W et al. Genetic diversity of OspC in a local population of Borrelia burgdorferi sensu stricto. Genetics 1999; 151:15-29.
106. Bey RF, Larson ME, Lowery DE et al. Protection of C3H/He mice from experimental Borrelia burgdorferi infection by immunization with a 110-kilodalton fusion protein. Infect Immun 1995; 63:3213-3217.
107. Nguyen TP, Lam TT, Barthold SW et al. Partial destruction of Borrelia burgdorferi within ticks that engorged on OspE- or OspF-immunized mice. Infect Immun 1994; 62(5):2079-84.
108. Fikrig E, Barthold SW, Marcantonio N et al. Roles of OspA, OspB, and flagellin in protective immunity to Lyme borreliosis in laboratory mice. Infect Immun 1992; 60(2):657-61.
109. Fikrig E, Barthold SW, Sun W et al. Borrelia burgdorferi P35 and P37 proteins, expressed in vivo, elicit protective immunity. Immunity 1996; 6:531-539.
110. Probert WS, LeFebvre RB. Protection of C3H/HeN mice from challenge with Borrelia burgdorferi through active immunization with OspA, OspB, or OspC, but not with OspD or the 83-kilodalton antigen. Inf Imm 1994; 62:1920-1926.
111. Feng S, Barthold SW, Telford SR et al. P55, an immunogenic but nonprotective 55-kilodalton Borrelia burgdorferi protein in murine Lyme disease. Infect Immun 1996; 64:363-365.

CHAPTER 14

Moraxella catarrhalis

Timothy F. Murphy

Introduction

The recognition of *Moraxella catarrhalis* in the past two decades as an important human respiratory tract pathogen has stimulated much interest in research on the organism. Recent work has unequivocally established *M. catarrhalis* as a common cause of otitis media and of lower respiratory tract infection in adults with chronic lung disease. Knowledge of the epidemiology of respiratory tract colonization by *M. catarrhalis* and an understanding of its antigenic structure is expanding rapidly. These observations along with the growing understanding of the human immune response to *M. catarrhalis* will form the basis of rational vaccine development. This chapter will review progress in the area and propose approaches which will lead to successful vaccine development to prevent infections caused by *M. catarrhalis*.

Infections Caused by *Moraxella catarrhalis*

Otitis Media

M. catarrhalis is an important cause of acute otitis media in children. Studies from many centers have been performed to elucidate the causes of otitis media. Culture of middle ear fluid obtained by tympanocentesis is the "gold standard" in identifying the etiology of acute otitis media. Based on cultures of middle ear fluid, *M. catarrhalis* is the third most common bacterial cause of otitis media. Table 1 shows the results of cultures of middle ear fluid from several studies over the past decade. Although some variability in the distribution of the three major bacterial pathogens among centers is seen, *M. catarrhalis* is recovered in cultures of up to one fourth of cases of acute otitis media.

Otitis media with effusion is characterized by the presence of middle ear fluid without symptoms of acute infection. The etiology of otitis media with effusion has been a matter of debate and confusion. While bacterial cultures are generally negative, recent studies involving analysis of middle ear fluid for the presence of bacterial DNA using the polymerase chain reaction has revealed that bacteria, including *M. catarrhalis*, appear to be an important cause of otitis media with effusion as well.[55,56,95,109]

Approximately three-fourths of all children experience an episode of otitis media by the age of three years. A subset of children, who are called "otitis prone", experience recurrent otitis media.[35] Recurrent otitis media is associated with a delay in speech and language development. Therefore, there is strong rationale for developing vaccines to prevent otitis media, particularly recurrent otitis media. A successful vaccine for bacterial otitis media will involve preventing infection caused by *Streptococcus pneumoniae*, nontypeable *Haemophilus influenzae* and *Moraxella catarrhalis*.

New Bacterial Vaccines, edited by Ronald W. Ellis and Bernard R. Brodeur.

Table 1. Causes of otitis media: results of tympanocentesis

Reference	Year	Location	% of Cases Caused by *Streptococcus pneumoniae*	*Haemophilus influenzae*	*Moraxella catarrhalis*
107	1990	Norway and Finland	28	16	16
46	1991	Dallas, Texas	29	30	15
63	1991	Cleveland, Ohio	25	27	11
36	1992	Buffalo, New York	19	35	18
31	1992	Philadelphia, Pennsylvania	48	20	23
23	1992	Galveston, Texas	39	34	18
91	1993	Galveston, Texas	29	37	15
6	1994	USA-five centers	39	27	14
47	1996	France	28	43	10
30	1998	Israel	28	45	7
13	2000	USA	52	33	11
14	2000	USA	39	39	12
65	2001	Finland	26	23	23

Lower Respiratory Tract Infections

M. catarrhalis is an important cause of lower respiratory tract infections in adults with chronic obstructive pulmonary disease (COPD).[25,34,64,82,104] COPD is characterized by intermittent exacerbations of the disease. A proportion of these exacerbations is caused by bacteria. Since *M. catarrhalis* can colonize the upper respiratory tract in the absence of acute infection, the presence of the organism in sputum does not establish the etiology of an exacerbation. Five lines of evidence indicate that *M. catarrhalis* causes exacerbations of COPD.

1. Some patients experience clinical evidence of lower respiratory tract infection and sputum Gram stain shows a predominance of intracellular and extracellular gram negative diplococci and culture reveals *M. catarrhalis.*
2. *M. catarrhalis* can be obtained in pure culture from patients with exacerbations using techniques which reliably reflect lower respiratory tract bacteriology, including transtracheal aspiration and bronchoscopy with the protected specimen brush.[41,79,90,94,106,117]
3. Administration of specific antimicrobial therapy directed at β-lactamase producing strains of *M. catarrhalis* results in clinical improvement after failure of β-lactam antibiotics.
4. Patients with clinical and laboratory evidence of *M. catarrhalis* infection develop new immune responses to their own isolate of M. catarrhalis.[8,20]
5. Acquisition of a new strain of *M. catarrhalis* is associated with the development of an exacerbation. Taken together, these lines of evidence indicate that *M. catarrhalis* is an important cause of exacerbations of COPD. Adults with COPD represent a population which would benefit from a vaccine to prevent respiratory tract infections caused by *M. catarrhalis.*

Other Infections

M. catarrhalis causes sinusitis in adults and children, and pneumonia in the elderly.[9,17,19,24,27,89,115,116] It has also been responsible for nosocomial outbreaks of respiratory tract infections, particularly in respiratory units, suggesting that the presence of a susceptible population contributed to the clusters.[10,28,77,80,92,93,100]

Epidemiology and Respiratory Tract Colonization

M. catarrhalis has been recovered exclusively from humans. Colonization of the upper respiratory tract with *M. catarrhalis* is common during infancy, with higher rates during winter months.[5,39,112,114] Substantial regional variation is seen in colonization rates. For example, a prospective study in Buffalo New York, USA, in which monthly nasopharyngeal cultures were performed, showed that two-thirds of infants were colonized by *M. catarrhalis* at some time during the first year of life and 78% were colonized at some time by the age of 2 years.[39] A similar study in Goteborg, Sweden revealed a colonization rate of approximately half that of the Buffalo study.[5] Another study involving infants in a rural Aboriginal community in Australia revealed that all infants were colonized by the age of 3 months.[71] Multiple factors are likely responsible for the variability in colonization rates including living conditions, hygiene, smoking rates among parents, genetic characteristics of the populations and others.

Nasopharyngeal colonization with middle ear pathogens, including *M. catarrhalis*, is associated with otitis media.[37,38,49] The presence of the organism in the nasopharynx has little diagnostic value in establishing the etiology of an individual episode of otitis media. However, the epidemiological association between colonization and otitis media is strong and otitis prone children are colonized at a higher rate. The precise relationship between nasopharyngeal colonization and otitis media is yet to be elucidated. The current data suggest that colonization by *M. catarrhalis* is a necessary first step in the pathogenesis of otitis media. However, colonization alone is not sufficient to cause otitis media. A second insult, such as a viral infection, in a colonized child may precipitate an episode of otitis media.

Colonization of the human respiratory tract with *M. catarrhalis* is a dynamic process. Studies which have employed molecular typing of isolates of *M. catarrhalis* collected as part of prospective studies reveal that strains are eliminated and acquired frequently.[67] This active turnover of strains of *M. catarrhalis* is observed both in children and in adults with chronic lung disease.

Immune Response to Infection

The literature on the immune response to *M. catarrhalis* is confusing and requires careful evaluation. Several features of studies immune responses to *M. catarrhalis* should be considered.

Absence of Animal Models of Infection

The mouse pulmonary clearance model which involves direct inoculation of *M. catarrhalis* into the lungs is being used to evaluate potential vaccine antigens (see below). While this model may provide useful data on the potential of vaccine antigens, it should be emphasized that this is a clearance model rather than a model of infection. Animals clear the bacteria within 24 hours and none develop respiratory tract infections suggestive of any of the forms seen in humans. Similarly, models of otitis media have not performed well with *M. catarrrhalis* because the bacterium appears to be cleared readily from the middle ear by the species of animals tested thus far.[7,26,32,45] In view of the observations that *M. catarrhalis* is an exclusively human pathogen and that humans appear to have a fundamentally different immune response compared to many laboratory animals, limited useful information has been learned from animal models about the immune response to infection due to *M. catarrhalis*.

Immune Response to Strain-Specific and Conserved Antigens

The sources of antigens used in immunoassays to study the human immune response to *M. catarrhalis* are of particular importance in interpreting the literature. Some studies have used a single strain, some studies have used mixtures of strains and some studies have used antigen preparations from homologous infecting strains to study the immune response following *M. catarrhalis* infection.[81,104] Different antigen preparations yield markedly different results. As information on the antigenic structure of outer membrane antigens of *M. catarrhalis* expands, the importance of considering immune responses to strain-specific determinants is becoming apparent. While using laboratory strains will allow the detection of antibodies to determinants which are shared among strains, using homologous infecting strains will detect immune responses to both common and strain-specific determinants. Several outer membrane antigens of *M. catarrhalis* show substantial antigenic heterogeneity among strains, emphasizing the importance of using homologous strains to detect strain-specific immune responses.

Immunoassays to Detect Antibodies to Surface Antigens

One goal of studying antibody responses to *M. catarrhalis* is to elucidate a protective immune response. Mechanisms by which antibodies may mediate a protective immune response include inhibition of binding to mucous membranes, complement mediated bactericidal activity, and opsonization for phagocytosis. Such antibodies must bind to the surface of the intact bacterium. Therefore, immunoassays which are likely to detect protective antibodies should measure antibodies to surface-exposed epitopes. Such immunoassays include functional assays (adherence, bactericidal and opsonophagocytosis assays), flow cytometry, adsorption assays, elution assays and whole cell radioimmunoprecipitation assays. In addition, assays such as ELISAs, immunofluorescence microscopy and immunoelectron microscopy can detect antibodies to surface epitopes when performed to allow antibodies to bind to nondenatured whole bacterial cells before fixation.

A large number of studies of the human immune response following *M. catarrhalis* infection have been performed using a variety of methods.[81,82,104] A correlate of protection from *M. catarrhalis* infection has yet to be identified. Identifying a correlate of protection will advance the field of vaccine development for *M. catarrhalis* significantly because such an observation will act as a guide for testing potential vaccine antigens. Analysis of samples from prospective studies of *M. catarrhalis* infection and colonization using immunoassays which are capable of detecting protective antibodies have the potential of elucidating a correlate of protection from infection.

Mucosal Immune Response

Since *M. catarrhalis* colonizes the human respiratory mucosal surface and causes mucosal infections, the mucosal immune response is likely important in a protective immune response. Several studies have established that antibodies to *M. catarrhalis* are present on the mucosal surface. Analysis of the systemic and mucosal antibody responses to outer membranes of homologous strains of *M. catarrhalis* following otitis media indicates that young children develop a mucosal response but do not consistently develop a systemic response.[40] *M. catarrhalis* which colonizes the nasopharynx of children is coated with IgA and IgG.[108] Interestingly, otitis prone children had significantly fewer IgA coated bacteria than did nonotitis prone children, suggesting the IgA to surface exposed epitopes is associated with relative protection from recurrent otitis media. Adults with COPD develop new mucosal IgA to surface exposed epitopes of the homologous isolates as detected by flow cytometry following exacerbations caused by *M. catarrhalis*.[8] Systemic and mucosal immune response occur independently of one another in this population. Characterizing the role of the mucosal immune response in protection from infection is an area of investigation which should receive high priority.

Animal Models

Animal models have provided useful data regarding the pathogenesis of infection and the immune response to infection for many bacterial infections. Furthermore, studies in animal models have been instrumental in the development of most successful vaccines to prevent bacterial infections. Therefore, much effort has been devoted toward the development of an animal model to study *M. catarrhalis*. As noted above, currently available models suffer from significant limitations as models of human infection. However, studies involving two of the models are providing potentially useful information in assessing vaccine antigens.

Table 2. Animal models to Study M. catarrhalis *infection*

Infection	Animal	Outcome Measurement	Observations	Refs.
Pulmonary clearance	Mouse	Rate of clearance from lungs following intrapulmonary challenge	*M. catarrhalis* is cleared in 24 hours	22,52,53,61,68,69, 75,87,111
Otitis media	Chinchilla	Signs of otitis and clearance of bacteria from middle ear	*M. catarrhalis* is cleared by 5 days	26,32,45
Systemic infection	SCID mouse	Clinical and post mortem findings	*M. catarrhalis* is not recovered from blood.	51
Colonization	Chinchilla	Colonization of upper airway	Intranasal inoculation readily colonizes the nasopharynx	7

Table 2 summarizes animal model systems which have been used to study *M. catarrhalis*. The mouse pulmonary clearance model has been used by several laboratories. Bacteria are instilled directly into the trachea and the clearance of viable bacteria from the lung is quantitated. *M. catarrhalis* is completely cleared from the lungs by 24 hours post challenge. The rate of clearance of bacteria in immunized animals compared to unimmunized animals is used as a measure of the efficacy of a potential vaccine antigen. Both systemic and mucosal routes of immunization with promising vaccine antigens are being evaluated in this model system.

The chinchilla has been used as a model of otitis media for *Streptococcus pneumoniae* and nontypeable *Haemophilus influenzae*. Unfortunately, when *M. catarrhalis* is instilled into the middle ear of chinchillas, the bacterium is cleared completely after 5 days.[26,32,45] The inability to establish otitis media in the chinchilla has thus far precluded the use of this model to study otitis media due to *M. catarrhalis*. By contrast, intranasal inoculation of *M. catarrhalis* readily colonizes the upper respiratory tract of chinchillas .[7] This colonization model may prove useful in elucidating immune responses involved in clearance of colonization.

Vaccine Development

Conjugating capsular polysaccharides to protein carriers has been used to develop highly successful vaccines for the prevention of infections caused by *H. influenzae* type b and *S. pneumoniae*. *M. catarrhalis* does not appear to express a capsule, so alternative antigens must be sought. Pili have been used successfully as vaccine antigens for other gram negative mucosal pathogens. *M. catarrhalis* expresses pili but they have not yet been purified or characterized and the gene which encodes pili has not yet been cloned. Studies to evaluate pili as a vaccine antigen for *M. catarrhalis* await this progress. The major focus of investigation thus far in identifying vaccine antigens has been on outer membrane proteins and lipooligosaccharide (LOS).

Characteristics of a Vaccine Antigen

In evaluating an outer membrane antigen as a potential vaccine candidate, several characteristics should be considered. First, the antigen should express epitopes which are available for antibody binding on the surface of the intact bacterium. As discussed above, if antibodies are going to block adherence, direct complement mediated killing or opsonize, then the antigen to which they are directed must be expressed on the bacterial surface. Molecules which are buried within the outer membrane and thus unavailable for antibody binding are not likely to generate protective antibodies.

A second important characteristic of a vaccine antigen is conservation among strains of the species. A successful vaccine will generate protective immune responses which are broadly cross reactive among all or most strains of *M. catarrhalis*. The ideal vaccine antigen would be identical among all strains. However, antigenic heterogeneity among strains could also be overcome by including a moderately conserved antigen from several selected strains in a vaccine preparation.

A third consideration is phase variation and expression of the vaccine antigen in vitro. If *M. catarrhalis* is able to turn off expression of an antigen (phase variation) to which antibodies are directed, those antibodies are not going to protect from infection. Similarly, it well known that bacteria alter the expression of surface molecules under different environmental conditions. A surface molecule which is expressed when the bacterium grows on artificial media but not when it grows in the human respiratory tract will not be a good vaccine antigen. Therefore, candidate vaccine antigens should be assessed carefully to determine whether they are expressed during human colonization and infection. Furthermore, once testing of a vaccine antigen begins by immunizing animals and eventually humans, the possibility that phase variation driven by immune selective pressure is occurring should be investigated.

A fourth consideration involves the immunogenicity of the antigen. In order for a vaccine to be effective, the antigen must be immunogenic in the target population. For example, the purified capsular polysaccharide of *H. influenzae* type b induces protective antibodies in adults but is not reliably immunogenic in infants under the age of 2 years. Since the majority of *H. influenzae* type b meningitis occurs in children under 18 months of age, the lack of immunogenicity in the target population was a major problem for the purified polysaccharide vaccine even though antibodies to the polysaccharide are protective. In the case of a vaccine for *M. catarrhalis*, it will be important that the vaccine be immunogenic in infants since a major goal of a vaccine is to prevent recurrent otitis media which usually has its onset in the first year of life. An advantage of proteins as vaccine antigens is that proteins are likely to be immunogenic in infants.

Finally, the candidate vaccine antigen must induce a protective immune response. For example, an outer membrane protein may be surface exposed, highly conserved among strains, constituitively expressed during infection and highly immunogenic. However, immunization with the antigen must induce protection from infection if the protein is to be an effective vaccine. Unfortunately, it is not possible to predict which antigens will induce protective immune responses at this time. The absence of a correlate of protection from *M. catarrhalis* infection is currently a major obstacle in assessing potential vaccine antigens. Serum bactericidal assays, opsonophagocytosis assays and the mouse pulmonary clearance model are being studied but none has shown a clear-cut correlation with a protective immune response in humans thus far. Identifying a correlate of protection is an area of high priority in the field of vaccine development for *M. catarrhalis*.

One approach to identifying potential vaccine antigens for bacterial pathogens has been to identify antigens to which humans make antibody following infection. Such an approach may be fruitful; however, one must be cautious in excluding antigens as effective vaccines based on the absence of a response following infection. The immune response following infection is likely to be different from the immune response following vaccination by a purified antigen in the presence of an adjuvant. A case in point is Lyme disease. Lyme disease does not induce an immune response to OspA, yet a vaccine containing OspA is effective in preventing infection.[72,110]

Candidate Vaccine Antigens

Table 3 lists outer membrane antigens of *M. catarrhalis* which have been considered as potential vaccine antigens, along with a brief summary of the current status of knowledge regarding selected characteristics of each. Several integral outer membrane proteins, adhesins

Table 3. ***Potential vaccine antigens of*** **Moraxella catarrhalis**

Outer Membrane Antigen	Molecular Mass (kDa)	Putative Function	Conservation Among Strains	Evidence of Protection	References
UspA1	88 (oligomer)[a]	Adhesin	Heterogeneous and conserved regions; phase varies	Bactercidal[b] Mouse clearance[c]	2,3,21,22,29, 53,57,66,70,78
UspA2	62 (oligomer)[a]	Involved in serum resistance	Heterogeneous and conserved regions	Bactericidal Mouse clearance	2,3,21,22,29, 53,78,101
200 kDa protein	200	Hemagglutinin	Unknown		42,43
MID	200	Binds IgD	Unknown		44
OMP CD	45[d]	Porin, binds mucin	Highly conserved	Bactericidal Mouse clearance	50,59,85-87,98 102,118
OMP E	50	Fatty acid transport	Highly conserved		11,12,83,84
Lipooligo- saccharide	2.5 - 4	Endotoxin	Moderately conserved	Bactericidal Mouse clearance	48,58,60,62, 96,97,113,121
		Proteins Involved in Iron Uptake			
TbpA	115-120	Transferrin transport	Unknown		73,120
TbpB (OMP B1)	80-85	Binds transferrin	Heterogeneous and conserved regions	Bactericidal Mouse clearance	18,73,74,76,88, 99,103,119,120
CopB (OMP B2)	80	Iron uptake	Heterogeneous in surface-exposed regions	Bactericidal Mouse clearance	1,4,52,54,105
LbpA	95-110	Binds lactoferrin	Unknown		15,16,33,120
LbpB	95-110	Binds lactoferrin	Variable, under study	Bactericidal	15,16,33 120

a. Molecular mass varies among strains
b. Antibodies to the antigen are bactericidal in vitro
c. Immunization with the antigen enhances clearance in the mouse pulmonary clearance model
d. OMP CD runs aberrantly (apparent molecular mass ~60 kDa) in SDS-P

and proteins involved in iron uptake are currently under study. In addition, a detoxified form of lipooligosaccharide conjugated to protein carriers is being studied. As noted in Table 3 some of these antigens may be limited by antigenic heterogeneity and phase variation. While several of the antigens induce bactericidal antibodies and enhance clearance in the mouse pulmonary clearance model, it is impossible to predict which, if any, will induce protective immune responses in humans. Since *M. catarrhalis* is an exclusively human pathogen and since the immune response in animals appears to be different from that of humans, it will be necessary to test potential vaccine in humans to draw meaningful conclusions regarding the likely efficacy of a vaccine under development.

Future Directions

Substantial progress has been made in the past decade in identifying putative vaccine antigens of *M. catarrhalis*. Emphasis should be placed in several areas to advance the field of vaccine development. 1) Elucidating the elements of a protective immune response and identifying a correlate of protection will facilitate the ability to evaluate candidate vaccines enormously. Delineating the immune response which will protect from otitis media and lower respiratory tract infections will serve as an important guide in vaccine development. 2) Emphasis should be placed on characterizing the mucosal immune response to *M. catarrhalis*. Such studies may lead to understanding the mechanisms by which strains are eliminated from the respiratory tract, invaluable information in developing vaccines to eradicate *M. catarrhalis* from the respiratory tract. 3) Candidate vaccine antigens should be tested in humans as soon as feasible. *M. catarrhalis* is an exclusively human pathogen and the human immune response is quite different from that of animals. Therefore, the most efficient approach to developing new vaccines is to carefully test putative vaccine antigens for safety and proceed to human testing once safety has been ensured. 4) Various delivery systems including mucosal immunization and novel adjuvants should be assessed in testing putative vaccine antigens for *M. catarrhalis*.

References

1. Aebi C, Cope LD, Latimer JL et al. Mapping a protective epitope of the CopB outer membrane protein of Moraxella catarrhalis. Infect Immun 1998; 66:540-8.
2. Aebi C, LaFontaine ER, Cope LD et al. Phenotypic effect of isogenic uspA1 and uspA2 mutations on Moraxella catarrhalis 035E. Infect Immun 1998; 66:3113-9.
3. Aebi C, Maciver I, Latimer JL et al. A protective epitope of Moraxella catarrhalis is encoded by two different genes. Infect Immun 1997; 65:4367-77.
4. Aebi C, Stone B, Beucher M et al. Expression of the CopB outer membrane protein by Moraxella catarrhalis is regulated by iron and affects iron acquisition from transferrin and lactoferrin. Infect Immun 1996; 64:2024-30.
5. Aniansson G, Alm B, Andersson B et al. Nasopharyngeal colonization during the first year of life. J Infect Dis 1992; 165(S1):S38-S42.
6. Aspin MM, Hoberman A, McCarty J et al. Comparative study of the safety and efficacy of clarithromycin and amoxicillin-clavulanate in the treatment of acute otitis media in children. J Pediatr 1994; 125:135-41.
7. Bakaletz LO, Murwin DM, Billy JM. Adenovirus serotype 1 does not act synergistically with Moraxella (Branhamella) catarrhalis to induce otitis media in the chinchilla. Infect Immun 1995; 63:4188-90.
8. Bakri F, Brauer AL, Sethi S et al. Systemic and mucosal antibody response to Moraxella catarrhalis following exacerbations of chronic obstructive pulmonary disease. J Infect Dis 2001; in press.
9. Barreiro B, Esteban L, Prats E et al. Branhamella catarrhalis respiratory infections. Eur Respir J 1992; 5:675-9.
10. Beaulieu D, Scriver S, Bergeron MG et al. Epidemiological typing of Moraxella catarrhalis by using DNA probes. J Clin Microbiol 1993; 31:736-9.
11. Bhushan R, Craigie R, Murphy. Molecular cloning and characterization of outer membrane protein E of Moraxella (Branhamella) catarrhalis. J Bacteriol 1994; 176:6636-43.
12. Bhushan R, Kirkham C, Sethi S et al. Antigenic characterization and analysis of the human immune response to outer membrane protein E of Branhamella catarrhalis. Infect Immun 1997; 65:2668-75.
13. Block SL, Hedrick JA, Kratzer J et al. Five-day twice daily cefdinir therapy for acute otitis media: microbiologic and clinical efficacy. Pediatr Infect Dis J 2000; 19(12S):S153-S158.
14. Block SL, McCarty JM, Hedrick JA et al. Comparative safety and efficacy of cefdinir vs amoxicillin/clavulanate for treatment of suppurative acute otitis media in children. Pediatr Infect Dis J 2000; 19:S159-S165.
15. Bonnah RA, Wong H, Loosmore SM et al. Characterization of Moraxella (Branhamella) catarrhalis lbpB, lpbA, and lactoferrin receptor orf3 isogenic mutants. Infect Immun 1999; 67:1517-20.
16. Bonnah RA, Yu R-H, Wong H et al. Biochemical and immunological properties of lactoferrin binding proteins from Moraxella (Branhamella) catarrhalis. Microb Pathogen 1998; 24:89-100.
17. Brorson J-E, Axelsson A, Holm SE. Studies on Branhamella catarrhalis (Neisseria catarrhalis) with special reference to maxillary sinusitis. Scand J Infect Dis 1976; 8:151-5.

18. Campagnari AA, Ducey TF, Rebmann CA. Outer membrane protein B1, an iron-repressible protein conserved in the outer membrane of Moraxella (Branhamella) catarrhalis, binds human transferrin. Infect Immun 1996; 64:3920-4.
19. Carr B, Walsh JB, Coakley D et al. Prospective hospital study of community acquired lower respiratory tract infection in the elderly. Respir Med 1991; 85:185-7.
20. Chapman AJ, Musher DM, Jonsson S et al. Development of bactericidal antibody during Branhamella catarrhalis infection. J Infect Dis 1985; 151:878-82.
21. Chen D, Barniak V, Van der Meid KR et al. The levels and bactericidal capacity of antibodies directed against the uspA1 and UspA2 outer membrane proteins of Moraxella (Branhamella) catarrhalis in adults and children. Infect Immun 1999; 67:1310-6.
22. Chen D, McMichael JC, van der Meid KR et al. Evaluation of purified UspA from Moraxella catarrhalis as a vaccine in a murine model after active immunization. Infect Immun 1996; 64:1900-5.
23. Chonmaitree T, Owen MJ, Patel JA et al. Effect of viral respiratory tract infection on outcome of acute otitis media. J Pediatr 1992; 120:856-62.
24. Choo PW, Gantz NM. Branhamella catarrhalis pneumonia with bacteremia. South Med J 1989; 82:1317-8.
25. Christensen JJ. Moraxella (Branhamella) catarrhalis: clinical, microbiological and immunological features in lower respiratory tract infections. APMIS 1999; 107(suppl):1-36.
26. Chung M-H, Enrique R, Lim DJ et al. Moraxella (Branhamella) catarrhalis-induced experimental otitis media in the chinchilla. Acta Otolaryngol. 1994; 114:415-22.
27. Collazos J, de Miguel J, Ayarza R. Moraxella catarrhalis bacteremic pneumonia in adults: two cases and review of the literature. Eur J Clin Microbiol Infect Dis 1992; 11:237-40.
28. Cook PP, Hecht DW, Snydman DR. Nosocomial Branhamella catarrhalis in a paediatric intensive care unit: risk factors for disease. J Hosp Infect 1989; 13:299-307.
29. Cope LD, LaFontaine ER, Slaughter CA et al. Characterization of the Moraxella catarrhalis uspA1 and uspA2 genes and their encoded products. J Bacteriol 1999; 181:4026-34.
30. Dagan R, Leibovitz E, Greenberg D et al. Early eradication of pathogens from middle ear fluid during antibiotic treatment of acute otitis media is associated with improved clinical outcome. Pediatr Infect Dis J 1998; 17:776-82.
31. DelBeccaro MA, Mendelman PM, Inglis AF et al. Bacteriology of acute otitis media: A new perspective. J Pediatr 1992; 120:81-4.
32. Doyle WJ. Animal models of otitis media: other pathogens. Pediatr Infect Dis J 1989; 8:S45-S47.
33. Du R-P, Wang Q, Yang Y-P et al. Cloning and expression of the Moraxella catarrhalis lactoferrin receptor genes. Infect Immun 1998; 66:3656-65.
34. Enright MC, McKenzie H. Moraxella (Branhamella) catarrhalis - clinical and molecular aspects of a rediscovered pathogen. J Med Microbiol 1997; 46:360-71.
35. Faden H. The microbiologic and immunologic basis for recurrent otitis media in children. Eur J Pediatr 2001; 160(7):407-13.
36. Faden H, Bernstein J, Stanievich J et al. Effect of prior antibiotic treatment on middle ear disease in children. Ann Otol Rhinol Laryngol 1992; 101:87-91.
37. Faden H, Brodsky L, Waz MJ et al. Nasopharyngeal flora in the first three years of life in normal and otitis-prone children. Ann Otol Rhinol Laryngol 1991; 100:612-5.
38. Faden H, Duffy L, Wasielewski R et al. Relationship between nasopharyngeal colonization and the development of otitis media in children. J Infect Dis 1997; 175:1440-5.
39. Faden H, Harabuchi Y, Hong JJ, Tonawanda/Williamsville Pediatrics. Epidemiology of Moraxella catarrhalis in children during the first 2 years of life: relationship to otitis media. J Infect Dis 1994; 169:1312-7.
40. Faden H, Hong J, Murphy TF. Immune response to outer membrane antigens of Moraxella catarrhalis in children with otitis media. Infect Immun 1992; 60:3824-9.
41. Fagon J-Y, Chastre J, Trouillet J-L et al. Characterization of distal bronchial microflora during acute exacerbation of chronic bronchitis. Am Rev Respir Dis 1990; 142:1004-8.
42. Fitzgerald M, Mulcahy R, Murphy S et al. A 200 kDa protein is associated with haemagglutinating isolates of Moraxella (Branhamella) catarrhalis. FEMS Immunol Med Microbiol 1997; 18:209-16.
43. Fitzgerald M, Mulcahy R, Murphy S et al. Transmission electron microscopy studies of Moraxella (Branhamella) catarrhalis. FEMS Immunol Med Microbiol 1999; 23:57-66.
44. Forsgren A, Brant M, Mollenkvist A et al. Isolation and characterization of a novel IgD-binding protein from Moraxella catarrhalis. J Immunol 2001; 167(4):2112-20.
45. Fulghum RS, Marrow HG. Experimental otitis media with Moraxella (Branhamella) catarrhalis. Ann Otol Rhinol Laryngol 1996; 105:234-41.
46. Gan VN, Kusmiesz H, Shelton S et al. Comparative evaluation of loracarbef and amoxicillin-clavulanate for acute otitis media. Antimicrob Agents Chemother 1991; 35:967-71.

47. Gehanno P, Lenoir G, Barry B et al. Evaluation of nasopharyngeal cultures for bacteriologic assessment of acute otitis media in children. Pediatr Infect Dis J 1996; 15:329-32.
48. Gu X-X, Chen J, Barenkamp SJ et al. Synthesis and characterization of lipooligosaccharide-based conjugates as vaccine candidates for Moraxella (Branhamella) catarrhalis. Infect Immun 1998; 66:1891-7.
49. Harabuchi Y, Faden H, Yamanaka N et al. Nasopharyngeal colonization with nontypeable Haemophilus influenzae and recurrent otitis media. J Infect Dis 1994; 170:862-6.
50. Harabuchi Y, Murakata H, Goh M et al. Serum antibodies specific to CD outer membrane protein of Moraxella catarrhalis, P6 outer membrane protein of nontypeable Haemophilus influenzae and capsular polysaccharides of Streptococcus pneumoniae in children with otitis media with effusion. Acta Otolaryngol.(Stockh) 1998; 118:826-32.
51. Harkness RE, Guimond MJ, McBey B-A et al. Branhamella catarrhalis pathogenesis in SCID and SCID/beige mice. APMIS 1993; 101:805-10.
52. Helminen ME, Maciver I, Latimer JL et al. A major outer membrane protein of Moraxella catarrhalis is a target for antibodies that enhance pulmonary clearance of the pathogen in an animal model. Infect Immun 1993; 61:2003-10.
53. Helminen ME, Maciver I, Latimer JL et al. A large, antigenically conserved protein on the surface of Moraxella catarrhalis is a target for protective antibodies. J Infect Dis 1994; 170:867-72.
54. Helminen ME, Maciver I, Paris M et al. A mutation affecting expression of a major outer membrane protein of Moraxella catarrhalis alters serum resistance and survival in vivo. J Infect Dis 1993; 168:1194-201.
55. Hendolin PH, Markkanen A, Ylikoski J et al. Use of multiplex PCR for simultaneous detection of four bacterial species in middle ear effusions. J Clin Microbiol 1997; 35:2854-8.
56. Hendolin PH, Paulin L, Ylikoski J. Clinically applicable multiplex PCR for four middle ear pathogens. J Clin Microbiol 2000; 38:125-32.
57. Hoiczyk E, Roggenkamp A, Reichenbecher M et al. Structure and sequence analysis of Yersinia YadA and Moraxella UspAs reveal a novel class of adhesins. EMBO 2000; 22:5989-99.
58. Holme T, Rahman M, Jansson P-E et al. The lipopolysaccharide of Moraxella catarrhalis. Structural relationships and antigenic properties. Eur J Biochem 1999; 265:524-9.
59. Hsiao CB, Sethi S, Murphy TF. Outer membrane protein CD of Branhamella catarrhalis: sequence conservation in strains recovered from the human respiratory tract. Microb Pathogen 1995; 19:215-25.
60. Hu WG, Chen J, Battey JF et al. Enhancement of clearance of bacteria from murine lungs by immunization with detoxified lipooligosaccharide from Moraxella catarrhalis conjugated to proteins. Infect Immun 2000; 68(9):4980-5.
61. Hu W-G, Chen J, Collins FM et al. An aerosol challenge mouse model for Moraxella catarrhalis. Vaccine 2000; 18:799-804.
62. Hu W-G, Chen J, McMichael JC et al. Functional characteristics of a protective monoclonal antibody against serotype A and C lipooligosaccharides from Moraxella catarrhalis. Infect Immun 2001; 69(3):1358-63.
63. Johnson CE, Carlin SA, Super DM et al. Cefixime compared with amoxicillin for treatment of acute otitis media. J Pediatr 1991; 119:117-22.
64. Karalus R, Campagnari A. Moraxella catarrhalis: a review of an important human mucosal pathogen. Microbes Infect 2000; 2(5):547-59.
65. Kilpi T, Herva E, Kaijalainen T et al. Bacteriology of acute otitis media in a cohort of Finnish children followed for the first two years of life. Pediatr Infect Dis J 2001; 20(7):654-62.
66. Klingman KL, Murphy TF. Purification and characterization of a high-molecular-weight outer membrane protein of Moraxella (Branhamella) catarrhalis. Infect Immun 1994; 62:1150-5.
67. Klingman KL, Pye A, Murphy TF et al. Dynamics of respiratory tract colonization by Moraxella (Branhamella) catarrhalis in bronchiectasis. Am J Respir Crit Care Med 1995; 152:1072-8.
68. Kyd J, John A, Cripps A et al. Investigation of mucosal immunisation in pulmonary clearance of Moraxella (Branhamella) catarrhalis. Vaccine 2000; 18:398-406.
69. Kyd JM, Cripps AW, Murphy TF. Outer membrane antigen expression by Branhamella catarrhalis influences pulmonary clearance. J Med Microbiol 1998; 47:159-68.
70. LaFontaine ER, Wagner NJ, Hansen EJ. Expression of the Moraxella catarrhalis UspA1 protein undergoes phase variation and is regulated at the transcriptional level. J Bacteriol 2001; 183(5):1540-51.
71. Leach AJ, Boswell JB, Asche V et al. Bacterial colonization of the nasopharynx predicts very early onset and persistence of otitis media in Australian Aboriginal infants. Pediatr Infect Dis J 1994; 13:983-9.

72. Luke CJ, Marshall MA, Zahradnik JM et al. Growth-inhibiting antibody responses of humans vaccinated with recombinant outer surface protein A or infected with Borrelia burgdorferi or both. J Infect Dis 2000; 181:1062-8.
73. Luke NR, Campagnari AA. Construction and characterization of Moraxella catarrhalis mutants defective in expression of transferrin receptors. Infect Immun 1999; 67:5815-9.
74. Luke NR, Russo TA, Luther N et al. The use of an isogenic mutant, constructed in Moraxella catarrhalis, to identify a protective epitope of OMP B1 defined by monoclonal antibody 11C6. Infect Immun 1999; 67(2):681-7.
75. Maciver I, Unhanand M, McCracken GH Jr et al. Effect of immunization on pulmonary clearance of Moraxella catarrhalis in an animal model. J Infect Dis 1993; 168:469-72.
76. Mathers KE, Goldblatt D, Aebi C et al. Characterisation of an outer membrane protein of Moraxella catarrhalis. FEMS Immunol Med Microbiol 1997; 19:231-6.
77. McKenzie H, Morgan MG, Jordens JZ et al. Characterisation of hospital isolates of Moraxella (Branhamella) catarrhalis by SDS-PAGE of whole-cell proteins, immunoblotting and restriction-endonuclease analysis. J Med Microbiol 1992; 37:70-6.
78. McMichael JC, Fiske MJ, Fredenburg RA et al. Isolation and characterization of two proteins from Moraxella catarrhalis that bear a common epitope. Infect Immun 1998; 66:4374-81.
79. Monso E, Ruiz J, Rosell A et al. Bacterial infection in chronic obstructive pulmonary disease. A study of stable and exacerbated outpatients using the protected specimen brush. Am J Respir Crit Care Med 1995; 152:1316-20.
80. Morgan MG, McKenzie H, Enright MC et al. Use of molecular methods to characterize Moraxella catarrhalis strains in a suspected outbreak of nosocomial infection. Eur J Clin Microbiol Infect Dis 1992; 11:305-12.
81. Murphy TF. Branhamella catarrhalis: epidemiology, surface antigenic structure, and immune response. Microbiol Rev 1996; 60:267-79.
82. Murphy TF. Branhamella catarrhalis: epidemiological and clinical aspects of a human respiratory tract pathogen. Thorax 1998; 53:124-8.
83. Murphy TF, Brauer AL, Yuskiw N et al. Antigenic structure of outer membrane protein E of Moraxella catarrhalis and construction and characterization of mutants. Infect Immun 2000; 68(11):6250-6.
84. Murphy TF, Brauer AL, Yuskiw N et al. Conservation of outer membrane protein E among strains of Moraxella catarrhalis. Infect Immun 2001; 69(6):3576-80.
85. Murphy TF, Kirkham C, Denardin E et al. Analysis of antigenic structure and human immune response to outer membrane protein CD of Moraxella catarrhalis. Infect Immun 1999; 67:4578-85.
86. Murphy TF, Kirkham C, Lesse AJ. The major heat-modifiable outer membrane protein CD is highly conserved among strains of Branhamella catarrhalis. Mol Microbiol 1993; 10:87-98.
87. Murphy TF, Kyd JM, John A et al. Enhancement of pulmonary clearance of Moraxella (Branhamella) catarrhalis following immunization with outer membrane protein CD in a mouse model. J Infect Dis 1998; 178:1667-75.
88. Myers LE, Yang Y-P, Du R-P et al. The transferrin binding protein B of Moraxella catarrhalis elicits bactericidal antibodies and is a potential vaccine antigen. Infect Immun 1998; 66:4183-92.
89. Nicotra B, Rivera M, Luman JI et al. Branhamella catarrhalis as a lower respiratory tract pathogen in patients with chronic lung disease. Arch Intern Med 1986; 146:890-3.
90. Ninane G, Joly J, Kraytman M. Bronchopulmonary infection due to Branhamella catarrhalis: 11 cases assessed by transtracheal puncture. Br Med J 1978; 1:276-8.
91. Owen MJ, Anwar R, Nguyen HK et al. Efficacy of cefixime in the treatment of acute otitis media in children. AJDC 1993; 147:81-6.
92. Patterson JE, Patterson TF, Farrel P et al. Evaluation of restriction endonuclease analysis as an epidemiologic typing system for Branhamella catarrhalis. J Clin Microbiol 1989; 27:944-6.
93. Patterson TF, Patterson JE, Masecar BL et al. A nosocomial outbreak of Branhamella catarrhalis confirmed by restriction endonuclease analysis. J Infect Dis 1988; 157:996-1001.
94. Pela R, Marchesani F, Agostinelli C et al. Airways microbial flora in COPD patients in stable clinical conditions and during exacerbations: a bronchoscopic investigation. Monaldi Arch Chest Dis 1998; 53:3-262.
95. Post JC, Preston RA, Aul JJ et al. Molecular analysis of bacterial pathogens in otitis media with effusion. JAMA 1995; 273:1598-604.
96. Rahman M, Holme T. Antibody response in rabbits to serotype-specific determinants in lipopolysaccharides from Moraxella catarrhalis. J Med Microbiol 1996; 44:348-54.
97. Rahman M, Jonsson A-B, Holme T. Monoclonal antibodies to the epitope α-Gal-(1-4)-β-gal-(1- of Moraxella catarrhalis LPS react with a similar epitope in type IV pili of Neisseria meningitidis. Microb Pathogen 1998; 24:299-308.

98. Reddy MS, Murphy TF, Faden HS et al. Middle ear mucin glycoprotein: purification and interaction with nontypable Haemophilus influenzae and Moraxella catarrhalis. Otolaryngol Head Neck Surg 1997; 116:175-89.
99. Retzer MD, Yu R-H, Schryvers AB. Identification of sequences in human transferrin that bind to the bacterial receptor protein, transferrin-binding protein B. Mol Microbiol 1999; 32:111-21.
100. Richards SJ, Greening AP, Enright MC et al. Outbreak of Moraxella catarrhalis in a respiratory unit. Thorax 1993; 48:91-2.
101. Ryan AF. Immune-mediated otitis media in an animal model. Ann Otol Rhinol Laryngol 1988; 97:24-7.
102. Sarwar J, Campagnari AA, Kirkham C et al. Characterization of an antigenically conserved heat-modifiable major outer membrane protein of Branhamella catarrhalis. Infect Immun 1992; 60:804-9.
103. Sethi S, Hill SL, Murphy TF. Serum antibodies to outer membrane proteins of Moraxella (Branhamella) catarrhalis in patients with bronchiectasis: identification of OMP B1 as an important antigen. Infect Immun 1995; 63:1516-20.
104. Sethi S, Murphy TF. Bacterial infection in chronic obstructive pulmonary disease in 2000. A state of the art review. Clin Microbiol Rev 2001; 14(2):336-63.
105. Sethi S, Surface JM, Murphy TF. Antigenic heterogeneity and molecular analysis of CopB of Branhamella (Moraxella) catarrhalis. Infect Immun 1997; 65:3666-71.
106. Soler N, Torres A, Ewig S et al. Bronchial microbial patterns in severe exacerbations of chronic obstructive pulmonary disease (COPD) requiring mechanical ventilation. Am J Respir Crit Care Med 1998; 157:1498-505.
107. Stenfors L-E, Raisanen S. Quantitative analysis of the bacterial findings in otitis media. J.Laryngol.Otol. 1990; 104:749-57.
108. Stenfors L-E, Raisanen S. Secretory IgA-,IgG- and C3b-coated bacteria in the nasopharynx of otitis-prone and nonotitis-prone children. Acta Otolaryngol 1993; 113:191-5.
109. Takada R, Harabuchi Y, Himi T et al. Antibodies specific to outer membrane antigens of Moraxella catarrhalis in sera and middle ear effusions from children with otitis media with effusion. Intl.J.Ped.Otorhinolaryngol. 1998; 46:185-95.
110. Thanassi WT, Schoen RT. The Lyme disease vaccine: conception, development, and implementation. Ann Intern Med 2000; 132:661-8.
111. Unhanand M, Maciver I, Ramilo O et al. Pulmonary clearance of Moraxella catarrhalis in an animal model. J Infect Dis 1992; 165:644-50.
112. Van Hare GF, Shurin PA, Marchant CD et al. Acute otitis media caused by Branhamella catarrhalis: biology and therapy. Rev Infect Dis 1987; 9:16-27.
113. Vaneechoutte M, Verschraegen G, Claeys G et al. Serological typing of Branhamella catarrhalis strains on the basis of lipopolysaccharide antigens. J Clin Microbiol 1990; 28:182-7.
114. Vaneechoutte M, Verschraegen G, Claeys G et al. Respiratory tract carrier rates of Moraxella (Branhamella) catarrhalis in adults and children and interpretation of the isolation of M. catarrhalis from sputum. J Clin Microbiol 1990; 28:2674-80.
115. Verghese A, Berk SL. Moraxella (Branhamella) catarrhalis. Infect Dis Clin No Amer 1991; 5:523-38.
116. Wald ER, Reilly JS, Casselbrant M et al. Treatment of acute maxillary sinusitis in childhood: a comparative study of amoxicillin and cefaclor. J Pediatr 1984; 104:297-302.
117. West M, Berk SL, Smith JK. Branhamella catarrhalis pneumonia. South Med J 1982; 75:1021-3.
118. Yang Y-P, Myers LE, McGuinness U et al. The major outer membrane protein, CD, extracted from Moraxella (Branhamella) catarrhalis is a potential vaccine antigen that induces bactericidal antibodies. FEMS Immunol Med Microbiol 1997; 17:187-99.
119. Yu R, Schryvers AB. The interaction between human transferrin and transferrin binding protein 2 from Moraxella (Branhamella) catarrhalis differs from that of other human pathogens. Microb Pathogen 1993; 15:433-45.
120. Yu R-H, Bonnah RA, Ainsworth S, Schryvers AB. Analysis of the immunological responses to transferrin and lactoferrin receptor proteins from Moraxella catarrhalis. Infect Immun 1999; 67:3793-9.
121. Zaleski A, Scheffler NK, Densen P et al. Lipooligosacchrdie P^k (Gal α1-4Galβ1-4GlC) epitope of Moraxella catarrhalis is a factor in resistance to bactericidal activity mediated by normal human serum. Infect Immun 2000; 68(9):5261-8.

CHAPTER 15

Neisseria meningitidis Vaccines

Carl E. Frasch and Margaret C. Bash

Summary

Meningococcal disease, both endemic and epidemic, remains a major cause of meningitis in many countries. Protective immunity is mediated primarily by bactericidal antibodies against the capsular polysaccharides as well as against outer membrane protein and lipopolysaccharide components. This article focuses on the new conjugate vaccines for serogroups A, C, Y and W135 as well as the latest approaches to development of group B vaccines. Group C meningococcal polysaccharide-protein conjugate vaccines have been used in the United Kingdom since November 1999 and are over 90% effective in both infants and children. Outer membrane protein vaccines have shown good efficacy against group B in individuals over 4 years of age, but most group B disease occurs in younger children. Newer group B vaccines are under development using new immunization regimens, individual outer membrane proteins and lipopolysaccharide conjugates. The problem of a universally effective group B vaccine may require new avenues of research.

Introduction

The focus of this chapter will be meningococcal conjugate vaccines for protection against serogroups A and C and protein vaccines for protection against serogroup B presented from a vaccine development perspective. A review of the history of meningococcal vaccine development was published in 1995.[1]

Neisseria meningitidis (the meningococcus) is a major cause of bacterial meningitis and remains a major public health problem in many countries. The WHO estimates that the world wide annual burden of meningococcal disease is approximately 300,000 to 350,000 cases. The incidence is much higher in many developing countries (about 25/100,000) compared to the US or Western Europe (1-4/100,000). In the United Kingdom (UK) meningococcal disease was the leading cause of death from invasive bacterial infections in teenagers and young adults prior to initiation of their meningococcal conjugate group C vaccination program. In the United States there are an estimated 3,000 cases per year, 95-97% of which are sporadic cases, mostly in young children. Unlike other causes of bacterial meningitis, the meningococcus remains a threat at all ages. The case-fatality rate in developed countries is approximately 10%, but up to 20% of survivors will have significant neurologic sequelae or limb loss from vascular complications.

Worldwide, essentially all meningococcal disease is caused by serogroups A, B, C, Y, and W135. The relative importance of each serogroup varies with geographic region; group A is currently a problem mostly in Africa, group C and Y accounts for two-thirds of the disease in the US, and group B causes up to 90% of meningococcal disease in some countries.

A combined polysaccharide (PS) vaccine has been available for over 20 years for protection of older children and adults against groups A, C, Y and W135. Development and use of this vaccine have been reviewed.[1-3]

New Bacterial Vaccines, edited by Ronald W. Ellis and Bernard R. Brodeur.

Immunobiology of Meningococcal Infection

Humans are the only natural host of *Neisseria meningitidis*, which normally colonizes the throat and nasopharynx. This colonization may lead to a carrier state; about 5 to 10% of adults at any given time are healthy carriers. This colonization may also lead to invasive disease. What determines carriage or disease? Many meningococci recovered from healthy carriers have very low pathogenic potential; only some strains are of high virulence, and expression of a capsular polysaccharide is required. Studies by Gotschlich et al[4] clearly show that only individuals lacking bactericidal antibodies against the encountered meningococcal strain go on to develop disease.

Prior to the development of antibiotics and effective vaccines, marked reductions in lethality were achieved using therapeutic sera. The success of this therapy demonstrated very early the central role of humoral antibody in protection against meningococcal bacteremia and meningitis.[1] The critical role of bactericidal antibodies has been further demonstrated in a number of ways. (a) The highest incidence of meningococcal disease occurs in individuals 6-12 months of age. This age group has the lowest bactericidal antibody levels. (b) Studies in US Army recruits in the mid- 1960's showed a direct correlation between susceptibility to meningitis and absence of serum bactericidal antibodies.[4] (c) Individuals deficient in complement components C5, C6, C7, or C8 have a significantly increased susceptibility to invasive meningococcal infection, even though they may have high levels of anti-meningococcal antibodies. (d) A correlation has been shown between the efficacy of meningococcal vaccines and induction and persistence of bactericidal antibodies. Thus, measurement of bactericidal antibody can serve as a surrogate for protective immunity. In the development of meningococcal vaccines, both PS-conjugate and outer membrane protein (OMP), it is of primary importance to demonstrate induction of bactericidal antibodies, though antibody responses will also be quantified by ELISA.

Immunological memory may also play an important role in protection against meningococcal disease. Induction of immunological priming for an anamnestic response has been well demonstrated using *Haemophilus influenzae* type b (Hib) and meningococcal conjugate vaccines.[5,6] The role of memory in providing long-term protection against meningococcal disease has not been shown but should not be very different from Hib, another cause of meningitis. Infants in the UK receive a Hib conjugate vaccine at 2, 3, and 4 months of age, but receive no booster immunization, and clear evidence of protection is evident to at least 6 years of age.[7]

Opsonophagocytosis has not been well studied, but is likely important in overall protection against meningococcal disease. Vaccination with the serogroup A and C PS induces opsonic antibody.[7a] Turbid CSF specimens from meningococcal patients have many polymorphonuclear leukocytes with internalized meningococci. Meningococci in phagolysosomes are rapidly killed. However, meningococci are protected from phagocytosis by their capsules in the absence of anticapsular or anti-outer membrane antibodies. Opsonic antibodies may be more important in protection against group B, whose capsular polysaccharide is virtually nonimmunogenic.

Meningococci colonize and invade the tonsillar tissue of the throat.[8] An intracellular niche for the meningococcus is consistent with the observation that only antibiotics (e.g., rifampicin) effective against intracellular pathogens will clear meningococcal carriage. An intracellular niche suggests that cellular immunity may also play a role in protection against meningococcal disease.

An additional virulence mechanism may be associated with the organism's ability to switch capsules. Meningococci of serogroups B, C, Y and W135 all express capsules containing sialic acid, and capsule switching between group B and group C strains have been confirmed.[9,10] Capsule switching can occur in vivo by horizontal transfer of the *Sia*D genes encoding polysialyltransferases. Presumably, the opportunity for capsule-switching arises from co-colonization of serogroup B and C strains in the human nasopharynx. A potential outcome of capsule switching is immune escape, but the military in many countries has routinely used the polysaccharide vaccine against group C, without observing increased group B disease.

Table 1. Published conjugation methods that have been used to produce meningococcal conjugate vaccines

Method	Saccharide Size	Carrier Protein	Spacer	Procedure	Used in Humans	Refs.
Reductive amination	Reduced	Tetanus toxoid	None	Aldehyde form of PS combined with protein in presence of cyanoborohydride	No	24, 25
Carbodiimide	Native	Tetanus toxoid	None	PS and protein combined in presence of carbodiimide, then blocked with ethanolamine	No	21, 26
Active ester [a]	Oligosaccharide	CRM_{197}	Adipic acid	Aminated reducing terminus of the oligosaccharide conjugated to protein by adipic acid $(NHS)_2$	Yes	27
Reductive amination	Reduced	CRM_{197}	None	Aldehyde form of saccharide combined with protein in presence of cyanoborohydride	Yes	6
Reductive amination	De-OAc PS [b]	Tetanus toxoid	None	Aldehyde form of PS combined with protein in presence of cyanoborohydride	Yes	24, 40

a. Used N-hydroxysuccinimide diester of adipic acid
b. De – Acetylylated PS only reported for Meningococcal group C

Meningococcal PS vaccines do not effectively stimulate the immune system in young children and are largely nonimmunogenic in infants. The exception is group A meningococcal PS which, for reasons not understood, is immunogenic in infants as young as 3 mo of age and is effective if used in young children in a two-dose immunization schedule.[11] However, infants do respond well to PS-conjugate vaccines. These are polysaccharide-protein hybrids formed by the covalent attachment of a protein through its amino groups to a chemically modified ("activated") PS. Attachment of the protein provides a number of T-cell epitopes that interact with CD4 helper T cells, greatly facilitating an antibody response to the attached polysaccharide. The T-helper-cell-dependent response to a conjugate vaccine results in both serum IgG antibodies and memory B cells, even in infants. Additionally, the immunogenicity of the PS conjugate, in contrast to the native PS, does not depend upon the size of the conjugated PS; conjugates prepared with either PS or oligosaccharides have similar immunogenicity (see Table 1).

Studies of conjugate vaccines in immunologically naïve individuals have shown that a conjugate can induce memory B cells without induction of circulating serum IgG. This was demonstrated in Finland using a subpotent Hib conjugate vaccine called PRP-D.[12] In the Finnish studies, some infants were nonresponders after three doses of PRP-D at 2, 4 and 6 mo of age. These nonresponder children received a 4th dose at 15 mo of age and responded with antibody levels far higher than could have been expected from primary immunization at 15 mo of age. The role of priming alone in protective immunity to meningococci remains unclear.

Strategies for New Vaccines

The existing quadrivalent PS vaccine is licensed for use in adults and children over 2 years of age. However, the immune response is age-dependent and adult-type antibody responses are not seen until *ca.* 10-12 years of age.[13,14] Monovalent group C conjugate vaccines, now licensed in several countries, should be used in children under 10 years of age when meningococcal immunization is considered necessary by public- health authorities. In the context of outbreak control, the PS vaccine is 85-90% effective in adults, and thus conjugate vaccination offers little added benefit for adults.

The vaccine strategy clearly needed for infants and children is a multivalent conjugate vaccine containing serogroups A, C, Y and W135, which is now under development. Some countries may wish to use an AC bivalent conjugate, while a group A monovalent conjugate may be best for epidemic control in Sub-Saharan Africa.

The vaccine strategy for protection against group B meningococcal disease is more complex and depends upon whether, from a public-health standpoint, the vaccine is for control of outbreaks or endemic disease. Outbreaks of group B meningococcal disease tend to be spread out over several years with levels ≥10 times endemic levels and is often due to a single antigenically stable clone. Endemic disease, by contrast, is due to a diverse population of group B strains. Development of an effective group B capsular PS vaccine would be the ideal solution, but the group B PS is not an effective immunogen because the PS is a homopolymer of sialic acid, a self-antigen identical to the polysialyl structures common on some mammalian tissues. A modified group B polysaccharide vaccine in which the N-acetyl groups have been replaced by N-propionyl groups is under development,[15] but such a vaccine will be difficult to prove safe. The major focus in group B meningococcal vaccine development therefore will be on use of noncapsular immunogens.

Meningococcal Conjugate Vaccines

Group C

Meningococcal PS vaccines elicit good bactericidal antibody responses in immunologically mature individuals and have been used effectively to control epidemics and localized outbreaks, as well as to protect military recruits and students. However, immunogenicity is age-related and, with the exception of group A, PSs fail to induce immunological memory.

Protection induced by the group C PS is age-dependent. An increased incidence of group C Meningococcal disease in the province of Quebec, Canada led to a mass immunization campaign beginning in December 1992 in 1.9 million people between the ages of 6 mo and 20 yr.[14] The group C PS provided no protection for children under 2 yr of age, and adult levels of protection were seen in vaccinated individuals by about 10-14 yr of age.

An additional problem with the group C PS vaccine is that reimmunization induces lower antibody concentrations compared to primary immunization. This hyporesponsiveness was evident in toddlers and adults when age-matched groups received either a second or primary group C PS immunization.[16,17] Hyporesponsiveness should not be a concern when the vaccine is being used for short- term protection as in military recruits or in localized outbreaks, and reimmunization with a conjugate vaccine overcomes the hyporesponsiveness.[18] The vaccine strategy for group C is to replace the PS vaccine with a conjugate when immunization of children or long-term protection is the goal.

Development of Conjugate Vaccines

The breakthrough demonstrating that conjugation of a complex bacterial PS to a protein carrier could induce a protective immune response in infants and young children was the publication by Schneerson et al in 1980 on a Hib conjugate vaccine.[19] The subsequent commercial development and licensure of several Hib conjugate vaccines has resulted in near eradication of Hib disease.[20]

Meningococcal PSs, like other bacterial PSs, cannot be chemically linked to a protein without first undergoing some chemical modification (activation). There are a number of approaches to activation of the PS (Table 1). Each mode of activation has the potential to alter important epitopes, even when relatively few sites are activated on the PS molecule. Periodate oxidation breaks carbon-carbon bonds in the PS, while the cyanylation and carbodiimide chemistries do not. Periodate activation of the group C meningococcal PS results in chain breakage generating smaller saccharide units with terminal aldehyde groups that will link the PS to the protein via reductive amination.

Initial studies on production and optimization of Meningococcal group C conjugates were reported by Beuvery [21 - 23] and Jennings,[24] well before commercialization of the Hib conjugates. Two differing conjugation methodologies were reported by these investigators for chemically linking the group C PS to a protein carrier.[22,24] The first approach used partially depolymerized PS which was activated by creation of terminal aldehyde groups through periodate oxidation. The reactive aldehydes then combined through reductive amination to free amino groups on the protein, mostly lysines, in the presence of sodium borohydride.[24] By this method activation occurred at one specific site on the group C PS. The second approach utilized the carbodiimide reaction to covalently link carboxylic groups in the high- molecular-weight PS to lysine amino groups on the carrier protein. By this method the activation sites were more random. While site-specific activation is attractive from a biochemical standpoint, the random activation may have less effect on the average upon individual PS epitopes.

Group C meningococcal conjugates prepared by reductive amination and by carbodiimide methods were evaluated in animals.[23,25] Importantly, the group C conjugate vaccine stimulated both T-cell-independent and T-cell-dependent responses upon initial immunization.[23] The PS must be covalently linked to the carrier protein to induce a T-cell-dependent antibody response. Beuvery showed that the amount of free PS in a conjugate should be minimized, but elimination was not necessary.[22,26]

The ability of the group C meningococcal conjugates to induce memory B cells in mice was demonstrated by the strong booster response resulting from reimmunization of primed animals with either the conjugate or PS.[26]

The first group A and group C meningococcal conjugates to be used in clinical trials were prepared by Chiron Vaccines and reported in 1992.[27] The conjugation method they developed was based upon selective terminal group activation of small oligosaccharides produced by mild acid hydrolysis and then coupling to a protein through a hydrocarbon spacer. They used the nontoxic mutant of diphtheria toxin, CRM 197, as the protein carrier. To activate the oligosaccharides for conjugation, an amino group was added to the end of the oligosaccharide, which was then reacted with the N-hydroxysuccinimide diester of adipic acid to create an active ester. This active ester then was covalently bound to lysine amino groups in the CRM 197 protein creating the conjugate.

The Chiron meningococcal group A and C conjugates were first evaluated in mice and rabbits and then in phase I clinical studies in adults.[27,28] A dose-response study was done in adults, comparing 5.5, 11, and 22 µg/mL of conjugated PS.[28] There was no statistical difference among the three vaccine dosages, and post-vaccination bactericidal titers in all the groups were higher than in a control group that received the PS vaccine. The conjugate was then evaluated in 18 to 24 month olds using a two-dose immunization series with either 5.5 or 11 µg/mL of PS per dose.[29,30] By either ELISA or bactericidal assay the antibody response to the two conjugate dosages were the same. By ELISA, after the second dose the group C conjugate induced antibody concentrations significantly higher than did the PS vaccine, but the group A conjugate only induced equivalent antibody levels compared to the PS vaccine. By bactericidal assay, the conjugate induced titers were 20-fold and 290-fold higher titers than that of the group A PS and C PS respectively. This vaccine was evaluated in Gambian infants using three different immunization schedules at a dosage level of 11 μg.[30] The immune response to the group C component was excellent, but the group A component was not more immunogenic than the A PS vaccine, and failed to prime for a booster response.

A critical observation from the toddler study was the poor correlation between antibody concentration and bactericidal titer.[29] This observation lead Granoff et al to develop a high-avidity meningococcal group C PS ELISA, which correlated much better with bactericidal titers.[31]

A second-generation Chiron meningococcal group C conjugate vaccine, in which small oligosaccharides were eliminated after size reduction and before conjugation, was evaluated in toddlers 12 to 23 months of age using two injections of 10 μg 2 mo apart.[17,32] This conjugate induced 20 μg/mL of antibody compared to 1.5 μg/mL for the PS control vaccine when antibody concentrations were measured using the high-avidity ELISA.[31] Similarly, bactericidal titers were significantly higher for the conjugate vaccine. The conjugate also induced immunologic memory, as shown by rechallenge using the PS vaccine 12 months after the second conjugate immunization.[31] The post-boost geometric mean antibody concentration was 69 μg/mL.

Use of Immunological Correlates

The meningococcus became the most common cause of invasive bacterial disease in young children in the United Kingdom following the near elimination of Hib disease by Hib vaccination.[33] The limited but encouraging clinical experience with the meningococcal conjugate vaccines described above led the UK in 1994 to invite clinical manufacturers to produce and clinically evaluate group C conjugate vaccines in UK children and infants for the control of meningococcal disease.

The UK Medicines Control Agency reasoned that since the relatively low burden of serogroup C disease made phase III clinical efficacy studies unfeasible, meningococcal conjugate vaccines would be licensed based upon their demonstrated immunogenicity rather than clinical efficacy.[34] The three vaccines that came to be licensed are shown in (Table 2). The rational behind their licensure was a) studies by Gotschlich et al[4] that demonstrated that serum bactericidal activity could be taken as an indicator of clinical protection against group C meningococcal disease; b) evidence for efficacy of the plain PS in children over 2 yr of age; c) evidence from clinical trials showing that group C conjugate vaccines were highly immunogenic, inducing bactericidal antibodies and immunological memory in all age groups; and d) the experience with Hib conjugate vaccines establishing the safety and advantages of conjugate vaccine technology.

For demonstration of immunogenicity in the UK the key serological correlate used was the serum bactericidal assay (SBA). The SBA has been done with either fresh human (hSBA) or baby rabbit (rSBA) sera as a source of complement.[35,36] Work in the 1960's by Gotschlich et al [4] indicated that presence of detectable bactericidal activity (titer ≥1:4) by hSBA predicted protection. Use of rabbit complement generally results in higher group C SBA titers than when human complement is used, and a rSBA titer of 1:128 strongly predicted hSBA titers of ≥1:8.[35] Recent comparisons of vaccine effectiveness in the UK and percent of children with different rSBA titers showed that a rSBA titer of ≥1:8 correlated best with percent disease reduction in vaccinated children.[33]

A series of studies were conducted in UK children to help define vaccine dosage, safety and immunization schedule.[6,37-40] From these studies the UK Medicines Control Agency decided upon a 10-μg dose, a three-dose series in infants and one dose in children 12 mo and older.[6,38] As with the Hib conjugate they chose not to give a booster dose.[33]

We will use the Wyeth-Lederle product to illustrate the clinical development process that was needed for UK licensure. After preliminary studies in adults the Wyeth-Lederle meningococcal group C conjugate vaccine (Meningitec) was evaluated in toddlers and infants.[6,37,38] The initial study in infants evaluated 2 μg and 10 μg dosages given at 2, 3 and 4 mo of age.

Table 2. Group C meningococcal conjugate vaccines presently licensed in the United Kingdom and other countries

Manufacturer	Trade Name	Date UK Approved	Type of PS	PS Dose	Carrier Protein	Dose of Protein
Wyeth-Lederle	Meningitec	Oct '99	Size reduced	10 µg	CRM_{197}	25 µg
Chiron	Menjugate	Mar '00	Oligosaccharide	10 µg	CRM_{197}	13 – 20 µg
Baxter Healthcare	NeisVac-C	July '00	Size reduced De- O Ac [a]	10 µg	Tetanus toxoid	10 – 20 µg

a. The isolated group C polysaccharide was De-O Acetylated.
This vaccine was produced by North American Vaccine, now Baxter Healthcare.

After 2 immunizations all infants had > 2 µg/mL of antibody, the third dose having little additional effect.[6] By 12 -14 months of age marked declines in antibody levels were seen, but levels remained above those of unimmunized toddlers. Interestingly, there was no significant difference after the primary immunization series between the two dosages, but the 2 µg-dose recipients had higher booster responses by both ELISA and rSBA. The 10-µg dose was chosen for further evaluation. A manufacturing lot consistency study was conducted comparing immunogenicity of two different full-scale lots to a smaller-scale pilot lot used in earlier clinical studies.[37] The antibody responses were assessed by ELISA and SBA, and no differences between lots were found. After three doses at 2, 3 and 4 mo of age all infants had ≥2 µg IgG/mL, and 95-98% had rSBA titers ≥1:32.

Richmond et al conducted a study in 12 – 18 month olds to see whether a single 10-µg dose would be sufficient for protection of children 12 mo and older and whether it primed the infants.[38] They found 83% of the toddlers had rSBA titers ≥1:32 one month post immunization. Ten µg of group C PS were administered 6 mo after the conjugate. Before the booster 66% of the Wyeth-Lederle-vaccinated toddlers still had rSBA titers of ≥1:32 and 100% did afterwards. In this study, a single 10-µg dose was sufficient for use in children 12 mo and older and induced immunological memory.

The Baxter meningococcal group C conjugate vaccine (Neisvac C) was unique in that it contained a de-O acetylated group C PS (see Table 2).[40] A recent study in the UK revealed that about 12 % of group C disease isolates were naturally O acetyl negative, with no difference in the case fatality rates in patients with O acetyl positive or negative strains.[41] A study of Neisvac C in infants demonstrated the vaccine to be highly immunogenic, inducing rSBA titers of ≥ 1:128 after doses 1, 2, and 3 in 89%, 96% and 100% of infants respectively.[40] In a toddler study comparing Neisvac C to two other UK-licensed group C conjugates, Neisvac C was statistically more immunogenic.[38]

The clear effectiveness of the meningococcal group C conjugate vaccines in the UK was a strong endorsement of the approach taken to utilize immunological criteria for licensure. The UK mass immunization of 15 – 17 year olds and infants, the age groups at greatest risk, began in November 1999. Other age groups were phased in as vaccine became available. As shown in (Table 2), the vaccines were phased in with the Wyeth-Lederle vaccine being the only vaccine used during the first 5 months. During the first year over 17 million children were immunized. In vaccinated individuals after 16 mo of follow up the effectiveness in toddlers was 88% (CI 67 – 95%) and in 15 –17 yr olds was 96 % (CI 85 –99%).[33] Overall, an 89% reduction in all group C meningococcal disease was seen, with no evidence of capsule switching.

Group A

Group A meningococcal disease is a major problem primarily in the Sub-Saharan region of Africa. In 1996 almost 190,000 cases occurred in this region of Africa, paralyzing medical care systems and exhausting international supplies of the A+C PS vaccine. Control of meningococcal disease in Africa poses significant problems, and prevention of endemic group A meningococcal disease will be more effective than outbreak control because the latter can prevent at most about 50% of the cases that would have occurred.[42] A meningitis threshold-rate approach has been used to trigger mass vaccination campaigns, but rapid implementation is hampered by difficulties of quickly obtaining and distributing the vaccine. A threshold of 10 cases/100,000 in one week in a region has been found sensitive in confirming an epidemic.[42] Such group A meningococcal epidemics last about 6-18 weeks, and thus a rapid response is critical.

There are two strategies for group A disease prevention as apposed to epidemic control. a) Apply the existing group A PS vaccine in young children. Robbins et al[43] have recommended two doses 2 mo apart starting at 3 mo of age, then additional doses at 2 yrs and upon entry into school. This immunization scheme is likely to be effective for the reasons elaborated by Robbins et al[44] but suffers from the problem of not fitting into the existing EPI infant immunization series and is not readily amendable to national immunization days, because of the need for multiple spaced immunizations. However, New Zealand did effectively control a group A outbreak even in young infants using a two dose PS immunization series.[11] b) Produce a group A conjugate vaccine that can be given as part of the EPI infant immunization program. Such a vaccine could then be readily used for booster immunization during national immunization days. A major problem is that a conjugate vaccine will be much more expensive than existing PS vaccine, and there has been little incentive for the major biologics manufacturers to produce such a vaccine, although some have been produced and clinically evaluated.[27,45]

The Global Alliance for Vaccines and Immunization (GAVI) announced a major grant from the Bill and Melinda Gates Foundation to manufacture a group A conjugate vaccine and conduct field trials (*GAVI Immunization Focus*, June 2001). Details of how such a vaccine will be produced and quality controlled have not been established. It is clear that the long-term problem for control of group A meningococcal disease in Africa will not be technical, but financial.

Vaccines for Group B

Most work on development of group B meningococcal vaccines has focused upon use of noncapsular surface components, and earlier work has been recently reviewed.[1-3] LPS depleted OMV vaccines have been evaluated in several million children and adults.

OMP Vaccine Efficacy Trials

Three efficacy studies of meningococcal outer membrane protein vaccines were conducted between 1987 and 1991: an outer membrane vesicle (OMV) vaccine produced by the Finlay Institute (VA-MENGO BC) was tested in Cuba, an OMV vaccine developed by the Norwegian National Institute of Public Health (NIPH) was tested in teenagers in Norway, and an outer membrane protein (OMP) vaccine developed by Walter Reed Army Institute of Research (WRAIR, Washington D.C.) was tested in Iquique, Chile.[46-48] Using a 2-dose regimen, these vaccines had between 57% and 83% protective efficacy in older children or teenagers. Little or no protective effect was seen in children under 4 years of age, which correlates with the lack of bactericidal antibody induction in young children.[49-51] In addition, an interim estimate of efficacy in the Norwegian vaccine trial showed 87% efficacy after 2 doses at 10 months, but efficacy dropped to 57% after 29 months, suggesting the need for a booster dose.[52]

Many subsequent studies have been conducted to examine the immunologic basis for protection following OMV vaccination, and the potential for improved responses in both children and adults. These studies show that OMV vaccination induced priming, and that boosting occurred following a third dose administered as late as 4 or 5 years after the primary series.[53-55]

The advantage of a third dose was confirmed in a randomized immunogenicity study in Iceland in which a booster dose at 10 months resulted in significantly increased bactericidal responses.[52] In addition to improved immunogenicity in adults, studies suggest that OMV vaccines may be effective in infants when administered as a three-dose series. Tappero et al showed that >90% of infants less than 1 year of age developed a ≥4-fold increase in SBA titer against the respective vaccine strain following a third dose. Although no SBA against the heterologous Chilean epidemic strain was seen in this age group, this study suggests that strain-specific protection in young infants may be achieved.[56]

Several studies of immune responses following immunization with OMP meningococcal vaccines have identified the class 1 (PorA) and the class 5 (Opc) proteins as important targets for bactericidal antibodies.[55,57] In Chilean infants, the SBA was almost exclusively PorA-dependent.[56] Although PorA appears to be the predominant immunogen, a more diverse response to OMPs is seen in adults following a booster immunization, including good anti-PorB responses.[52,55,57]

Persistence of epidemic group B meningococcal disease in New Zealand caused by a B 4:P1.7b,4 strain will provide an opportunity to directly examine the effects of increased dosing on efficacy in young children and infants using a targeted OMV vaccine. If efficacy is shown in young children, it will prove the utility of OMV vaccines in the context of epidemic disease caused predominantly by a single strain type.

New OMV Vaccines

Several mechanisms, in addition to increased dosing schedules, are being investigated to improve the magnitude or the breadth of the response to OMV vaccines. These include changes in route of administration, changes in growth conditions to modify expression of surface antigens and genetic engineering to modify the protein and lipooligosaccharide (LOS) constituents of the OMV.

Intranasal (i.n.) administration of meningococcal OMV may offer the advantages of stimulating local mucosal immune responses and eliminating the need to remove LOS from the preparation. I.n. administration of 10 times the intramuscular (i.m.) dose of the NIPH OMV vaccine without aluminum hydroxide adjuvant resulted in both mucosal IgA responses and systemic bactericidal responses.[58] Native outer membrane vesicles (NOMV) containing a similar concentration of LOS to intact outer membranes were safely administered to volunteers by i.n. metered dose spray.[59] In this study, SBA titers to homologous and some heterologous strains were observed. Absorption studies indicated that the SBA was related to both OMP and LOS antigens. Although encouraging, the need for relatively high doses and the low proportion of responders are problems that will need to be overcome.

Iron-regulated proteins, particularly transferring binding proteins (Tpb) A and B, are of interest as vaccine candidates. These proteins are surface-exposed and stimulate antibody formation during natural infection.[60,61] Following three doses of the Norwegian OMV vaccine, which was not produced to contain elevated levels of iron regulated protein, antibodies to the Tbp proteins were detected, but no significant contribution to the bactericidal activity of serum could be found.[62] Studies of recombinant TpbB has shown the development of bactericidal antibodies in mice, and immunization with TbpA conferred protection in a mouse sepsis model.[63,64] Thus, iron binding proteins may be important components of group B vaccines, and OMV produced under iron limiting conditions to enhance the expression of these proteins are under investigation as vaccines.[65]

The recognition that PorA is responsible for a large portion of the bactericidal antibody response following natural infection or vaccination with OMP, has led to many investigations regarding ways to utilize PorA as a vaccine. Recombinant PorA has been expressed in *E. coli*, and several mechanisms for using peptides corresponding to the protective epitopes of PorA as immunogens have been investigated.[66-68] Maintenance of the native conformation of PorA is important for stimulating functional antibodies, and OMV from genetically-engineered meningococcal strains have proven much more immunogenic than recombinant PorA vaccines.[69] A hexavalent PorA vaccine composed of OMV from two strains that are capsule- and PorB-deficient and express three different PorA proteins has been tested in adults, toddlers and infants.[70-72] This vaccine induces bactericidal antibody to all PorA serosubtypes contained in the vaccine, especially following three doses and a booster in infants. However, there has been a consistent observation of immundominance of some PorA proteins resulting in decreased antibodies to other PorA serosubtypes.[73] Another problem; bactericidal responses are restricted to strains containing PorA that are highly homologous to the types included in the vaccine. In some cases, minor sequence variations in the regions encoding the epitopes results in complete loss of bactericidal activity.[74]

LOS As a Vaccine

About 80% of invasive group B and C strains have the L3,7,9 LOS immunotype, compared to 25% of healthy carrier isolates.[75] Antibodies to the LOS are bactericidal, making LOS a logical vaccine candidate.[76] Several modifications of LOS have been investigated in the context of OMV vaccines. In a study of OMV-conjugated meningococcal B PS vaccines, a large portion of the bactericidal activity was attributed to anti-LOS antibodies that were inhibited by L3,7,9 LOS.[76] OMV with added detoxified LOS has been prepared and studied in animals.[77] Another promising approach to the development of LOS vaccines is to conjugate the LOS or Lipid A depleted LOS to protein carriers, but no meningococcal LOS conjugates have yet been clinically evaluated.[3]

Studies of Other Individual Components

NspA is a low molecular weight, surface exposed protein that has been shown to elicit antibodies that are cross-reactive with a variety of meningococcal strains.[3,82] Although highly conserved, this protein may vary in its accessibility to antibody binding.[80] PorB, a porin protein similar to PorA, is less immunogenic, but has been shown to contribute to the bactericidal responses in as many as 25% of individuals who respond to OMV vaccines, and may be important in opsonophagocytosis.[78-80] This protein, unlike PorA, has no identified mechanism for decreased expression. OpC, an adhesion protein, has clearly been identified as the target of bactericidal antibodies, but is not always expressed.

Group B PS As a Vaccine

The PS of group B *N. meningitidis* has been investigated as a vaccine candidate, and an extensive discussion of this work can be found.[3] In the native form, the group B PS is poorly immunogenic because of its being a self-antigen chemically identical to a carbohydrate on human cells, and conjugation of the PS to protein does not overcome this. Jennings et al modified the group B PS by N-propionylation, and this modified PS conjugated to protein continues to be studied as a vaccine candidate.[82] Concern remains regarding the ability to adequately evaluate the safety of such vaccines. However, since some epitopes of the group B PS are not present in the human N-CAM molecule, efforts to develop an immunogen that consists only of noncross-reactive epitopes continues.[83]

Genomics As a Vaccine Approach

One of the most exciting new areas in the field of vaccine development has been the availability of entire genome sequences from a number of organisms. The genome sequence of group B meningococcal strain MC58 was reported in March 2000 along with the description of a new approach for vaccine development.[84] "Reverse vaccinology," described by Rappuoli and coworkers, is the process of antigen identification that begins with computer analysis of sequence data. Using sequence analysis to predict open reading frames that likely coded for surface exposed proteins, 350 regions were identified, expressed recombinantly and examined as immunogens. Seven candidates that were immunogenic also stimulated bactericidal responses, and several of these appear to be highly conserved amongst a diverse set of meningococcal strains. Further work with these newly identified antigens is anticipated.

Prospects for the Next Five Years

Within the next 5 years meningococcal conjugate vaccines will largely replace the PS vaccines. Monovalent group C conjugate vaccines have been licensed in the UK, Canada and a number of other countries, and conjugates for groups A, Y and W135 are in clinical development. One or more of the meningococcal conjugates may be combined with pneumococcal and Hib conjugate vaccines to produce a combination vaccine against meningitis.

New group B OMP vaccines will have been used in large-scale effectiveness trials in New Zealand and elsewhere, and multivalent PorA vaccines may be in routine use in some European countries. However, two questions will still remain. How do we prevent endemic group B meningococcal disease caused by diverse populations of strains, and will long-term use of a vaccine that stimulates primarily PorA-based protection result in either antigenic drift of PorA, or an increased occurrence of strains that have a diminished or absent expression of PorA? In light of the tremendous explosion of technologic advances in the area of genomics and proteomics, it is likely that these questions will be addressed by multiple component vaccines, produced either as combination subunit vaccines or as OMV vaccines engineered and produced to enhance the expression of particular surface proteins. These vaccines will utilize both the antigens identified in earlier vaccines, as described above, and novel antigens, perhaps those identified "in-silico".

References

1. Frasch CE. Meningococcal vaccines: Past, present and future. In: Cartwright K, ed. Meningococcal Disease. New York: Wiley, 1995:245-83.
2. Peltola H. Meningococcal vaccines - Current status and future possibilities. Drugs 1998; 55:347-66.
3. Zollinger WD. New and improved vaccines against meningococcal disease. In: Levine MM, Woodrow GC, Kaper JB, eds. New Generation Vaccines. 2nd ed. New York: Marcel Dekker, 1997:469-88.
4. Goldschneider I, Gotschlich EC, Artenstein MS. Human immunity to the meningococcus. II. Development of natural immunity. J Exp Med 1969; 129:1327-48.
5. Granoff DM, Holmes SJ, Osterholm MT et al. Induction of immunologic memory in infants primed with Haemophilus influenzae type b conjugate vaccines. J Infect Dis 1993; 168:663-71.
6. Richmond P, Borrow R, Miller E et al. Meningococcal serogroup C conjugate vaccine is immunogenic in infancy and primes for memory. J Infect Dis 1999; 179:1569-72.
7. Booy R, Kroll JS. Is Haemophilus influenzae finished? J Antimicrob Chemother 1997; 40:149-53.

7a. Roberts RB. The relationship between group A and group C meningococcal polysaccharides and serum opsonins in man. J Exp Med 1970; 131:499-513.

8. Sim RJ, Harrison MM, Moxon ER et al. Underestimation of meningococci in tonsillar tissue by nasopharyngeal swabbing. Lancet 2000; 356:1653-4.
9. Swartley JS, Marfin AA, Edupuganti S et al. Capsule switching of Neisseria meningitidis. Proc Natl Acad Sci USA 1997; 94:271-6.
10. Vogel U, Claus H, Frosch M. Rapid serogroup switching in Neisseria meningitidis. N Engl J Med 2000; 342:219-20.
11. Lennon D, Gellin B, Hood D et al. Successful intervention in a Group A meningococcal outbreak in Auckland, New Zealand. Pediatr Infect Dis J 1992; 11:617-23.
12. Käyhty H, Peltola H, Eskola J et al. Immunogenicity of Haemophilus influenzae oligosaccharide-protein and polysaccharide-protein conjugate vaccination of children at 4, 6, and 14 months of age. Pediatrics 1989; 84:995-9.
13. Maslanka SE, Tappero JW, Plikaytis BD et al. Age-dependent Neisseria meningitidis serogroup C class-specific antibody concentrations and bactericidal titers in sera from young children from Montana immunized with a licensed polysaccharide vaccine. Infect Immun 1998; 66:2453-9.
14. De Wals P, De Serres G, Niyonsenga T. Effectiveness of a mass immunization campaign against serogroup C meningococcal disease in Quebec. J Amer Med Assoc 2001; 285:177-81.

15. Pon RA, Lussier M, Yang QL et al. N-propionylated group B meningococcal polysaccharide mimics a unique bactericidal capsular epitope in group B Neisseria meningitidis. J Exper Med 1997; 185:1929-38.
16. Granoff DM, Gupta RK, Belshe RB et al. Induction of immunologic refractoriness in adults by meningococcal C polysaccharide vaccination. J Infect Dis 1998; 178:870-4.
17. MacDonald NE, Halperin SA, Law BJ et al. Induction of immunologic memory by conjugated vs plain meningococcal C polysaccharide vaccine in toddlers - A randomized controlled trial. J Amer Med Assoc 1998; 280:1685-9.
18. Richmond P, Kaczmarski E, Borrow R et al. Meningococcal C polysaccharide vaccine induces immunologic hyporesponsiveness in adults that is overcome by meningococcal C conjugate vaccine. J Infect Dis 2000; 181:761-4.
19. Schneerson R, Barrera O, Sutton A et al. Preparation, characterization, and immunogenicity of Haemophilus influenzae type b polysaccharide protein conjugates. J Exp Med 1980; 152:361-76.
20. Bisgard KM, Kao A, Leake J et al. Haemophilus influenzae invasive disease in the United States, 1994-1995: Near dissappearance of a vaccine-preventable childhood disease. Emerging Infect Dis 1998; 4:1-14.
21. Beuvery EC, Rossum FV, Nagel J. Comparison of the induction of immunoglobulin M and G antibodies in mice with purified pneumococcal type 3 and meningococcal group C polysaccharides and their protein conjugates. Infect Immun 1982; 37:15-22.
22. Beuvery EC, Miedema F, Delft RV et al. Preparation and Immunochemical characterization of meningococcal group C polysaccharide-tetanus toxoid conjugates as a new generation of vaccines. Infect Immun 1983; 40:39-45.
23. Beuvery EC, Miedema F, Delft RV et al. Vaccine potential of meningococcal group C polysaccharide-tetanus toxoid conjugate. J Infect 1983; 6:247-55.
24. Jennings HJ, Lugowski C. Immunochemistry of groups A, B, and C meningococcal polysaccharide-tetanus toxoid conjugates. J Immunol 1981; 127:1011-8.
25. Beuvery EC, Roy R, Kanhai V et al. Characteristics of two types of meningococcal group C polysaccharide conjugates using tetanus toxoid as protein carrier protein. Dev Biol Stand 1986; 65:197-204.
26. Beuvery EC, Delft RV, Miedema F et al. Immunological evaluation of meningococcal group C polysaccharide-tetanus toxoid conjugate in mice. Infect Immun 1983; 41:609-17.
27. Costantino P, Viti S, Podda A et al. Development and phase 1 clinical testing of a conjugate vaccine against meningococcus A and C. Vaccine 1992; 10:691-8.
28. Anderson EL, Bowers T, Mink CM et al. Safety and immunogenicity of meningococcal A and C polysaccharide conjugate vaccine in adults. Infect Immun 1994; 62:3391-5.
29. Lieberman JM, Chiu SS, Wong VK et al. Safety and immunogenicity of a serogroups A/C Neisseria meningitides oligosaccharide-protein conjugate vaccine in young children - A randomized controlled trial. J Amer Med Assoc 1996; 275:1499-503.
30. Twumasi Jr PA, Kumah S, Leach A et al. A trial of a group A plus group C meningococcal polysaccharide- protein conjugate vaccine in African infants. J Infect Dis 1995; 171:632-8.
31. Granoff DM, Maslanka SE, Carlone GM et al. A modified enzyme-linked immunosorbent assay for measurement of antibody responses to meningococcal C polysaccharide that correlate with bactericidal responses. Clin Diagn Lab Immunol 1998; 5:479-85.
32. Granoff DM, Forrest B, Rappuoli R. Meningococcal polysaccharide-protein conjugate vaccines. Int J Infect Dis 1997; 1:152-7.
33. Miller E, Salisbury D, Ramsey M. Planning, registration, and implementation of an immunization campaign against meningococcal serogroup C disease in the UK: a success story. Vaccine 2001; 20:S58-67.
34. Feavers IM. Meningococcal vaccines and vaccine development. In: Pollard AJ, Maidan MCJ, eds. Meningococcal Vaccines: Methods and Protocols. New York: Humana Press, 2001:1-22.
35. Borrow R, Andrews N, Goldblatt D et al. Serological basis for use of meningococcal serogroup C conjugate vaccines in the United Kingdom: Reevaluation of correlates of protection. Infect Immun 2001; 69:1568-73.
36. MacLennan JM, Shackley F, Heath PT et al. Safety, immunogenicity, and induction of immunologic memory by a serogroup C meningococcal conjugate vaccine in infants - A randomized controlled trial. J Amer Med Assoc 2000; 283:2795-801.
37. Bramley JC, Hall T, Finn A et al. Safety and immunogenicity of three lots of meningococcal serogroup C conjugate vaccine administered at 2, 3 and 4 months of age. Vaccine 2001; 19:2924-31.

38. Richmond P, Borrow R, Goldblatt D et al. Ability of 3 different meningococcal C conjugate vaccines to induce immunologic memory after a single dose in UK toddlers. J Infect Dis 2001; 183:160-3.
39. Choo S, Zuckerman J, Goilav C et al. Immunogenicity and reactogenicity of a group C meningococcal conjugate vaccine compared with a group A + C meningococcal polysaccharide vaccine in adolescents in a randomised observer-blind controlled trial. Vaccine 2000; 18:2686-92.
40. Richmond P, Borrow R, Findlow J et al. Evaluation of de-O-acetylated meningococcal C polysaccharide-tetanus toxoid conjugate vaccine in infancy: Reactogenicity, immunogenicity, immunologic priming, and bactericidal activity against O-acetylated and de-O-acetylated serogroup C strains. Infect Immun 2001; 69:2378-82.
41. Borrow R, Longworth E, Gray SJ et al. Prevalence of de-O-acetylated serogroup C meningococci before the introduction of meningococcal serogroup C conjugate vaccines in the United Kingdom. FEMS Immunol Med Microbiol 2000; 28:189-91.
42. Lewis R, Nathan N, Diarra L et al. Timely detection of meningococcal meningitis epidemics in Africa. Lancet 2001; 358:287-93.
43. Robbins JB, Schneerson R, Gotschlich EC. A rebuttal: epidemic and endemic meningococcal. meningitis in sub-Saharan Africa can be prevented now by routine immunization with group A meningococcal capsular polysaccharide vaccine. Pediatr Infect Dis J 2000; 19:945-53.
44. Robbins JB, Towne DW, Gotschlich EC et al. "Love's labours lost": failure to implement mass vaccination against group A meningococcal meningitis in sub-Saharan Africa. Lancet 1997; 350:880-2.
45. Campagne G, Garba A, Fabre P et al. Safety and immunogenicity of three doses of a Neisseria meningitidis A+C diphtheria conjugate vaccine in infants from Niger. Pediatr Infect Dis J 2000; 19:144-50.
46. Sierra GVG, Campa HC, Varcacel NM et al. Vaccine against group B Neisseria meningitidis: Protection trial and mass vaccination results in Cuba. NIPH Ann 1991; 14:195-210.
47. Bjune G, Hoiby EA, Gronnesby JK et al. Effect of outer membrane vesicle vaccine against group B meningococcal disease in Norway. Lancet 1991; 338:1093-6.
48. Boslego J, Garcia J, Cruz C et al. Efficacy, safety, and immunogenicity of a meningococcal group B (15:P1.3) outer membrane protein vaccine in Iquique, Chile. Vaccine 1995; 13:821-30.
49. Noronha CP, Struchiner CJ, Halloran ME. Assessment of the direct effectiveness of BC meningococcal vaccine in Rio de Janeiro, Brazil: A case-control study. Int J Epidemiol 1995; 24:1050-7.
50. De Moraes JC, Perkins BA, Camargo MCC et al. Protective efficacy of a serogroup B meningococcal vaccine in Sao Paulo, Brazil. Lancet 1992; 340:1074-8.
51. Milagres LG, Ramos SR, Sacchi CT et al. Immune response of Brazilian children to a Neisseria meningitidis serogroup B outer membrane protein vaccine: Comparison with efficacy. Infect Immun 1994; 62:4419-24.
52. Perkins BA, Jonsdottir K, Briem H et al. Immunogenicity of two efficacious outer membrane protein-based serogroup B meningococcal vaccines among young adults in Iceland. J Infect Dis 1998; 177:683-91.
53. Milagres LG, Gorla MCO, Rebelo MC et al. Bactericidal antibody response to Neisseria meningitidis serogroup B in patients with bacterial meningitis: effect of immunization with an outer membrane protein vaccine. FEMS Immunol Med Microbiol 2000; 28:319-27.
54. Wedege E, Hoiby EA, Rosenqvist E et al. Immune responses against major outer membrane antigens of Neisseria meningitidis in vaccinees and controls who contracted meningococcal disease during the Norwegian serogroup B protection trial. Infect Immun 1998; 66:3223-31.
55. Rosenqvist E, Hoiby EA, Wedege E et al. Human antibody responses to meningococcal outer membrane antigens after three doses of the Norwegian group B meningococcal vaccine. Infect Immun 1995; 63:4642-52.
56. Tappero JW, Lagos R, Ballesteros AM et al. Immunogenicity of 2 serogroup B outer-membrane protein meningococcal vaccines - A randomized controlled trial in Chile. Journal of the American Medical Association 1999; 281:1520-7.
57. Milagres LG, Gorla MCA, Sacchi CT et al. Specificity of bactericidal antibody response to serogroup B meningococcal strains in Brazilian children after immunization with an outer membrane vaccine. Infect Immun 1998; 66:4755-61.

58. Haneberg B, Dalseg R, Wedege E et al. Intranasal administration of a meningococcal outer membrane vesicle vaccine induces persistent local mucosal antibodies and serum antibodies with strong bactericidal activity in humans. Infect Immun 1998; 66:1334-41.
59. Drabick JJ, Brandt BL, Moran EE et al. Safety and immunogenicity testing of an intranasal group B meningococcal native outer membrane vesicle vaccine in healthy volunteers. Vaccine 1999; 18:160-72.
60. Ala'Aldeen DAA, Borriello SP. The meningococcal transferrin-binding proteins 1 and 2 are both surface exposed and generate bactericidal antibodies capable of killing homologous and heterologous strains. Vaccine 1996; 14:49-53.
61. Gorringe AR, Borrow R, Fox AJ et al. Human antibody response to meningococcal transferrin binding proteins: Evidence for vaccine potential. Vaccine 1995; 13:1207-12.
62. Rosenqvist E, Hoiby EA, Wedege E et al. Human antibody responses to meningococcal outer membrane antigens after three doses of the Norwegian group B meningococcal vaccine. Infect Immun 1995; 63:4642-52.
63. Rokbi B, Mignon M, Maitre-Wilmotte G et al. Evaluation of recombinant transferrin-binding protein B variants from Neisseria meningitidis for their ability to induce cross-reactive and bactericidal antibodies against a genetically diverse collection of serogroup B strains. Infect Immun 1997; 65:55-63.
64. West D, Reddin K, Matheson M et al. Recombinant Neisseria meningitidis transferrin binding protein A protects against experimental meningococcal infection. Infect Immun 2001; 69:1561-7.
65. Fukasawa LO, Gorla MCO, Schenkman RPF et al. Neisseria meningitidis serogroup C polysaccharide and serogroup B outer membrane vesicle conjugate as a bivalent meningococcus vaccine candidate. Vaccine 1999; 17:2951-8.
66. Ward SJ, Scopes D, Christodoulides M et al. Expression of Neisseria meningitidis class 1 porin as a fusion protein in Escherichia coli: The influence of liposomes and adjuvants on the production of a bactericidal immune response. Microb Pathog 1996; 21:499-512.
67. Hoogerhout P, Donders EMLM, Van Gaans-van den Brink JAM et al. Conjugates of synthetic cyclic peptides elicit bactericidal antibodies against a conformational epitope on a class 1 outer membrane protein of Neisseria meningitidis. Infect Immun 1995; 63:3473-8.
68. Sardinas G, Gonzalez S, Garay HE et al. Anti-PorA antibodies elicited by immunization with peptides conjugated to P64k. Biochem Biophys Res Commun 2000; 277:51-4.
69. Peeters CCAM, Claassen IJTM, Schuller M et al. Immunogenicity of various presentation forms of PorA outer membrane protein of Neisseria meningitidis in mice. Vaccine 1999; 17:2702-12.
70. Peeters CCAM, Rümke HC, Sundermann LC et al. Phase I clinical trial with a hexavalent PorA containing meningococcal outer membrane vesicle vaccine. Vaccine 1996; 14:1009-15.
71. De Kleijn ED, De Groot R, Labadie J et al. Immunogenicity and safety of a hexavalent meningococcal outer-membrane-vesicle vaccine in children of 2-3 and 7-8 years of age. Vaccine 2000; 18:1456-66.
72. Cartwright K, Morris R, Rümke H et al. Immunogenicity and reactogenicity in UK infants of a novel meningococcal vesicle vaccine containing multiple class 1 (PorA) outer membrane proteins. Vaccine 1999; 17:2612-9.
73. De Kleijn ED, De Groot R, Lafeber AB et al. Immunogenicity and safety of monovalent P1.7h, 4 meningococcal outer membrane vesicle vaccine in toddlers: comparison of two vaccination schedules and two vaccine formulations. Vaccine 2000; 19:1141-8.
74. Martin SL, Borrow R, Van der Ley P et al. Effect of sequence variation in meningococcal PorA outer membrane protein on the effectiveness of a hexavalent PorA outer membrane vesicle vaccine. Vaccine 2000; 18:2476-81.
75. Jones DM, Borrow R, Fox AJ et al. The lipooligosaccharide immunotype as a virulence determinant in Neisseria meningitidis. Microb Pathog 1992; 13:219-24.
76. Zollinger WD, Moran EE, Devi SJN et al. Bactericidal antibody responses of juvenile rhesus monkeys immunized with group B Neisseria meningitidis capsular polysaccharide-protein conjugate vaccines. Infect Immun 1997; 65:1053-60.
77. Milagres LG, Brandileone MCC, Sacchi CT et al. Antibody studies in mice of outer membrane antigens for use in an improved meningococcal B and C vaccine. FEMS Immunol Med Microbiol 1996; 13:9-17.
78. Martin D, Cadieux N, Hamel J et al. Highly conserved Neisseria meningitidis surface protein confers protection against experimental infection. J Exper Med 1997; 185:1173-83.

79. Cadieux N, Plante M, Rioux CR et al. Bactericidal and cross-protective activities of a monoclonal antibody directed against Neisseria meningitidis NspA outer membrane protein. Infect Immun 1999; 67:4955-9.
80. Moe GR, Tan SQ, Granoff DM. Differences in surface expression of NspA among Neisseria meningitidis group B strains. Infect Immun 1999; 67:5664-75.
81. Delvig AA, Wedege E, Caugant DA et al. A linear B-cell epitope on the class 3 outer-membrane protein of Neisseria meningitidis recognized after vaccination with the Norwegian group B outer-membrane vesicle vaccine. Microbiology 1995; 141:1593-600.
82. Pon RA, Lussier M, Yang QL et al. N-propionylated group B meningococcal polysaccharide mimics a unique bactericidal capsular epitope in group B Neisseria meningitidis. J Exper Med 1997; 185:1929-38.
83. Granoff DM, Bartoloni A, Ricci S et al. Bactericidal monoclonal antibodies that define unique meningococcal B polysaccharide epitopes that do not cross-react with human polysialic acid. J Immunol 1998; 160:5028-36.
84. Pizza M, Scarlato V, Masignani V et al. Identification of vaccine candidates against serogroup B meningococcus by whole-genome sequencing. Science 2000; 287:1816-20.

Chapter 16

A Vaccine for Nontypable *Haemophilus influenzae*

Allan W. Cripps and Jennelle M. Kyd

Summary

Nontypable *H. influenzae* (NTHI) is a common commensal of the upper respiratory tract residing in both the nasopharynx and the posterior oropharynx. It is one of the leading causative bacterial pathogens of otitis media (OM) in children and serious urogenital, neonatal and mother-infant infections. It is also the cause of significant morbidity in patients with pulmonary diseases such as cystic fibrosis and chronic obstructive pulmonary disease. NTHI colonizes the respiratory tract through adherence to the mucous and epithelial cells. It has several bacterial surface components that have the capacity to facilitate adherence and interactions between the bacterium and epithelial cells, setting the stage for the cycle of inflammation. Whole killed cell or bacterial extracts have been investigated in human trials providing results that demonstrate the potential for a vaccine to protect against infection. Several lead candidate antigens have been proposed based on studies in animal models but have yet to be formulated for human trials. The composition of a vaccine requires that the antigens be conserved among strains, immunogenic and protective against infection and that the delivery of the vaccine results in the relevant immune response, probably a balance of specific cellular and humoral responses.

NTHI Infections and Disease

H. influenzae

H. influenzae are small Gram negative pleomorphic bacilli first described in 1892 by Richard Pfeiffer,[1] who mistakenly attributed this organism as being the causative agent for the influenza outbreak in Europe in 1889-1892. The microbe's requirement for blood in the growth media and its association with influenza led the classification committee of the Society of American Bacteriologists to taxonomically classify the bacillus as *H. influenzae*.[2] With the establishment in 1933[3] that influenza was caused by a virus, effort was directed at determining the pathogenic nature of the microbe that is commensally carried in up to 85% of healthy adults.[4] It was not until the early 1950s that the significance of nontypable isolates in chest infections was accepted (reviewed in ref. 5).

The genus name Haemophilus is now reserved for bacilli that have a requirement for one or both of the blood components haemin (X factor) and NAD (V factor). *H. influenzae* is dependent on both factors. *H. influenzae* exists as six serotypes (a-f) which possess a polysaccharide (Ps) capsule and a nonserotype form that lacks the capsule (nontypeable). Both serotypeable and nontypeable *H. influenzae* (NTHI) may be further classified into eight biotypes on the basis of growth–independent rapid tests for indole, urease and ornithine decarboxylase production.[6] There are now many techniques for investigating microbial phenotypes and genotypes.[7]

New Bacterial Vaccines, edited by Ronald W. Ellis and Bernard R. Brodeur.

Extensive studies have been performed to establish whether a relationship exists among serotype, biotype, genotype, distribution and the virulence of the strains.[8-13] More recent advances in molecular biology have only reinforced earlier studies indicating the significant diversity within the NTHI populations. It is apparent that certain strains are more virulent.[9,12,14,15] However, specific phenotypes or genotypes, individual genes or loci associated with disease-associated strains have not been conclusively identified in any studies.

The Disease Burden

NTHI is a common commensal of the upper respiratory tract, residing in both the nasopharynx and the posterior oropharynx. In healthy subjects, NTHI has been reported to be present on the pharynx in up to 80% of children and 40% of adults. However, in developing countries such as Papua New Guinea, a 100% carriage rate is observed within three months of life.[16] NTHI is commonly identified as the causative infectious agent in 25-37% of acute and chronic otitis media (OM)[17,18] and similarly high incidence rates for sinusitis and acute conjunctivitis in otherwise healthy subjects.

NTHI is one of the leading causative bacterial pathogens of OM in children. It accounts for ~20-30% of episodes of acute OM and >40% of cases of OM with effusion.[19] While the level of colonization correlates with the frequency of NTHI OM,[20] there appears to be no relationship between recent acquisition of strains and the occurrence of disease. In addition, the early colonization of infants by NTHI correlates with the onset and persistence of episodes of OM.[20,21] The strains associated with disease derive from a variety of genotypes[8] and most of the eight biotypes,[22] although biotypes I, II and III are the most prevalent (reviewed in ref. 19).

NTHI also has been reported as the cause of serious urogenital, neonatal and mother-infant infections. Biotype IV predominates in these infections.[23] Studies of such isolates by electrophoretic typing,[22] rDNA restriction fragment length polymorphism patterns and genomic DNA-DNA hybridization[24] suggest the existence of a distinct clonal group responsible for these infections. A number of strains investigated in this particular cryptic genospecies displayed abundant peritrichous piliation that preferentially adhered to cultured HeLa cells of genital origin.[25] However, it should be noted, that not all of these infections are biotype IV.

NTHI infections are also a significant cause of morbidity in patients with pulmonary diseases such as cystic fibrosis and chronic obstructive pulmonary disease (COPD). NTHI is responsible for up to 57% of acute infection exacerbations in COPD.[26] In extensive studies of patients with COPD, Butt and colleagues demonstrated that during an infective episode, NTHI isolated from sputum was essentially restricted to Biotypes I-IV. Biotypes III and IV were more likely to be present throughout the year, whilst biotypes I and II were more commonly identified in sputum in autumn and spring (see ref. 6, authors' unpublished observations). Quantitative bacteriological studies of sputum demonstrate that when NTHI was present, it accounted for >95% of the total bacterial count. NTHI was present in 26% of sputum specimens.[6,27]

Invasive NTHI disease is less common than serotypeable *H. influenzae*, particularly serotype *b*. NTHI has been reported as a significant cause of pneumonia in children in developing countries,[28,29] in the elderly,[30] and in patients with COPD.[28,31] NTHI bacteremia is mostly associated with pneumonia.[32,33]

NTHI infections are associated with substantial financial and nonfinancial costs to communities. A recent study in the United States determined that 60% of children were diagnosed with at least one OM episode within the first 3 years.[34] By extrapolation from Colorado's Medicaid data, Bondy and colleagues were able to determine that the USA national expenditure on OM for children under 14 years of age was ~$4 billion in 1992 and extrapolated to ~$5 billion in 1998, with 40% of this going to children aged between 1 and 3 years. These figures did not include estimates for nonmedically related costs, such as lost work-time by parents.

It is not just infections in children that are a burden to the community, but the incidence rate of infections in sufferers of chronic bronchitis and emphysema is also significant. There are an estimated 14 million people in the USA with chronic bronchitis and 2 million with emphysema.[35] It is the exacerbations of bacterial infections, such as caused by NTHI, that are responsible for much of the morbidity and mortality in these people. These respiratory conditions result in ~10 million medical-practitioner visits and ~2 million hospitalizations per year with an estimated financial burden of $11 billion in direct health care costs and ~$5 billion in indirect costs.

It is difficult to obtain accurate figures on the worldwide cost, let alone the misery that NTHI infections inflict on humanity. If the limited data available from the USA are any indication, then a vaccine is long overdue.

Adherence of NTHI to the Human Respiratory Epithelium

The first step towards colonization of the respiratory tract is adherence of the microbe to the epithelium. NTHI not only has the ability to adhere to respiratory epithelial cells, but also to the protective mucous coat bathing the epithelium.[36] Several proteins have been reported as adhesins and assisting the bacteria in colonisation.

Adherence to Mucin

The mechanism by which NTHI specifically binds to mucin in the human respiratory tract requires better definition. Both pili[37] and outer membrane proteins (OMPs), e.g., P2 and P5[38,39] have been reported to mediate binding of the bacteria to mucin. Mucin binding has been reported to be mediated through the sialic acid residues on mucin.[38] Recently Kubiet et al[37] re-examined the role of hemagglutinating pili in binding to human tracheobronchial mucin and demonstrated convincingly that NTHI strains with pili were able to bind to mucin better than their nonpiliated derivatives. However, given that only about one third of NTHI isolates contain a fimbria gene cluster[40-42] most do not bear fimbria. Hence this adherence mechanism to both mucin and epithelial cells is probably a less important virulence factor for NTHI compared with other adherence mechanisms.

This aside, it is clear that NTHI can bind to human mucin through a number of adhesins that enable the microbe to establish an initial presence in the respiratory tract and to subsequently colonize the epithelium. This process would be considerably exacerbated in situations where the mucocillary escalator was impaired for any reason. However, in healthy individuals there would be efficient mucocillary clearance, so mucin-binding properties would only provide an advantage when this clearance is impeded.

Adherence to the Respiratory Epithelium

Fimbria Mediated

NTHI isolates that bear fimbria have been shown to be similar to those found on serotypeable *H. influenzae* isolates, i.e., binding to oropharyngeal epithelial cells is mediated through sialyl ganglioside receptors.[43] The genes *hifA* to *hifE* located on the chromosome between *purE* and *pepN* comprise the fimbria gene cluster, with *hifA* encoding the subunit that binds to the ganglioside receptor.[40,44] The LKP fimbria associated with this adherence when expressed on the bacteria will agglutinate human erythrocytes expressing the AnWj antigen.[45] The fimbriae on NTHI strains vary in expression levels due to the insertions or deletions within the gene cluster, although the organization of this gene cluster is well conserved.[40] The changes in composition of these fimbria elements do not seem to influence infection.

Fimbria Independent

Adherence to the respiratory epithelium can be mediated by a member of the nonfimbria proteins, such as Hia (*H. influenzae* adhesin),[42,46] Hap (Haemophilus adhesin and penetration),[47,48] OapA (opacity-associated protein A),[49] P5 (OMP P5),[50,51] and the high-molecular-weight surface proteins HMW1 and HMW2.[52,53] Hap, OapA and P5 adhesins are present on all isolates so far examined whilst expression of HMW1, HMW2 and Hia varies, with Hia present on only 20-30% of isolates.

Hap is a 155-kD protein which has significant sequence similarity to *H. influenzae* serine-type IgA1 proteases.[54] While the mechanism by which Hap facilitates adherence and entry into cells is unknown, St Geme has hypothesized[55] that Hap may also be important in pathogenesis through proteolytic activity once the bacterium becomes intracellular.

OapA is a 47-kD protein responsible for the transparent colony phenotype of *H. influenzae*.[56] The mechanism by which OapA mediates adhesin to epithelial cells is unknown.[49]

P5 is a 37-kD heat-modifiable OMP.[57] P5 has been reported as a fimbrin protein,[50,51] but more recent studies[58] demonstrated that P5 forms a β-barrel structure analogous to OMPA, with no evidence of a coiled-coil structure. Hill et al[59] have shown that P5 adherence to epithelial cells can be mediated through the carcinoembryonic antigen family of cell adhesin molecules (CEACAMS), specifically CEACAM1. This group has also reported that binding to CEACAM1 was not dependent on carbohydrate residues on CEACAM1 molecules[59] but that P5 interacts primarily with CEACAM1 by protein-protein interactions.[60]

Hia is a 115-kD adhesin protein that has significant sequence homology with surface protein Hsf of *H. influenzae* type b strains[61] and similar binding characteristics.[55] The *Hia* and *Hsf* genes are alleles of the same locus. However, the *hia* gene is not in all NTHI strains.

HMW1 and HMW2 have received a great deal of attention over the last decade and are present in 75-80% of unrelated NTHI isolates.[42,62,63] Although there is significant similarity in the predicted amino acid sequences of HMW1 and HMW2, these adhesin molecules are characterised by distinct epithelial cell binding specificities and are not expressed by all NTHI strains.[64] HMW1 has a high level of adherence to epithelial cells, specifically recognizing a sialylated glycoprotein, which is inhibited by dextran sulfate and heparin.[47,65,66] On the other hand, HMW2 has a low level of adherence to epithelial cells.[64] The specific receptor for HMW2 on epithelial cells is unknown. Despite large antigenic diversity shown by HMW proteins, their adherence patterns (HMW1-or HMW2-like) are conserved.[14] A greater percentage of NTHI isolates from patients with OM express HMW adhesins than those isolates obtained from healthy carriers.[42,62,64] While van Schilfgaarde et al reported a similar finding for NTHI isolates from the sputum of patients with COPD (in contrast to the OM isolates), these isolates were not more adherent to epithelial cell lines than isolates obtained from healthy carriers.[14] The authors hypothesized that an alternative adherence mechanism may be important in COPD patients. In this context, Gorter et al have shown that neutrophil defensins released by PMNs and consequently present in the sputum of patients with COPD are capable of enhancing adherence of NTHI to human bronchial epithelial cells in a concentration-dependent manner.[67]

In addition to these proteins, lipooligosaccharide (LOS) components can bind to cell receptors. The ability of NTHI to bind to human cells through different adhesins provides several options for the microorganism to successfully colonise the host. This process would be considerably exacerbated in the situation where the mucocillary escalator was impaired for any reason.

The Pathogenesis of Haemophilus Disease

Studies of the pathogenesis of NTHI disease are limited to the airways, particularly the lung and middle ear. Hallmarks of NTHI infections at these mucosal sites are acute inflammation and polymorph accumulation. NTHI probably establishes itself in the first instance by its ability to adhere to mucin. The early events leading to respiratory inflammation are most likely to occur as a result of cellular interactions between the bacteria and respiratory epithelial cells and the subsequent release of inflammatory mediators. Several studies have shown that NTHI can penetrate and reside between and beneath epithelial cells,[31,39,41,47,49,57,62,68,69] although the exact mechanisms by which NTHI penetrates the epithelium are still being defined. NTHI produces not only several adherence proteins, some of which can bind extracellular matrix components (e.g., laminin, fibronectin and collagens)[70] it also binds plasminogen, hence potentiating penetration of the basement membrane.[71] There are potentially multiple mechanisms by which the interaction between the bacterium and the epithelial cells can commence the inflammatory cascade and aid paracytosis of the bacterium. Incubation of whole NTHI cells and purified NTHI LOS have been shown to induce the secretions of TNFα, IL-6, IL-8 and MCP-1 (all very potent pro-inflammatory cytokines) as well as intercellular adhesion molecule-1 (ICAM-1).[72,73] LOS is reported to bind membrane-bound CD14 to initiate cell signalling.[74] Since CD14 is not a transmembrane protein, toll-like receptors act as transmembrane co-receptors to initiate intracellular signalling.[75] However, human respiratory epithelial cells lack CD14 receptors to bind LOS. Other receptors that recently have been shown to interact with LOS are the PAF (platelet activating factor) receptor on human bronchial epithelial cells[76] and MD-2.[77] The latter forms a complex with toll-like receptor 4.

Whole NTHI cells induced greater responses than purified NTHI LOS, indicating other NTHI modulins play a role in adherence and the inflammatory cascade. These early interactions between the bacterium and epithelial cells set the stage for the cycle of inflammation, particularly in patients where the mucocillary escalator is impaired. However, it should be noted that, adhesions such as HMW1, HMW2, Hap, Hia and pili do not enhance IL-8 or IL-6 secretion.[73]

Little is known about the pathogenesis of NTHI in the ear. In an excellent review, Klein[78] identified 15 host and environment risk factors for "otitis prone" children. In addition to these risk factors, Faden has suggested that OM-prone children have a subtle immune deficiency[79] as they are less able to mount specific antibody responses[80] and lymphoproliferative responses to NTHI antigens.[81] In children and adults in the Eastern Highlands of Papua New Guinea, where there is endemic heavy airway colonization from early in life,[16] it has been suggested that a state of "high zone" tolerance to NTHI exists at the mucosal level.[82]

The evidence emerging from different studies supports the concept that NTHI can modulate the host immune response. In addition to that described above, NTHI activates NF-κB,[83] a transcriptional regulator of multiple host defence genes involved in immune and inflammatory responses including those encoding cytokines and chemokines.[84] Activation of NF-κB is mediated by toll-like receptor-2 on human epithelial cells, and data support a role for the major OMP P6 in this activation, resulting in IL-1β, IL-8 and TNFα expression.[83]

Vaccination Strategies for Nontypeable *Haemophilus influenzae*

It is now generally accepted that NTHI infections remain a major cause of morbidity and mortality despite the widespread availability of antibiotics. As a consequence, there is little debate that the burden of NTHI disease justifies the development of a vaccine. However, major challenges exist for vaccinologists in its development.

First, NTHI predominantly exists as a commensal on mucosal surfaces, particularly the airways. What changes the host-parasite relationship to favour the parasite? The only common criteria would appear to be damage of the mucosal surface. In COPD, impairment of the mucocillary escalator function by exposure to cigarette smoke or other chemical irritants sets up an environment in the lung where bacteria are not rapidly cleared from the airways. Inflammation in OM resulting from a previous viral infection may allow bacteria, such as NTHI, to ascend the eustachian tube and establish infection in the middle ear. However, it is not always possible to identify these predisposing insults to the mucosal surface prior to NTHI infection.

Secondly, NTHI is genetically highly diverse and, to date, no typing system has been able to determine any genetic markers to differentiate between NTHI isolates capable of causing diseases from those that are carried as part of the natural flora. At this stage, it has to be assumed that all NTHI isolates have the capacity to be pathogenic.

Thirdly, NTHI has evolved an impressive array of evading host defences (reviewed in ref. 85 and ref. 19). From the vaccine development perspective, it is the microbes' ability to undergo phase variation, whereby the bacteria is able to reversibly modify antigen expression, e.g., LOS,[86] HMW1 and HMW2,[65] which creates one of the greatest challenges. NTHI is also able to undergo antigenic drift whereby the microbe can irreversibly change surface antigenic structures through amino-acid substitutions, for example with IgA1 protease and P2.[87,88]

Therefore, the challenge remains to identify antigens that can be considered for human trials. The key performance criteria for these antigens are that the antigen is conserved across the genus, it must induce immune mechanisms to protect against initial colonization in acute infections and overcome chronic infection, while not enhancing tissue damage at the site of infection; and the induced immune response must overcome the immuno-modulatory and immune-evasion capabilities of the bacteria.

Animal infection models for NTHI have been well established for acute and chronic lung infections and acute OM in the rat.[89-91] In the chinchilla, models have been established for nasopharyngeal colonisation and OM.[92] These models are used to investigate pathogenic mechanisms and immune responses and are valuable tools for vaccine development.

Before the availability of the *H. influenzae* Rd genome,[93] most NTHI antigens were identified in their native form from the bacteria. Despite this being a very time-consuming approach, a number of lead vaccine antigens were demonstrated to be efficacious in animal models of infection. Since the availability of the Rd genome, "genomic mining" has become more popular. However, it is too early to determine the impact of this approach on the number of NTHI vaccine candidates available for trial.

The general strategy for NTHI has been to use the animal models available to assess whole-killed NTHI cell preparations, bacterial extracts, purified native or recombinant proteins and peptides as potential vaccine candidates. Both mucosal and parenteral immunization routes have been studied. On the basis of protection, these studies have focused attention on several antigens as lead vaccine candidates.[94,95] Such studies have also generated a substantial amount of data on the mechanisms of immune protection against NTHI lung infection.

In the following section, we review what we consider to be the current lead antigens with vaccine potential for NTHI. We have included a section on killed whole-cell and bacterial extracts that have been studied most extensively in human trials.

Potential Vaccine Candidates

Whole Killed Cell and Bacterial Extracts

NTHI killed whole-cell preparations have been predominantly used in formulations either alone, with other bacteria as a polybacterial mix, or as a bacterial extract with other bacterial extracts. The rationale behind this approach was to access the common mucosal immune system whereby immune responses are induced in the lymphoid aggregates of the small intestine, the Peyer's patches, and lymphocytes selectively migrate from the intestine to other mucosal sites, such as the respiratory tract, where an effector response occurs.

During the 1980s, six oral immunization clinical trials were undertaken of a whole killed cell formulation.[96-102] In these studies 10^{11} formalin-killed NTHI were prepared into an enteric-coated tablet containing 25 mg sodium tauroglycochate. Three courses of tablets were given at 0, 28 and 56 days. Each course consisted of two tablets taken before breakfast each day for three consecutive days. The patients were monitored for periods of up to one year. The investigators concluded that protection against acute recurrent episodes of bronchitis was achieved but varied with the prevalence of NTHI colonization. A reduction in bacterial load was shown in all studies. Bacterial load was determined by the incidence of throat colonization and/or quantitative or semiquantitative bacteriology of sputum samples. The reduction of bacterial load was relatively short, except in one study where the reduction persisted over the 12-month observation period. An oral vaccine "Bronchostat" was produced as a result of these studies but is no longer commercially available. A recent Cochrane Review of these studies has been conducted.[103] Analysis of the six trials confirmed this vaccine reduced the number and severity of exacerbations within 3-6 months of vaccination and that NTHI carriage was lower in the vaccinated group and at three and six months after vaccination.

A bacterial extract preparation Broncho-Vaxom® (also known as Broncho-Munal, Ommunal, Imocur and OM-85BV; OM Pharma, Geneva, Switzerland) has also been extensively studied.

This product is administered orally as capsules, with each capsule containing a lyophilized extract from the following bacteria, *Streptococcus pneumoniae, Klebsiella pneumoniae, Klebsiella ozaenae, H. influenzae, Staphylococcus aureus, Streptococcus pyogenes, Streptococcus viridans* and *Moraxella catarrhalis*. One capsule is administered daily for ten consecutive days for three months. Clinical trials have demonstrated efficacy in a number of infection scenarios where NTHI is acknowledged as one of the causative agents, such as respiratory tract infections in children,[104,105] acute exacerbations in patients with chronic bronchitis,[106,107] and sinusitis in adults.[108] Unfortunately, these studies have not been accompanied by any comprehensive bacteriology to demonstrate the effect of this preparation on NTHI carriage.

Despite the considerable volume of research that has been conducted to define the mechanisms of mucosal immunity induced by these preparations, precise mechanisms remain unclear. No clear correlate of immune protection has emerged. Studies in an animal model of acute infection have shown that there is a more rapid but controlled nonspecific inflammatory response in the lung within the first four hours of infection, compared to nonimmune animals. By 24 hours, there is a significant infiltration of $CD8^+$ T cells, some $CD4^+$ T cells and B cells.[109] Wallace et al[110] demonstrated that it was possible to transfer immunity from immune animals to naïve recipients with immune T cells.

Our studies have shown that the efficacy of mucosal immunization is significantly influenced by vaccination site (see ref. 111 and authors' unpublished data). Using a protective antigen OMP26[111,112] or whole killed cells, intratracheal (IT) immunization did not result in clearance of the lung infection, whereas a combined gut priming with an IT boost regime did. Both regimes induced similar levels of specific IgA antibody in the lungs but differed in the IgG isotypes. The gut/lung regime produced both IgG1 and IgG2a antibodies, suggesting a balanced Th1 and Th2 response, whereas the lung-only regime was dominated by an IgG2a response, suggesting polarization towards a Th1 response. Interestingly, studies on the oral bacterial extract Broncho-Vaxom® demonstrated that oral administration of the preparation to neonatal rats resulted in an enhanced postnatal maturation of Th1 function, thus balancing the Th1/Th2 ratio, which is innately Th2 polarized in the neonate.[113]

Clinical studies also have demonstrated that these formulations are able to stimulate NTHI-specific cellular responses. Oral immunization of healthy subjects with a killed whole cell formulation or a polybacterial mix[114] induced an enhanced antigen-driven proliferative response in peripheral blood lymphocytes and increased the precursor frequency of *H. influenzae* antigen-specific cells determined by limiting dilution analysis. The polybacterial mix induced greater responses than the monobacterial preparation. The polybacterial mix also increased the frequency of IL-2 receptors on blood lymphocytes.

The role of specific antibody in protection against NTHI infections still requires clarification. In the animal models, mucosal immunization with whole killed cells causes a significant increase in IgA and to a lesser extent IgG and IgM.[115] However, correlation with protection is not consistent. Using killed whole-cell NTHI, one study has reported correlation between the level of specific antibody and enhanced pulmonary clearance of NTHI,[116] while a second has not.[115] Wallace et al[115] hypothesized that the predominant IgA response was anti-inflammatory. However, while a polyclonal IgA response probably occurs, specific IgA is produced in response to oral immunization. Studies using Broncho-Vaxom® on mice have also demonstrated significant increases in IgA levels in gut and lung secretions following immunization.[117]

The results of antibody studies in humans using these preparations are inconsistent. A killed whole-cell NTHI oral vaccine did not stimulate an enhanced IgA response in saliva[96], although the vaccine was efficacious. On the other hand, Broncho-Vaxom®[118] and a killed whole-cell polybacterial vaccine containing 1.5×10^9 *H. influenzae* type *b* both significantly increased IgA levels in saliva. In the latter study, the antibody response was demonstrated to be specific against an antigen prepared from a NTHI isolate (author's personal communication, refs. 118, 119). To complicate the role of antibody further, Cripps et al[120] demonstrated that in chronic bronchitis, patients with high levels of specific antibody had greater infection and mortality rates.

Whether or not these preparations protect against NTHI disease may well be dose-dependent. Clancy and colleagues [97] demonstrated that a killed whole-cell formulation containing $1.8x10^{12}$ killed *H. influenzae* was highly efficacious in reducing the number of acute episodes of bronchitis compared with another monobacterial mix containing $3x10^{10}$ *H. influenzae* per course and polybacterial mix containing $3x10^{10}$ and $1x10^{10}$ killed *H. influenzae.* Suitable delivery systems for oral immunization remain a major impediment to the development of oral vaccines. While killed whole-cell and extract preparations have shown very promising results, there remains reluctance with respect to their widespread use.[121,122] The studies conducted to date should stimulate further studies on the optimization of formulations (particularly for killed whole-cell preparations), specificity of the responses (particularly for extracts), and mechanisms of protective immunity against NTHI induced at mucosal sites where NTHI is pathogenic.

Vaccine Antigens

The identification of potential vaccine candidates for an NTHI vaccine has been a significant challenge. Many antigens have been studied including OMPs, adherence factors and modified LOS. One major problem is the heterogeneity of many of these antigens among strains. The vaccine candidate antigen composition requires the antigens to be conserved between strains, immunogenic and protective against infection. The assessment of the last two criteria is usually dependent upon animal model studies.

This section will report on some of the antigens evaluated as vaccine candidates. The NTHI outer membrane is typical of a Gram negative bacteria[123] and most of the antigens reported to date as showing potential to protect against infection have been located on the outer membrane. There is a long list that include P6 (16-kD lipoprotein that appears to be highly conserved),[124] P5 fimbriae (heat-modifiable protein),[50] P4 (28-to 30-kD lipoprotein that has a conserved surface-exposed region),[125] protein D (42-kD protein with an affinity for binding human IgD),[126] P2 (the major porin protein),[127] modified LOS,[128] a group of 120- to 125-kD proteins,[129] and OMP26 (26-kD protein).[112,130]

OMP26 is a highly-conserved protein[130] that significantly clears both lung[112,130] and middle-ear infections[95] in animal studies. The mechanism by which clearance of infection is achieved post-immunization remains unclear. However, our studies have shown that antibody alone is not the key factor.[111] This protein has been one of the most efficacious antigens evaluated in our laboratory[131] and recently has been investigated in the chinchilla model of OM with equally promising protection (unpublished data).

The P5-fimbria protein has been an interesting antigen. This protein has four surface-exposed loops that appear quite heterogeneous[58] but which has a role in adherence.[38] Studies in the rat and chinchilla models have found this antigen is protective,[132,133] particularly when the vaccine is based on the loop 3. The sequence patterns for the loop can be divided into three groups.[134] Three peptides have been designed for this region (LB1-1, LB1-2 and LB1-3). The mechanism by which this antigen protects against infection appears to be antibody-mediated since both active immunization and passive transfer of anti-LB1 sera significantly reduced the severity and incidence of OM in chinchillas.[134,135] Vaccination with these peptides requires conjugation to another protein or peptide that can provide T-cell help. Studies have shown that these peptides confer protection when conjugated to either the promiscuous T-cell epitope from the measles virus protein or to lipoprotein D (the lipoprotein form of NTHI protein D that contains fatty acids linked to the N-terminal cysteine residue).[132,134]

Protein D or lipoprotein D is a 42-kD protein that appears highly antigenically conserved across strains.[126,136,137] The acylated form of the protein D is more immunogenic.[138] Parenteral immunization with lipoprotein D yielded higher IgG and IgA titers and greater bactericidal activity against NTHI than did immunization with protein D. However, this immunization did not protect rats from developing OM.[138] Similar results were obtained for parenteral immunization in the chinchilla model, where there was no significant protection from infection, but there was a slight reduction in the clearance rate of the bacteria from the middle ear.[134]

Mucosal immunization with lipoprotein D in rat models of lung and middle ear infections did show significantly enhanced clearance of infection, indicating that more than an antibody response is required for protection, as found also for OMP26.[95]

Another highly conserved OMP is P6, a peptidoglycan-associated lipoprotein[124] that is one of the major proteins expressed on the bacterial surface. Both humoral and cellular immune responses to P6 seem to correlate with susceptibility to OM in children.[80,81] In addition, antibody to P6 from human sera[139] and following animal immunization[140] has been shown to be bactericidal. In the chinchilla model, P6 was not protective when used in combined vaccination with P4 and PCP,[141] whereas some protection was achieved in another study where P6 was used alone.[140] Mucosal immunization of rats with P6 was found to be highly effective in clearing both homologous and heterologous lung infections.[90] Similar results for mucosally delivered P6 have recently been reported in a mouse model of otitis media.[142] Subsequent studies on the relevance of the differences in clearance of infection between parenteral and mucosal immunization have suggested that induction of both T- and B-cell responses to P6 are important (authors' unpublished data).

Two of the most abundant components on the bacterial surface are LOS and the porin protein P2. LOS is a virulence factor with certain oligosaccharide epitopes known to contribute to pathogenesis.[86] However, this oligosaccharide structure is subject to significant phase variation of its epitopes, resulting in substantial heterogeneity within a single strain.[143] Phase variation occurs as a result of frame shifts in repeat regions of the genes encoding the proteins involved in the biosynthesis of LOS and affects the invasive character of the bacterium.[144] These shifts result in differences in the addition of phosphorylcholine to LOS and alter the antibody-mediated reactivity.[145] Studies by Gu and coworkers have investigated the vaccine potential of detoxified LOS conjugates and have shown that vaccine-induced antibodies to the LOS showed a significant level of protection against NTHI OM in chinchillas.[146,147] An LOS vaccine would certainly be advantageous for disease prevention. However, the significant heterogeneity of the LOS both within and between strains does pose a major limitation. P2, as one of the most abundant proteins on the surface, is also limited in potential as a vaccine candidate because of heterogeneity. Rats mucosally immunized with P2 in the respiratory infection model significantly cleared the bacteria following homologous NTHI challenge.[148] In this study, the mechanism of immune clearance of infection was found to relate to the induced T- and B-cell responses. A P2 vaccine would need to direct the immune response to a highly conserved and protective epitope. A recent report has indicated that a region of loop 6 may be a suitable peptide-based antigen.[149]

Our group has investigated many proteins in a rat model of infection. Apart from those already described, these studies have included P1, P4, transferrin-binding protein b, D15 and several other minor proteins.[131,150] None of these have provided the same level of protection as OMP26, lipoprotein D, LB1-conjugates or P6. The only other major proteins considered as vaccine antigens are HMW1, HMW2 and Hia. However, these antigens have limitations due to both between strain heterogeneity and differences in expression. The effectiveness of such a vaccine or the mechanisms required for immune protection using these antigens have yet to be reported.

Conclusions and Future Directions

It is our opinion that the lead antigens for an NTHI vaccine are P6, conserved epitopes of P2, OMP26 and the P5 peptides (LB1-1, LB1-2 and LB1-3). The paucity of human studies on these antigens makes it difficult to predict further the requirement of a single antigen or optimal antigen mix that will result in the best efficacy. Data from animal studies suggest a requirement for complex humoral and cellular responses; however, mechanisms of induced immunity and correlates of protection in humans require investigation. It is important that immunogenicity studies be conducted in humans for these lead antigens. Selection of one or two vaccine candidates will enable the development of a parenteral NTHI vaccine. It would be ideal if this were in combination with antigens from *M. catarrhalis* and *S. pneumoniae*, which are capable of causing a similar disease spectrum as NTHI. Care will need to be taken to ensure that the immune response generated by parenteral immunization induces a balanced Th1/Th2 response at mucosal surfaces. The need for this balanced response has been demonstrated by oral immunization studies.

There has been significant work conducted on NTHI killed whole cells, polybacterial mixes and polybacterial extracts containing NTHI as oral vaccines. Two formulations, a monobacterial vaccine containing 1.8 x 10^{12} per course and Broncho-Vaxom® have demonstrated significant efficacy in NTHI infections. Although further studies are required to optimise dosage (monobacterial preparations) and determine the specificity of responses (Broncho-Vaxom®), these preparations should not be overlooked as safe and effective oral NTHI vaccines. The different studies presented in this chapter demonstrate the potential for a vaccine to protect against NTHI infection.

References

1. Pfeiffer R. Vorlaufige mittheilungen ber die errenger der influenza. Deutsche medizinische Wochenschrift 1892; 18:28.
2. Winslow CEA, Broadhurst J, Buchanan RE. The families and genera of the bacteria. Final report of the Society of American Bacteriologists on characterization and classification of beacterial types. J Bacteriol 1920; 5:191-229.
3. Smith W, Hale JH, O'Callaghan. Haem utilisation and nitrate reduction by Haemophilus influenzae. J Path Bact 1933; 65:229-238.
4. Turk DC, May JR. Haemophilus influenzae as a pathogen. In: Haemophilus influenzae: Its clinical importance. First ed. English Universities Press, 1967:24-26.
5. May JR. Chemotherapy of chronic bronchitis and allied disorders. 2nd ed. London: English Universities Press, 1972.
6. Butt HL, Clancy RL, Cripps AW et al. Bacterial colonization of the respiratory tract in chronic bronchitis. Aust NZ J Med 1990; 20:35-38.
7. van Belkum A, Struelens M, de Visser A et al. Role of genomic typing in taxonomy, evolutionary genetics, and microbial epidemiology. Clin Microbiol Rev 2001; 14:547-60.
8. Dhooge I, Vaneechoutte M, Claeys G et al. Turnover of Haemophilus influenzae isolates in otitis-prone children. Int J Pediatr Otorhinolaryngol 2000; 54:7-12.
9. van Alphen L, Caugant DA, Duim B et al. Differences in genetic diversity of nonecapsulated Haemophilus influenzae from various diseases. Microbiol 1997; 143:1423-1431.
10. Smith-Vaughan HC, Sriprakash KS, Leach AJ et al. Low genetic diversity of Haemophilus influenzae type b compared to nonencapsulated H. influenzae in a population in which H. influenzae is highly endemic. Infect Immun 1998; 66:3403-9.
11. Harper JJ, Tilse MH. Biotypes of Haemophilus influenzae that are associated with noninvasive infection. J Clin Microbiol 1991; 29:2539-2542.
12. Quentin R, Goudeau A, Wallace RJ Jr et al. Urogenital, maternal and neonatal isolates of Haemophilus influenzae: Identification of unusually virulent serologically non-typable clone families and evidence for new Haemophilus species. J Gen Microbiol 1990; 136:1203-1209.
13. Weinberg GA, Lehmann D, Tupasi TE et al. Diversity of outer membrane protein profiles of nontypable Haemophilus influenzae from children from Papua New Guinea and the Philipines. Rev Infect Dis 1990; 12:1017-1020.
14. van Schilfgaarde M, van Ulsen P, Eijk P et al. Characterization of adherence of nontypeable Haemophilus influenzae to human epithelial cells. Infect Immun 2000; 68:4658-4665.
15. Claesson BA, Lagergard T, Trollfors B. Antibody response to outer membrane of noncapsulated Haemophilus influenzae isolated from the nasopharynx of children with pneumonia. Pediatr Infect Dis J 1991; 10.104-108.
16. Gratten M, Gratten H, Poli A et al. Colonisation of Haemophilus influenzae and Streptococcus pneumoniae in the upper respiratory tract of neonates in Papua New Guinea: primary acquisition, duration of carriage, and relationship to carriage in mothers. Biol Neonate 1986; 50:114-20.
17. Giebink GS. Immunoprophylaxis of otitis media. Adv Exp Med Biol 1991; 303:149-58.
18. Harabuchi Y, Faden H, Yamanaka N et al. Nasopharyngeal colonization with nontypeable Haemophilus influenzae and recurrent otitis media. J Infect Dis 1994; 170:862-866.
19. St Geme III JW. The pathogenesis of nontypeable Haemophilus influenzae otitis media. Vaccine 2001; 19:S41-S50.

20. Faden H, Duffy L, Wasielewski R et al. Relationships between nasopharyngeal colonization and the development of otitis media in children. J Infect Dis 1997; 175:1440-1445.
21. Leach AJ, Boswell JB, Asche V et al. Bacterial colonisation of the nasopharynx predicts very early onset and persistence of otitis media in Australian Aboriginal infants. Pediatr Infect Dis J 1994; 13:983-989.
22. Cote S, Sanschagrin F, Dargis M et al. Molecular typing of Haemophilus influenzae using a DNA probe and multiplex PCR. Mol Cell Probes 1994; 8:23-37.
23. Wallace RJ, Jr., Baker CJ, Quinones FJ et al. Nontypable Haemophilus influenzae (biotype 4) as a neonotal, maternal, and genital pathogen. Rev Infect Dis 1983; 5:123-136.
24. Quentin R, Martin C, Musser JM et al. Genetic characterization of a cryptic genospecies of Haemophilus causing urogenital and neonatal infections. J Clin Microbiol 1993; 31:1111-6.
25. Rosenau A, Sizaret PY, Musser JM et al. Adherence to human cells of a cryptic Haemophilus genospecies responsible for genital and neonatal infections. Infect Immun 1993; 61:4112-8.
26. Schafer H, Ewig S. Acute exacerbations in chronic obstructive pulmonary disease (COPD)—microbial patterns and risk factors. Monaldi Arch Chest Dis Oct; 2000; 55:415-9.
27. Gump DW, Phillips CA, Forsyth BR et al. Role of infection in chronic bronchitis. Am Rev Respir Dis 1976; 113:465-74.
28. Shann F. Etiology of severe pneumonia in children in developing countries. Pediatr Infect Dis 1986; 5:247-52.
29. Weinberg GA, Ghafoor A, Ishaq Z et al. Clonal analysis of Hemophilus influenzae isolated from children from Pakistan with lower respiratory tract infections. J Infect Dis 1989; 160:634-43.
30. Berk SL, Holtsclaw SA, Wiener SL et al. Nontypeable Haemophilus influenzae in the elderly. Arch Intern Med 1982; 142:537-9.
31. Musher DM, Kubitschek KR, Crennan J et al. Pneumonia and acute febrile tracheobronchitis due to Haemophilus influenzae. Ann Int Med 1983; 99:444-450.
32. Wallace RJ, Jr, Musher DM, Septimus EJ et al. Haemophilus influenzae infections in adults: Characterization of strains by serotypes, biotypes, and β lactamase production. J Infect Dis 1981; 144:101-106.
33. Deulofeu F, Nava JM, Bella F et al. Prospective epidemiological study of invasive Haemophilus influenzae disease in adults. Eur J Clin Microbiol Infect Dis 1994; 13:633-8.
34. Bondy J, Berman S, Glazner J et al. Direct expenditures related to otitis media diagnoses: extrapolations from a pediatric medicaid cohort. Pediatrics 2000; 105:E72.
35. Vital and Health Statistics Series 10, No. 200. In: National Center for Health Statistics, Center for Disease Control, USA, 1996.
36. Wilson R, Read R, Cole P. Interaction of Haemophilus influenzae with mucus, cilia, and respiratory epithelium. J Infect Dis 1992; 165(suppl 1):S100-102.
37. Kubiet M, Ramphal R. Adhesion of nontypeable Haemophilus influenzae from blood and sputum to human tracheobronchial mucins and lactoferrin. Infect Immun 1995; 63:899-902.
38. Reddy MS, Bernstein JM, Murphy TF et al. Binding between outer membrane proteins of nontypeable Haemophilus influenzae and human nasopharyngeal mucin. Infect Immun 1996; 64:1477-1479.
39. Reddy MS, Murphy TF, Faden HS et al. Middle ear mucin glycoprotein: purification and interaction with nontypeable Haemophilus influenzae and Moraxella catarrhalis. Otolaryngol-Head Neck Surg 1997; 116:175-180.
40. Geluk F, Eijk PP, van Ham SM et al. The fimbria gene cluster of nonencapsulated Haemophilus influenzae. Infect Immun 1998; 66:406-417.
41. Gilsdorf JR, Chang HY, McCrea KW et al. Comparison of hemagglutinating pili of Haemophilus influenzae type b with similar structures of nontypeable Haemophilus influenzae. Infect Immun 1992; 60:374-379.
42. Krasan GP, Cutter D, Block SL et al. Adhesin expression in matched nasopharyngeal and middle ear isolates of nontypeable Haemophilus influenzae from children with acute otitis media. Infect Immun 1999; 67:449-454.
43. van Alphen L, Broek Geelen-van der, Blaas L et al. Blocking of fimbria-mediated adherence of Haemophilus influenzae by sialyl gangliosides. Infect Immun 1991; 59:4473-4477.
44. van Ham SM, van Alphen L, Mooi FR et al. Contribution of the major and minor subunits to fimbria-mediatedadherence of Haemophilus influenzae to human epithelial cells and erythrocytes. Infect Immun 1995; 63:4883-9.
45. van Alphen L, Poole J, Geelen L et al. The erythrocyte and epithelial cell receptors for Haemophilus influenzae are expressed independently. Infect Immun 1987; 55:2355-8.
46. Barenkamp SJ, St Geme III JW. Identification of a second family of high-molecular-weight adhesion proteins expressed by nontypeable Haemophilus influenzae. Mol Microbiol 1996; 19:1215-1223.

47. St Geme III JW, Morena MLdl, Falkow S. A Haemophilus influenzae IgA protease-like protein promotes intimate interaction with human epithelial cells. Mol Microbiol 1994; 14:217-233.
48. Hendrixson DR, St Geme III JW. The Haemophilus influenzae Hap serine protease promotes adherence and microcolony formation, potentiated by a soluble host protein. Mol Cell 1998; 2:841-50.
49. Prasadarao NV, Lysenko E, Wass CA et al. Opacity-associated protein A contributes to the binding of Haemophilus influenzae to chang epithelial cells. Infect Immun 1999; 67:4153-60.
50. Sirakova T, Kolattukudy PE, Murwin D et al. Role of fimbriae expressed by nontypeable Haemophilus influenzae in pathogensis of and protection against otitis media and relatedness of the fimbrin subunit to outer membrane protein A. Infect Immun 1994; 62:2002-2020.
51. Novotny LA, Jurcisek JA, Pichichero ME et al. Epitope mapping of the outer membrane protein P5-homologous fimbrin adhesin of nontypeable Haemophilus influenzae. Infect Immun 2000; 68:2119-2128.
52. Barenkamp SJ, Leininger E. Cloning, expression and DNA sequence analysis of genes encoding nontypeable Haemophilus influenzae high-molecular-weight surface-exposed proteins related to hemagglutinin of Bordetella pertussis. Infect Immun 1992; 60:1302-1313.
53. St Geme III JW, Falkow S, Barenkamp SJ. High-molecular-weight proteins of nontypable Haemophilus influenzae mediate attachment to human epithelial cells. Proc Natl Acad Sciences USA 1993; 90:2875-2879.
54. Hendrixson DR, de la Morena ML, Stathopoulos C et al. Structural determinants of processing and secretion of the Haemophilus influenzae hap protein. Mol Microbiol 1997; 23:505-18.
55. St Geme III JW. Insights into the mechanism of respiroatory tract colonization by nontypeable Haemophilus influenzae. Pediatr Infect Dis J 1997; 116:931-935.
56. Weiser JN, Chong ST, Greenberg D et al. Identification and characterization of a cell envelope protein of Haemophilus influenzae contributing to phase variation in colony opacity and nasopharyngeal colonization. Mol Microbiol 1995; 17:555-64.
57. Munson RS, Jr., Grass S, West R. Molecular cloning and sequence of the gene for outer membrane protein P5 of Haemophilus influenzae. Infect Immun 1993; 61:4017-4020.
58. Webb DC, Cripps AW. Secondary structure and molecular analysis of interstrain variability in the P5 outer-membrane protein of non-typable Haemophilus influenzae isolated from diverse anatomical sites. J Med Microbiol 1998; 47:1059-1067.
59. Hill DJ, Toleman MA, Evans DJ et al. The variable P5 proteins of nontypeable Haemophilus influenzae target human CEACAM1. Mol Microbiol 2001; 39:850-862.
60. Virji M, Evans D, Griffith J et al. Carcinoembryonic antigens are targeted by diverse strains of typable and non-typable Haemophilus influenzae. Mol Microbiol 2000; 36:784-95.
61. St Geme III JW, Cutter D, Barenkamp SJ. Characterization of the genetic locus encoding Haemophilus influenzae type b surface fibrils. J Bacteriol 1996; 178:6281-7.
62. Barenkamp SJ, St Geme III JW. Identification of surface-exposed B-cell epitopes on high molecular-weight adhesion proteins of nontypeable Haemophilus influenzae. Infect Immun 1996; 64:3032-7.
63. St Geme III JW. Molecular determinants of the interaction between Haemophilus influenzae and human cells. Am. J. Respir. Crit Care Med 1996; 154:S192-S196.
64. St Geme III JW, Grass S. Secretion of the Haemophilus influenzae HMW1 and HMW2 adhesins involves a periplasmic intermediate and requires the HMWB and HMWC proteins. Mol Microbiol 1998; 27:617-630.
65. St Geme III JW, Kumar VV, Cutter D et al. Prevalence and distribution of the hmw and hia genes and the HMW and Hia adhesins among genetically diverse strains of nontypable Haemophilus influenzae. Infect Immun 1998; 66:364-8.
66. Noel GJ, Barenkamp SJ, III JWSG et al. High-molecular-weight surface-exposed proteins of Haemophilus influenzae mediate binding to macrophages. J Infect Dis 1994; 169:425-429.
67. Gorter AD, Eijk PP, van Wettering S et al. Stimulation of the adherence of Haemophilus influenzae to human lung epithelial cells by antimicrobial neutrophil defensins. J Infect Dis 1998; 178:1067-1074.
68. Noel GJ, Love DC, Mosser DM. High-molecular-weight proteins of nontypeable Haemophilus influenzae mediate bacterial adhesion to cellular proteoglycans. Infect Immun 1994; 62:4028-4033.
69. Moller LVM, Timens W, van der Bij W et al. Haemophilus influenzae in lung explants of patients with end-stage pulmonary disease. Am J Respir Critical Care Med 1998; 157(950-956).
70. Virkola R, Brummer M, Rauvala H et al. Interaction of fimbriae of Haemophilus influenzae type b with heparin-binding extracellular matrix proteins. Infect Immun 2000; 68:5696-5701.
71. Lahteenmaki K, Virkola R, Pouttu R et al. Bacterial plasminogen receptors: in vitro evidence for a role in degradation of the mammalian extracellular matrix. Infect Immun 1995; 63:3659-64.

72. Khair OA, Davies RJ, Devalia JL. Bacterial-induced release of inflammatory mediators by bronchial epithelial cells. Eur Respir J 1996; 9:1913-1922.
73. Clemans DL, R.J.Bauer, Hanson JA et al. Induction of proinflammatory cytokines from human respiratory epithelial cells after stimulation by nontypeable Haemophilus influenzae. Infect Immun 2000; 68:4430-4440.
74. Tobias PS, Soldau K, Gegner JA et al. Lipopolysaccharide binding protein-mediated complexation of lipopolysaccharide with soluble CD14. J Biol Chem 1995; 270:10482-8.
75. da Silva Correia J, Soldau K, Christen U et al. Lipopolysaccharide is in close proximity to each of the proteins in its membrane receptor complex. transfer from CD14 to TLR4 and MD-2. J Biol Chem 2001; 276:21129-35.
76. Swords WE, Buscher BA, ver Steeg Ii K et al. Nontypeable Haemophilus influenzae adhere to and invade human bronchial epithelial cells via an interacting of lipooligosaccharide with the PAF receptor. Mol Microbiol 2000; 37:13-27.
77. Viriyakosol S, Tobias PS, Kitchens RL et al. MD-2 binds to bacterial lipopolysaccharide. J Biolog Chem 2001; 276:38044-51.
78. Klein JO. The burden of otitis media. Vaccine 2000; 19:S2-S8.
79. Faden H. The microbiologic and immunologic basis for recurrent otitis media in children. Eur J Pediatr 2001; 160:407-413.
80. Yamanaka N, Faden H. Local antibody response to P6 of nontypable Haemophilus influenzae in otitis-prone and normal children. Acta Otolaryngology 1993; 113:524-529.
81. Kodama H, Faden H. Cellular immunity to the P6 outer membrane protein of nontypeable Haemophilus influenzae. Infect Immun 1995; 63:2467-2472.
82. Clancy RL, Cripps AW, Yeung S et al. Salivary and serum antibody responses to Haemophilus influenzae infection in Papua New Guinea. PNG Med J 1987; 30:271-276.
83. Shuto T, Xu H, Wang B et al. Activation of NF-kB by nontypeable Hemophilus influenzae is mediated by toll-like receptor 2-TAK1-dependent NIK-IKK a /b-IkBa and MKK3/6-p38 MAP kinase signaling pathways in epithelial cells. Proc Nat Acad Sci USA 2001; 98:8774-8779.
84. Hatada EN, Krappmann D, Scheidereit C. NF-kappaB and the innate immune response. Curr Opin Immunol 2000; 12:52-8.
85. Foxwell AR, Kyd JM, Cripps AW. Nontypeable Haemophilus influenzae: pathogenesis and prevention. Microbiol Mol Biol Rev 1998; 62:294-308.
86. Maskell DJ, Szabo MJ, Butler PD et al. Molecular biology of phase-variable lipopolysaccharide biosynthesis by Haemophilus influenzae. J Infect Dis 1992; 165(S1):S90-2.
87. Lomholt H, van Alphen L, Kilian M. Antigenic variation of immunoglobulin A1 proteases among sequential isolates of Haemophilus influenzae from healthy children and patients with chronic obstructive pulmonary disease. Infect Immun 1993; 61:4575-4581.
88. Duim B, Dankert J, Jansen HM et al. Genetic analysis of the diversity in outer membrane P2 of non-encapsulated Haemophilus influenzae. Microbial Pathogenesis 1993; 14:451-462.
89. Wallace FJ, Clancy RL, Cripps AW. An animal model demonstration of enhanced clearance of nontypable Haemophilus influenzae from respiratory tract after antigen stimulation of gut-associated lymphoid tissue. Am Rev Respir Dis 1989; 140:311-316.
90. Kyd JM, Dunkley ML, Cripps AW. Enhanced respiratory clearance of nontypeable Haemophilus influenzae following mucosal immunization with P6 in a rat model. Infect Immun 1995; 63:2931-2940.
91. Magnuson K, Hermansson A, Melhus A et al. The tympanic membrane and middle ear mucosa during non-typeable Haemophilus influenzae and Haemophilus influenzae type b acute otitis media: a study in the rat. Acta Otolaryngology 1997; 117:396-405.
92. Giebink GS. Otitis media: the chinchilla model. Microbial Drug Resist 1999; 5:57-72.
93. Fleischmann RD, Adams MD, White O et al. Whole-genome random sequencing and assembley of Haemophilus influenzae Rd. Science 1995; 269:496-512.
94. Kyd J, Cripps A. Identifying vaccine antigens and assessing delivery systems for the prevention of bacterial infections. J Biotechnol 2000; 83:85-90.
95. Poolman JT, Bakaletz L, Cripps A et al. Developing a nontypeable Haemophilus influenzae (NTHi) vaccine. Vaccine 2000; 19(S1):S108 - S115.
96. Clancy RL, Cripps AW, Muree-Allen K et al. Oral immunisation with killed Haemophilus influenzae for protection against acute bronchitis in chronic obstructive pulmonary disease. Lancet 1985; ii:1395-1397.
97. Clancy R, Cripps A, Pang G et al. The paradox of immunisation against Haemophilus influenzae-related endobronchitis: protection restricted to ingestion of "non adjuvenated" vaccine. In: Mestecky J, McGhee J, eds. Recent Advances in Mucosal Immunology. Vol. 216B. New York: Plenum Press, 1987:1759-1764.

98. Clancy RL, Cripps AW, Gebeski V. Protection against recurrent acute bronchitis after oral immunization with killed Haemophilus influenzae. Med J Aust 1990; 152:413-416.
99. Clancy RL, Cripps AW. Specific protection against acute bronchitis associated with nontypeable Haemophilus influenzae. J Infect Dis 1992; 165(suppl 1):S194-S195.
100. Lehmann D, Coakley KJ, Coakley CA et al. Reduction in the incidence of acute bronchitis by an oral Haemophilus influenzae vaccine in patients with chronic bronchitis in the highlands of Papua New Guinea. Am Rev Respir Dis 1991; 144:324-330.
101. Clancy RL, Pang G, Dunkley G et al. Control of bacterial colonisation of the respiratory tract mucosa in man. In: Husband AJ, Beagley KW, Clancy RL et al eds. Mucosal Solutions: Advances in mucosal immunology. Vol I. Sydney: University of Sydney, 1997:261-268.
102. Tandon MK, Gebski V. A controlled trial of a killed Haemophilus influenzae vaccine for prevention of acute exacerbations of chronic bronchitis. Aust NZ J Medicine 1991; 21:427-432.
103. Foxwell AR, Cripps AW. Haemophilus influenzae oral vaccination against acute bronchitis. Cochrane Database Syst Rev 2000; 2:CD001958.
104. Gutiérrez-Tarango MD, Berber A. Efficacy of a bacterial extract (OM-85 BV) in preventing recurrent respiratory tract infections in susceptible children. Clin Drug Invest 1997; 13:76-84.
105. Gutiérrez-Tarango MD, Berber A. Safety and efficacy of two courses of OM-85 BV in the prevention of respiratory tract infections in children during 12 months. Chest 2001; 119:1742-48.
106. Orcel B, Delclaux B, Baud M et al. Oral immunization with bacterial extracts for protection against acute bronchitis in elderly institutionalized patients with chronic bronchitis. Eur Respir J 1994; 7:446-452.
107. Collet JP, Shapiro S, Ernst P et al. Effects of an immunostimulating agent on acute exacerbations and hospitalizations in patients with chronic obstructive pulmonary disease. Am J Respir Crit Care Med 1997; 156:1719-1724.
108. Heintz B, Schlenter WW, Kirsten R et al. Clinical efficacy of Broncho-Vaxom® in adult patients with chronic purulent sinusitis—a multicentric, placebo-controlled, double-blind study. Int J Clin Pharmacol Ther Toxicol 1989; 27:530-534.
109. Foxwell AR, Kyd JM, Karupiah G et al. CD8+ T cells have an essential role in pulmonary clearance of nontypeable Haemophilus influenzae following mucosal immunisation. Infect Immun 2001; 69:2636-2642.
110. Wallace FJ, Cripps AW, Clancy RL et al. A role for intestinal T lymphocytes in bronchus mucosal immunity. Immunol 1991; 74:68-73.
111. Kyd JM, Cripps AW. Nontypeable Haemophilus influenzae: Challenges in developing a vaccine. J Biotechnol 1999; 73:103-108.
112. Kyd JM, Cripps AW. Potential of a novel protein, OMP26, from nontypeable Haemophilus influenzae to enhance pulmonary clearance in a rat model. Infect Immun 1998; 66:2272-2278.
113. Bowman LM, Holt PG. Selective enhancement of systemic Thuimmunity in immunologically immature rats with an orally administered bacterial extract. Infect Immun 2001; 69:3719-3727.
114. Pang GT, Yeung S, Clancy RL et al. Induction of antigen-reactive and IL-2 receptor bearing cells following oral immunisation in humans. In: Mestecky J, McGhee J, eds. Recent Advances in Mucosal Immuno logy. Vol 216B. New York: Plenum Press, 1987: 1731-1739.
115. Wallace FJ, Witt CS, Clancy RL et al. Protection against non-typeable Haemophilus influenzae following sensitization of gut associated lymphoid tissue: Role of specific antibody and phagocytes. Immunol Cell Biol 1995; 73:258-265.
116. Hansen EJ, Hart DA, McGehee JL et al. Immune enhancement of pulmonary clearance of nontypable Haemophilus influenzae. Infect Immun 1988; 56:182-190.
117. Bosch A, Lucena F, Pares R et al. Bacterial immunostimulant (Broncho-Vaxom) versus levamisole on the humoral immune response in mice. J Immunopharm 1983; 5:107-116.
118. Puigdollers JM, Rodes Serna G, Hernandez del Rey L et al. Immunoglobulin production in man stimulated by an orally administered bacterial lysate. Respiration 1980; 40:142-149.
119. Clancy RL, Cripps AW, Husband AJ et al. Specific immune response in the respiratory tract after administration of an oral polyvalent bacterial vaccine. Infect Immun 1983; 39:491-6.
120. Cripps AW, Clancy RL, Murree-Allen K et al. Quantitation of isotype specific Haemophilus influenzae antibody in serum and saliva of normal subjects and chronic bronchitis. Asian Pac J Allergy Immunol 1986; 4:5-11.
121. Anthonisen NR. OM-85 BV for COPD. Am J Respir Crit Care Med 1997; 156:1713-1714.
122. Ekberg-Jansson A, Larrson S, Löfdahl C-G. Preventing exacerbations on chronic bronchitis and COPD. BMJ 2001; 322:12591260.
123. Loeb MR, Smith DH. Outer membrane protein composition in disease isolates of Haemophilus influenzae: pathogenic and epidemiological implications. Infect Immun 1980; 30:709-717.

124. Nelson MB, Munson RS Jr, Apicella MA et al. Molecular conservation of the P6 outer membrane among strains of Haemophlius influenzae: analysis of antigenic determinants, gene sequences, and restriction fragment length polymorphisms. Infect Immun 1991; 59:2658-2663.
125. Green BA, Farley JE, Quinn-Dey T et al. The e (P4) outer membrane protein of Haemophilus influenzae: Biologic activity of anti-e serum and cloning and sequencing of the structural gene. Infect Immun 1991; 59:3191-3198.
126. Akkoyunlu M, Ruan M, Forsgren A. Distribution of Protein D, an immunoglobulin D-binding protein in Haemophilus strains. Infect Immun 1991; 59:1231-1238.
127. Haase EM, Yi K, Morse GD et al. Mapping of bactericidal epitopes on the P2 porin protein of nontypeable Haemophilus influenzae. Infect Immun 1994; 62:3712-3722.
128. Gu XX, Sun J, Jin S et al. Detoxified lipooligosaccharide from nontypeable Haemophilus influenzae conjugated to proteins confers protection against otitis media in chinchillas. Infect Immun 1997; 65:4488-93.
129. Barenkamp SJ. Immunization with high-molecluar-weight adhesion proteins of nontypeable Haemophilus influenzae modifies experimental otitis media in chinchillas. Infect Immun 1996; 64:1246-1251.
130. El-Adhami W, Kyd JM, Bastin DA et al. Characterisation of the gene for OMP26 from nontypeable Haemophilus influenzae and immune responses to the recombinant protein. Infect Immun 1999; 67:1935-1942.
131. Kyd JM, Cripps AW. Towards a protein vaccine for nontypeable Haemophilus influenzae. Clin Infect Dis 1999; 28:238.
132. Bakaletz LO, Leake ER, Billy JM et al. Relative immunogenicity and efficacy of two synthetic chimeric peptides of fimbrin as vaccinogens against nasopharyngeal colonization by nontypeable Haemophilus influenzae in the chinchilla. Vaccine 1997; 15:955-961.
133. Webb DC, Cripps AW. A P5 peptide that is homologous to peptide 10 of OprF from Pseudomonas aeruginosa enhances clearance of nontypeable Haemophilus influenzae from acutely infected rat lung in the absence of detectable peptide-specific antibody. Infect Immun 2000; 68:377-381.
134. Bakaletz LO, Kennedy B-J, Novotny LA et al. Protection against development of otitis media induced by nontypeable Haemophilus influenzae by both active and passive immunization in a chinchilla model of virus-bacterium infection. Infect Immun 1999; 67:2746-2762.
135. Kennedy B-J, Novotny LA, Jurcisek JA et al. Passive transfer of antiserum specific for immunogens derived from a nontypeable Haemophilus influenzae adhesin and lipoprotein D prevents otitis media after heterologous challenge. Infect Immun 2000; 68:2756-2765.
136. Janson H, Heden LO, Forsgren A. Protein D, the immunoglobulin D-binding protein of Haemophilus influenzae, is a lipoprotein. Infect Immun 1992; 60:1336-1342.
137. Song X-M, Forsgren A, Janson H. The gene encoding protein D (hyp) is highly conserved among Haemophilus influenzae type b and nontypeable strains. Infect Immun 1995; 63:696-699.
138. Akkoyunlu M, Melhus A, Capiau C et al. The acylated form of protein D of Haemophilus influenzae is more immunogenic than the non-acylated form and elicits an adjuvant effect when it is used as a carrier conjugated to polyribosyl ribitol phosphate. Infect Immun 1997; 65:5010-5016.
139. Murphy TF, Bartos LC, Rice PA et al. Identification of a 16,600-Dalton outer membrane protein on nontypable Haemophilus influenzae as a target for human serum bactericidal antibody. J Clin Invest 1986; 78:1020-1027.
140. DeMaria TF, Urwin DM, Leake ER. Immunization with outer membrane protein P6 from nontypeable Haemophilus influenzae induces bactericidal antibody and affords protection in the chinchilla model of otitis media. Infect Immun 1996; 64:5187-5192.
141. Green BA, Vazquez ME, Zlotnick GW et al. Evaluation of mixtures of purified Haemophilus influenzae outer membrane proteins in protection against challenge with nontypable H. influenzae in the chinchilla otitis media model. Infect Immun 1993; 61:1950-1957.
142. Sabirov A, Kodama S, Hirano T et al. Intranasal immunization enhances clearance of nontypeable Haemophilus influenzae and reduces stimulation of tumor necrosis factor alpha production in the murine model of otitis media. Infect Immun 2001; 69:2964-2971.
143. Kimura A, Hansen EJ. Antigenic and phenotypic variation of Haemophilus influenzae type b lipooligosaccharide and their relationship to virulence. Infect Immun 1986; 51:69-79.
144. Weiser JN, Williams, Moxon ER. Phase-variable lipopolysaccharide structures enhance the invasive capacity of Haemophilus influenzae. Infect Immun 1990; 58:3455-3457.
145. Weiser JN, Pan N, McGowan KL et al. Phosphorylcholine on the lipopolysaccharide of Haemophilus influenzae contributes to persistence in the respiratory tract and sensitivity to serum killing mediated by C-reactive protein. J Exp Med 1998; 187:631-40.
146. Wu TH, Gu XX. Outer membrane proteins as a carrier for detoxified lipooligosaccharide conjugate vaccines for nontypeable Haemophilus influenzae. Infect Immun 1999; 67:5508-5513.

147. Sun J, Chen J, Cheng Z et al. Biological activities of antibodies elicited by lipooligosaccharide based-conjugate vaccines of nontypeable Haemophilus influenzae in an otitis media model. Vaccine 2000; 18:1264-1272.
148. Kyd JM, Cripps AW. Modulation of antigen-specific T and B cell responses influence bacterial clearance of nontypeable Haemophilus influenzae from the lung in a rat model. Vaccine 1996; 14:1471-1478.
149. Neary JM, Yi KY, Karalus RJ et al. Antibodies to loop 6 of the P2 porin protein of nontypeable Haemophilus influenzae are bactericidal against multiple strains. Infect Immun 2001; 69:773-778.
150. Webb DC, Cripps AW. Immunization with recombinant transferrin binding protein B enhances clearance of nontypeable Haemophilus influenzae from the rat lung. Infect Immun 1999; 67:2138-2144.

Chapter 17

Vaccines for *Pseudomonas aeruginosa*

Gregory P. Priebe and Gerald B. Pier

Pseudomonas aeruginosa causes a wide variety of serious infections, particularly in the critically ill,[1,2] the immunocompromised,[3,4] and those with cystic fibrosis.[5] It also causes community-acquired bacterial ulcerative keratitis of the eye, particularly in users of extended-wear contact lenses.[6,7] In the setting of nosocomial pneumonia, the isolation of *P. aeruginosa* has a strikingly high attributable mortality.[8] The prevalence and importance of *P. aeruginosa* in human infections, coupled with the intrinsic antibiotic resistance due to the low permeability of the outer membrane[9] and the presence of multiple drug efflux pumps,[10] confer a pressing need for effective vaccines. A large variety of antigenic targets and delivery methods have been used in many preclinical studies of *P. aeruginosa* vaccines, and there has also been a number of actual human trials. The failure to have an effective vaccine at this time point can be attributed to a large number of factors. The overwhelming issues appear to encompass the wide variety of often redundant virulence factors that render ineffective approaches that target a single or even a few bacterial products; the antigenic and immunogenic properties of the major target of protective immunity, the O antigen of the lipopolysaccharide (LPS); the ability of the organism to have both extracellular and intracellular stages; and an incomplete understanding of the variation in production of antigens at different sites of infection and at different times during the infectious process, particularly as manifest by clinical isolates. This review discusses many of the strategies pursued to date in the quest for an effective vaccine for *P. aeruginosa*. A diagrammatic representation of the bacterium is presented in (Fig. 1) and helps to categorize the various *P. aeruginosa* antigens that have been used as vaccine targets.

Secreted Products: Exotoxin A, Alkaline Protease, Elastase

Early studies of *P. aeruginosa* virulence factors described exotoxin A as a secreted ADP-ribosyltransferase.[11,12] Exotoxin A was shown to be important for pathogenesis in a number *P. aeruginosa* infection models.[13,14] However, unlike the experience with diphtheria and tetanus toxoids as vaccines, vaccine strategies using exotoxin A alone have not shown significant and consistent protective efficacy in animal models of *P. aeruginosa* infection.[15-17] Most of the positive results have come from using high-exotoxin A-producing strains for vaccine evaluation, whereas demonstration of efficacy against typical clinical isolates has not been shown. Nevertheless, a detoxified version of exotoxin A has been used extensively as a carrier protein for a number of other antipseudomonal vaccines as well as for vaccines against other pathogens, notably staphylococci.[18]

Alkaline protease and elastase are two proteases secreted by *P. aeruginosa*. Both are thought to play significant role in localized tissue damage in the lung, eye, or burn wound.[19-21] Active immunization with the alkaline protease combined with exotoxin A was shown to protect neutropenic mice from death due to gut-derived bacteremia with a single strain of *P. aeruginosa*, although immunization with either component alone or with elastase had no benefit.[22] A recombinant, mutated inactivated elastase was also found to protect mice from IP challenge with a single *P. aeruginosa* strain (IFO 3455), with increase in LD_{50} by 27- to 69-fold.[23] Sokol

New Bacterial Vaccines, edited by Ronald W. Ellis and Bernard R. Brodeur.

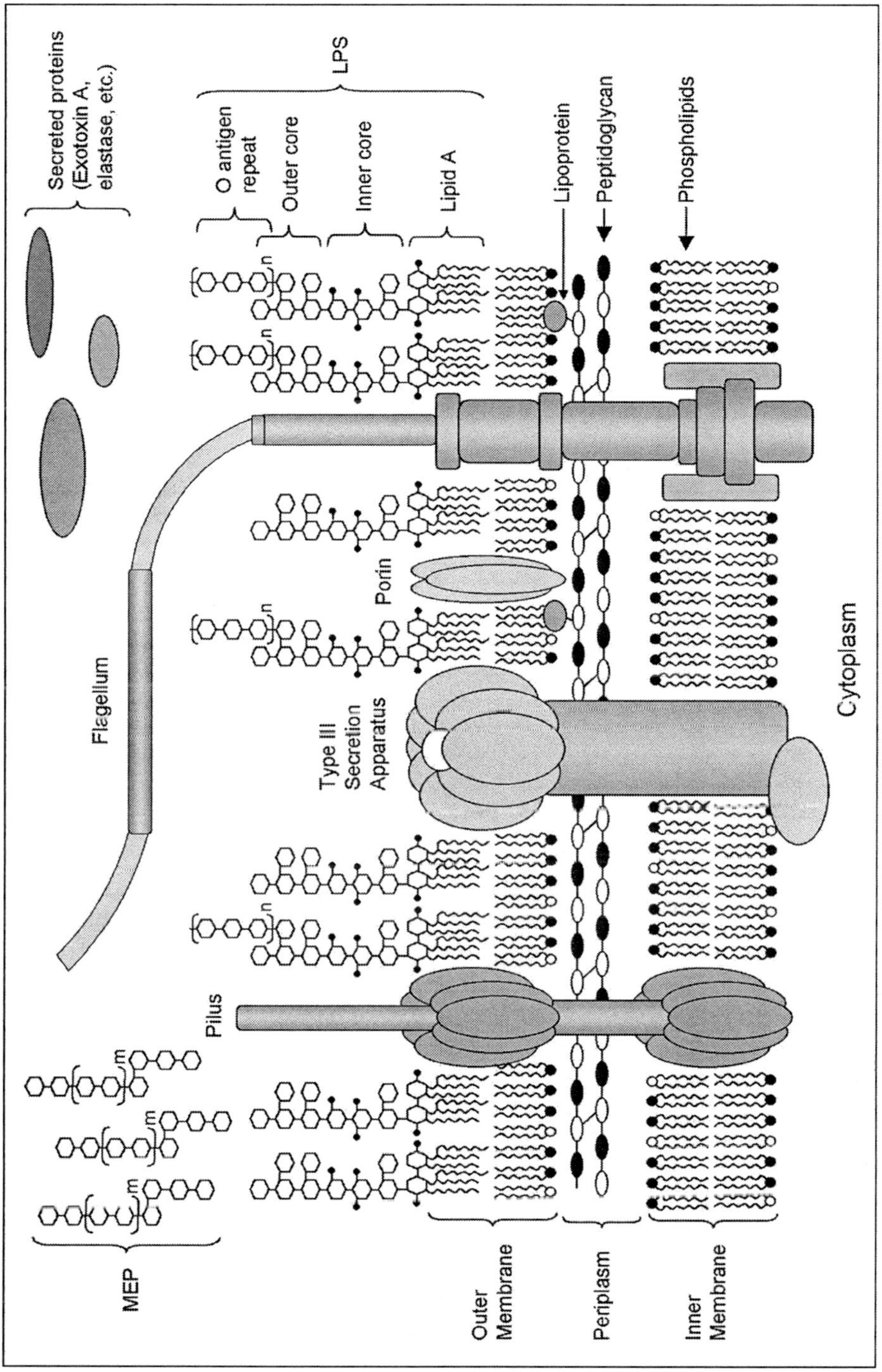

Figure 1. Schematic representation of the *P. aeruginosa* cell wall and secreted products highlighting potential vaccine targets. Abbreviations: LPS, lipopolysaccharide; MEP, mucoid expolysaccaride.

et al immunized rats with elastase peptides conjugated to KLH or TT and found in the rat agar bead chronic lung infection model that immunization with one of the peptide conjugates lead to less histopathological injury in the lung compared with controls. Again, the vaccine was studied using only one *P. aeruginosa* and one *Burkholderia cepacia* strain.[24]

LPS

The LPS of *P. aeruginosa* (Fig. 1) is similar to that of other Gram negative bacteria in that it contains three main regions – namely a lipid A backbone, the core (often divided into inner core and outer core, with the inner core attached to lipid A), and the O antigen (also known as O side chain or termed "B band" polysaccharide by some authors[25]). The O antigen is made up of di- to pentasaccharide repeating units and is heterogeneous in length. *P. aeruginosa* strains may be either LPS smooth, in which 5-15% of the LPS cores are substituted with long O side chains, or LPS rough, in which the LPS contains few, short, or no O side chains.[26,27] *P. aeruginosa* differs from Gram negative enteric bacteria in that an LPS-smooth strain has O side chains on less than 15% of the LPS molecules, with the majority of LPS molecules terminating with the outer core moieties.[26] Recent studies have indicated that *P. aeruginosa* strains actually produce two related glycoforms of the core oligosaccharide.[28] One of these appears to carry the site of attachment for the O side chain whereas the other glycoform is not substituted (Gerald B. Pier, unpublished observations).

Strains isolated from environmental sources and from acutely infected patients are usually LPS smooth and thereby serum resistant. In contrast, *P. aeruginosa* strains that cause chronic lung infections in cystic fibrosis (CF) patients are usually LPS rough and serum sensitive, although the initial infecting strain is LPS smooth.[29] It should be noted that although strains of *P. aeruginosa* infecting CF patients produce a rough LPS they also elaborate large quantities of an exopolysaccharide called mucoid exopolysaccharide (MEP) or alginate, an acetylated version of seaweed alginic acid. It is thought that MEP production substitutes for LPS O side chains in protecting the organism against complemented-mediated host defenses.

Based on chemical and serologic variations, the LPS O antigens of *P. aeruginosa* are currently classified into 20 serogroups, with many serogroups possessing subtype strains having subtle variations in the O antigen. Thus, there are over 30 subtypes (also called chemotypes) based on variable LPS O antigen chemical structures.[30-32] As an example, the O2 serogroup (which is also known as serogroup O2/O5/O16) is probably the most complex. Table 1 depicts the chemical structures of the O antigens of the 7 prototypic serogroup O2 subtype strains, most of which have O antigen repeats containing a related trisaccharide repeat unit. It has been suggested that in fact all of these related strains can produce the same, basic trisaccharide repeat unit, and that modifications that include O-acetylation, monosaccharide epimerization and variation in linkages that distinguish the subtypes may actually be post-synthetic modifications. This view is supported by structural analysis of the O antigen of several of the O2 strains, where the overall LPS molecular structures are comprised of mixed repeat units.[28] If this is the case, then it may be possible that in the presence of protective antibody to one variant structure, strains producing an altered structure that does not bind the antibody will be selected for. Furthermore, lysogenizing bacteriophage can mediate serogroup conversion of *P. aeruginosa* by altering O antigen biosynthesis.[33,34] There may be additional variability produced in vivo during infection that could further complicate our understanding of this situation. Thus, while the chemical composition of most of the LPS components made in vitro is known, use of these data for vaccine development is hampered by the lack of knowledge of the macromolecular structure and antigenic diversity that the organism undergoes during infection.

For many years, it has been clear that high-level immunity to infections due to LPS-smooth *P. aeruginosa* can be mediated by antibodies to the LPS O antigen.[35] A particularly striking illustration of the remarkably potent protective efficacy of LPS-based vaccines was seen in animal trials evaluating a *P. aeruginosa* outer membrane protein (OMP) F vaccine.[36] The OMP F preparation contained a low, but highly immunogenic dose of LPS, such that controls needed

Table 1. Structure of the related LPS O antigen trisaccharide repeat units found among members of the* P. aeruginosa *serogroup O2/O5/O16 strains

Strain	Subtype Epitope	Structure[a]
170003	2a,2b	-4)-β-D-Man(2NAc3N)A-(1-4)-β-D-Man(NAc)2-A(1-3)-β-D-FucNAc- (1- 3 | C=NHCH$_3$
IATS O16	2a, 2b,2e	-4)-β-D-Man(2NAc3N)A-(1-4)-β-D-Man(NAc)2-A(1-3)-β-D-FucNAc- (1- 3 | **4 |** C=NHCH$_3$ **OAc**
Fisher IT-3	2a,2c	-4)-β-D-Man(2NAc3N)A-(1-4)-α-**L-Gul**(NAc)2A-(1-3)-β-D-FucNAc- (1- 3 | C=NHCH$_3$
PAO1	2a,2d	-4)-β-D-Man(2NAc3N)A-(1-4)-β-D-Man(NAc)2A-(1-3)-α-D-FucNAc- (1- 3 | C=NHCH$_3$
170006	2a,2d,2e	-4)-β-D-Man(2NAc3N)A-(1-4)-α-**L-Gul**(NAc)2A-(1-3)-α-D-FucNAc- (1- 3 | C=NHCH$_3$
170007[b]	2a,2d,2f	-4)-β-D-Man(2NAc3N)A-(1-4)-β-D-Man(NAc)2A-(1-3)-α-D-FucNAc- (1- 3 | **4 |** C=NHCH$_3$ **OAc** -4)-α-**L-Gul**(2NAc3N)A-(1-4)-β-D-Man(NAc)2A-(1-3)-α-D-FucNAc-(1- 3 | 4 | C=NHCH$_3$ OAc
Fisher IT-7	-2a, ?	4)-α-**L-Gul**(2NAc3N)A-(1-4)-β-D-Man(NAc)2A-(1-3)-α-D-FucNAc-(1 3 | C=NHCH$_3$

[a]**Bold faced** type indicates features of a structure that distinguish it from a related structure of the same serogroup.
[b]The lower structure is also part of O-antigen of strain 170007; about 2:1 ratio of uper and lower structures.
Abbreviations: FucNAc, 2-acetamido-2,6-dideoxygalactose (N-acetyl fucosamine); Man(NAc)2A, 2,3 diacetamido-2,3-dideoxymannuronic acid; Man(2NAc3N)A, 2-acetamido-3-acetamidino-2,3 dideoxymannuronic acid; Gul(NAc)2A, 2,3-diacetamido-2,3-dideoxyguluronic acid; OAc, O-acetyl group.

to receive a comparable amount of LPS from the source-strain for the OMP F, strain PAO1.[36] The OMP F vaccine itself protected between 30% and 95% of burned mice against challenge doses up to 2 x 10^6 CFU (8 LD_{50}s) of 6 different *P. aeruginosa* serogroups. However, mice challenged with strain PAO1, which were also immune to the LPS O antigen of this strain, resisted a challenge dose of 3 x 10^{11} CFU, 5-6 orders of magnitude above the LD_{50} of this strain.[36] No other *P. aeruginosa* antigen has even come close to this level of protection in animal studies.

LPS-specific vaccine efforts began in the 1970s and focused on a heptavalent vaccine called Pseudogen (Parke Davis and Co.) prepared from LPS of seven different *P. aeruginosa* serogroups that were referred to as immunotypes. These 7 immunotypes appeared to comprise the range of LPS antigens found among the vast majority of strains causing infections. This vaccine was extensively studied in humans and showed some efficacy in nonrandomized trials among adult cancer and burn patients in preventing fatal infections from *P. aeruginosa*.[37,38] However, not surprisingly, there was significant toxicity associated with this LPS-based vaccine, and studies in patients with leukemia and cystic fibrosis showed no benefit.[39,40]

A general feature of studies using LPS as vaccine antigens is that protective epitopes have proven to be poorly immunogenic, while nonprotective or minimally protective O antigen epitopes often elicit the best immune responses. Although O antigen-based vaccines can elicit antibodies that are protective in animal models, this protection is generally seen only when the strains used to isolate the vaccine antigen are used in the challenge studies.[41-44] Broad-based protection against other strains, even subtypes within the same serogroup, is not reliably generated.[45,46] With these observations in mind, an O antigen-based vaccine would need to be more than 20-valent (probably more than 30-valent). However, efforts by our laboratory to make even a divalent vaccine have highlighted a potential problem with this approach — when related O antigens (in the form of purified high-molecular-weight O-polysaccharide) from strains within the same serogroup were combined, the opsonic-antibody response to each individual component was diminished.[45] The basis for this appears to be an antigenic-competition phenomenon that reduces the ability of B cells bearing surface IgM for the proper epitopes to be fully engaged.

Studies by Cryz and colleagues have shown that an octavalent O antigen-exotoxin A conjugate vaccine engendered opsonic antibody responses only against strains used to manufacture the vaccine and did not protect humans at risk for nosocomial *P. aeruginosa* infections after passive transfer of IgG isolated from vaccinated individuals.[42,47,48] While the basis for this negative outcome cannot be known, one possibility is that the octavalent vaccine did not elicit protective antibody against a sufficient number of *P. aeruginosa* serotypes. The octavalent O antigen-exotoxin A conjugate vaccine has been reported to show some encouraging efficacy in preventing colonization of cystic fibrosis with *P. aeruginosa* — after 6 years of clinical follow-up, 15/20 (75%) of historical age-matched controls and 8/23 (35%) of immunized subjects were classified as infected ($p = 0.022$).[49]

Immunotherapeutic strategies using components of LPS other than the O antigen have also been pursued. The core portion of *P. aeruginosa* LPS consists of two regions, an inner core containing phosphorylated L-glyero-D-*manno*-heptose and 3-deoxy-D-*manno*-octulosonic acid (KDO) and an outer core containing N-acetyl galactosamine substituted with alanine, glucose and rhamnose.[28,50-52] Subtle differences have been found between strains of different serogroups such as phosphorylation pattern and acetylation,[50,52] which could affect immunogenicity and protective efficacy. A human IgM monoclonal antibody with specificity for the outer core region was shown to protect mice from IP challenge with clinical isolates of *P. aeruginosa* of several different serogroups, and this protection correlated with opsonophagocytic activity.[53] However, the method of using IP administration of the monoclonal antibody coincident with IP administration of the inoculum suggests a rapid, but local clearance of the organisms in the peritoneum by antibodies in the peritoneum, raising questions regarding the true in vivo protective efficacy.

P. aeruginosa LPS contains an additional polysaccharide antigen known as the A band or common polysaccharide antigen (CPA).[54] CPA is common to most serogroups and is composed of a polymer of D-rhamnose monosaccharides. It appears that both O antigen and CPA are attached to the same lipid A/LPS core,[55] although others have disputed this.[54] A conjugate vaccine of a synthetic version of CPA conjugated to BSA showed no protective efficacy after passive immunotherapy in a mouse model of acute infection.[56]

Overall, while antibodies to LPS O antigens clearly mediated the best protective immunity to acute *P. aeruginosa* infections in almost all animal models studied,[16,41,44] correlates with human resistance to infection[57] and has shown tantalizing potential as a protective antigen in human clinical trials,[37,38] there have been many obstacles to making an LPS-based vaccine. The principal problem appears to be the variation in chemical, and thus serologic, O antigen structure, which impacts on both the diversity of the protective epitopes and the ability to produce nontoxic vaccines that elicit the needed spectrum of antibodies that are going to be protective against a majority of *P. aeruginosa* strains.

Mucoid Exopolysaccharide (MEP)

With the goal of protecting patients with CF from the ravages of chronic infection with mucoid *P. aeruginosa*, a number of investigators have focused on the MEP coat of *P. aeruginosa* characteristic of these mucoid strains. MEP is an acetylated polymer of β-(1-4) linked mannuronic and guluronic acids, with the ratios of mannuronic and guluronic acids and the degree of acetylation of the mannuronic acid hydroxyl groups varying among strains.[58,59] Interestingly, for a single strain, the ratio of mannuronic to guluronic acid appears fairly stable under a variety of growth conditions, whereas the degree of acetylation is more variable. How this affects the ability to generate protective immunity, and whether it provides the organism with an ability to avoid antibody-mediated host defenses is not known.

Animal studies conducted in 1990 showed that active and passive immunotherapeutic strategies that provide opsonic antibodies to MEP can protect mice and rats from chronic lung infection with mucoid *P. aeruginosa* encased in agar beads.[60] Others have also found that an MEP vaccine improves bacterial clearance in a similar rat model of chronic pneumonia.[61] A single MEP antigen appears capable of eliciting opsonic, thus potentially protective, antibodies against a large number of mucoid strains,[60] but whether sufficient titers to this putative common antigen can be provoked by a single vaccine component remains unclear. Interestingly, among a small subset of older (>12 years, by which time 60-80% of CF patients are chronically infected with mucoid *P. aeruginosa*), uninfected CF patients (approximately 5% of all patients), naturally acquired, MEP-specific opsonic antibodies are routinely present.[5,62] This contrasts to the chronically infected CF patients in whom the antibody response to MEP is composed almost entirely of nonopsonic antibodies.[5,62] These nonopsonic antibodies are also found in virtually all humans, indicating a common source of antigenic material. One conclusion of these studies was that in the presence of preexisting, nonopsonic antibodies to MEP, it was very difficult to produce opsonic antibodies to a different epitope. Thus, while a small percentage of CF patients fortuitously produce opsonic, MEP-specific, and apparently protective antibodies, most do not, possibly due to the near universal presence of naturally acquired, nonopsonic antibodies to MEP.

Studies in mice have supported this conclusion. Immunization of mice with high doses of purified MEP (50 μg) elicits only nonopsonic antibodies to mucoid *P. aeruginosa* whereas immunization with lower doses (1-10 μg) elicits both opsonic and nonopsonic antibodies. When mice are first immunized with a 50 μg dose of MEP and respond with only nonopsonic antibodies, follow-up immunizations with low doses (1-10 μg) of MEP that otherwise elicit opsonic antibodies in naïve mice did not do so.[63] The mechanism for this appears to be that in the presence of preexisting nonopsonic antibody, B cells with membrane IgM specific for the protective, opsonic epitopes of MEP bind the antigen after immunization and become targets for killing by $CD8^+$ cytotoxic T lymphocytes (CTL) via an antibody-dependent cytotoxicity mechanism.[64] The preexisting nonopsonic antibodies sensitize the CTL by binding to Fc receptors that are expressed on activated CTL, allowing the CTL to find the free, nonopsonic epitopes on the MEP bound to the B cell surface and kill the target B cell. Whether such a mechanism accounts for the poor human immune response to the protective epitopes on MEP is not known. Nonetheless, this work indicates that the successful chronic infection of the CF lung by mucoid *P. aeruginosa* proceeds in the presence of the inability of most CF patients to produce opsonic antibodies to MEP.

Human studies of a purified MEP vaccine have demonstrated that the antigen is safe and immunogenic under some circumstances. When a purified MEP vaccine was tested in humans at doses of 1-150 μg, it was well tolerated but only a minority (2 of 23) of vaccinees responded with long-lived (>6 month) increases in opsonic antibody titer.[65] Interestingly, continued studies of MEP vaccines in mice suggested that if only the highest molecular-weight polymers of

MEP were used in the vaccine, then opsonic antibodies could be generated in the presence of preexisting nonopsonic antibodies.[63] Thus, a second lot of MEP vaccine composed of only the highest molecular weight polymers of MEP was produced for human trials, and this vaccine was evaluated over a 10-250 μg dose range. Overall, the high molecular weight MEP vaccine provoked an opsonic antibody response in human volunteers of 30%, with 90% of men receiving 100 μg responding with opsonic antibody. Subsequently a comparable third lot was manufactured for administration to humans who would serve as plasma donors for manufacturing of intravenous immunoglobulin G (IVIgG) preparation for testing in infected CF patients. When given to hundreds of volunteers the vaccine was again safe but poorly immunogenic — only 35% of vaccines responded with measurable opsonic antibody, and for many of these the titers were quite low. Nonetheless, plasma was harvested from the putative "high responders" and manufactured into a hyperimmune IVIgG preparation that was administered monthly for one year to infected CF patients in a double-blind clinical trial. Controls received human serum albumin IV. After 1 year, an interim analysis showed no benefit, and the trial was halted. The negative results of this trial could reasonably be attributed to the overall low titer of the hyperimmune IVIgG preparation that was administered to many patients with fairly advanced disease, encompassing long-term, high level infection with mucoid *P. aeruginosa.* Under these circumstances there was unlikely to be any benefit from such a therapy. The negative results of that trial underscore the low immunogenicity of native MEP preparations and the pressing need for better MEP-based vaccines. Recent work suggests that the difference in the opsonic and nonopsonic antibodies is their epitope specificity – opsonic antibodies are directed towards the acetylated epitopes of MEP while nonopsonic antibodies are specific for the nonacetylated epitopes.[66] In addition, conjugation of MEP to carrier proteins appears to dramatically increase its immunogenicity.[67] These findings suggest avenues for design of more immunogenic MEP-based vaccines.

Outer Membrane Proteins (OMPs)

A number of *P. aeruginosa* vaccine strategies have focused on outer membrane proteins (OMPs), particularly OMPs F[36,68-76] and I,[69,77-79] both of which are antigenically conserved in all strains.[80] As noted above, some of the initial studies of OMPs as vaccines were convoluted by contamination of OMP preparations with low, but highly immunogenic levels of LPS. Nonetheless, these preparations did show some evidence of protection against strains expressing an LPS heterologous to that from which the OMP F was purified (strain PAO1). Efficacy was demonstrated using the OMP F vaccine in both a mouse IP challenge model[71] and a rat chronic lung infection model.[72] As controls received comparable amounts of the contaminating, heterologous PAO1 LPS, this vaccine indicated some efficacy against a range of *P. aeruginosa* strains representing the most common serogroups. Using two different versions of recombinant fusion proteins of OMPs F and I, von Specht and colleagues have shown that active immunization can protect neutropenic mice and passive immunization can protect SCID mice, both against a challenge dose 1000-fold above the LD_{50}.[73,74] Hughes et al used synthetic peptides of OMP F conjugated to KLH to immunize mice intranasally and found significant protection against acute pneumonia caused by a single strain.[75] Furthermore, a DNA vaccine encoding OMP F administered intradermally via "gene gun" demonstrated protection in a mouse model of chronic pulmonary infection with reduction in the presence of severe macroscopic lesions as well as in the number of bacteria present in the lungs,[76] although these workers were also performing challenges with only a single strain. Recombinant OMP I[79,81] and an F-I fusion protein[69] have advanced to human trials and have been shown to be well tolerated.

A *P. aeruginosa* vaccine called CFC-101 (CheilJedang Corp., Ichon, Korea) containing OMPs with molecular weights of 10-100 kDa from 4 *P. aeruginosa* strains of Fisher-Devlin immunotypes (IT) 1, 2, 3, and 6 has been extensively tested in animals and humans.[82-86] This vaccine contains less than 20 ng of LPS per mg protein. When CFC-101 was given to burn patients, the pooled antisera had modest opsonophagocytic killing activity (the highest killing percentage was 64%, with most sera mediating killing of ≤50%) and protected mice against IP challenge with a strain used to produce some of the components of the vaccine. However, the protection was not significantly different from that seen with serum from burn patients who received the control placebo vaccine.[85] This OMP-based vaccine was also used in a double-blind, placebo-controlled trial in burn patients of whom 19 received placebo and 76 received various doses and schedules of the CFC-101 vaccine.[86] In that trial, antibody levels to the vaccine antigens rose by 2.3-fold in the placebo group and 4.9 fold in the vaccine group. There was only 1 *P. aeruginosa* bacteremia (in the placebo group). The detection rate of *P. aeruginosa* in blood using nested PCR was significantly lower among immunized patients than placebo patients (6.1 vs. 40.0%, P<0.001). However, the clinical significance of a positive PCR for *P. aeruginosa* is unclear. Furthermore, the follow-up of patients in the trial was incomplete, analysis was not by intention-to-treat, and there were no data regarding clinical outcomes. Even more troubling are the exclusion from analysis and lack of further comment about or evaluation of a patient in the vaccine group who developed "an acute pulmonary complication" 3 days after the first injection. CFC-101 is similar to another vaccine called *P. aeruginosa* vaccine (PV) that was prepared from 4 strains (IT-1, 2, 6, and 7) using nearly identical methods to that for CFC-101.[87] Plasma from volunteers immunized with PV was reported to have some benefit in a case series of children and adults with *P. aeruginosa* infections not responding to conventional therapy.[88] The uncontrolled nature of that trial and the scant clinical data reported raise questions regarding the true efficacy of anti-PV immune plasma, as does the lack of follow-up studies.

An interesting although somewhat crude vaccine preparation called PEV-01 (Wellcome Research Laboratories) was prepared in the 1970s and extensively studied in animals and humans. PEV-01 was an EDTA-glycine extract of viable cells from each of 16 *P. aeruginosa* serogroups. Thus, it contained large amounts of both LPS and OMPs. PEV-01 conferred significant protection in mice against fatal *P. aeruginosa* infections when challenged with one of the strains included in the vaccine.[89] Vaccination with PEV-01 also protected guinea pigs from acute pneumonia caused by two clinical isolates from different serogroups, although both serogroups were contained in the vaccine.[90] When given to burned children and adults in India either actively or passively (as a hyperimmune globulin isolated from vaccinated volunteers) in a randomized trial, there was improved survival, particularly in the passively immunized children (mortality 0 of 18 versus 9 of 42 in controls).[91] However, MacIntyre et al showed the protective efficacy in mice was attributable to the LPS component of the vaccine, not the OMP component.[92] The PEV-01 vaccine was not further pursued for unclear reasons, and it is reasonable to conclude that it was more of an LPS-based protective immunogen than an OMP-based one.

Flagella

Motility was found to be particularly important in the pathogenesis of burn infections,[93] and *P. aeruginosa* produces only two serologically distinct types of flagella.[94] Using the burned mouse model, Holder and coworkers showed that active immunization with purified flagella protected mice from death when both flagella types were included in the vaccine.[95] A vaccine based on purified flagella has been produced and tested in humans (IMMUNO vaccine), and it appears to be safe and immunogenic.[96,97] A trial of the protective efficacy of this vaccine in CF patients is being carried out by Doering and colleagues in Europe, but the outcome will not be available until late 2002.[96] A flagellin-specific IgM monoclonal antibody, which recognized only 31% of clinical isolates, was shown to protect burned mice from death, and the protection was correlated in vitro with diminished *P. aeruginosa* motility.[98] A similar flagella-directed mAb also protected neutropenic mice from gut-derived *P. aeruginosa* sepsis[99] and from pneumonia,[100] but the protection from pneumonia was realized only when the mice also received an antibiotic.

Overall, flagella antigens appear to be very promising vaccine candidates, or at least a component of a multivalent anti-*P. aeruginosa* vaccine. Recent studies confirm a limited serologic and genetic diversity of *P. aeruginosa* flagella antigens.[101] Positive results in the European trial in CF patients will likely provide a large boost to the attractiveness of this vaccine approach. However, production of flagella can be variable; Luzar and Montie showed that chronically-infecting, mucoid *P. aeruginosa* strains from CF patients did not make flagella, making antigenic phase variation a potential confounding factor in developing a flagella-based vaccine.[102] The cap protein of flagella, the product of the *fliD* gene, mediates adherence of *P. aeruginosa* to mucin and is associated with a related major flagella protein produced from the *fliC* gene.[103] Studies to date with the flagella vaccines have not attributed protective efficacy to a particular component of the flagella structure, and it may be important to know this for further vaccine work with this antigen.

Pili

The type IV pili of *P. aeruginosa* are involved both in twitching motility and in attachment of *P. aeruginosa* to epithelial cells.[104,105] A synthetic, disulfide-linked pilin-C-terminal peptide was conjugated to tetanus toxin and found to modestly protect mice from challenge with a heterologous strain after active immunization.[106] This synthetic peptide was based on a relatively conserved region of the C terminus of the pilin monomer and was chosen as a target for vaccine development since this region appeared to mediate bacterial binding to mucins and epithelial cells. However, further studies have not been reported. The use of pili as vaccines is further confounded by results from the recent report of the crystal structure of the pilin monomer.[107] This report indicated that the C-terminal peptide was unlikely to be a surface structure on the outer side of the pilin, but was buried in the molecule's interior. While it is conceivable that this epitope is exposed upon contact with target receptors, the lack of this epitope on the pilin surface makes it unlikely to be a reasonable target for protective antibody.

Components of the Type III Secretion System

The type III secretion systems in Gram negative rods are involved in the translocation of toxic effector proteins into the cytoplasm of eukaryotic cells,[108] and this mechanism appears to be a major component of virulence.[109] Hence, neutralization of this toxicity should theoretically reduce the pathology generated by *P. aeruginosa* infection. The main effector proteins of the *P. aeruginosa* type III secretion system are the ADP-ribosyltransferases ExoS and ExoT and the adenylate cyclase ExoY, which are thought to disrupt host signal transduction.[110,111] Another component, with a high level of cytotoxicity, is the ExoU protein.[112,113] Interestingly, *exoS* and *exoU* appear to be mutually exclusive; *P. aeruginosa* strains have either one or the other.[109] The type III secretion system has been shown to be a significant virulence factor in murine models of *P. aeruginosa* burn infections[114] and in animal models of pneumonia and septic shock.[115,116]

In order to translocate the enzymatic or toxic type III secretion system effectors into target cells, Gram negative organisms with this system have to assemble additional proteins on the bacterial and target-cell surfaces. One of these is the PcrV component of the type III secretion system of *P. aeruginosa*, which is the homologue of another protein described in the type III secretion system of *Yersinia*. PcrV is primarily a translocation protein and, in *Yersinia*, seems to be a structural component that determines pore size of the type III secretion apparatus.[117] PcrV was over-expressed in *E. coli* and used for active and passive immunization studies in which significant protection against lung injury and death was seen in a mouse model of acute pneumonia.[118] Efficacy in this study did not extend much beyond a challenge dose that was only 10-fold above the LD_{50}, and only one strain (PA103) that is particularly virulent in mouse lung infections was evaluated. Therapeutic administration of anti-PcrV IgG or its $F(ab')_2$ fragments was recently shown to improve hemodynamic parameters and decrease lung injury and bacteremia in a rabbit model of pneumonia and septic shock.[119] Active immunization with PcrV also enhanced survival in the burned mouse model although was not effective against strains producing high levels of exotoxin A.[120] While much more remains to be done with this antigen, particularly extending its protective efficacy to a range of clinical isolates, the encouraging results to date suggest that the PcrV antigen may be a key component to an effective *P. aeruginosa* vaccine.

Other Aspects of Immunity to *P. aeruginosa*

Antitoxic immunity to secreted products of *P. aeruginosa* have, in general, shown poor protective efficacy. Antibody mediated immunity, particularly to LPS O antigens, has repeatedly been shown to be the predominant form of protection against *P. aeruginosa.* However, the inability to harness the protective efficacy of LPS O antigen-elicited antibodies into an effective, broadly protective vaccine using either LPS itself,[37] purified, immunogenic high-molecular weight O antigens[46] or O-antigen conjugate vaccines[48] suggests that other approaches are likely needed to try to elicit protective titers of LPS-specific antibodies to a sufficiently high percentage of clinical isolates. Antibody-mediated immunity to nonLPS-based antigens indicate the potential for generating protection using a limited number of antigens that are effective against a range of heterologous LPS serogroups, but the protection afforded by these vaccines has, as a rule, been of comparatively low potency. One potential conclusion from these findings is that antibody-mediated immunity may be insufficient for full-fledged immunity to *P. aeruginosa* and there might be an important role for cell-mediated immunity (CMI) in the control of these infections.

A potential biologically-relevant basis for a role for CMI has come from recent evidence indicating that *P. aeruginosa* readily enters lung and corneal epithelial cells during in vitro infection of cell cultures and in vivo infection of mice.[121,122] Of great interest is the finding that this cellular invasion is mediated by bacterial interactions with the cystic fibrosis transmembrane conductance regulator (CFTR).[123-125] The *CFTR* gene is, of course, mutated in patients with CF and the lack of a functional CFTR protein in airway epithelial cells has been proposed to be the basis for hypersusceptibility of CF patients to *P. aeruginosa* infection.[121,123,124] Not only does an intracellular phase of *P. aeruginosa* infection indicate a target for CMI effectors, but this may also be an important avenue for generating CMI, suggesting that effective vaccines may need to include a mechanism for inducing CMI. It has become increasingly clear in the past few years that immunogenic antigens are picked up from apoptotic cells following microbial uptake by these cells. The apoptotic cells are ingested by local dendritic cells (DCs) that then travel to regional lymphoid organs and process and present microbial antigens to T lymphocytes.[126,127] Bhardwaj and coworkers have shown that human DCs can ingest apoptotic cells, present antigens derived from these apoptotic cells to $CD8^+$ T cells, and stimulate potent cytotoxic T lymphocyte (CTL) responses.[128] In fact, a single injection of autologous antigen-pulsed dendritic cells rapidly generates specific $CD4^+$ and $CD8^+$ T cell responses in humans.[129] Following CFTR-mediated ingestion of *P. aeruginosa* by epithelial cells, an apoptotic response eventually ensues.[130-132] These cells may be a source of antigens for activation of *P. aeruginosa*-specific CMI. Thus, these new findings that *P. aeruginosa* induces apoptosis of infected epithelial cells indicate not only a need but a potential means to generate effective CMI.

Cytolysis of *P. aeruginosa*-infected cells by CTL might not alone be able to curtail the infection if viable organisms are released. However, human CTL have been found to possess granulysin, a granule-associated antimicrobial peptide with activity against many microbes, including bacterial pathogens.[133] Although a murine homologue of granulysin has not been described, similar effectors are likely to exist in the mouse. Indeed, recent evidence suggests that CTL clones derived from mice immunized with the *M. tuberculosis* 65-kD heat shock protein antigen can kill *M. tuberculosis* via a granule-derived factor.[134]

Specific T cell activity against Gram negative bacilli has been well documented in murine models of infections caused by *Salmonella enterica* serovar Typhimurium[135] and *Bordetella pertussis*[136] and in human infections caused by *Helicobacter pylori*.[137] In the realm of *P. aeruginosa* infections, a number of investigations have demonstrated T cell-mediated control in rodent models. In a series of 13 papers published in the late 1980s and early 1990s,[138-151] Markham and collaborators reported that a carbohydrate antigen (in the form of high-molecular-weight LPS O-antigen polysaccharide) could elicit *P. aeruginosa*-specific T cells capable of killing the organism in vitro and protecting neutropenic mice against infection. In the final paper of that series,[143] it was shown that cytophilic anti-LPS IgG on the T cell surface mediated immunity by an ADCC mechanism. Other studies have observed T cell-mediated control of *P. aeruginosa* using paraformaldehyde-killed *P. aeruginosa* as a vaccine given to rats orally or injected into Peyer's patches. These studies demonstrated that $CD4^+$ T cells conferred resistance to *P. aeruginosa* pneumonia.[152,153]

Protective *P. aeruginosa*-derived T cell epitopes have not been defined, although studies in humans in the early 1980s reported that the alkaline phosphatase of *P. aeruginosa*, a secreted protein, was the principle antigen recognized by clones of T cells derived by stimulation of peripheral blood mononuclear cells of healthy volunteers.[154] It should also be noted that other secreted products of *P. aeruginosa*, including ExoS and pyocyanin, have been shown to alter T lymphocyte function, with ExoS inducing proliferation[155] and apoptosis,[156] and pyocyanin stimulating proliferation at low concentrations but inhibiting proliferation at high concentrations.[157] The implications of these types of analysis are not clear.

Several investigators have focused on comparing susceptibility to *P. aeruginosa* infection in various strains of inbred mice prone to produce either a T-helper type 1 (T_H1) response (characterized by secretion of IFN-γ) or a T-helper type2 (T_H2) response (characterized by production of interleukin (IL)-4 and IL-10 cytokines). Stevenson and coworkers recently reported on results following generation of *P. aeruginosa*-specific $CD4^+$ T cell clones from lymph nodes and lungs of both C57BL/6 and BALB/c mice immunized either subcutaneously or intratracheally with heat-killed *P. aeruginosa*.[158] All the T-cell clones they isolated were T-cell receptor (TCR)-$\alpha\beta^+$. As expected, the T cell clones from the C57BL/6 mice displayed a T_H1 pattern of cytokine production, while those from BALB/c mice evinced a T_H2 pattern. These investigators had previously observed that the T_H1 C57BL/6 mice were more susceptible than the (T_H2) BALB/c mice to chronic bronchopulmonary infection with mucoid *P. aeruginosa* strain 508 enmeshed in agar beads[159] Lungs from the T_H1-prone C57BL/6 mice in this model showed extensive neutrophilic inflammation while those from the T_H2-prone BALB/c mice had very mild granulomatous inflammation.[160]

The situation is more complex, however, since others have found that T_H1-responding C3H/HeN mice were **less** susceptible to a similar *P. aeruginosa* lung infection than T_H2-responding BALB/c mice and the C3H/HeN mice were **more** likely to have normal lung histopathology.[161] That study used a different strain of *P. aeruginosa* (PAO 597, IATS O5, a mucoid derivative of strain PAO1) and did not report the IL-10 levels in the different mouse strains to confirm a bias to a particular T_H type. Thus, while the character of the T cell response is probably critical in determining the balance between minimal collateral tissue damage versus immune-mediated tissue destruction, the categorization of T_H1 versus T_H2 responses may be overly simplified. Indeed, several animal studies have suggested that the T_H2-associated cytokine IL-10 may be the most important factor in protecting lung tissue from damage during pneumonia caused by *P. aeruginosa* strains,[115,162] although one of the studies used a cytotoxic strain that produced the ExoU protein via the type III secretion system.[112,116] Further evidence of the complexity of these systems is that the T_H1-associated cytokine IFN-γ was found in another study to be necessary as a cofactor in mediating the protective effect of the T_H2-cytokine IL-10.[162]

Cell-mediated immunity also appears to play a role, although possibly detrimental, in corneal infections due to *P. aeruginosa*. Hazlett and coworkers observed that strains of inbred mice prone to T_H1 responses (C57BL/6 background) were **more** susceptible to late corneal perforation than strains prone to T_H2 responses (BALB/c background).[163] A cellular infiltrate of $CD4^+$ and $CD8^+$ T cells, some staining positive for the IL-2 receptor (CD25), was noted only in the more susceptible T_H1 responders. The T cell-associated susceptibility to perforation appeared to be mediated by $CD4^+$ T cells, as shown by the lack of an effect on pathology in CD8 knockout mice and in studies using in vivo depletion of T cells with either anti-CD4 or anti-CD8 monoclonal antibodies. In these studies it was reported that CD4-depletion improved pathology while the CD8 depletion had no effect.[164]

The seemingly conflicting roles of T cells in the lung versus the eye might be explained by the so-called "immune privileged" status of the eye and the role of apoptotic pathways mediated by the factors Fas (CD95) and its ligand, Fas ligand (CD95L). Epithelial and endothelial cells in the cornea constitutively express CD95L in order to eliminate CD95-expressing T cells entering that tissue, to prevent potentially destructive effects of immune T cells.[165,166] In contrast, in the lung, these pathways of T cell-mediated apoptosis likely involves CTL expressing CD95L to induce cell death by cross linking CD95 on the surface of target cells such as infected lung epithelial cells. However, effector CTL also express CD95, making them susceptible to CD95L-mediated cytolysis if this ligand is expressed by the target cell. Thus, the cells resident in the eye that constitutively produce CD95L are able to kill potentially destructive CTL before collateral damage to the sensitive tissues of the eye ensues. In the anterior chamber of the eye, CD95L-induced apoptosis of invading T cells has also been shown to stimulate IL-10 production by the apoptotic T cells with subsequent induction of T_H2 responses and, thereby, minimization of immune-mediated tissue damage.[167]

In the lung, Grassme et al have shown a critical role for expression of both CD95 and CD95L in resistance to *P. aeruginosa* pneumonia and sepsis.[132] Using mice defective in either CD95 or CD95L they showed both strains had low apoptosis in lung epithelial cells and a consequent rapid development of pneumonia and sepsis in the deficient animals compared to wild-type controls. Again this study suggests a CD95-CD95L interaction in the lung during *P. aeruginosa* infection may be a critical component of effective resistance to infection. Interestingly, a recent study reported increased expression of CD95L in the airway epithelial cells of CF humans,[168] but the significance of this finding has not been determined.

The importance of cellular immunity in the pathogenesis and control of *P. aeruginosa* infections is also suggested by several reports of defective cellular immunity to *P. aeruginosa* in patients with cystic fibrosis, although the etiology and consequences of these abnormalities are unclear. Studies in the 1970s, prior to the identification of the CF gene, found that T cell responses to gentamicin-killed *P. aeruginosa* were absent in CF patients with advanced disease despite strong responses to T-cell mitogens and to other bacterial antigens such as heat-killed *Staphylococcus aureus*, Group A Streptococcus, and *H. influenzae*.[169,170] Other investigators reported that CF patients, regardless of severity of lung disease or colonization with *P. aeruginosa*, had significantly lower percentage of overall $CD4^+$ T cells and had T cells that displayed decreased allogeneic T cell-mediated cytotoxic responses.[171] The defective T cell responses found in CF patients might be related to an intrinsic defect in CF lymphocytes. Indeed, a Cl^- conductance due to CFTR is present in both T and B lymphocytes,[172] is cell-cycle specific (maximal in G_1), is activated by nitric oxide,[173] and is defective in lymphocytes from CF patients, a state correctable by transfection of isolated lymphocytes with wild-type CFTR.[174] The physiologic relevance of CFTR expression in lymphocytes is unknown, although Cl^- transport in general has been shown to be involved in lymphocyte activation and CTL activity. Gardner and colleagues have also shown that human $CD4^+$ T cell clones from CF patients secreted 45% less IL-10 than normal T cells after activation with Con A or anti-CD3 antibody plus phorbol esters and hypothesized that defective IL-10-mediated inflammatory effects might contribute to sustained inflammation in CF airways.[175,176] Despite these data regarding intrinsic defects in CF T cells, it is difficult to rationalize how such defects could account for the high specificity of infection by *P. aeruginosa* in CF patients.

Vaccine Approaches to Elicit Antibody-Mediated and Cell-Mediated Immunity

Dendritic Cell-Based Immunization

Recent work by Crystal and coworkers has focused on using isolated dendritic cells (DCs) to deliver *P. aeruginosa* antigens and stimulate immunity.[177-180] In the initial studies,[177] unmodified bone marrow-derived DCs were incubated with *P. aeruginosa* in vitro and then administered intravenously to syngeneic mice. Upon lung challenge with the immunizing strain (PAO1) using the agar bead model, unimmunized control mice and mice that had previously received naive DC or DC stimulated with commercially-prepared LPS or *E. coli* cells died within 72 h. In contrast, 45% of mice receiving *P. aeruginosa*-pulsed DC survived. Studies with knockout mice suggested that $CD4^+$ T cells but not $CD8^+$ T cells were important for this protection. The LD_{50} in their infection model was not indicated, so the potency of protection is unclear.

In other experiments,[178,179] these workers used DCs expressing the CD40 ligand (CD40L) following transfection with DNA for this surface protein. They found that *P. aeruginosa*-specific antibodies and protection against lung infection with the immunizing strain (agar-bead encased) could be generated without $CD4^+$ T cell help.[178] The protection could be transferred by immune serum or by adoptive transfer of immune splenic B cells (including into CD4 knockout mice). Again, the potency of protection was not assessed, although there are indications that the protective efficacy of unmodified DCs was not very high since challenge of the empty vector control group with a dose 4-fold above that used in the unmodified DC experiments[177] resulted in no protection. The CD40L on the DCs is thought to interact with CD40 on B cells to generate humoral immunity without T cell help.[181-183] The protection after immunization with CD40L-expressing DCs pulsed with *P. aeruginosa* could extend to a strain not used for immunization,[179] but these assessments were limited by the fact that only two challenge strains were evaluated (PAO1 and a serogroup O3 isolate called PA514 from a CF patient). Further studies by the same group demonstrated that immunization with *P. aeruginosa*-pulsed DCs transfected with DNA encoding macrophage-derived chemokine (MDC), a T_H2 T cell chemoattractant, elicited high levels of serum anti-*P. aeruginosa* antibodies and protection from a lethal respiratory challenge, including significant but not absolute cross-protection against different strains.[180] This protective immunity could be transferred by immune serum or by adoptive transfer of immune splenocytes, which required $CD4^+$ T cells, B cells, and IL-4, but not $CD8^+$ T cells and IL-12

While these DC-based vaccine strategies have revealed some important insights into how DCs can present *P. aeruginosa* antigens and elicit immunity, the vaccine potential of this approach seems impractical, as one would need to isolate and grow DC from potential vaccinees, pulse them with *P. aeruginosa*, and then inject them into the DC donors. Furthermore, if transfection with CD40L or MCP DNA is needed, this would further complicate this approach and might even be harmful, potentially causing a CD40L-mediated lymphoproliferative disorder[184] or lung disease[185] or MCP-mediated atopic disease.[186]

Live, Attenuated Vaccines

To explore the humoral and cellular immunity generated by the intracellular phase of *P. aeruginosa* infections, we and collaborators have recently designed live, attenuated *P. aeruginosa* vaccine strains that we postulated could exploit both the extracellular and intracellular phases of infection and elicit a broadly protective immune response, including both antibody and potent cellular immune effectors. The approach was based on producing mutations in the *aroA* gene, which encodes an enzyme essential for the synthesis of aromatic amino acids (5-enolpyruvylshikimate 3-phosphate synthase of the shikimate pathway). In the absence of these amino acids, such as occurs in host tissues, the organisms cannot grow. This approach has been utilized with several other pathogens, including *Salmonella* species[187] and *Aeromonas hydrophila*,[188] for the production of live, attenuated vaccine strains. In fact, in the *Salmonella enterica* serovar Typhimurium system, *aroA* deletants have been used as delivery vehicles to vaccinate mice against plasmid-encoded foreign proteins, with subsequent generation of broad cellular immunity against the encoded antigen.[189,190] Although single *aroA* deletants in *Salmonella enterica* serovar Typhi retain sufficient virulence to make them unacceptable as human vaccines, the intrinsically lower virulence of *P. aeruginosa* for healthy humans was predicted to allow single *aroA* deletants to be sufficiently attenuated to permit study in animal models.

To produce *aroA* deletants in *P. aeruginosa*, we used a gene replacement system based on the Flp recombinase to construct an unmarked *aroA* deletion mutant of the *P. aeruginosa* serogroup O2/O5 strain PAO1.[191] The resultant *aroA* deletion mutant of PAO1 is designated PAO1Δ*aroA*. The *aroA* deletion was confirmed by both PCR and failure of the mutant to grow on minimal media lacking aromatic amino acids.

When evaluated for safety and immunogenicity in mice, PAO1Δ*aroA* could be applied either intranasally (IN) or IP at doses up to 5 X 10^9 CFU per mouse without adverse effects. No dissemination of PAO1Δ*aroA* to blood, liver, or spleen was detected after IN application, and histological evidence of pneumonia was minimal.

Intranasal immunization of mice and rabbits elicited high titers of IgG to whole bacterial cells and to heat-stable bacterial antigens of all seven prototypic *P. aeruginosa* serogroup O2/O5 strains. The mouse antisera mediated potent phagocytic killing of most of the prototypic serogroup O2/O5 strains, while the rabbit antisera mediated phagocytic killing of several serogroup-heterologous (i.e., nonO2/O5) strains in addition to killing all O2/O5 strains. Following IN immunization with PAO1Δ*aroA*, mice were challenged IN with a recombinant version of *P. aeruginosa* strain PAO1, whose virulence was increased 50-fold by transforming the strain with plasmid pUCP19exoUspcU to produce the ExoU cytotoxin.[116] PAO1Δ*aroA* immunized mice were fully protected against challenge when compared with 100% mortality of those similarly immunized with *E. coli* HB101. IP immunization was also completely protective against challenge with PAO1(pUCP19exoUspcU) . Currently this and other *aroA* mutant strains of *P. aeruginosa* are being further evaluated for safety and to determine the mechanisms of immunity elicited by them. If safe and effective, a multivalent cocktail of live attenuated *P. aeruginosa* strains covering the gamut of protective antigens may be an approach that can be tried in humans.

Considerations and Conclusions

In all of the vaccine development work considered so far, the focus has been on identifying protective antigens and finding an effective and safe means to generate immunity. Almost all of the studies have been in animals and the few human studies conducted to date have either been failures,[48] inconclusive,[37,38] or not followed up.[91,192] Underlying these situations is likely the complexity of developing a vaccine for both a nosocomial pathogen and a related, but with a distinct phenotype, pathogen for CF patients. Probably two of the most vexing issues are simply the numbers of patients needed to conduct a clinical trial and the issue of who will be vaccinated and what will be the outcome. In the nosocomial setting active vaccination is unlikely to be practical since the target population, patients in intensive care units, cannot be identified sufficiently ahead of time. Also, many of these patients are immunocompromised and thus likely to be poorly responsive to vaccines. While a passive therapeutic approach may seem feasible, it is unlikely that a broad enough spectrum of antibodies to protective antigens can be reasonably produced in a cost effective manner using either IVIgG or human monoclonal antibodies with current technology. If CMI is needed for full immunity against pneumonia and sepsis, then an active vaccination approach is mandated since there are no current means to adoptively transfer CMI in humans. Finally, many patients at risk for *P. aeruginosa* infection have severe underlying disease and determining a reduction in mortality attributable to *P. aeruginosa* infection is not straightforward. Increased survival of these patients may be short lived in the face of their underlying disease, and there are clear ethical dilemmas associated with use of therapies that only prolong life by a short amount.

In the setting of CF it may be more reasonable to pursue a vaccination program if one targets patients diagnosed at an early age prior to onset of much lung damage. Expanded use of diagnostic tests for CF in newborns increases the likelihood of identifying candidates for vaccination. The current trial of a flagella vaccine in CF points out the feasibility of this approach.[96] Concerns here are principally focused on two issues: safety and a reasonable outcome measure. Beyond the usual safety considerations for any vaccine, in CF much of the pathology is due to immune-mediated inflammation. A vaccine that fails to provide protection but elicits antibodies that exacerbate inflammation could be more detrimental then doing nothing. In terms of outcome measures, the course of CF lung disease is highly variable and many patients do quite well in spite of being colonized and infected with *P. aeruginosa*. While the outcome in the flagella vaccine trial will be the rate of positive throat cultures for *P. aeruginosa*, this measure may not give any indication of a desired effect — decreased morbidity and increased life expectancy. The former outcome is difficult to measure as there are many factors to consider, although likely factors could be effect on the forced expiratory volume in one second (FEV_1), hospitalizations, density of *P. aeruginosa* in sputum, and use of antibiotics. Increased life expectancy is essentially impossible to determine in a clinical trial as it would take well over 30 years to document an increase in the current life expectance of about 31 years.[193] Increasing use of routine antibiotic administration to CF patients once they have become infected with *P. aeruginosa* would further complicate the outcome measures. There is no consensus on what outcome measure for a *P. aeruginosa* vaccine trial in CF should be.

Another issue is simply one of numbers. Obviously, the higher the protective efficacy of a vaccine the smaller numbers of patients would need to be enrolled in a clinical trial. Many of the vaccines investigated to date show only modest efficacy in animals and the most potent ones, LPS O antigens and MEP, have been problematic in their own right. The clinical trial of the LPS-based IVIgG passive therapy for *P. aeruginosa* infection in ICU patients was halted because the number of patients needed to demonstrate an effect was simply too large.[48] A vaccine efficacy of much less than 60% would probably not be acceptable, although one could argue that in CF efficacy as low as 30-40% could be considered to be a positive outcome. But with lower efficacy rates the number of patients needed in the trial increases dramatically. In one recent study on the use of inhaled tobramycin in CF, 520 patients with an average age of 21 were enrolled to achieve an increase in FEV_1 of 10%, a decrease of 0.8 $\log_{10}$ CFU *P. aeruginosa* in the sputum, and a 26% (95 percent confidence interval, 2 to 43 percent) decrease in hospitalizations.[194] If comparable numbers of very young CF patients were needed for similar outcomes in a vaccine trial, this would mean identifying over half of the CF patients less than one year old in the U.S., vaccinating them and following them for 5 or more years before the control group will show significant enough pathology to be different from the vaccine group. There are of course many other practical considerations for a vaccine trial for *P. aeruginosa*, but the preeminent ones are who to vaccinate and what will be a desirable outcome measure.

The need and desire for an effective *P. aeruginosa* vaccine is clear. The practicality of getting there is not. Many candidate antigens exist and sorting out which ones are worthy of investing in expensive clinical trials is a formidable task. Another consideration may be something as simple as ownership of intellectual rights and patent protection — companies may be more willing to invest in a trial of less promising vaccines if they have a better patent protection for that vaccine. Nonetheless a large array of candidate antigens has been identified, newer means of delivery to produce broad-based immunity are being developed, and at least one vaccine clinical trial in CF patients is proceeding. Particularly in this latter setting an effective vaccine is needed. Success will be hard to judge but as experience accumulates in defining the course of CF lung disease and preventing and treating *P. aeruginosa* infection, it is expected that improvements in quality of life and life expectancy will begin to be seen, and vaccine interventions that lead to similar positive changes in outcome could be validated based on the effectiveness outcomes derived from these other various approaches.

References

1. Richards MJ, Edwards JR, Culver DH et al. Nosocomial infections in medical intensive care units in the United States. National Nosocomial Infections Surveillance System. Crit Care Med 1999; 27(5):887-892.
2. Foca M, Jakob K, Whittier S et al. Endemic Pseudomonas aeruginosa infection in a neonatal intensive care unit. N Engl J Med 2000; 343(10):695-700.
3. Elishoov H, Or R, Strauss N et al. Nosocomial colonization, septicemia, and Hickman/Broviac catheter-related infections in bone marrow transplant recipients. A 5-year prospective study. Medicine 1998; 77(2):83-101.
4. Afessa B, Green B. Bacterial pneumonia in hospitalized patients with HIV infection: the Pulmonary Complications, ICU Support, and Prognostic Factors of Hospitalized Patients with HIV (PIP) Study. Chest 2000; 117(4):1017-1022.
5. Parad RB, Gerard CJ, Zurakowski D et al. Pulmonary outcome in cystic fibrosis is influenced primarily by mucoid Pseudomonas aeruginosa infection and immune status and only modestly by genotype. Infect Immun 1999; 67(9):4744-4750.
6. Schein OD, Glynn RJ, Seddon JM et al. The relative risk of ulcerative keratitis among users of daily-wear and extended-wear soft contact lenses. N Engl J Med 1989; 321:773-778.
7. Poggio EC, Glynn RJ, Schein OD et al. The incidence of ulcerative keratitis among users of daily-wear and extended-wear soft contact lenses. N Engl J Med 1989; 321:779-783.
8. Rello J, Rue M, Jubert P et al. Survival in patients with nosocomial pneumonia: impact of the severity of illness and the etiologic agent. Crit Care Med 1997; 25(11):1862-1867.
9. Hancock RE, Woodruff WA. Roles of porin and beta-lactamase in beta-lactam resistance of Pseudomonas aeruginosa. Rev Infect Dis 1988; 10(4):770-775.
10. Poole K, Krebes K, McNally C et al. Multiple antibiotic resistance in Pseudomonas aeruginosa: Evidence for involvement of an efflux operon. J Bacteriol 1993; 175(22):7363-7372.
11. Liu PV. Exotoxins of Pseudomonas aeruginosa I. Factors which influence the production of exotoxin A. J Infect Dis 1973; 128:506-513.
12. Snell K, Holder IA, Leppla SA et al. Role of exotoxin and protease as possible virulence factors in experimental infections with Pseudomonas aeruginosa. Infect Immun 1978; 19:839-845.
13. Bartell PF, Orr TE, Garcia M. The lethal events in experimental Pseudomonas aeruginosa infection of mice. J Infect Dis 1968; 118(2):165-172.
14. Stieritz DD, Holder IA. Experimental studies of the pathogenesis of Pseudomonas aeruginosa infection: Evidence for the in-vivo production of a lethal toxin. J Med Micro 1978; 11(2):101-109.
15. Pavlovskis OR, Edman DC, Leppla SH et al. Protection against experimental Pseudomonas aeruginosa infection in mice by active immunization with exotoxin A toxoids. Infect Immun 1981; 32(2):681-689.
16. Cryz SJ, Jr., Furer E, Germanier R. Passive protection against Pseudomonas aeruginosa infection in an experimental leukopenic mouse model. Infect Immun 1983; 40(2):659-664.
17. Cryz SJ, Jr., Furer E, Germanier R. Protection against Pseudomonas aeruginosa infection in a murine burn wound sepsis model by passive transfer of antitoxin A, antielastase, and antilipopolysaccharide. Infect Immun 1983; 39(3):1072-1079.
18. Fattom AI, Sarwar J, Ortiz A et al. A Staphylococcus aureus capsular polysaccharide (CP) vaccine and CP-specific antibodies protect mice against bacterial challenge. Infect Immun 1996; 64(5):1659-1665.
19. Wretlind B, Pavlovskis OR. The role of proteases and exotoxin A in the pathogenicity of Pseudomonas aeruginosa infections. Scand J Infect Dis Suppl 1981; 29:13-19.
20. Wretlind B, Pavlovskis OR. Pseudomonas aeruginosa elastase and its role in Pseudomonas infections. Rev Infect Dis 1983; 5 Suppl 5:S998-S1004.
21. Blackwood LL, Stone RM, Iglewski BH et al. Evaluation of Pseudomonas aeruginosa exotoxin A and elastase as virulence factors in acute lung infection. Infect Immun 1983; 39(1):198-201.
22. Matsumoto T, Tateda K, Furuya N et al. Efficacies of alkaline protease, elastase and exotoxin A toxoid vaccines against gut-derived Pseudomonas aeruginosa sepsis in mice. J Med Micro 1998; 47(4):303-308.
23. Kawamoto S, Shibano Y, Fukushima J et al. Site-directed mutagenesis of glu-141 and his-223 in Pseudomonas aeruginosa elastase: Catalytic activity, processing, and protective activity of the elastase against Pseudomonas infection. Infect Immun 1993; 61:1400-1405.
24. Sokol PA, Kooi C, Hodges RS et al. Immunization with a Pseudomonas aeruginosa elastase peptide reduces severity of experimental lung infections due to P. aeruginosa or Burkholderia cepacia. J Infect Dis 2000; 181(5):1682-1692.

25. Rocchetta HL, Burrows LL, Lam JS. Genetics of O-antigen biosynthesis in Pseudomonas aeruginosa. Microbiol Mol Biol Rev 1999; 63(3):523-553.
26. Wilkinson SG. Composition and structure of lipopolysaccharides from Pseudomonas aeruginosa. Rev Infect Dis 1983; 5Supp5:S941-S947.
27. Rivera M, Bryan LE, Hancock RE et al. Heterogeneity of lipopolysaccharides from Pseudomonas aeruginosa: Analysis of lipopolysaccharide chain length. J Bacteriol 1988; 170(2):512-521.
28. Sadovskaya I, Brisson JR, Thibault P et al. Structural characterization of the outer core and the O-chain linkage region of lipopolysaccharide from Pseudomonas aeruginosa serotype O5. Eur J Biochem 2000; 267(6):1640-1650.
29. Hancock RE, Mutharia LM, Chan L et al. Pseudomonas aeruginosa isolates from patients with cystic fibrosis: A class of serum-sensitive, nontypeable strains deficient in lipopolysaccharide O side chains. Infect Immun 1983; 42(1):170-177.
30. Knirel YA. Polysaccharide antigens of Pseudomonas aeruginosa. CRC Crit Rev Microbiol 1990; 17:273-304.
31. Knirel YA, Vinogradov EV, Kocharova NA et al. The structure of O-specific polysaccharides and serological classification of Pseudomonas aeruginosa (a review). Acta Microbiol Hung 1988; 35(1):3-24.
32. Stanislavsky ES, Lam JS. Pseudomonas aeruginosa antigens as potential vaccines. FEMS Micro Rev 1997; 21(3):243-77.
33. Kuzio J, Kropinski AM. O-antigen conversion in Pseudomonas aeruginosa PAO1 by bacteriophage D3. J Bacteriol 1983; 155(1):203-212.
34. Newton GJ, Daniels C, Burrows LL et al. Three-component-mediated serotype conversion in Pseudomonas aeruginosa by bacteriophage D3. Mol Microbiol 2001; 39(5):1237-1247.
35. Fisher MW, Devlin HB, Gnabski F. New immunotype schema for Pseudomonas aeruginosa based on protective antigens. J Bacteriol 1969; 98:835-836.
36. Matthews-Greer JM, Gilleland HE, Jr. Outer membrane protein F (porin) preparation of Pseudomonas aeruginosa as a protective vaccine against heterologous immunotype strains in a burned mouse model. J Infect Dis 1987; 155(6):1282-1291.
37. Alexander JW, Fisher MW, MacMillan BG. Immunological control of Pseudomonas infection in burn patients: a clinical evaluation. Arch Surgery 1971; 102(1):31-35.
38. Young LS, Meyer RD, Armstrong D. Pseudomonas aeruginosa vaccine in cancer patients. Ann Intern Med 1973; 79(4):518-527.
39. Haghbin M, Armstrong D, Murphy ML. Controlled prospective trial of Pseudomonas aeruginosa vaccine in children with acute leukemia. Cancer 1973; 32(4):761-766.
40. Pennington JE, Reynolds HY, Wood RE et al. Use of a Pseudomonas aeruginosa vaccine in pateints with acute leukemia and cystic fibrosis. Am J Med 1975; 58(5):629-636.
41. Cryz SJ, Jr., Furer E, Germanier R. Protection against fatal Pseudomonas aeruginosa burn wound sepsis by immunization with lipopolysaccharide and high-molecular-weight polysaccharide. Infect Immun 1984; 43(3):795-799.
42. Cryz SJ, Jr., Furer E, Sadoff JC et al. Production and characterization of a human hyperimmune intravenous immunoglobulin against Pseudomonas aeruginosa and Klebsiella species. J Infect Dis 1991; 163(5):1055-1061.
43. Pier GB, Pollack M. Isolation, structure, and immunogenicity of Pseudomonas aeruginosa immunotype 4 high-molecular-weight polysaccharide. Infect Immun 1989; 57(2):426-431.
44. Pier GB, Thomas D, Small G et al. In vitro and in vivo activity of polyclonal and monoclonal human immunoglobulins G, M, and A against Pseudomonas aeruginosa lipopolysaccharide. Infect Immun 1989; 57(1):174-179.
45. Hatano K, Pier GB.Complex serology and immune response of mice to variant high-molecular-weight O polysaccharides isolated from Pseudomonas aeruginosa serogroup O2 strains. Infect Immun 1998; 66(8):3719-3726.
46. Hatano K, Boisot S, DesJardins D et al. Immunogenic and antigenic properties of a heptavalent high-molecular-weight O-polysaccharide vaccine derived from Pseudomonas aeruginosa. Infect Immun 1994; 62(9):3608-3616.
47. Cryz SJ, Jr., Sadoff JC, Furer E. Octavalent Pseudomonas aeruginosa O-polysaccharide-toxin A conjugate vaccine. Micro Pathogen 1989; 6(1):75-80.
48. Donta ST, Peduzzi P, Cross AS et al. Immunoprophylaxis against Klebsiella and Pseudomonas aeruginosa infections. The Federal Hyperimmune Immunoglobulin Trial Study Group. J Infect Dis 1996; 174(3):537-43.
49. Cryz SJ, Jr., Lang A, Rudeberg A et al. Immunization of cystic fibrosis patients with a Pseudomonas aeruginosa O-polysaccharide-toxin A conjugate vaccine. Behring Inst Mitt 1997; (98):345-349.

50. Masoud H, Sadovskaya I, de Kievit T et al. Structural elucidation of the lipopolysaccharide core region of the O-chain-deficient mutant strain A28 from Pseudomonas aeruginosa serotype 06 (International Antigenic Typing Scheme). J Bacteriol 1995; 177(23):6718-6726.
51. Sadovskaya I, Brisson JR, Lam JS et al. Structural elucidation of the lipopolysaccharide core regions of the wild-type strain PAO1 and O-chain-deficient mutant strains AK1401 and AK1012 from Pseudomonas aeruginosa serotype O5. Eur J Biochem 1998; 255(3):673-684.
52. Knirel YA, Bystrova OV, Shashkov AS et al. Structural analysis of the lipopolysaccharide core of a rough, cystic fibrosis isolate of Pseudomonas aeruginosa. Eur J Biochem 2001; 268(17):4708-4719.
53. Terashima M, Uezumi I, Tomio T et al. A protective human monoclonal antibody directed to the outer core region of Pseudomonas aeruginosa lipopolysaccharide. Infect Immun 1991; 59(1):1-6.
54. Rivera M, McGroarty EJ. Analysis of a common-antigen lipopolysaccharide from Pseudomonas aeruginosa. J Bacteriol 1989; 171:2244-2248.
55. Hatano K, Goldberg JB, Pier GB. Pseudomonas aeruginosa lipopolysaccharide: evidence that the O side chains and common antigens are on the same molecule. J Bacteriol 1993; 175(16):5117-5128.
56. Makarenko TA, Kocharova NA, Edvabnaya LS et al. Immunological studies of an artificial antigen with specificity of a common polysaccharide antigen of Pseudomonas aeruginosa. FEMS Immunol Med Micro 1993; 7(3):251-256.
57. Pollack M, Young LS. Protective activity of antibodies to exotoxin A and lipopolysaccharide at the onset of Pseudomonas aeruginosa septicemia in man. J Clin Invest 1979; 63:276-286.
58. Russell NJ, Gacesa P. Chemistry and biology of the alginate of mucoid strains of Pseudomonas aeruginosa in cystic fibrosis. Mol Aspects Med 1988; 10(1):1-91.
59. Sherbrock-Cox V, Russell NJ, Gacesa P. The purification and chemical characterisation of the alginate present in extracellular material produced by mucoid strains of Pseudomonas aeruginosa. Carbohydr Res 1984; 135(1):147-154.
60. Pier GB, Small GJ, Warren HB. Protection against mucoid Pseudomonas aeruginosa in rodent models of endobronchial infections. Science 1990; 249(4968):537-540.
61. Johansen HK, Espersen F, Cryz SJ, Jr. et al. Immunization with Pseudomonas aeruginosa vaccines and adjuvant can modulate the type of inflammatory response subsequent to infection. Infect Immun 1994; 62(8):3146-3155.
62. Pier GB, Saunders JM, Ames P et al. Opsonophagocytic killing antibody to Pseudomonas aeruginosa mucoid exopolysaccharide in older noncolonized patients with cystic fibrosis. New Engl J Med 1987; 317(13):793-798.
63. Garner CV, DesJardins D, Pier GB. Immunogenic properties of Pseudomonas aeruginosa mucoid exopolysaccharide. Infect Immun 1990; 58(6):1835-1842.
64. Pier GB, Takeda S, Grout M et al. Immune complexes from immunized mice and infected cystic fibrosis patients mediate murine and human T cell killing of hybridomas producing protective, opsonic antibody to Pseudomonas aeruginosa. J Clin Invest 1993; 91(3):1079-1087.
65. Pier GB, DesJardin D, Grout M et al. Human immune response to Pseudomonas aeruginosa mucoid exopolysaccharide (alginate) vaccine. Infect Immun 1994; 62(9):3972-3979.
66. Pier GB, Coleman F, Grout M et al. Role of alginate O acetylation in resistance of mucoid Pseudomonas aeruginosa to opsonic phagocytosis. Infect Immun 2001; 69(3):1895-1901.
67. Sood RK, Salem NK, Fuller S et al. Sythesis and immunogenicity in mice of mucoexopolysaccharide -diphtheria toxoid (MEP-DTd) conjugate. In: Abstracts of the 34th Intersciences Conference on Antimicrobial Agents and Chemotherapy 1994; 23.
68. Brennan FR, Jones TD, Gilleland LB et al. Pseudomonas aeruginosa outer-membrane protein F epitopes are highly immunogenic in mice when expressed on a plant virus. Microbiology 1999; 145(Pt 1):211-220.
69. Mansouri E, Gabelsberger J, Knapp B et al. Safety and immunogenicity of a Pseudomonas aeruginosa hybrid outer membrane protein F-I vaccine in human volunteers. Infect Immun 1999; 67(3):1461-1470.
70. Matthews-Greer JM, Robertson DE, L.B. G et al. Pseudomonas aeruginosa outer membrane protein F produced in Escherichia coli retains vaccine efficacy. Curr Microbiol 1990; 20:171-175.
71. Gilleland HE, Jr., Parker MG, Matthews JM et al. Use of a purified outer membrane protein F (porin) preparation of Pseudomonas aeruginosa as a protective vaccine in mice. Infect Immun 1984; 44(1):49-54.
72. Fox CW, Campbell GD, Jr., Anderson WM et al. Preservation of pulmonary function by an outer membrane protein F vaccine. A study in rats with chronic pulmonary infection caused by Pseudomonas aeruginosa. Chest 1994; 105(5):1545-1550.
73. von Specht BU, Knapp B, Muth G et al. Protection of immunocompromised mice against lethal infection with Pseudomonas aeruginosa by active or passive immunization with recombinant P.

aeruginosa outer membrane protein F and outer membrane protein I fusion proteins. Infect Immun 1995; 63(5):1855-1862.
74. Knapp B, Hundt E, Lenz U et al. A recombinant hybrid outer membrane protein for vaccination against Pseudomonas aeruginosa. Vaccine 1999; 17(13-14):1663-1666.
75. Hughes EE, Gilleland HE, Jr. Ability of synthetic peptides representing epitopes of outer membrane protein F of Pseudomonas aeruginosa to afford protection against P. aeruginosa infection in a murine acute pneumonia model. Vaccine 1995; 13(18):1750-1753.
76. Worgall S, Kikuchi T, Singh R et al. Protection against Pseudomonas aeruginosa chronic lung infection in mice by genetic immunization against outer membrane protein F (OprF) of P. aeruginosa. Infect Immun 2001; 69(7):4521-4527.
77. Toth A, Schodel F, Duchene M et al. Protection of immunosuppressed mice against translocation of Pseudomonas aeruginosa from the gut by oral immunization with recombinant Pseudomonas aeruginosa outer membrane protein I expressing Salmonella dulbin. Vaccine 1994; 12(13):1215-1221.
78. Duchene M, Barron C, Schweizer A et al. Pseudomonas aeruginosa outer membrane lipoprotein I gene: molecular cloning, sequence, and expression in Escherichia coli. J Bacteriol 1989; 171(8):4130-4137.
79. Finke M, Duchene M, Eckhardt A et al. Protection against experimental Pseudomonas aeruginosa infection by recombinant P. aeruginosa lipoprotein I expressed in Escherichia coli. Infect Immun 1990; 58:2241-2244.
80. Mutharia LM, Nicas TI, Hancock RE. Outer membrane proteins of Pseudomonas aeruginosa serotype strains. J Infect Dis 1982; 146(6):770-779.
81. von Specht BU, Lucking HC, Blum B et al. Safety and immunogenicity of a Pseudomonas aeruginosa outer membrane protein I vaccine in human volunteers. Vaccine 1996; 14(12):1111-1117.
82. Jang IJ, Kim IS, Park WJ et al. Human immune response to a Pseudomonas aeruginosa outer membrane protein vaccine. Vaccine 1999; 17(2):158-168.
83. Lee NG, Ahn BY, Jung SB et al. Human anti-Pseudomonas aeruginosa outer membrane proteins IgG cross-protective against infection with heterologous immunotype strains of P. aeruginosa. FEMS Immunol Med Micro 1999; 25(4):339-347.
84. Lee NG, Jung SB, Ahn BY et al. Protection of mice against P. aeruginosa infections by large-scale affinity-purified human IgG specific to P. aeruginosa outer membrane proteins. Vaccine 1999; 18(7-8):665-674.
85. Lee NG, Jung SB, Ahn BY et al. Immunization of burn-patients with a Pseudomonas aeruginosa outer membrane protein vaccine elicits antibodies with protective efficacy. Vaccine 2000; 18(18):1952-1961.
86. Kim DK, Kim JJ, Kim JH et al. Comparison of two immunization schedules for a Pseudomonas aeruginosa outer membrane proteins vaccine in burn patients. Vaccine 2001; 19(9-10):1274-83.
87. Stanislavsky ES, Edvabnaya LS, Bandman OA et al. Experimental studies on the protective efficacy of a Pseudomonas aeruginosa vaccine. Vaccine 1989; 7:562-566.
88. Stanislavsky ES, Balayan SS, Sergienko AI et al. Clinicoimmunological trials of Pseudomonas aeruginosa vaccine. Vaccine 1991; 9(7):491-494.
89. Miler JM, Spilsbury JF, Jones RJ et al. A new polyvalent Pseudomonas vaccine. J Med Microbiol 1977; 10(1):19-27.
90. Pennington JE, Pier GB. Efficacy of cell wall Pseudomonas aeruginosa vaccines for protection against experimental pneumonia. Rev Infect Dis 1983; 5Supp5:S852-S857.
91. Jones RJ, Roe EA, Gupta JL. Controlled trial of Pseudomonas immunoglobulin and vaccine in burn patients. Lancet 1980; 2(8207):1263-1265.
92. MacIntyre S, Lucken R, Owen P. Smooth lipopolysaccharide is the major protective antigen for mice in the surface extract from IATS serotype 6 contributing to the polyvalent Pseudomonas aeruginosa vaccine PEV. Infect Immun 1986; 52(1):76-84.
93. Sato H, Okinaga K, Saito H. Role of pili in the pathogenesis of Pseudomonas aeruginosa burn infection. Microbiol Immunol 1988; 32(2):131-139.
94. Montie TC, Anderson TR. Enzyme-linked immunosorbent assay for detection of Pseudomonas aeruginosa H (flagellar) antigen. Eur J Clin Microbiol Infect Dis 1988; 7:256-260.
95. Holder IA, Naglich JG. Experimental studies of the pathogenesis of infections due to Pseudomonas aeruginosa: Immunization using divalent flagella preparations. J Trauma 1986; 26:118-122.
96. Doering G, Dorner F. A multicenter vaccine trial using the Pseudomonas aeruginosa flagella vaccine IMMUNO in patients with cystic fibrosis. Behring Inst Mitt 1997; (98):338-44.
97. Doering G, Pfeiffer C, Weber U et al. Parenteral application of a Pseudomonas aeruginosa flagella vaccine elicits specific anti-flagella antibodies in the airways of healthy individuals. Am J Resp Crit Care Med 1995; 151(4):983-5.

98. Ochi H, Ohtsuka H, Yokota S et al. Inhibitory activity on bacterial motility and in vivo protective activity of human monoclonal antibodies against flagella of Pseudomonas aeruginosa. Infect Immun 1991; 59(2):550-554.
99. Matsumoto T, Tateda K, Miyazaki S et al. Effect of antiflagellar human monoclonal antibody on gut-derived Pseudomonas aeruginosa sepsis in mice. Clin Diag Lab Immunol 1999; 6(4):537-541.
100. Oishi K, Sonoda F, Iwagaki A et al. Therapeutic effects of a human antiflagella monoclonal antibody in a neutropenic murine model of Pseudomonas aeruginosa pneumonia. Antimicrob Agents Chemother 1993; 37(2):164-170.
101. Arora SK, Dasgupta N, Lory S et al. Identification of two distinct types of flagellar cap proteins, FliD, in Pseudomonas aeruginosa. Infect Immun 2000; 68(3):1474-1479.
102. Luzar MA, Montie TC. Avirulence and altered physiological properties of cystic fibrosis strains of Pseudomonas aeruginosa. Infect Immun 1985; 50(2):572-576.
103. Arora SK, Ritchings BW, Almira EC et al. The Pseudomonas aeruginosa flagellar cap protein, FliD, is responsible for mucin adhesion. Infect Immun 1998; 66(3):1000-1007.
104. Saiman L, Prince A. Pseudomonas aeruginosa pili bind to asialo-GM1 which is increased on the surface of cystic fibrosis epithelial cells. J Clin Invest 1993; 92:1875-1880.
105. Comolli JC, Waite LL, Mostov KE et al. Pili binding to asialo-GM1 on epithelial cells can mediate cytotoxicity or bacterial internalization by Pseudomonas aeruginosa. Infect Immun 1999; 67(7):3207-3214.
106. Cachia PJ, Glasier LM, Hodgins RR et al. The use of synthetic peptides in the design of a consensus sequence vaccine for Pseudomonas aeruginosa. J Peptide Res 1998; 52(4):289-299.
107. Hazes B, Sastry PA, Hayakawa K et al. Crystal structure of Pseudomonas aeruginosa PAK pilin suggests a main-chain-dominated mode of receptor binding. J Mol Biol 2000; 299(4):1005-1017.
108. Cornelis GR, Van Gijsegem F. Assembly and function of type III secretory systems. Annu Rev Microbiol 2000; 54:735-774.
109. Roy-Burman A, Savel RH, Racine S et al. Type III protein secretion is associated with death in lower respiratory and systemic Pseudomonas aeruginosa infections. J Infect Dis 2001; 83(12): 1767-1774.
110. Frank DW. The exoenzyme S regulon of Pseudomonas aeruginosa. Mol Micro 1997; 26(4):621-629.
111. Yahr TL, Vallis AJ, Hancock MK et al. ExoY, an adenylate cyclase secreted by the Pseudomonas aeruginoas type III system. Proc Nat Acad Sci 1998; 95(23):13899-13904.
112. Finck-Barbancon V, Goranson J, Zhu L et al. ExoU expression by Pseudomonas aeruginosa correlates with acute cytotoxicity and epithelial injury. Mol Micro 1997; 25(3):547-557.
113. Hauser AR, Kang PJ, Engel JN. PepA, a secreted protein of Pseudomonas aeruginosa, is necessary for cytotoxicity and virulence. Mol Micro 1998; 27(4):807-818.
114. Holder IA, Neely AN, Frank DW. Type III secretion/intoxication system important in virulence of Pseudomonas aeruginosa infections in burns. Burns 2001; 27(2):129-130.
115. Kurahashi K, Kajikawa O, Sawa T et al. Pathogenesis of septic shock in Pseudomonas aeruginosa pneumonia. J Clin Invest 1999; 104(6):743-750.
116. Allewelt M, Coleman FT, Grout M et al. Acquisition of expression of the P. aeruginosa ExoU cytotoxin leads to increased bacterial virulence in a murine model of acute pneumonia and systemic spread. Infect Immun 2000; 68:3998-4004.
117. Holmstrom A, Olsson J, Cherepanov P et al. LcrV is a channel size-determining component of the Yop effector translocon of Yersinia. Mol Micro 2001; 39(3):620-632.
118. Sawa T, Yahr TL, Ohara M et al. Active and passive immunization with the Pseudomonas V antigen protects against type III intoxication and lung injury. Nature Med 1999; 5(4):392-398.
119. Shime N, Sawa T, Fujimoto J et al. Therapeutic administration of anti-PcrV F(ab')(2) in sepsis associated with Pseudomonas aeruginosa. J Immunol 2001; 167(10):5880-5886.
120. Holder IA, Neely AN, Frank DW. PcrV immunization enhances survival of burned Pseudomonas aeruginosa-infected mice. Infect Immun 2001; 69(9):5908-5910.
121. Pier GB, Grout M, Zaidi TS et al. Role of mutant CFTR in hypersusceptibility of cystic fibrosis patients to lung infections. Science 1996; 271(5245):64-67.
122. Sawa T, Ohara M, Kurahashi K et al. In vitro cellular toxicity predicts Pseudomonas aeruginosa virulence in lung infections. Infect Immun 1998; 66(7):3242-3249.
123. Pier GB, Grout M, Zaidi TS. Cystic fibrosis transmembrane conductance regulator is an epithelial cell receptor for clearance of Pseudomonas aeruginosa from the lung. Proc Nat Acad Sci 1997; 94(22):12088-12093.
124. Pier GB, Grout M, Zaidi TS et al. How mutant CFTR may contribute to Pseudomonas aeruginosa infection in cystic fibrosis. Am J Resp Crit Care Med 1996; 154(4 Pt 2):S175-S182.

125. Zaidi TS, Lyczak J, Preston M et al. Cystic fibrosis transmembrane conductance regulator-mediated corneal epithelial cell ingestion of Pseudomonas aeruginosa is a key component in the pathogenesis of experimental murine keratitis. Infect Immun 1999; 67(3):1481-1492.
126. Kupiec-Weglinski JW, Austyn JM, Morris PJ. Migration patterns of dendritic cells in the mouse. Traffic from the blood, and T cell-dependent and -independent entry to lymphoid tissues. J Exp Med 1988; 167(2):632-645.
127. Banchereau J, Briere F, Caux C et al. Immunobiology of dendritic cells. Ann Rev Immunol 2000; 18:767-811.
128. Albert ML, Sauter B, Bhardwaj N. Dendritic cells acquire antigen from apoptotic cells and induce class I-restricted CTLs. Nature 1998; 392(6671):86-89.
129. Dhodapkar MV, Steinman RM, Sapp M et al. Rapid generation of broad T-cell immunity in humans after a single injection of mature dendritic cells. J Clin Invest 1999; 104(2):173-180.
130. Cannon CL, Stopak K, Pier GB. Defective apoptosis of lung cells expressing mutant CFTR after infection with Pseudomonas aeruginosa. In: North American Cystic Fibrosis Meeting; 1999.
131. Hauser AR, Engel JN. Pseudomonas aeruginosa induces type-III-secretion-mediated apoptosis of macrophages and epithelial cells. Infect Immun 1999; 67(10):5530-5537.
132. Grassme H, Kirschnek S, Riethmueller J et al. CD95/CD95 ligand interactions on epithelial cells in host defense to Pseudomonas aeruginosa. Science 2000; 290(5491):527-530.
133. Stenger S, Hanson DA, Teitelbaum R et al. An antimicrobial activity of cytolytic T cells mediated by granulysin. Science 1998; 282(5386):121-125.
134. Silva CL, Lowrie DB. Identification and characterization of murine cytotoxic T cells that kill Mycobacterium tuberculosis. Infect Immun 2000; 68(6):3269-3274.
135. Lo WF, Ong H, Metcalf ES et al. T cell responses to Gram-negative intracellular bacterial pathogens: a role for CD8+ T cells in immunity to M. tuberculosis infection and the involvement of MHC class Ib molecules. J Immunol 1999; 162(9):5398-5406.
136. Leef M, Elkins KL, Barbic J et al. Protective immunity to Bordetella pertussis requires both B cells and CD4(+) T cells for key functions other than specific antibody production. J Exp Med 2000; 191(11):1841-1852.
137. Wang J, Fan X, Lindholm C et al. Helicobacter pylori modulates lymphoepithelial cell interactions leading to epithelial cell damage through Fas/Fas ligand interactions. Infect Immun 2000; 68(7):4303-4311.
138. Markham RB, Pier GB. Characterization of the antibody response in inbred mice to a high-molecular-weight polysaccharide from Pseudomonas aeruginosa immunotype 1. Infect Immun 1983; 41(1):232-236.
139. Markham RB, Goellner J, Pier GB. In vitro T cell-mediated killing of Pseudomonas aeruginosa. I. Evidence that a lymphokine mediates killing. J Immunol 1984; 133(2):962-968.
140. Markham RB, Pier GB, Goellner JJ et al. In vitro T cell-mediated killing of Pseudomonas aeruginosa. II. The role of macrophages and T cell subsets in T cell killing. J Immunol 1985; 134(6):4112-4117.
141. Markham RB, Pier GB, Powderly WG. Suppressor T cells regulating the cell-mediated immune response to Pseudomonas aeruginosa can be generated by immunization with anti-bacterial T cells. J Immunol 1988; 141(11):3975-3979.
142. Markham RB, Powderly WG. Exposure of mice to live Pseudomonas aeruginosa generates protective cell-mediated immunity in the absence of an antibody response. J Immunol 1988; 140:2039-2045.
143. Markham RB, Pier GB, Schreiber JR. The role of cytophilic IgG3 antibody in T cell-mediated resistance to infection with the extracellular bacterium, Pseudomonas aeruginosa. J Immunol 1991; 146(1):316-320.
144. Markham RB, Pier GB. Immunologic basis for mouse protection provided by high-molecular-weight polysaccharide from immunotype 1 Pseudomonas aeruginosa. Rev Infect Dis 1983; 5Supp5:S957-S962.
145. Pier GB, Markham RB. Induction in mice of cell-mediated immunity to Pseudomonas aeruginosa by high molecular weight polysaccharide and vinblastine. J Immunol 1982; 128(5):2121-2125.
146. Pier GB, Markham RB, Eardley D. Correlation of the biologic responses of C3H/HEJ mice to endotoxin with the chemical and structural properties of the lipopolysaccharides from Pseudomonas aeruginosa and Escherichia coli. J Immunol 1981; 127(1):184-191.
147. Powderly WG, Pier GB, Markham RB. In vitro T cell-mediated killing of Pseudomonas aeruginosa. IV. Noneresposiveness in polysaccharide-immunized BALB/c mice is attributable to vinblastine-sensitive suppressor T cells. J Immunol 1986; 137(6):2025-2030.
148. Powderly WG, Pier GB, Markham RB. T lymphocyte-mediated protection against Pseudomonas aeruginosa infection in granulocytopenic mice. J Clin Invest 1986; 78(2):375-380.

149. Powderly WG, Pier GB, Markham RB. In vitro T cell-mediated killing of Pseudomonas aeruginosa. III. The role of suppressor T cells in nonresponder mice. J Immunol 1986; 136(1):299-303.
150. Powderly WG, Pier GB, Markham RB. In vitro T cell-mediated killing of Pseudomonas aeruginosa. V. Generation of bactericidal T cells in nonresponder mice. J Immunol 1987; 138(7):2272-2277.
151. Powderly WG, Schreiber JR, Pier GB et al. T cells recognizing polysaccharide-specific B cells function as contrasuppressor cells in the generation of T cell immunity to Pseudomonas aeruginosa. J Immunol 1988; 140(8):2746-2752.
152. Dunkley ML, Clancy RL, Cripps AW. A role for CD4+ T cells from orally immunized rats in enhanced clearance of Pseudomonas aeruginosa from the lung. Immunology 1994; 83(3):362-369.
153. Dunkley ML, Cripps AW, Clancy RL. Immunity to respiratory Pseudomonas aeruginosa infection: P. aeruginosa-specific T cells arising after intestinal immunization. Adv Exp Med Biol 1995; 371B:755-759.
154. Parmely MJ, Iglewski BH, Horvat RT. Identification of the principal T lymphocyte-stimulating antigens of Pseudomonas aeruginosa. J Exp Med 1984; 160(5):1338-1349.
155. Mody CH, Buser DE, Syme RM et al. Pseudomonas aeruginosa exoenzyme S induces proliferation of human T lymphocytes. Infect Immun 1995; 63(5):1800-1805.
156. Bruno TF, Woods DE, Mody CH. Exoenzyme S from Pseudomonas aeruginosa induces apoptosis in T lymphocytes. J Leukocyte Biol 2000; 67(6):808-816.
157. Ulmer AJ, Pryjma J, Tarnok Z et al. Inhibitory and stimulatory effects of Pseudomonas aeruginosa pyocyanine on human T and B lymphocytes and human monocytes. Infect Immun 1990; 58(3):808-815.
158. Kondratieva TK, Kobets NV, Khaidukov SV et al. Characterization of T cell clones derived from lymph nodes and lungs of Pseudomonas aeruginosa-susceptible and resistant mice following immunization with heat-killed bacteria. Clin Exp Immunol 2000; 121(2):275-282.
159. Stevenson MM, Kondratieva TK, Apt AS et al. In vitro and in vivo T cell responses in mice during bronchopulmonary infection with mucoid Pseudomonas aeruginosa. Clin Exp Immunol 1995; 99:98-105.
160. Tam M, Snipes GJ, Stevenson MM. Characterization of chronic bronchopulmonary Pseudomonas aeruginosa infection in resistant and susceptible inbred mouse strains. Am J Resp Cell Mol Biol 1999; 20(4):710-719.
161. Moser C, Johansen HK, Song Z et al. Chronic Pseudomonas aeruginosa lung infection is more severe in Th2 responding BALB/c mice compared to Th1 responding C3H/HeN mice. APMIS 1997; 105(11):838-842.
162. Sawa T, Corry DB, Gropper MA et al. IL-10 improves lung injury and survival in Pseudomonas aeruginosa pneumonia. J Immunol 1997; 159(6):2858-2866.
163. Hazlett LD, McClellan S, Kwon B et al. Increased severity of Pseudomonas aeruginosa corneal infection in strains of mice designated as Th1 versus Th2 responsive. Invest Ophth Vis Sci 2000; 41(3):805-810.
164. Kwon B, Hazlett LD. Association of CD4+ T cell-dependent keratitis with genetic susceptibility to Pseudomonas aeruginosa ocular infection. J Immunol 1997; 159(12):6283-6290.
165. Griffith TS, Brunner T, Fletcher SM et al. Fas ligand-induced apoptosis as a mechanism of immune privilege. Science 1995; 270(5239):1189-1192.
166. Stuart PM, Griffith TS, Usui N et al. CD95 ligand (FasL)-induced apoptosis is necessary for corneal allograft survival. J Clin Invest 1997; 99(3):396-402.
167. Gao Y, Herndon JM, Zhang H et al. Anti-inflammatory effects of CD95 ligand (FasL)-induced apoptosis. J Exp Med 1998; 188(5):887-896.
168. Durieu I, Amsellem C, Paulin C et al. Fas and Fas ligand expression in cystic fibrosis airway epithelium. Thorax 1999; 54(12):1093-1098.
169. Sorensen RU, Stern RC, Polmar SH. Cellular immunity to bacteria: Impairment of in vitro lymphocyte responses to Pseudomonas aeruginosa in cystic fibrosis patients. Infect Immun 1977; 18(3):735-740.
170. Sorensen RU, Stern RC, Polmar SH. Lymphocyte responsiveness to Pseudomonas aeruginosa in cystic fibrosis: Relationship to status of pulmonary disease in sibling pairs. J Pediatr 1978; 93(2):201-205.
171. Knutsen AP, Slavin RG, Roodman ST et al. Decreased T helper cell function in patients with cystic fibrosis. Int Arch Allergy Appl Immunol 1988; 85(2):208-212.
172. Chen JH, Schulman H, Gardner P. A cAMP-regulated chloride channel in lymphocytes that is affected in cystic fibrosis. Science 1989; 243(4891):657-660.
173. Dong YJ, Chao AC, Kouyama K et al. Activation of CFTR chloride current by nitric oxide in human T lymphocytes. EMBO J 1995; 14(12):2700-2707.

174. Krauss RD, Bubien JK, Drumm ML et al. Transfection of wild-type CFTR into cystic fibrosis lymphocytes restores chloride conductance at G1 of the cell cycle. Embo J 1992; 11(3):875-883.
175. Moss RB, Bocian RC, Hsu YP et al. Reduced IL-10 secretion by CD4+ T lymphocytes expressing mutant cystic fibrosis transmembrane conductance regulator (CFTR). Clin Exp Immunol 1996; 106(2):374-388.
176. Moss RB, Hsu YP, Olds L. Cytokine dysregulation in activated cystic fibrosis (CF) peripheral lymphocytes. Clin Exp Immunol 2000; 120(3):518-525.
177. Worgall S, Kikuchi T, Singh R et al. Protection against pulmonary infection with Pseudomonas aeruginosa following immunization with P. aeruginosa-pulsed dendritic cells. Infect Immun 2001; 69(7):4521-4527.
178. Kikuchi T, Worgall S, Singh R et al. Dendritic cells genetically modified to express CD40 ligand and pulsed with antigen can initiate antigen-specific humoral immunity independent of CD4+ T cells. Nature Med 2000; 6(10):1154-1159.
179. Kikuchi T, Hackett NR, Crystal RG. Cross-strain protection against clinical and laboratory strains of Pseudomonas aeruginosa mediated by dendritic cells genetically modified to express CD40 ligand and pulsed with specific strains of Pseudomonas aeruginosa. Hum Gene Ther 2001; 12(10):1251-1263.
180. Kikuchi T, Crystal RG. Antigen-pulsed dendritic cells expressing macrophage-derived chemokine elicit Th2 responses and promote specific humoral immunity. J Clin Invest 2001; 108(6):917-927.
181. Dubois B, Vanbervliet B, Fayette J et al. Dendritic cells enhance growth and differentiation of CD40-activated B lymphocytes. J Exp Med 1997; 185(5):941-951.
182. Dubois B, Massacrier C, Vanbervliet B et al. Critical role of IL-12 in dendritic cell-induced differentiation of naive B lymphocytes. J Immunol 1998; 161(5):2223-2231.
183. Van Kooten C, Banchereau J. CD40-CD40 ligand: a multifunctional receptor-ligand pair. Adv Immunol 1996; 61:1-77.
184. Brown MP, Topham DJ, Sangster MY et al. Thymic lymphoproliferative disease after successful correction of CD40 ligand deficiency by gene transfer in mice. Nature Med 1998; 4(11):1253-1260.
185. Wiley JA, Geha R, Harmsen AG. Exogenous CD40 ligand induces a pulmonary inflammation response. J Immunol 1997; 158(6):2932-2938.
186. Gonzalo JA, Pan Y, Lloyd CM et al. Mouse monocyte-derived chemokine is involved in airway hyperreactivity and lung inflammation. J Immunol 1999; 163(1):403-411.
187. Stocker BA. Auxotrophic M. tuberculosis typhi as live vaccine. Vaccine 1988; 6(2):141-145.
188. Hernanz Moral C, Flano del Castillo E, Lopez Fierro P et al. Molecular characterization of the Aeromonas hydrophila aroA gene and potential use of an auxotrophic aroA mutant as a live attenuated vaccine. Infect Immun 1998; 66(5):1813-1821.
189. Poirier TP, Kehoe MA, Beachey EH. Protective immunity evoked by oral administration of attenuated aroA Salmonella typhimurium expressing cloned streptococcal M protein. J Exp Med 1988; 168:25-32.
190. Lo-Man R, Langeveld JPM, Deriaud E et al. Extending the CD4+ T-Cell epitope specificity of the Th1 immune response to an antigen using a Salmonella enterica serovar Typhimurium delivery vehicle. Infect Immun 2000; 68(6):3079-3089.
191. Priebe GP, Brinig MM, Hatano K et al. Construction and characterization of a live, attenuated aroA deletion mutant of Pseudomonas aeruginosa as a candidate intranasal vaccine. Infect Immun 2002; 70(3):1507-1517.
192. Jones RJ, Roe EA, Gupta JL. Controlled trials of a polyvalent Pseudomonas vaccine in burns. Lancet 1979; 2(8150):977-82.
193. Cystic Fibrosis Foundation. Cystic Fibrosis Foundation Patient Registry 2000 Annual Report. Bethesda, MD; September, 2001.
194. Ramsey BW, Pepe MS, Quan JM et al. Intermittent administration of inhaled tobramycin in patients with cystic fibrosis. Cystic Fibrosis Inhaled Tobramycin Study Group. N Engl J Med 1999; 340(1):23-30.

Chapter 18

Staphylococcus aureus Vaccine

Jean C. Lee

Summary

Staphylococcus aureus is frequently isolated from both hospital-acquired and community-acquired infections, and the emergence of antibiotic resistance among clinical isolates has made treatment of staphylococcal infections difficult. This scenario has sparked renewed interest in the development of a vaccine for individuals at high risk for staphylococcal infections. As part of the effort to develop a multicomponent vaccine against *S. aureus*, several vaccine candidates are being evaluated in clinical trials or in animal models of infection. The most promising candidates to date include the capsular polysaccharides type 5 and 8, the adhesins (fibronectin-binding protein, collagen-binding protein, and fibrinogen-binding protein [clumping factor]), and a nontoxic alpha-toxin mutant.

Introduction

Staphylococcus aureus is an important bacterial pathogen that is responsible for a diverse spectrum of human infections. Superficial infections caused by this microbe include impetigo, cellulitis, and folliculitis, whereas more invasive staphylococcal infections include osteomyelitis, septic arthritis, pneumonia, bacteremia, and endocarditis. *S. aureus* infections are often nosocomial, but reports of community-acquired infections have increased. Because of the emergence of antibiotic-resistant staphylococcal strains, including the recent identification of isolates with reduced susceptibility to glycopeptide antibiotics, alternative strategies for the prevention and treatment of staphylococcal infections are needed.

The development of an *S. aureus* vaccine has the potential to reduce the morbidity and mortality associated with staphylococcal infections, decrease the number of hospitalizations and the length of stay for patients, provide long-term protection for patients at risk for staphylococcal infections, and deal with the ominous threat of pathogenic staphylococci resistant to all available antibiotics. Nonetheless, defining the situations wherein one would use staphylococcal vaccines is problematic. Because most humans exhibit a high level of innate resistance to staphylococcal infections, it would be difficult to justify an active vaccination program aimed at the general population. A likely target group for active vaccination would be individuals needing medical care that increases their risk for staphylococcal infections: patients facing surgery that is scheduled sufficiently far in advance for a vaccine to induce protective immunity, receiving long-term or permanent foreign-body implants, or facing chemotherapy or other treatments likely to lower their innate immunity and increase their risk for staphylococcal infection. Health-care workers likely to be colonized with antibiotic-resistant staphylococci and individuals working in professions with increased risks for burn or wound injuries such as soldiers, fire fighters, and police officers are a subset of the population for whom vaccination against staphylococci might be indicated. Table 1 provides a more comprehensive list of population groups that are at increased risk for *S. aureus* infections and might be suitable candidates for immunization. The list includes patients with a variety of predisposing factors and groups

New Bacterial Vaccines, edited by Ronald W. Ellis and Bernard R. Brodeur.

Table 1. Potential candidates for active or passive immunization against S. aureus infections

Surgical patients	Premature neonates	Diabetics
Intravenous drug users	Immunocompromised individuals	Patients with prosthetic implants
Peritoneal dialysis patients	Firefighters	Law enforcement agents
Military personnel	Hospital personnel	Hemodialysis patients

at risk for trauma. Nasal carriage of *S. aureus* is a risk factor for acquisition of staphylococcal infection; thus a vaccine that would prevent nasal carriage of *S. aureus* would benefit hospital personnel as well as their patients.

Since the likelihood of a staphylococcal infection increases substantially following injury or the sudden onset of illness, active vaccination may not be feasible for short-term protection against infection. Passive therapy with immune globulin preparations derived from plasma donors immunized with a vaccine may increase specific immunity rapidly. Immunocompromised hosts or neonates may not be able to mount their own immune response to a vaccine and could benefit from passive infusion of biologically active antibodies. Any therapeutic agent must not only be cost-effective but should also diminish antibiotic use. Administration of an immune globulin could provide short-term protection against *S. aureus* during hospitalization, particularly in cases with only a moderate risk of infection, such as the use of temporary in-dwelling vascular access devices or surgery.

Major challenges that must be addressed in *S. aureus* vaccine development include determining which clinical situations warrant vaccination, defining strategies that make the most effective use of active and passive vaccination, and deciding which clinical outcomes most clearly document vaccine efficacy. Optimal target antigens to incorporate in a vaccine must be identified, the immune effector(s) providing effective protection against the infection and its consequences must be defined, and whether a cost-effective immunotherapeutic reagent can be produced must be determined. Progress toward the development of a vaccine to protect against *S. aureus* has been limited by a poor understanding of what constitutes a protective host immune response to this microbe. Humans possess a high degree of innate immunity to staphylococcal infections, and antibodies to *S. aureus* cell wall constituents and exoproteins are widespread in healthy humans. Nonetheless, evidence that recovery from *S. aureus* infections confers immunity to subsequent episodes of staphylococcal diseases is lacking.

Ongoing efforts to design an *S. aureus* vaccine have targeted known virulence factors of this organism. These factors are listed in (Table 2)and include staphylococcal surface proteins, polysaccharides, exoproteins, and toxins elaborated by this pathogen. Whether some combination of purified *S. aureus* components can be included in a vaccine that will provide broad range protection against staphylococcal infections is the challenge faced by researchers in this field. Studies to date have focussed on the use of single or, in the case of capsular polysaccharides, dual-component *S. aureus* vaccines. The results of the most current studies are summarized below.

Capsular Polysaccharide (CP)

CPs elaborated by many pathogenic bacteria are important virulence factors, and antibodies directed toward capsular antigens are often protective against infections induced by encapsulated microbes. Several published reports have indicated that antibodies elicited to *S. aureus* CPs are protective in animal models of experimental staphylococcal infection. Because CPs are

Table 2. Potential virulence determinants of* S. aureus *that could be targeted for vaccine production

Cell-Associated Components	Exoenzymes	Exotoxins
Protein A	Coagulase	Leukocidin
Capsular polysaccharide	Hyaluronate lyase	Enterotoxins (A To E, G To P)
Peptidoglycan	Lipase	Exfoliative Toxin
Poly-N-acetyl glucosamine or Polysaccharide intercellular adhesin	Nuclease	Toxic shock syndrome toxin-1
Adhesins for	Proteases	Alpha toxin
Fibronectin		Beta toxin
Fibrinogen		Gamma toxin
Collagen		Delta toxin
Elastin		
Vitronectin		
Thrombospondin		
Plasmin		
von Willebrand factor		

poorly immunogenic and generally elicit a T-cell-independent antibody response, Fattom et al[1] conjugated the most prevalent *S. aureus* CP types (serotypes 5 and 8; Fig. 1) to recombinant *Pseudomonas aeruginosa* exotoxoid A (rEPA). The conjugate vaccines were highly immunogenic in mice and humans and induced antibodies that opsonized encapsulated *S. aureus* for phagocytosis. [1,2] Antibodies elicited by immunization with the CP5 and CP8 conjugate vaccines were protective in a mouse model of *S. aureus* lethality and disseminated infection. [3] Similarly, intraperitoneal (i.p.) administration of antibodies to the conjugate vaccine protected rats against infection in a catheter-induced model of staphylococcal endocarditis if the animals were challenged by the i.p. route. [4]

Active Immunization of Humans with the CP5/CP8 Conjugate Vaccines

Fattom and colleagues at Nabi (Boca Raton, FL) have prepared conjugates of CP5 and CP8 linked to rEPA that are intended for commercial use. The CP8-rEPA and CP5-rEPA conjugate vaccines were evaluated for safety and immunogenicity in 70 healthy adult volunteers. [2] Neither conjugate caused significant local or systemic reactions in the volunteers. The conjugate vaccines induced CP-specific IgM and IgG antibodies. A second injection six weeks later did not have a booster effect. The authors suggested that the initial vaccination behaved more like a booster than a primary dose in these subjects because of their low levels of prevaccination anti-CPs antibodies.

Nabi combined the CP5- and CP8-conjugate vaccines into a bivalent vaccine called StaphVAX™ that is intended for immunization of humans at high risk for *S. aureus* infection. They conducted a phase II, double-blinded, placebo-controlled clinical study of StaphVAX in ~230 patients receiving chronic ambulatory peritoneal dialysis, who are at high risk of staphylococcal disease. The patients were actively immunized with StaphVAX, and their antibody responses and infection rates were monitored. The vaccine elicited only mild local or systemic symptoms. The results of this trial indicated that the vaccine dose of 25 μg of each CP was suboptimal in these patients. Their antibody responses to the vaccine were weak, and the immunized patients had infection rates similar to those of nonimmunized patients.

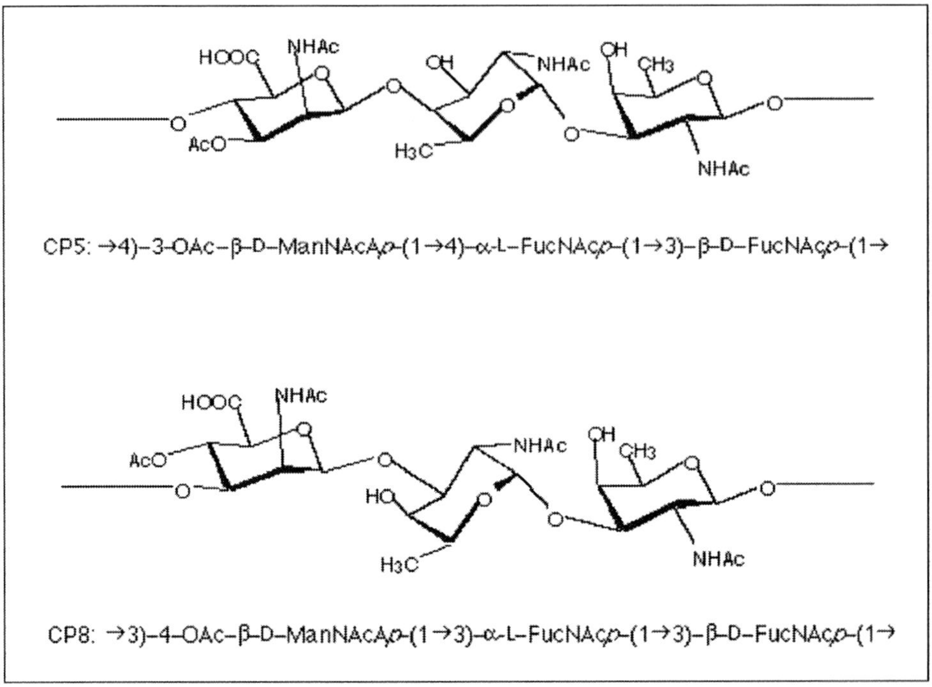

Figure 1. Structural composition of serotype 5 and 8 capsular polysaccharides. OAc, O-acetyl; ManNAcA, N-acetyl mannosaminuronic acid; FucNAc, N-acetyl fucosamine.

In subsequent phase II clinical trials, 32 volunteers with end-stage renal disease and 29 healthy controls were injected twice (6 weeks apart) with 25 μg of CP5-rEPA or the bivalent conjugate vaccine (25 μg each of CP5 and CP8 linked to rEPA). The vaccines elicited only mild local or systemic symptoms in both populations [5] (and G. Horwith, personal communication). Four weeks after the second dose of vaccine, 23 of 24 healthy volunteers and 14 of 17 patients in one study responded to the immunization with a four-fold or greater increase in preimmunization levels of specific IgG and IgM antibody. However, the IgG and IgM levels of the patients were only ~50% of those achieved by the healthy controls at all postimmunization intervals. The monovalent and bivalent vaccines did not contain any adjuvant. Data from animal studies indicate that enhanced immunogenicity may be achieved by incorporating an adjuvant such as monophosphoryl lipid A.[6]

Phase III Clinical Trial of the CP5/CP8/rEPA Vaccine

Between 1998 and 2000, a phase III clinical trial to evaluate the efficacy of StaphVAX was conducted at the Kaiser Permanente Vaccine Study Center in California.[7] This randomized, double-blinded, placebo-controlled study was designed to assess safety, immunogenicity, and ability to prevent bacteremia in patients with end-stage renal disease receiving hemodialysis. Approximately 1800 patients were enrolled in 73 hemodialysis centers. Half of the patients were administered a placebo, and the other half were immunized with Nabi's bivalent StaphVAX (100 μg each of CP5 and CP8 conjugated to an equal weight of rEPA). Patients receiving hemodialysis are at high risk for staphylococcal infection, with 3 to 4 of every 100 patients infected with *S. aureus* per year. In this clinical trial, the patients were monitored for culture-proven *S. aureus* bacteremia. There were no significant differences in the number of deaths in the vaccine and control groups, and none of the deaths were considered related to the vaccine.

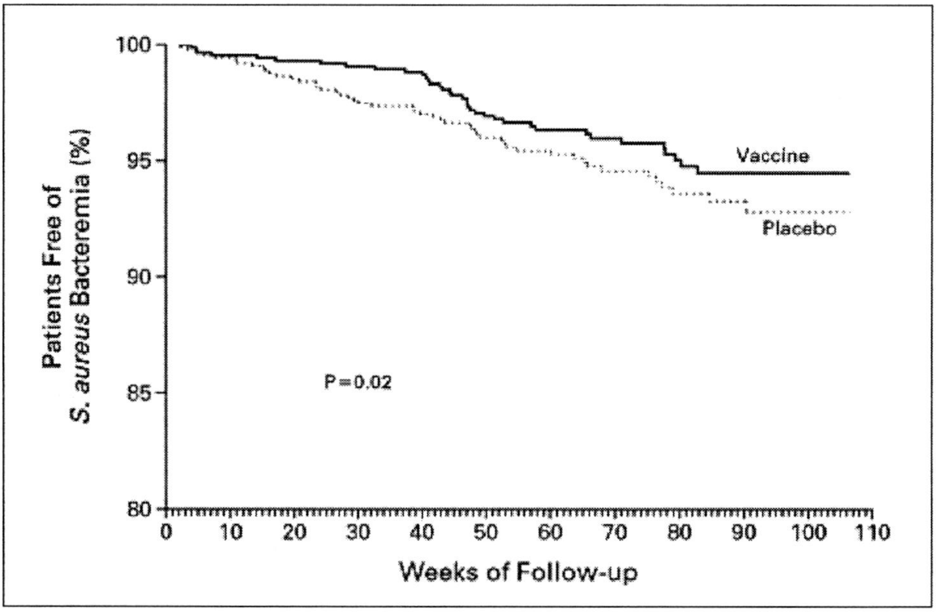

Figure 2. Kaplan - Meier Survival Curves for S. aureus bacteremia. The P value is for the difference between the two group during weeks 3 to 40. There was no statistically differences between the groups during weeks 3-54. Permission from: Shinefield H et al. N Engl J Med 2002; 346(7):491-496. ©2002 Massachusetts Medical Society. All Rights Reserved.

As shown in Figure 2, at the end of the study period (54 weeks), the vaccine reduced the incidence of bacteremia in the study population by only 26% (not significant). It was notable that the vaccine efficacy at 40 weeks was 57% (p = 0.02). However, after that time period, the antibody levels in the vaccinated patients declined, mirroring the decline in efficacy of the vaccine. StaphVAX was the first staphylococcal vaccine to reach clinical trials, and a second phase II clinical trial is planned. Fattom and his colleagues are hopeful that StaphVAX will provide better protection in other populations, such as patients who will undergo elective surgery and are at risk of systemic infection with *S. aureus*.

Passive Immunization of Humans with Antibodies to CPs

Another goal of Nabi is to immunize healthy people with StaphVAX to generate an immunoglobulin product with high levels of antibodies to *S. aureus* CP5 and CP8. Polyclonal antibodies have been purified from the plasma of healthy vaccinees. In passive immunization studies, the IgG antibody generated in this fashion, referred to as StaphGAM^{TM}, is administered to patients who are at immediate risk for staphylococcal infection. The circulating half-life of such antibodies is estimated to be 14-21 days.[8] Twenty-nine very-low-birth-weight infants, who are at high risk for staphylococcal infection, were enrolled in a phase I/II safety and pharmacokinetics study conducted between 1998 and 1999 at the University of Texas. Subjects, who were stratified by weight (0.5-1.0 and 1.0-1.5 kg), were administered two injections of AltaStaph two weeks apart. Three dosage levels (500, 750 and 1000 μg/kg) of AltaStaph were administered, and the safety of each level was assessed before escalation to the next dosage level. All doses were well tolerated. Additional trials with AltaStaph are planned to test its efficacy as a prophylactic agent to prevent bacteremia. In addition, Nabi hopes to evaluate the therapeutic effect of AltaStaph as an adjunct to antibiotics in patients with documented *S. aureus* infection (G. Horwith, personal communication).

Poly-N-Acetyl Glucosamine (Polysaccharide Intercellular Adhesin)

McKenney et al [9] identified a new surface-associated *S. aureus* polysaccharide (Ps) that was poorly expressed in vitro but could be detected by serologic methods on organisms recovered from infections. The Ps has been given several names, including poly-N-succinyl β-1-6 glucosamine and Ps intercellular adhesin. [10] The succinyl groups on the polymer have recently been shown to be an artifact of the acid hydrolysis protocol used to solubilize the Ps for analysis by nuclear magnetic resonance. The correct structure is a variably N-acetylated polymer of β-1-6 glucosamine.[11] The protective efficacy of immunization with the glucosamine polymer was evaluated in a murine model of renal abscess formation. Mice immunized with three 100-μg Ps doses (5-6 days apart) before bacterial challenge showed significant reductions in the cfu of *S. aureus* per gram of kidney compared with mice immunized with an irrelevant Ps. Mice passively immunized with rabbit antibodies to the polymer before i.v. challenge with *S. aureus* and again 18 hours after challenge also were protected against renal infection and showed lower mortality than animals injected with antiserum to an irrelevant Ps. Because a similar Ps (capsular Ps/adhesin) is also elaborated by many isolates of coagulase-negative staphylococci, a vaccine to the β-1-6 glucosamine Ps might target both coagulase-positive and coagulase-negative staphylococci. Previous studies showed that the Ps adhesin was effective in laboratory animals as a vaccine against infections caused by coagulase-negative staphylococci.[12,13]

Protein Vaccines

S. aureus produces a variety of cell wall-associated proteins that interact with extracellular matrix proteins of the host. These staphylococcal adhesins have been dubbed "microbial cell surface components recognizing adhesive matrix molecules" (MSCRAMMS). Staphylococcal proteins that bind to fibronectin, fibrinogen, and collagen (Fig. 3) have been investigated as components of vaccines to protect against experimental *S. aureus* infections in laboratory animals.

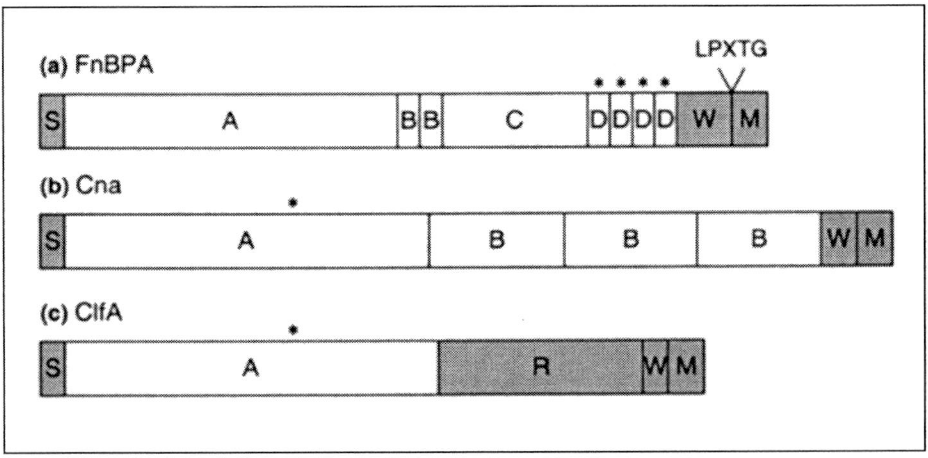

Figure 3. Structural organization of the MSCRAMM proteins (a) FnBpA; (b) Cna; (c) ClfA of *S. aureus*. "S" represents the signal sequence; "R" represents Ser-Asp dipeptide repeats; "W" represents the wall-spanning region; and "M" represents the membrane-spanning region and positively charged residues. The positions of the LPXTG motif and the A-, B-, C- and D-domains are indicated. Asterisks indicate ligand-biding domains. Adapted with permission from: Foster T, Höök M. Trends Microbiol 1998;6:484-488. ©1998 Elsevier Science.

Fibronectin-Binding Proteins

Most *S. aureus* strains carry two fibronectin-binding proteins (FnBps) arranged in tandem on the bacterial chromosome. The binding motifs within FnBpA (and also FnBpB) consist of three repeat regions (37-38 amino acids long) designated D1-3 (Fig. 2). The D-repeats of FnBpA and FnBpB are highly homologous. Schennings et al[14] prepared a fusion protein by cloning the *lacZ* gene encoding beta-galactosidase (gal) in frame with the D1-3 repeat region of the *S. aureus fnbA*. Rats were immunized with the gal-FnBP in Freund's complete adjuvant, and the resulting antibodies blocked the in vitro binding of *S. aureus* to immobilized fibronectin. Immunization with the fusion protein provided modest protection against experimental endocarditis in rats compared with nonimmunized animals. Likewise, mice immunized with gal-FnBp (with Freund's adjuvant) showed fewer cases of severe mastitis than did control mice (immunized with adjuvant alone), and fewer bacteria were recovered from the mammary glands of vaccinees than from those of control mice.[15]

In a more recent study by Brennan et al,[16] a truncated form of the D2 peptide (amino acids 1-30) derived from *S. aureus* FnBpB was expressed on the surface of the icosahedral cowpea mosaic virus (CPMV). Mice and rats were immunized subcutaneously (s.c.) with the recombinant plant virus-based recombinant vaccine (CPMV-D) with adjuvant. All of the mice produced high titers of FnBp D2-specific IgG2a and IgG2b and little IgG1. Antibodies to CPMV-D inhibited the binding of *S. aureus* to purified fibronectin, but the opsonic activity of these antibodies against *S. aureus* was not assessed. To determine whether antibodies to the recombinant CPMV-D particles provided protection against *S. aureus* infection, Rennermalm et al[17] immunized rats s.c. on days 0, 14 and 28 with either 250-500 µg of CPMV-D or 150-500 µg of CPMV alone, both with the adjuvant QS-21. Protection against staphylococcal infection was evaluated in a coupled model of arthritis/endocarditis. A corticosteroid was injected into the right temporomandibular joint, and *S. aureus* was injected intravenously (i.v.). As a result, the rats developed septic arthritis in the joint and a continuous low-grade bacteremia. One week later, the rats were catheterized to induce the development of vegetations on the aortic valve. The animals were sacrificed 24 hours later, and the vegetations, mandibular joints and kidneys were homogenized and cultured quantitatively. The number of bacteria recovered from infected joints (~$10^{6.5}$ cfu *S. aureus*) was similar for the two groups, but the median cfu/valve ($10^{3.2}$) for animals immunized with CPMV-D was ~10^3-fold lower than that for control animals given virus alone. The numbers of *S. aureus* cultured from the kidneys of immunized rats ($10^{7.2}$ cfu) was only '10-fold lower than the number in control rats ($10^{8.2}$ cfu).

In a separate study[18] rats and mice were immunized intranasally (i.n.) with purified recombinant CPMV-D. The nonreplicating recombinant viral particles induced high titers of FnBP-specific IgG in the rodent sera. Peptide-specific IgA and IgG could also be detected in the bronchial, intestinal, and vaginal lavage fluids. The collective results of this group of studies demonstrate the potential of FnBP and plant virus-based vaccines to elicit partial protection against *S. aureus* infections.

Collagen-Binding Protein

The staphylococcal collagen-binding protein (Cna) is present on 30% to 60% of *S. aureus* strains and represents an important virulence factor in the pathogenesis of staphylococcal septic arthritis, endocarditis, and keratitis.[19-21] Immunization with purified Cna did not protect rats against staphylococcal endocarditis.[14] However, Nilsson et al[22] demonstrated that vaccination with the domain A fragment of the *S. aureus* collagen adhesin (Cna-A) protected mice against sepsis-induced death. Mice were injected s.c. with 100 µg of protein (in Freund's complete adjuvant) and with two booster doses (without adjuvant). Mice immunized with the recombinant protein or BSA were challenged i.v. with 2 x 10^7 cfu of the Cna-positive *S. aureus* strain Phillips. After 14 days, mortality in the group vaccinated with Cna-A was only 13%, compared with 87% in the control group immunized with BSA. Among mice given a sublethal inoculum (6 x 10^6 cfu), the control animals exhibited a significant decrease in their body weight compared with the Cna-A-immunized mice, but there was no significant decrease in the development of septic arthritis between the two groups of animals. The investigators demonstrated that the protective effect against *S. aureus*-induced lethality was antibody mediated by passive immunization of naïve mice with rat antibodies to the collagen adhesin. Compared with mice given antibodies to BSA, mice passively immunized with Cna-A antibodies were protected against sepsis-induced death.

Fibrinogen-Binding Proteins

S. aureus produces a number of cell-associated proteins that bind to fibrinogen. Two of the best-characterized proteins are clumping factor A and B (ClfA and ClfB). ClfA has been shown to be critical for staphylococcal virulence in rodent models of endocarditis[23] and septic arthritis.[24] Josefsson et al[24] actively immunized mice with 30 μg of either BSA or the purified binding region A of ClfA (rClfA40-559) emulsified in Freund's complete adjuvant. Ten days later the animals were boosted with antigen prepared in Freund's incomplete adjuvant. The immunized mice were challenged i.v. with the homologous *S. aureus* strain Newman 10 days after the second immunization. Mice immunized with rClfA40-559 had less severe arthritis and weight reduction than did the BSA-immunized group of mice. However, the numbers of *S. aureus* recovered from the infected kidneys and joints was not significantly different between the two groups of animals. A reduction in *S. aureus*-induced arthritis was also observed in mice passively administered anti-rClfA40-559 immunoglobulin.

Additional animals were vaccinated with rClfA40-559 or BSA and challenged with heterologous *S. aureus* strains 601 (methicillin-resistant) or LS-1 (a mouse isolate). Mortality induced by strain 601 was reduced by rClfA immunization (11%) compared to BSA immunization (50%; p = 0.06). However, there was no protection against arthritis or weight loss when the animals were challenged with *S. aureus* strain LS-1. Additional studies are warranted to determine whether immunization with recombinant ClfA fragments will elicit broad-range protection against staphylococcal infections.

In unpublished studies, Bayer and colleagues evaluated whether antibodies to ClfA would protect rabbits in a catheter-induced model of *S. aureus* endocarditis. Rabbits were immunized four times with 50-100 μg of a recombinant peptide encompassing the ligand-binding domain A of ClfA adsorbed to alum or alum alone. The rabbits were catheterized and challenged i.v. 24 hours later with 8×10^4 cfu of a methicillin-resistant *S. aureus* isolate (strain 67-0). The ClfA-immunized rabbits had significantly fewer staphylococci in their blood, vegetations, and kidneys compared with control animals. In a related study, scientists at Inhibitex evaluated the ability of a ClfA-specific monoclonal antibody (MAb) to protect mice against lethality in an i.v. challenge model of infection. The animals were passively immunized with 0.3 mg of purified MAb 12-9 (IgG1) 18 h prior to challenge with 2×10^9 cfu of *S. aureus* 67-0. Seven days after bacterial challenge, 70% of the mice treated with 12-9 MAb survived as compared with only 30% of the animals given an isotype control MAb (Joseph Patti, personal communication).

Toxoids

Alpha Toxoid

Alpha toxin, a poreforming and hemolytic exoprotein produced by most strains of *S. aureus*, is a major staphylococcal virulence determinant. Human cells that demonstrate a high susceptibility to the lethal effects of this toxin include platelets, endothelial cells, and monocytes. Antibodies raised to alpha toxin detoxified with formaldehyde have been shown to protect monkeys against the toxic and lethal actions of purified alpha toxin.[25] However, animals immunized with alpha toxoid and challenged with live bacteria are not generally protected from infection with alpha toxin-producing strains of *S. aureus*, although the clinical severity of their disease may be less than that in nonimmunized controls.[15,26-28] Menzies and Kernodle[29] constructed a nontoxic alpha toxin mutant by replacing a histidine with a leucine at amino acid 35

(H35L toxoid). The investigators demonstrated that passive immunization of mice with rabbit antiserum to this toxoid protected the animals against lethality induced by i.p injection of purified alpha toxin. Mice given preimmune serum died 2-4 hours after challenge, whereas animals given immune serum were alive at 24 hours (when the experiment was terminated). Antibodies to the H35L toxoid also prevented the lethality at 24 h induced by an alpha toxin-overproducing strain of *S. aureus*. However, two of the six surviving mice developed intraabdominal abscesses 10 days after challenge.

Enterotoxins (Superantigens)

S. aureus produces a wide variety of superantigen exoproteins, including toxic shock syndrome toxin-1, exfoliative toxins A and B, and enterotoxins A to P. The native proteins would not be appropriate vaccine components since superantigens act as potent oligoclonal T-cell activators, resulting in the massive release of cytokines. Administration of the native molecules would likely disturb the homeostasis of the immune system and possibly result in tissue damage, septic shock, or death. However, mutant forms of the enterotoxin proteins devoid of their superantigenic properties may still express antigenic determinants that could be the target of neutralizing antibodies. Nilsson et al[30] generated a genetically modified staphylococcal enterotoxin A (SEA) mutated in a hydrophobic loop dominating the interface with the MHC class II locus. Mice were injected with 1-3 doses of recombinant SEA (10 μg) emulsified in Freund's adjuvant. The mice were inoculated i.v. with 5-8 x 10^7 cfu of an SEA-producing *S. aureus* 1-5 weeks after the last immunization. In three separate experiments, mice injected with the recombinant protein showed a significantly higher survival rate than mice immunized with BSA. Passive administration of SEA-specific rat antibodies to naïve mice also protected the animals against lethality due to staphylococcal sepsis. After 5 days, however, the differences in survival between the two groups of mice diminished, suggesting that additional doses of antibody might be necessary to extend the protection afforded by passive immunization.

Similarly, Lowell et al[31] demonstrated that immunization with a formalinized staphylococcal enterotoxin B (SEB) toxoid formulated with meningococcal outer membrane protein proteosomes was immunogenic in mice. Proteosome-toxoid delivered i.n. or intramuscularly (i.m.) afforded protection against lethal challenge with purified SEB delivered by the parenteral or respiratory route to D-galactosamine-sensitized mice. In a subsequent study Lowell et al[32] immunized nonhuman primates i.m. with the same proteosome-toxoid vaccine. Booster doses were administered by either the i.m. or intratracheal route. One month after the last immunization, the primates were challenged by the aerosol route with 15 times the 50% lethal dose (LD_{50}) of purified SEB. Aerosol exposure to SEB results in gastrointestinal symptoms, lethargy, shock, and death in naïve animals. However, the proteosome-SEB toxoid vaccine protected 100% of monkeys against severe symptomatology and death due to aerosolized SEB intoxication. LeClaire et al[33] passively transferred chicken anti-SEB antibodies to rhesus monkeys before SEB exposure or 4 hours after the animals were exposed to ~5 LD_{50} of aerosolized SEB. Eight of 8 monkeys administered antibodies to SEB survived, whereas the control animals that received no antibodies died.

Staphylococcal enterotoxins that are devoid of their superantigenic properties may be useful vaccine candidates for protection against superantigens used as potential biological warfare agents. However, the many different superantigens produced by this organism and the variability that exists between strains limit the utility of these toxins as constituents of a multicomponent staphylococcal vaccine.

Conclusion

Interest in the development of new approaches for the prevention of staphylococcal infections is a result of the worldwide dissemination of multiresistant strains of *S. aureus* and the increasing role of this microorganism in both nosocomial and community-acquired staphylococcal infections. The ideal vaccine against *S. aureus* would induce antibodies to prevent bacterial adherence, promote opsonophagocytic killing by leukocytes, and neutralize toxic exoproteins produced by the bacterium. Many impediments to the design of an effective staphylococcal vaccine exist, including the multitude of staphylococcal virulence determinants (i.e., adhesins, exoenzymes and exotoxins) and the complex pathways by which *S. aureus* regulates these factors. An evaluation of the experimental data from animal vaccine trials suggests that viable options for constituents of a multicomponent *S. aureus* vaccine would include one or more of the adhesins (fibronectin-binding protein, collagen-binding protein, and fibrinogen-binding protein [clumping factor]), a nontoxic alpha toxin mutant, CP5, and CP8. With the recent release to the public of the *S. aureus* genomic sequence and its ongoing analysis, it is likely that new targets for vaccine development will be unveiled and tested in the near future. Other avenues of investigation worth pursuing include the delivery of therapeutic agents such as the autoinducing peptides that target the regulatory network that controls expression of staphylococcal virulence determinants. These agents and vaccines may be useful adjuncts to antibiotic therapy for *S. aureus* infections.

Acknowledgment

Research in my laboratory is supported by NIH research grants AI 290 40 and AI 44136.

References

1. Fattom A, Schneerson R, Szu SC et al. Synthesis and immunologic properties in mice of vaccines composed of Staphylococcus aureus type 5 and type 8 capsular polysaccharides conjugated to Pseudomonas aeruginosa exotoxin A. Infect Immun 1990; 58(7):2367-2374.
2. Fattom A, S R, Watson DC et al. Laboratory and clinical evaluation of conjugate vaccines composed of Staphylococcus aureus type 5 and type 8 capsular polysaccharides bound to Pseudomonas aeruginosa recombinant exoprotein A. Infect Immun 1993; 61(3):1023-1032.
3. Fattom AI, Sarwar J, Ortiz A et al. A Staphylococcus aureus capsular polysaccharide (CP) vaccine and CP-specific antibodies protect mice against bacterial challenge. Infect Immun 1996; 64 (5):1659-1665.
4. Lee JC, Park J-S, Shepherd SE et al. Protective efficacy of antibodies to the Staphylococcus aureus type 5 capsular polysaccharide in a modified model of endocarditis in rats. Infect Immun 1997; 65:4146-4151.
5. Welch PG, Fattom A, Moore J et al. Safety and immunogenicity of Staphylococcus aureus type 5 capsular polysaccharide-Pseudomonas aeruginosa recombinant exoprotein A conjugate vaccine in patients on hemodialysis. J Amer Soc Nephrol 1996; 7(2):247-253.
6. Fattom A, Li X, Cho YH et al. Effect of conjugation methodology, carrier protein, and adjuvants on the immune response to Staphylococcus aureus capsular polysaccharides. Vaccine 1995; 13 (14):1288-1293.
7. Shinefield H, Black S, Fattom A et al. Use of a Staphylococcus aureus conjugate vaccine in patients receiving hemodialysis. N Engl J Med 2002; 346(7):491-496.
8. Naso R, Fattom A. Polysaccharide conjugate vaccines for the prevention of gram-positive bacterial infections. Adv Exp Med Biol 1996; 397:133-140.
9. McKenney D, Pouliot KL, Wang Y et al. Broadly protective vaccine for Staphylococcus aureus based on an in vivo-expressed antigen. Science 1999; 284:1523-1527.
10. Cramton SE, Gerke C, Schnell NF et al. The intercellular adhesion (ica) locus is present in Staphylococcus aureus and is required for biofilm formation. Infect Immun 1999; 67(10):5427-5433.
11. Maira-Litrán T, Kropec A, Abeygunawardana C et al. Immunochemical properties of the staphylococcal poly-N-acetyl glucosamine surface polysaccharide. Infect Immun 2002; 70(8):4433-4440.
12. Kojima Y, Tojo M, Goldmann DA et al. Antibody to the capsular polysaccharide/adhesin protects rabbits against catheter related bacteremia due to coagulase-negative staphylococci. J Infect Dis 1990; 162:435-441.
13. Takeda S, Pier GB, Kojima Y et al. Protection against endocarditis due to Staphylococcus epidermidis by immunization with capsular polysaccharide/adhesin. Circulation 1991; 84:2539-2546.
14. Schennings T, Heimdahl A, Coster K et al. Immunization with fibronectin binding protein from Staphylococcus aureus protects against experimental endocarditis in rats. Microb Pathogen 1993; 15(3):227-236.
15. Mamo W, Jonsson P, Flock J-I et al. Vaccination against Staphylococcus aureus mastitis: immunological response of mice vaccinated with fibronectin-binding protein (FnBP-A) to challenge with S. aureus. Vaccine 1994; 12(11):988-992.

16. Brennan FR, Jones TD, Longstaff M et al. Immunogenicity of peptides derived from a fibronectin-binding protein of S. aureus expressed on two different plant viruses. Vaccine 1999; 17(15-16):1846-1857.
17. Rennermalm A, Li Y, Bohaufs L et al. Antibodies against a truncated Staphylococcus aureus fibronectin- binding protein protect against dissemination of infection in the rat. Vaccine 2001; 19(25-26):3376-3383.
18. Brennan FR, Bellaby T, Helliwell SM et al. Chimeric plant virus particles administered nasally or orally induce systemic and mucosal immune responses in mice. J Virol 1999; 73(2):930-938.
19. Patti JM, Bremell T, Krajewska-Pietrasik D et al. The Staphylococcus aureus collagen adhesin is a virulence determinant in experimental septic arthritis. Infect Immun 1994; 62:152-161.
20. Rhem MN, Lech EM, Patti JM et al. The collagen-binding adhesin is a virulence factor in Staphylococcus aureus keratitis. Infect Immun 2000; 68(6):3776-3779.
21. Hienz SA, Schennings T, Heimdahl A et al. Collagen binding of Staphylococcus aureus is a virulence factor in experimental endocarditis. J Infect Dis 1996; 174:83-88.
22. Nilsson I-M, Patti JM, Bremell T et al. Vaccination with a recombinant fragment of collagen adhesin provides protection against Staphylococcus aureus-mediated septic death. J Clin Invest 1998; 101(12):2640-2649.
23. Moreillon P, Entenza JM, Francioli P et al. Role of Staphylococcus aureus coagulase and clumping factor in pathogenesis of experimental endocarditis. Infect Immun 1995; 63(12):4738-4743.
24. Josefsson E, Hartford O, O'Brien L et al. Protection against experimental Staphylococcus aureus arthritis by vaccination with clumping factor A, a novel virulence determinant. J Infect Dis 2001; 184(12):1572-1580.
25. Bhakdi S, Mannhardt U, Muhly M et al. Human hyperimmune globulin protects against the cytotoxic action of staphylococcal alpha-toxin in vitro and in vivo. Infect Immun 1989; 57:3214-3220.
26. Adlam C, Ward PD, McCartney AC et al. Effect of immunization with highly purified alpha- and beta-toxins on staphylococcal mastitis in rabbits. Infect Immun 1977; 17(2):250-256.
27. Ekstedt RD. Immunity to the staphylococci. In: Cohen JO, ed. The staphylococci. New York: Wiley-Interscience, 1972:385-418.
28. Hume EB, Dajcs JJ, Moreau JM et al. Immunization with alpha-toxin toxoid protects the cornea against tissue damage during experimental Staphylococcus aureus keratitis. Infect Immun 2000; 68(10):6052-6055.
29. Menzies BE, Kernodle DS. Passive immunization with antiserum to a nontoxic alpha-toxin mutant from Staphylococcus aureus is protective in a murine model. Infect Immun 1996; 64(5):1839-1841.
30. Nilsson IM, Verdrengh M, Ulrich RG et al. Protection against Staphylococcus aureus sepsis by vaccination with recombinant staphylococcal entertoxin A devoid of superantigenicity. J Infect Dis 1999; 180:1370-1373.
31. Lowell GH, Kaminski RW, Grate S et al. Intranasal and intramuscular proteosome-stahylococcal enterotoxin B (SEB) toxoid vaccines: immunogenicity and eficacy against lethal SEB intoxication in mice. Infect Immun 1996; 64(5):1706-1713.
32. Lowell GH, Colleton C, Frost D et al. Immunogenicity and efficacy against lethal aerosol staphylococcal entertoxin B challenge in monkeys by intramuscular and respiratory delivery of proteosome-toxoid vaccines. Infect Immun 1996; 64(11):4686-4693.
33. LeClaire RD, Hunt RE, Bavari S. Protection against bacterial superantigen staphylococcal enterotoxin B by passive vaccination. Infect Immun 2002; 70(5):2278-2281.

Chapter 19

Streptococcus pneumoniae Vaccines

James C. Paton and David E. Briles

Abstract

Almost sixty years after the advent of penicillin, *Streptococcus pneumoniae* (the pneumococcus) continues to cause more deaths from invasive infections (pneumonia, meningitis and bacteremia) than any other bacterium. It is also the most common cause of acute otitis media in children, which, although less serious, is a major contributor to morbidity and a significant cost to health-care systems. Management of pneumococcal (Pn) disease is also being complicated by an alarming increase in the prevalence of penicillin- and multiple drug-resistant strains and the lack of an efficacious broadly protective vaccine. Vaccines developed to date have been directed against the type-specific polysaccharide (Ps) capsule. Anti-capsular antibodies are highly protective against homologous Pn serotypes, but purified Ps vaccines are poorly immunogenic in high-risk groups such as young children and the elderly. Moreover, protection is serotype-specific, and the existing formulation covers only 23 of the 90 known Pn types. Recently licensed Ps-protein conjugate vaccine formulations are much more immunogenic and protective in infants, but they are very expensive and serotype coverage is even more restricted. Therefore, new vaccines based on protein antigens common to all Pn types may provide a more broadly efficacious and cost-effective alternative.

Introduction

S. pneumoniae is a major human pathogen, causing high morbidity and mortality throughout the world. It causes invasive diseases such as pneumonia, meningitis and bacteremia, as well as less serious but highly prevalent infections such as otitis media (OM) and sinusitis. Children under 2 years and adults over 65 years of age are particularly susceptible to Pn disease. Other high-risk groups include persons with functional or anatomical asplenia, those with underlying medical conditions such as chronic cardiovascular, pulmonary, renal or liver disease, and immunocompromised individuals (particularly those with HIV infection).

S. pneumoniae is the single most common cause of community-acquired pneumonia and has become the most common cause of meningitis in many regions, particularly those in which vaccination has reduced the incidence of *Haemophilus influenzae* type b (Hib) infection. Determining the true burden of Pn disease is complicated by difficulties in establishing an etiological diagnosis, particularly in cases of non-bacteremic pneumonia. Nevertheless, the pneumococcus is conservatively estimated to kill >1 million children under the age of 5 years each year in developing countries, thereby accounting for 20-25% of all deaths in this age group.[1,2] Even in developed countries, where effective antimicrobial therapy is readily accessible, morbidity and mortality from Pn disease is substantial. For example, in the United States there are approximately 500,000 cases of Pn pneumonia, 50,000 cases of bacteremia and 3,000 cases of Pn meningitis each year, collectively resulting in an estimated 40,000 deaths.[2-4] *S. pneumoniae* is also the single most common cause of OM, which in the USA results in over 24 million visits to pediatricians each year, and more prescriptions for antibiotics than any other infectious

New Bacterial Vaccines, edited by Ronald W. Ellis and Bernard R. Brodeur.

disease.[4,5] Thus, OM has a significant impact on health-care costs in developed countries, and estimates for USA exceed $5 billion per annum.[5]

For the past 50 years antibiotics have been the principal weapon in the fight against Pn disease. Clinical isolates of *S. pneumoniae* were universally and exquisitely sensitive to penicillin in the first two decades after its introduction. However, strains with reduced susceptibility to penicillin (MIC >0.1 μg/mL) were detected in the late 1960s and since then have steadily increased in prevalence throughout the world. The problem is greatest in areas in which the use of antibiotics has been poorly regulated, and rates of resistance to β-lactams may exceed 50% of isolates.[6] Moreover, the degree of resistance has been increasing as a consequence of accumulation of multiple mutations in penicillin-binding protein genes, resulting in strains with high-level penicillin-resistance (MIC ≥ 2 μg/mL). Penicillin-resistant pneumococci are also often resistant to one or more other classes of antibiotics, such as tetracycline, erythromycin, chloramphenicol, cotrimoxazole and extended spectrum cephalosporins, and multiply-resistant clones of *S. pneumoniae* have spread globally.[7] The increasing prevalence of penicillin- and multiply-resistant pneumococci is complicating management of patients with suspected Pn disease, particularly those with meningitis. In developed countries this is necessitating the use of more expensive alternative antimicrobials, but this option is not available in poorer parts of the world. There also have been several reports from the US and Europe of cases of Pn meningitis caused by strains resistant to virtually all antimicrobials except vancomycin.[8] Vancomycin resistance is now common in Enterococci; *S. pneumoniae*, a naturally transformable organism, may acquire the genes encoding this capacity. Infections caused by such an organism could be essentially untreatable.

The potential contribution of immunoprophylaxis to the control of Pn disease was recognized in the early 20th century. Early trials of killed whole cell vaccines yielded inconclusive results. Although interest fluctuated in the decades that followed, the steady increase in knowledge of the immunobiology of Pn disease enabled a rational approach to vaccine design. Nevertheless, as we enter the 21st century, the continued high global morbidity and mortality associated with Pn disease, and the increasing threat posed by antibiotic-resistant strains, underscore the need for a more effective vaccination strategy against this organism. In this chapter we will summarize the current status of Pn vaccine development, the strengths and weaknesses of existing approaches, and future prospects.

Polysaccharide Vaccines

An important feature of *S. pneumoniae* is its capacity to produce a Ps capsule, which is structurally distinct for each of the 90 known serotypes of the organism. The capsule is considered to be the sine qua non of pneumococcal virulence.[3] All fresh clinical isolates are encapsulated, and spontaneous non-encapsulated (rough) derivatives of such strains are avirulent. The precise manner in which the Ps contributes to virulence is not fully understood, although it is known to have strong anti-phagocytic properties in non-immune hosts. The majority of Ps serotypes are negatively charged at physiological pH, and this may directly cause interference of interactions with phagocytes and complement (C'). Pn cell wall teichoic acid (also known as C-polysaccharide) is capable of activating the alternative C' pathway. In addition, antibodies to this and other cell surface constituents, which are found in most adult human sera, may result in activation of the classical C' pathway, as does interaction of the teichoic acid with C-reactive protein. However, the capsule forms an inert shield, which appears to prevent interaction of either the Fc region of IgG or C3b fixed to deeper cell surface structures from interacting with receptors on phagocytic cells.[9] Pneumococci belonging to different Ps serotypes vary in their capacity to resist phagocytosis in vitro and their polysaccharides also differ in their immunogenicity.[10] This accounts in large part for the fact that certain Pn types are far more commonly associated with human disease than are others.[3] Otherwise isogenic pneumococci expressing different Ps serotypes, generated by in vitro or in vivo transformation, also exhibit marked differences in virulence for mice.[11,12] However, within a given strain and serotype, virulence of *S. pneumoniae* is directly related to capsular thickness.[3]

The immunogenicity of Pn Ps was recognized in the late 1920s, and a well-constructed trial of a quadrivalent Ps vaccine in US military recruits during World War II demonstrated a high degree of protection against pneumonia caused by vaccine serotypes.[13] The protection imparted by Ps vaccines is largely a result of binding of specific antibody to the capsule, resulting in opsonization and rapid clearance of invading pneumococci. However, in the above study, vaccinees were also partially protected against nasopharyngeal colonization by Pn types included in the formulation. Invasive Pn disease is almost invariably preceded by nasopharyngeal colonization. Although only a minority of such carriers develops frank disease, they are an important reservoir of infection. Thus, the capacity to reduce Pn carriage is a highly desirable vaccine trait, as it is likely to reduce transmission of disease in the community, thereby conferring a degree of protection upon non-vaccinees.

The success of the quadrivalent vaccine trial led to the commercial production of two hexavalent Ps vaccines in the late 1940s. However, this coincided with the introduction of penicillin and other antibiotics, which at the time appeared to be spectacularly effective against the pneumococcus. As a result the vaccines were not utilized to any great extent and eventually were withdrawn from the market.[14] Nevertheless, it subsequently became clear that prompt and appropriate antibiotic therapy could not be relied upon to prevent death from invasive Pn disease in certain high-risk patient groups. The continued high morbidity and mortality rekindled interest in Ps vaccines, and further trials were conducted in healthy young adults (South African miners) who had high attack rates of Pn pneumonia and bacteremia. Multivalent formulations were shown to be ~80% effective in preventing invasive Pn disease caused by vaccine serotypes.[4,14] A 14-valent PS vaccine was licensed in 1977, and coverage was expanded to 23 types in 1983. This latter formulation includes types 1, 2, 3, 4, 5, 6B, 7F, 8, 9N, 9V, 10A, 11A, 12F, 14, 15B, 17F, 18C, 19A, 19F, 20, 22F, 23F and 33F.[4]

A number of additional trials have been conducted in older adults since the introduction of the Ps vaccines (reviewed in refs. 4 and 15). Comparisons of the results of the different studies are complicated by differences in study design and clinical criteria, but they have tended to show somewhat lower efficacy rates (usually ~60%), particularly in elderly recipients, the immunocompromized, and those with underlying chronic diseases. Nevertheless, controversy surrounding the efficacy of PS vaccines for preventing Pn pneumonia has continued, particularly since some prospective randomized trials in older adults failed to demonstrate any protection whatsoever.[16,17] In spite of this, the vaccine is recommended for all persons aged >65 years, and those <65 belonging to other high-risk groups (those with functional or anatomical asplenia, chronic cardiovascular or pulmonary disease, alcoholism, chronic liver disease, immunocompromized individuals, etc.).[4] Ps vaccines are not recommended for children aged <2 years, even though they are a particularly high-risk group, because efficacy has not been demonstrated in clinical trials.

The likely explanation for the failure of the vaccine in young children is the poor immunogenicity of many of the component Ps antigens. Children < 2 years of age can mount an adequate antibody response to some types (e.g., type 3), but responses are particularly poor for the Ps types which most commonly cause invasive disease in children, namely 6A/B, 14, 18C, 19F and 23F.[18] Indeed, responses to these types are weak up to the age of 5 years and do not reach adult levels until 8-10 years of age.[19] Elderly adults also exhibit weaker and more transient antibody responses compared with younger adults to some of these Ps serotypes, and this undoubtedly accounts for the poorer clinical efficacy in this age group referred to above.[15]

Ps is referred to as a "thymus-independent type-2" antigen, which activates B lymphocytes independently of $CD4^+$ cells by directly binding and cross-linking antigen receptors on the B-cell surface. This process is distinct from that induced by protein antigens and involves co-stimulation by CD21 (type 2 C' receptor) after binding of C3d (generated by activation of the alternative C' pathway by PS). Neonatal B lymphocytes express low levels of CD21, which may explain the hyporesponsiveness to Ps during infancy.[20] Ps antigens do not induce immunological memory, and antibodies produced are mainly of the IgG_2 subclass. Even in healthy adults, antibody levels begin to decline about 1 year post-vaccination and for many types return to preimmunization levels after about 5 years.[15] Interestingly, Musher et al[21] have recently reported that healthy individuals varied markedly in their capacity to mount an antibody response to various Pn Ps serotypes and that this was controlled genetically and inherited in a codominant pattern. Thus, a subset of the adult population may be refractory to immunization with Pn Ps vaccines.

The other principal weakness of Ps vaccines is that the induced protection is strictly serotype-dependent. As mentioned above, the current vaccine formulation includes Ps purified from 23 of the 90 known Pn serotypes, and clinical trials have confirmed that it provides negligible cover against non-vaccine serotypes. Fortunately, not all types are equally prevalent, and the formulation was determined with reference to available data on the distribution of types causing invasive disease in adults and children.[22] Most of these data emanated from the US or Europe, and the 23 included serotypes currently account for ~90% of invasive Pn infections in these regions. However, there are geographical and temporal differences in the serotype distribution of disease-causing pneumococci, and the existing formulation may cover as little as ~60% of strains in parts of Asia.[23] Moreover, serotype prevalence data are scanty for many developing countries, and vaccine coverage in these regions is uncertain.

Some Ps types in the vaccine (e.g., 6B) are known to elicit antibodies that cross-react with structurally-related Ps types that are not included (in this example type 6A). Type 6A and 6B pneumococci are both important causes of invasive disease in children, but the vaccine was formulated with the expectation that the cross-reacting antibodies would provide cross-protection.[22] However, this assumption may be incorrect, as the cross-reacting antibodies appear to be of low avidity and function poorly in in vitro opsonophagocytic assays against the heterologous type. More recent clinical trials are also strongly suggestive of a lack of adequate cross-protection.[15]

The inevitable conclusion that must be drawn from the above is that, notwithstanding the high protective efficacy in healthy adults, existing Ps vaccines have suboptimal efficacy in groups who are most at risk from life-threatening invasive Pn disease. The combination of incomplete protection against included serotypes and variation in serotype distribution affecting vaccine coverage will undoubtedly attenuate the overall global impact of Ps vaccines. Nevertheless, even a 50%-effective vaccine will prevent countless deaths in groups for whom the Ps vaccine is currently recommended, and so until a better alternative is available, its continued use must be vigorously encouraged. Urgent efforts are required, however, to develop vaccines that are efficacious in young children, for whom the existing PS vaccine provides little demonstrable clinical benefit.

Polysaccharide-Protein Conjugate Vaccines

A possible solution to the poor immunogenicity of Ps in young children emanated from the seminal work of Avery and Goebel,[24] who reported in 1931 that chemical conjugation of type 3 Pn Ps to a protein carrier massively increased its immunogenicity in rabbits. The significance of these early studies was recognized by Schneerson et al,[25] who synthesized Hib PS-protein conjugates to overcome the poor Ps immunogenicity in children. This led to the development of the Hib conjugate vaccine, which has dramatically reduced morbidity and mortality from invasive Hib disease where widely utilized in many parts of the world.[26] The spectacular success of the Hib conjugate has encouraged development of multivalent pneumococcal Ps-protein conjugate vaccines, the first generation of which are now licensed in several countries. Conjugation to a protein carrier converts the Ps into a T-cell-dependent antigen. The Ps is thought to react with receptors on B cells, which then internalize the conjugate, process it, and present peptide fragments in association with Class II MHC molecules to peptide-specific T-cells. Memory responses are generated, and primed B-cells can be boosted either with conjugate or free Ps.[15]

Development of Pn Ps-protein conjugate vaccines has been considerably more complex than was the case with Hib, owing to the multiplicity of disease-causing serotypes. A number of parameters that influence immunogenicity of conjugate antigens need to be optimized for each type, including the molecular size of the Ps component, the carrier protein, the Ps:carrier ratio, and the method used to covalently link the two components. In view of this developmental complexity, the number of serotypes that can be included is by necessity less than in the PS vaccine. However, the conjugate vaccines are principally designed to prevent invasive disease and OM in young children, for whom the range of disease-causing serotypes is more restricted than in adults.

Conjugate vaccines developed to date by various manufacturers are either 7-, 9- or 11-valent, use different cross-linking chemistries, and employ a range of carriers such as tetanus or diphtheria toxoids, the diphtheria toxin derivative CRM_{197}, or outer membrane proteins from *Neisseria meningitidis* group B or non-typable *H. influenzae*. The 7-valent formulation includes types 4, 6B, 9V, 14, 18C, 19F and 23F, and it is estimated that this would cover ~60-90% of pediatric infections based on North American and European seroprevalence studies.[27] The 9-valent vaccine includes these same types with the addition of types 1 and 5, which, although uncommon in Europe and North America, are important causes of invasive pediatric disease in other geographic regions. Indeed, a ten-year study of the seroprevalence of pneumococci causing invasive disease in children in Southern Israel indicated that inclusion of these two types would increase coverage from 41% to 67% in Jewish children and from 22% to 63% in Bedhouin children.[28] Types 3 and 7F were also included in the 11-valent formulation.

These conjugate vaccines are typically administered as a course of three injections at 2, 4 and 6 months of age, followed by a booster of either conjugate or Ps vaccine at 12-15 months. Several clinical studies have demonstrated that they are well tolerated by infants and elicit strong, boostable antibody responses. A large study of the 7-valent vaccine in Northern California demonstrated 97% protection against invasive (bacteremic) disease caused by vaccine types.[29] A Finnish study designed to test the protective efficacy of the same vaccine against OM, which included microbiological analysis of middle ear fluid from all suspected cases, demonstrated a 57% reduction in infections caused by vaccine types.[30] This figure is similar to the 67% reduction in OM caused by vaccine types reported in the Californian study, although microbiological analysis had been confined to spontaneously draining ears.[29]

Although the degree of type-specific protection imparted by the conjugate vaccine was less spectacular against OM as compared to invasive disease, this outcome was not unexpected, as higher antibody concentrations are probably required for prevention of the former. Nevertheless, the prevalence of Pn OM is such that even a partially protective vaccine would prevent a very large number of cases. Interestingly, in the Finnish study the vaccine also reduced the number of OM episodes caused by pneumococci belonging to non-included types such as 6A and 19A, which cross-react with vaccine types (6B and 19F, respectively) by 51%.[30] This occurred even though antibodies to type 6B PS elicited by the conjugate have been shown to have weaker in vitro opsonophagocytic activity against type 6A pneumococci relative to type 6B strains.[31]

A major concern emanating from the Finnish study, however, was the finding that OM caused by non-vaccine serotypes increased by ~33%.[30] This finding was also not unexpected. In previous trials conducted in the Gambia,[32] South Africa[33] and Israel[34] the conjugate vaccine significantly reduced nasopharyngeal carriage of vaccine types in children, but this was offset at least partially by an increase in carriage of non-vaccine types, many of which were known to be capable of causing disease.

Nasopharyngeal carriage of *S. pneumoniae* is generally accepted as a prerequisite for Pn disease, and serotypes being carried usually correlate with those causing disease in a community. Carriers are the major source for transmission of pneumococci, and communities with high rates of carriage also have high attack rates of Pn disease. Carriage rates are high in young children, particularly in developing countries, where infants acquire pneumococci (presumably from their colonized mothers) in the first few days of life. Individuals may be colonized by multiple Pn strains or serotypes and these presumably compete (with each other and perhaps with other microflora) for occupation of the nasopharyngeal niche.[35] Detection of multiple Pn serotypes in nasopharyngeal cultures is technically difficult if one strain is significantly outnumbered. Thus, it is hard to determine the extent to which "replacement carriage" observed in a conjugate vaccine recipient is a result of acquisition of new Pn types not previously present, or facilitated detection of a pre-existing non-vaccine serotype whose numbers have increased after elimination of interference from vaccine types. However, regardless of the mechanism, replacement carriage does appear to translate into increased disease caused by non-vaccine serotypes.[30]

S. pneumoniae strains undoubtedly differ in their capacity to colonize the nasopharynx, as well as in their capacity to cause either OM or invasive disease once carriage has been established. These differences have a multifactorial basis and depend upon capsular serotype as well as upon other ill-defined virulence traits. This accounts for the non-uniform distribution and relative prevalence of the 90 Pn serotypes as well as for the existence of highly successful widely distributed clones, some of which are multidrug-resistant. Molecular analysis of one such highly transmissible, multiply resistant strain (Spanish type 23F clone) demonstrated that pneumococci are capable of switching serotype by recombinational exchange of capsule biosynthesis loci in vivo.[36] It is easy to see how antibiotic therapy would facilitate such exchanges between co-colonizing sensitive and resistant strains; DNA released from the sensitive strain would directly transform the resistant type, enabling it to assume the serotype of the donor.

Most, but by no means all, serotype exchanges in resistant pneumococci detected to date have been from one vaccine type to another vaccine type, presumably because the other vaccine types are also commonly carried.[37] However, increased colonization by non-vaccine types due to use of the conjugate vaccines will increase the likelihood of in vivo transformation of multiply-resistant pneumococci to non-vaccine serotypes. Introduction of the conjugate vaccines will also provide direct selective pressure for acquisition of non-vaccine serotype capsule loci by highly virulent Pn clones that hitherto had expressed a vaccine-type capsule.

The impact of widespread use of conjugate vaccines on the complex biology of Pn disease is difficult to predict. The full effect of the vaccine on serotype prevalence may take many years to become apparent and will vary from region to region depending upon levels of endemic carriage and rates of vaccine utilization. In well-vaccinated populations, disease caused by vaccine types will be markedly reduced, and reduction of carriage of vaccine types will undoubtedly provide a degree of homotypic herd immunity. In the short term, the vaccine may also help to control the spread of antibiotic-resistant pneumococci, because they are more prevalent in children (the principal target population) than in adults, and the majority of such isolates belong to vaccine serotypes.

However, these major clinical benefits may be ephemeral. As vaccine use grows, so too will the rate of nasopharyngeal carriage of non-vaccine types. In turn, this will increase the likelihood of transmission of non-vaccine-serotype pneumococci to others in the community, including vaccinees, further increasing overall carriage rates of such strains. Capsule-type switching also may facilitate vaccine escape and enable the spread of antibiotic resistance to a broader range of serotypes than is currently the case. Continued surveillance of the serotype distribution of disease-causing pneumococci will be essential. Inclusion of additional conjugated Ps in the formulation may be required if non-vaccine types become too prevalent.

There are limits, however, on just how many capsular types can be accommodated. Polyvalent Ps-protein conjugate vaccines are very expensive to produce, and the addition of further Ps types or periodic reformulation to take account of altered serotype prevalence will add further to this cost. This may place the vaccine even further out of the reach of many developing countries, whose need for effective Pn vaccines is greatest. In countries that can afford them, conjugate vaccines are likely to have a major impact upon the burden of Pn disease in the short term, but their overall efficacy is likely to diminish with time, necessitating ongoing investment in development of alternative vaccination strategies capable of eliciting more broad-based and affordable protection.

Purified Protein Vaccines

The known and potential shortcomings of the Ps and Ps-conjugate vaccines have prompted extensive research aimed at developing vaccines based on proteins that contribute to virulence and are common to all serotypes. Such vaccines should be highly immunogenic and elicit immunological memory in infants and young children, who respond well to T-dependent protein antigens. High level protein expression generally can be engineered in recombinant *E. coli*, enabling large-scale production at relatively low cost, resulting in vaccines that are more affordable, particularly for developing countries. A number of candidate Pn protein antigens have been examined for vaccine potential, as discussed below.

Pneumolysin

Pneumolysin was the first Pn protein to be proposed as a vaccine antigen.[38] It is a potent 53-kD thiol-activated pore-forming cytolysin produced by virtually all Pn strains. In addition to its cytotoxic properties, this bifunctional toxin can directly activate the classical C' pathway (with a concomitant reduction in serum opsonic activity) by binding to the Fc region of human IgG. In vitro studies using purified toxin have demonstrated that pneumolysin has a variety of detrimental effects on cells and tissues, which undoubtedly contribute to the pathogenesis of disease (reviewed in ref. 39). These properties include inhibition of the bactericidal activity of leukocytes, blockade of proliferative responses and Ig production by lymphocytes, reduction of ciliary beating of human respiratory epithelium, and direct cytotoxicity for respiratory endothelial and epithelial cells. Thus, pneumolysin may function in pathogenesis by interfering with both phagocytic and ciliary clearance of pneumococci, by blocking humoral immune responses, and by aiding penetration of host tissues.[39]

Pneumolysin is also capable of direct induction of inflammatory responses,[40] and injection of purified pneumolysin into rat lungs induces severe lobar pneumonia, indistinguishable histologically from that seen when virulent pneumococci are injected.[41] Additional insights into the role of pneumolysin in pathogenesis have been gained by studies of the behavior of defined pneumolysin-negative mutants of *S. pneumoniae* in a number of animal models. Such strains have significantly reduced virulence in mouse models of sepsis and pneumonia.[42] Intranasal challenge with these mutants results in a less severe inflammatory response, a reduced rate of multiplication within the lung, a reduced capacity to injure the alveolar-capillary barrier and a delayed onset of bacteremia, compared with the wild type strain.[39] Additional site-directed mutagenesis studies have shown that both the cytotoxic and C'-activation properties of the toxin contribute to the pathogenesis of Pn pneumonia.[43,44]

Although native pneumolysin is a protective immunogen in mice, it is not suitable as a human vaccine antigen because of its toxicity. To overcome this, the pneumolysin gene has been mutated in regions essential for its cytotoxic and/or C'-activation properties, resulting in expression of non-toxic but immunogenic "pneumolysoids", which are easily purified from recombinant *E. coli* expression systems.[45] Pneumolysin is a highly conserved protein, and extensive analysis of genes from a wide range of serotypes has detected negligible variation in deduced amino acid sequence, auguring well for broad coverage. Indeed, immunization of mice with a pneumolysoid carrying a Trp_{433}-Phe mutation resulting in >99.5% reduction in cytotoxicity (designated PdB) provided a significant degree of protection against all nine tested serotypes.[46]

Humans are known to mount an antibody response to pneumolysin as a result of natural exposure to *S. pneumoniae*, and a recent study has shown that purified human anti-pneumolysin IgG also passively protects mice from challenge with virulent pneumococci.[47] Thus, it is anticipated that the various pneumolysoids will be immunogenic in humans. However, pneumolysoid may not provide a sufficient degree of protection to be effective as a stand-alone vaccine antigen. Pneumolysin is not displayed on the Pn surface; it is located in the cytoplasm and is released into the external milieu when pneumococci undergo spontaneous autolysis in some strains[48] as well as by an as-yet-uncharacterized export mechanism in others.[49] Antibodies to pneumolysin are presumed to impart protection by neutralization of the biological properties of the toxin, thereby impeding the kinetics of infection, rather than by stimulating opsonophagocytic clearance of the invading bacteria. Thus, protein-based vaccines combining pneumolysoid with Pn surface proteins capable of eliciting opsonic antibodies would be expected to be more effective.

Pneumococcal Surface Protein A (PspA)

PspA is a variable, but cross-reactive protein that is expressed on the surface of all tested pneumococci.[50,51] PspA has been shown to be able to elicit cross-protective antibodies against strains producing diverse PspAs.[52,53] Strains of pneumococci in which PspA has been genetically deleted or inactivated are less virulent than wild-type strains.[54,55] An important virulence function of PspA relates to its ability to inhibit complement deposition on pneumococci through the alternative pathway.[54,56] Studies with mice have demonstrated that the presence of PspA significantly inhibits the depletion of C' from the serum of infected mice.[54] PspA also binds to lactoferrin.[57,58] The significance of this binding is not clear, but it appears not to be a mechanism for the acquisition of iron by pneumococci.[59] Under some circumstances, apolactoferrin is able to kill pneumococci and other bacteria.[60] When concentrations of lactoferrin are limiting, the presence of surface PspA can protect the bacteria (Mirza and Briles, manuscript in preparation).

PspA is among a group of 12 choline-binding Pn proteins. These proteins are able to bind the phosphocholine residues on lipoteichoic acids or teichoic acids of the cell membrane and cell wall.[61-63] PspA and PspC (described below) are attached to the bacterial surface by their choline-binding domains,[62,64] which consist of 9-10 highly conserved 20-amino-acid choline-binding repeats near the C-terminal end of the molecule.[65,66] Just N-terminal to the choline binding domain is a proline-rich domain that can be as long as 80⁺ amino acids and comprises at least 20% prolines.[65-67] The N-terminal end of the molecule usually contains from ~300-400 amino acids that make a highly charged largely α-helical structure, which is thought to be an anti-parallel coiled-coil.[67,68] Although there may be some protection-eliciting epitopes in the proline-rich region,[69] the bulk of the protective epitopes of PspA lie in the α-helical part of the molecule.[70] Studies with two different PspA types have revealed that the most cross-protective region is the 100 amino acids that are most C-terminal in the α-helical region;[70] this region has been called the B region.[67]

By comparing the sequence diversity within the B-region and the cross-reactivity of immune sera to PspA, it has been possible to divide PspAs into three families.[51,67] PspAs within families differ by no more than 40% of their amino acids within the B region. The difference can be 60⁺% between families.[67] Over 95% of pneumococci express one or more PspAs of families 1 or 2.[51,67]

In recent studies, human volunteers were immunized with a family-1 recombinant PspA from strain Rx1. The induced antibodies were able to passively protect mice against type 3, 6A and 6B strains regardless of whether they expressed family 1 or 2 PspAs. These results make it likely that a successful PspA vaccine for humans need not contain more than a few different PspA molecules.[53,71]

Intranasal immunization with full-length native PspA, using the cholera toxin B subunit (CTB) as an adjuvant, elicits strong protection in mice against nasal carriage of *Streptococcus pneumoniae.*[72] Intranasal immunization with a recombinant N-terminal fragment of PspA containing the first 302 amino acids also elicits protection against carriage, but may be less efficacious than immunization with full-length PspA.[73-74] Mucosal immunization also elicited strong systemic antibody responses and was able to protect against intraperitoneal, intravenous, or intrapulmonary challenge with virulent *S. pneumoniae.*[72,74,75]

Systemic immunization with PspA elicits high systemic levels of antibody, but little or no mucosal antibody and no detectable protection against nasal carriage.[72] However, systemic immunization with PspA was able to elicit measurable protection against lung infection as well as sepsis. The best protection against lung infection was observed with a combination of PspA and pneumolysin.[52]

Pneumococcal Surface Protein C (PspC) / Choline Binding Protein A (CbpA)

Another choline-binding protein (PspC) has also been shown to be able to elicit protection against invasive disease and carriage. PspC has choline-binding and repeat regions that are within the variability seen for PspA. In fact, the *pspC* gene was first identified using a probe for *pspA*, and at the time was predicted to likely encode another protective antigen. The first sequence of this gene was deposited in Gene Bank in September 1996 under the name *pspC*.[76] The molecule was independently identified through its ability to bind choline (designated CbpA)[63] and the secretory component of IgA (designated SpsA).[77-79] The molecule also has been shown to interact with the C' system through its ability to bind C3[80] and factor H.[81-83] PspC/CbpA/SpsA has been reported to play a role in adherence and cell invasion.[63] The latter is thought to occur through interaction with the secretory component associated with the polymeric immunoglobulin receptor pIgR.[79]

PspC is present on ~75% of Pn strains.[69,77] The N-terminal half of PspC shares homology with an allelic protein Hic,[82] which together with PspC appear to be present on virtually all pneumococci (Susan Hollingshead, personal communication). Hic lacks a choline-binding domain and instead is assumed to bind to the Pn cell wall through its LPXTG motif.[82] Hic and PspC both bind to factor H, a C' regulatory protein.[81,82] Very recent studies with PspC have demonstrated that in the presence of factor H, PspC/Hic can inhibit C' activation and decrease phagocytosis.[82,83] Thus, both PspA and PspC/Hic can affect C' activation, but by different mechanisms.

PspC is maximally produced by pneumococci in the transparent phase.[63] Pneumococci in the transparent phase are much more efficient at carriage than those in the opaque phase which are better suited to invasion.[84] The phase switch is an apparently random event, with all cultures containing at least a small fraction of bacteria in each phase. It has been shown that mutations in PspC can have a deleterious effect on carriage.[85] Even though PspC is produced in the largest amounts during carriage, it may also play a role in invasive disease. This is apparent from studies showing that the lack of PspA and PspC[85] or pneumolysin and PspC[86] can have greater effects on invasive virulence than the lack of either protein by itself.

Immunization of mice with PspC has been shown to be highly protective against intravenous or intraperitoneal challenge with *S. pneumoniae*.[69,87] However, at least some of this protection appears to be due to cross-reaction of antibodies to PspC with PspA.[69]

Pneumococcal Surface Antigen A (PsaA)

Another candidate vaccine antigen is PsaA, a highly conserved 37-kD surface protein produced by all pneumococci tested. It was thought initially to be an adhesin based on sequence homology with putative lipoprotein adhesins of oral streptococci, but it is actually the metal-binding lipoprotein component of an ATP-binding cassette (ABC) transport system with specificity for Mn^{2+}.[88] Defined *psaA*-negative mutants of *S. pneumoniae* are virtually avirulent for mice and exhibit markedly reduced adherence in vitro to human type II pneumocytes.[89] This is presumed to be a consequence of a requirement for Mn as a cofactor or for regulation of expression of other virulence factors (e.g., adhesins), and/or growth retardation due to an inability to scavenge this metal in vivo. Immunization of mice with purified PsaA has been shown to confer partial protection, although it is less efficacious than either pneumolysoid or PspA in an intraperitoneal challenge model.[90] The dimensions of PsaA (~7 nm at its longest axis)[91] are such that, if it is anchored to the outer face of the cell membrane via its N-terminal lipid moiety, it is unlikely to be exposed on the outer surface of the pneumococcus. Thus, the observed protection is presumably due to in vivo blockade of ion transport, which necessitates diffusion of antibody through the capsule and cell wall layers. Penetration of antibody may be influenced by thickness of the capsule, which may be up-regulated during invasive infection. In contrast, pneumococci colonizing the nasopharynx are thought to down-regulate capsule expression, thereby facilitating interaction between surface adhesins and the host mucosa. Consistent with this hypothesis, intranasal immunization of mice with PsaA has been shown to significantly reduce the level of nasopharyngeal carriage of *S. pneumoniae*, as will be discussed later.[73]

Other Pneumococcal Proteins

The release of the *S. pneumoniae* genome sequence by The Institute for Genome Research (TIGR) in 1997 was a watershed event in the quest for additional pneumococcal vaccine antigens. Whereas previous studies had identified individual proteins as virulence factors, usually by studying the behavior of gene knock-out mutants in animal models, access to the genome sequence permitted targeting of entire families of genes encoding proteins with recognizable structural features.[92] The choline-binding proteins referred to above are good examples of this approach. Although several members of this family previously had been identified by conventional techniques (e.g., elution from the cell surface with choline), a search of the genome sequence identified a total of 12 functional genes encoding proteins with choline-binding motifs. Site-specific mutagenesis then was used to demonstrate that several of the novel choline-binding proteins were involved in in vitro adherence to epithelial cells, nasopharyngeal colonization or sepsis, thereby identifying them as vaccine candidates.[93] Another large-scale study identified potential surface-exposed proteins by examination of the genome sequence for open reading frames (ORFs) with motifs associated with transport, cell-wall anchorage, or choline binding, as well as for those with similarity to known virulence factors in other bacteria. This identified >100 genes, which then were expressed in *E. coli*, enabling purification of the respective proteins (or fragments thereof). Five of these, including two choline-binding proteins (LytB and LytC), were demonstrated to be protective immunogens in a mouse model, although the degree of protection observed was marginally less than that observed using PspA which was used as a control antigen.[94] One of the novel protective proteins (PhtA) contained five copies of an unusual histidine-triad motif (HXXHXH). Examination of the genome sequence revealed three additional related ORFs, each with five or six copies of the motif, and immunization with two of these (PhtB and PhtD) also protected mice against some but not all tested Pn challenge strains.[95] Another recent study demonstrated that the metal-binding lipoprotein components of two ABC iron transporters (PiuA and PiaA), which had previously been shown to contribute to virulence, also elicited protection against systemic challenge in mice.[96]

Thus, there is a considerable array of Pn proteins that exhibit potential as vaccine antigens. To a large extent these have been characterized in different laboratories, and protective immunogenicity has been assessed in different animal models using different challenge strains. Only a few direct comparative protection studies have been performed, and so it is very difficult to determine which of these proteins provides the strongest protection against the widest variety of Pn strains.

Combination Protein Vaccines

Virtually all of the Pn proteins under consideration as vaccine antigens are directly or indirectly involved in the pathogenesis of pneumococcal disease. Mutagenesis of some combinations of virulence factor genes, e.g., those encoding pneumolysin and either PspA or PspC, or PspA and PspC, has been shown to synergistically attenuate virulence in animal models, implying that the respective proteins function independently in the pathogenic process.[85,86] This strongly suggests that immunization with combinations of these antigens might provide additive protection. Moreover, there may be differences in the relative protective capacities of the individual antigens against particular strains, particularly for surface-exposed antigens that exhibit some degree of sequence variation. Thus, a combined Pn protein vaccine may elicit a higher degree of protection against a wider variety of strains than any single antigen. To date only a limited number of combination experiments have been performed. Of these, the combination of pneumolysoid PdB and PspA clearly provides enhanced protection against systemic infection and pneumonia, whereas the combination of PspA and PsaA provides additive protection against carriage.[52,73,90] Additional comparative studies of the protective efficacy of the better characterized proteins as well as the more recently identified vaccine candidates (both singly and in combination) are required to enable informed decisions on the formulation of a protein-based Pn vaccine.

Consideration also should be given to using protein antigens as supplements to Ps-protein conjugate vaccines. Incorporation of one or more group-common proteins may reduce significantly the problems associated with limited serotype coverage and replacement carriage associated with the conjugate vaccines, although the problem of high cost remains. Pneumolysin has also been proposed as an alternative carrier in Ps-protein conjugate vaccines, and conjugates of the pneumolysoid PdB with type 19F Ps have been shown to be highly immunogenic and protective in mice.[45,97] In a more recent study, a similar detoxified pneumolysin derivative was shown to be a very effective carrier protein in a quadrivalent conjugate vaccine formulation including Ps types 6B, 14, 19F and 23F.[98] Use of pneumolysin, or other suitable pneumococcal proteins as conjugate vaccine carriers also may minimize any problems associated with overuse of existing carrier proteins.

Mucosal Vaccination Strategies

Given the pivotal role of nasopharyngeal colonization in transmission and as a precursor of Pn disease, vaccination strategies specifically designed to elicit mucosal immune responses may be more efficacious than parenteral immunization for certain antigens, particularly those implicated in colonization. To date this has been examined in animal models using direct intranasal administration of vaccine formulations (killed whole cells or purified antigens) with a strong mucosal adjuvant such as cholera toxin (CT) the related *E. coli* heat-labile enterotoxin (LT) or cytokines such as IL-1, IL-12, or GM-CSF.[74,99] Use of CT and LT holotoxins as adjuvants in human vaccine formulations is somewhat controversial, owing to their reactogenicity. However, significant mucosal adjuvant activity resides in the B subunits of CT and LT, and these are much less reactogenic, although there are residual concerns because of their capacity to bind to GM_1 receptors on olfactory nerve endings.

Intranasal administration of heat-killed type 4 pneumococci resulted in strong humoral and mucosal responses to type 4 Ps and protection from homologous challenge.[100] Similar anti-Ps responses in mice have been achieved using Ps conjugated to either CTB or an LT derivative.[101,102] On the other hand, use of killed non-encapsulated pneumococci has been shown to prevent nasopharyngeal carriage of type 6B pneumococci in a mouse model and to protect rats from intrathoracic challenge with virulent type 3 pneumococci.[103] This latter study is a further demonstration of non-serotype-dependent protection achieved using non-PS antigens. As discussed previously, intranasal immunization of mice with purified PspA or PsaA also has been shown to significantly reduce nasopharyngeal colonization. PsaA elicited stronger immune responses and was more protective than PspA, but immunization with a combination of PsaA and PspA provided a much greater degree of protection against colonization than either antigen alone.[73]

An alternative means of eliciting mucosal immune responses involves oral administration of live recombinant carrier bacteria expressing Pn antigens. Recombinant attenuated Salmonellae expressing pneumolysoid,[104] PspA[105] or both these antigens as well as PsaA[106] have been constructed and shown to elicit mucosal and humoral antibody responses in mice. Expression of type 3 PS has also been achieved in *Lactococcus lactis*, which has been proposed as an alternative carrier for vaccine antigens.[107] However, the mechanism of biosynthesis of this Ps serotype is much simpler than those of all other clinically significant Ps types and requires expression of only a small number of genes.[108] Expression of the other much larger Ps biosynthesis loci in heterologous bacteria may be extremely difficult, and any such live vaccines would also suffer from the disadvantages of serotype-dependent protection and poor immunogenicity of Ps antigens in high risk groups.

DNA Vaccines

A further strategy under consideration for prevention of pneumococcal disease is the use of DNA vaccines. This involves injection (usually intramuscularly) of naked plasmid DNA carrying genes encoding protective antigens under the control of a eukaryotic promoter. The DNA is taken up by host cells, and the antigens are expressed in vivo. This approach has been used for a variety of viral, bacterial and protozoan pathogens, and such vaccines are attractive because they are potentially cheap to produce on a large scale. DNA vaccines usually elicit both humoral and cell-mediated immune responses, and although protection against *S. pneumoniae* is generally considered to be antibody-dependent, the role (if any) of cell-mediated immune responses has not been investigated to any significant extent. A recent study reported construction of a DNA vaccine plasmid encoding the α-helical N-terminal half of PspA (the region which contains the cross-protective epitopes).[109] This DNA vaccine induced strong antibody responses in mice and conferred long-lasting protection against both homologous and heterologous challenge strains. Another study demonstrated that DNA vaccine constructs directing expression of either the C-terminal two-thirds of PspA or PsaA elicited significant antibody responses in mice to the respective protein, although protection against challenge was not examined.[110] The DNA vaccines preferentially elicited IgG2a antibodies, and spleen cells from vaccinated mice secreted elevated levels of γ-interferon, consistent with priming of Th1 immunity. In contrast, antibody responses to vaccination with the purified proteins were primarily of the IgG1 isotype, consistent with a Th2 response.[110]

Use of DNA vaccine delivery systems for Ps antigens is extremely problematic, not only because of the multiplicity of serotypes but also because the genetic loci encoding Ps biosynthesis are very large, comprising up to 20 or more genes for each PS type.[108] The latter problem has been circumvented by using phage display technology and a monoclonal antibody to type 4 Ps to identify a peptide mimic capable of eliciting an anti-Ps response. An oligonucleotide encoding this peptide was then inserted into a DNA vaccine vector and this elicited an anti-type 4 antibody response in mice.[111] It remains to be seen whether such antibodies are protective against challenge with type 4 pneumococci and whether peptide mimics can be developed for a sufficient number of the other Ps serotypes.

Concluding Remarks

The ongoing high global morbidity and mortality associated with Pn disease and the complications caused by increasing rates of resistance to antimicrobials has underpinned extensive efforts in recent years to develop more effective Pn vaccination strategies. These efforts have benefited from a better understanding of the mechanisms of pathogenesis of Pn disease and the advances made possible by the advent of recombinant DNA technology and access to genome sequence data. The polyvalent Ps vaccines have prevented many deaths from invasive disease in recipients belonging to those patient groups for whom this vaccine is currently recommended. The newer Ps-protein conjugate formulations also will confer a very high degree of protection on young children against included serotypes and may also have an impact on prevalence of drug-resistant strains. However, there is now general acceptance that this vaccination approach is not without its drawbacks, and as explained above, the initially substantial clinical benefits that are expected to be derived from widespread use of conjugate vaccines may diminish with time. It will take many years for the overall impact of conjugate vaccines on disease burden and the population biology of *S. pneumoniae* to become apparent. At the very least, use of the conjugate vaccines will buy time for development of cheaper, non-serotype-specific vaccines based on combinations of protein antigens. It must be emphasized, however, that the success of these protein vaccines is not dependent upon real or perceived failure of the conjugates. Rather, the two approaches should be viewed as complementary, each having an important role to play in global prevention of pneumococcal disease. Neither should development of parenteral protein vaccines impede future research on mucosal- or DNA-based delivery systems, which may further improve presentation of protective antigens to the immune system, thereby optimizing host responses.

References

1. Broome C. Meningococcal and pneumococcal disease vaccines. In: Progress of Vaccine Research and Development - 1996. Geneva: World Health Organization (document WHO/VRD/GEN/96.02), 1996:28-32.
2. Klein DL. Pneumococcal disease and the role of conjugate vaccines. In: Tomasz A, ed. Streptococcus pneumoniae Molecular Biology and Mechanisms of Disease. New York: Mary Ann Liebert Inc., 2000:467-477.
3. Austrian R. Some observations on the pneumococcus and on the current status of pneumococcal disease and its prevention. Rev Infect Dis 1981; 3(Suppl.):S1-S17.
4. Centers for Disease Control and Prevention. Prevention of pneumococcal disease: recommendations of the Advisory Committee on Immunization Practices (ACIP). MMWR 1997; 46(RR-8):1-24.
5. Klein JO. The burden of otitis media. Vaccine 2001; 19:S2-S8.
6. Klugman KP. Pneumococcal resistance to antibiotics. Clin Microbiol Rev 1990; 3:171-196.
7. McGee L, Klugman KP, Tomasz A. Serotypes and clones of antibiotic-resistant pneumococci. In: Tomasz A, ed. Streptococcus pneumoniae Molecular Biology and Mechanisms of Disease. New York: Mary Ann Liebert Inc., 2000: 375-379.
8. Klugman KP. Epidemiology, control and treatment of multiresistant pneumococci. Drugs 1996; 52(Suppl 2):42-46.
9. Musher DM. Infections caused by Streptococcus pneumoniae: clinical spectrum, pathogenesis, immunity and treatment. Clin Infect Dis 1992; 14:801-809.
10. van Dam JEG, Fleer A, Snippe H. Immunogenicity and immunochemistry of Streptococcus pneumoniae capsular polysaccharides. Antonie van Leeuwenhoek 1990; 58:1-47.
11. Kelly T, Dillard JP, Yother J. Effect of genetic switching of capsular type on virulence of Streptococcus pneumoniae. Infect Immun 1994; 62:1813-1819.
12. Nesin M, Ramirez M, Tomasz A. Capsular transformation of a multidrug-resistant Streptococcus pneumoniae in vivo. J Infect Dis 1998; 177:707-713.
13. MacLeod CM, Hodges R, Heidelberger M et al. Prevention of pneumococcal pneumonia by vaccination. J Exp Med 1945; 82:445-465.
14. Austrian R. Pneumococcal otitis media and pneumococcal vaccines, a historical perspective. Vaccine 2001; 19:S71-S77.
15. Briles DE, Paton JC, Nahm MH et al. Immunity to Streptococcus pneumoniae. In: Cunningham MW, Fujinami RS, eds. Effects of Microbes on the Immune System. Philadelphia: Lippincott Williams and Wilkins, 1999:263-280.
16. Simberkoff MS, Cross AP, Al-Ibrahim M et al. Efficacy of pneumococcal vaccine in high-risk patients: results of a Veterans Administration cooperative study. N Engl J Med 1986; 315:1318-1327.
17. Ortqvist A, Hedlund J, Burman L-A et al. Randomised trial of 23-valent pneumococcal capsular polysaccharide vaccine in prevention of pneumonia in middle-aged and elderly people: Swedish pneumococcal vaccine group study. Lancet 1998; 351:399-403.
18. Douglas RM, Paton JC, Duncan SJ et al. Antibody response to pneumococcal vaccination in children younger than five years of age. J Infect Dis 1983; 148:131-137.
19. Paton JC, Toogood IR, Cockington R et al. Antibody response to pneumococcal vaccine in children aged 5 to 15 years. Am J Dis Child 1986; 140:135-138.
20. Rijkers GT, Sanders EA, Breukels MA et al. Infant B cell responses to polysaccharide determinants. Vaccine 1998; 16:1396-1400.
21. Musher DM, Watson DA, Baughn RE. Genetic control of the immunological response to pneumococcal capsular polysaccharides. Vaccine 2001; 19:623-627.
22. Robbins JB, Austrian R, Lee CJ et al. Considerations for formulating the second-generation pneumococcal capsular polysaccharide vaccine with emphasis on the cross-reactive types within groups. J Infect Dis 1983; 148:1136-1159.
23. Lee CJ, Banks SD, Li JP. Virulence, immunity and vaccine related to S. pneumoniae. Crit Rev Microbiol 1991; 18:89-114.

24. Avery OT, Goebel WF. Chemo-immunological studies on conjugated carbohydrate-proteins. V. The immunological specificity of an antigen prepared by combining the capsular polysaccharide of type III pneumococcus with foreign protein. J Exp Med 1931; 54:437-447.
25. Schneerson R, Barrera O, Sutton A et al. Preparation, characterization, and immunogenicity of Haemophilus influenzae type b polysaccharide-protein conjugates. J Exp Med 1980; 152:361-376.
26. Robbins JB, Schneerson R, Anderson P et al. Prevention of systemic infections, especially meningitis, caused by Haemophilus influenzae type b. J Am Med Assoc 1996; 276:1181-1185.
27. Eskola J. Polysaccharide-based pneumococcal vaccines in the prevention of acute otitis media. Vaccine 2001; 19:S78-S82.
28. Fraser D, Givon-Lavi N, Bilenko N et al. A decade (1989-1998) of pediatric invasive pneumococcal disease in 2 populations residing in 1 geographical location: implications for vaccine choice. Clin Infect Dis 2001; 33:421-427.
29. Black S, Shinefield H, Fireman B et al. Efficacy, safety and immunogenicity of heptavalent pneumococcal conjugate vaccine in children. Northern California Kaiser Permanente Vaccine Study Center Group. Pediatr Infect Dis J 2000; 19:187-195.
30. Eskola J, Kilpi T, Palmu A et al. Efficacy of a pneumococcal conjugate vaccine against acute otitis media. N Engl J Med 2001; 344:403-409.
31. Vakevainen M, Eklund C, Eskola J et al. Cross-reactivity of antibodies to type 6B and 6A polysaccharides of Streptococcus pneumoniae evoked by pneumococcal conjugate vaccine in infants. J Infect Dis 2001; 184:789-793.
32. Obaro SK, Adegbola RA, Banya WAS et al. Carriage of pneumococci after pneumococcal vaccination. Lancet 1996; 348:271-272.
33. Mbelle N, Huebner RE, Wasas AD et al. Immunogenicity and impact on nasopharyngeal carriage of a nonavalent pneumococcal conjugate vaccine. J Infect Dis 1999; 180:1171-1176.
34. Dagan R. Effect of vaccine on antibiotic resistant S. pneumoniae (PNC) carriage and spread. Second International Symposium on Pneumococci and Pneumococcal Disease. Sun City, South Africa, March 19-23 2000; Abstract O72.
35. Lipsitch M, Dykes JK, Johnson SE et al. Competition among Streptococcus pneumoniae for intranasal colonization in a mouse model. Vaccine 2000; 18:2895-2901.
36. Coffey TJ, Enright MC, Daniels M et al. Recombinational exchanges at the capsular polysaccharide biosynthetic locus lead to frequent serotype changes among natural isolates of Streptococcus pneumoniae. Mol Microbiol 1998; 27:73-84.
37. Spratt BG, Greenwood BM. Prevention of pneumococcal disease by vaccination: does serotype replacement matter. Lancet 2000; 356:1210-1211.
38. Paton JC, Lock RA, Hansman DJ. Effect of immunization with pnuemolysin on survival time of mice challenged with Streptococcus pneumoniae. Infect Immun 1983; 40:548-552.
39. Paton JC. The contribution of pneumolysin to the pathogenicity of Streptococcus pneumoniae. Trends Microbiol. 1996; 4:103-106.
40. Houldsworth S, Andrew PW, Mitchell TJ. Pneumolysin stimulates production of TNFa and IL-1b by human mononuclear phagocytes. Infect Immun 1994; 62:1501-1503.
41. Feldman C, Munro NC, Jeffrey DK et al. Pneumolysin induces the salient histological features of pneumococcal infection in the rat lung in vivo. Am. J. Respir. Cell Mol. Biol. 1991; 5: 416-423.
42. Berry AM, Yother J, Briles DE et al. Reduced virulence of a defined pneumolysin-negative mutant of Streptococcus pneumoniae. Infect Immun 1989; 57:2037-2042.
43. Berry AM, Alexander JE, Mitchell TJ et al. Effect of defined point mutations in the pneumolysin gene on the virulence of Streptococcus pneumoniae. Infect Immun 1995; 63: 1969-1974.
44. Rubins JB, Charboneau D, Fasching C et al. Distinct roles for pneumolysin's cytotoxic and complement activities in the pathogenesis of pneumococcal pneumonia. Am J Respir Crit Care Med 1996; 153:1339-1346.
45. Paton JC, Lock RA, Lee C-J et al. Purification and immunogenicity of genetically obtained pneumolysin toxoids and their conjugation to Streptococcus pneumoniae type 19F polysaccharide. Infect Immun 1991; 59: 2297-2304.
46. Alexander JE, Lock RA, Peeters CCAM et al. Immunization of mice with pneumolysin toxoid confers a significant degree of protection against at least nine serotypes of Streptococcus pneumoniae. Infect Immun 1994; 62: 5683-5688.
47. Musher DM, Phan HM, Baughn RE. Protection against bacteremic pneumococcal infection by antibody to pneumolysin. J Infect Dis 2001; 183:827-830.
48. Berry AM, Lock RA, Hansman D et al. Contribution of autolysin to the virulence of Streptococcus pneumoniae. Infect Immun 1989; 57: 2324-2330.
49. Balachandran P, Hollingshead SK, Paton JC et al. The autolytic enzyme LytA of Streptococcus pneumoniae is not responsible for releasing pneumolysin. J Bacteriol 2001; 183: 3108-3116.

50. Crain MJ, Waltman WD, Turner JS et al. Pneumococcal surface protein A (PspA) is serologically highly variable and is expressed by all clinically important capsular serotypes of Streptococcus pneumoniae. Infect Immun 1990;58: 3293-3299.
51. Coral MCV, Fonseca N, Castaneda E et al. Families of pneumococcal surface protein A (PspA) of Streptococcus pneumoniae invasive isolates recovered from Colombian children. Emerging Infect Dis 2001;7: 832-836.
52. Briles DE, Nabors GS, Brooks-Walter A et al. The potential for using protein vaccines to protect against otitis media caused by Streptococcus pneumoniae. Vaccine 2001;19:S87-S95.
53. Briles DE, Hollingshead SK, King J et al. Immunization of humans with rPspA elicits antibodies, which passively protect mice from fatal infection with Streptococcus pneumoniae bearing heterologous PspA. J Infect Dis 2000;182: 1694-1701.
54. Tu A-HT, Fulgham RL, McCory MA et al. Pneumococcal surface protein A (PspA) inhibits complement activation by Streptococcus pneumoniae. Infect Immun 1999; 67: 4720-4724.
55. McDaniel LS, Yother J, Vijayakumar M et al. Use of insertional inactivation to facilitate studies of biological properties of pneumococcal surface protein A (PspA). J Exp Med 1987; 165: 381-394.
56. Abeyta M. Pneumococcal surface protein A and capsular polysaccharide in virulence of Streptococcus pneumoniae. Microbiology. Birmingham, Alabama: University of Alabama at Birmingham 1999
57. Hammerschmidt S, Bethe G, Remanen P et al. Identification of pneumococcal surface protein A as a lactoferrin-binding protein of Streptococcus pneumoniae. Infect Immun 1999; 67: 1683-1687.
58. Hakansson A, Roche H, Mirza S et al. Characterization of the binding of human lactoferrin to pneumococcal surface protein A (PspA). Infect Immun 2001; 69: 3372-3381.
59. Tai SS, Lee CJ, Winter RE. Hemin utilization is related to virulence of Streptococcus pneumoniae. Infect Immun 1993; 61: 5401-5405.
60. Bullen JJ, Griffiths E. Iron and Infection. 2nd ed New York: John Wiley & Sons1999.
61. Briese T, Hakenbeck R. Interaction of the pneumococcal amidase with lipoteichoic acid and choline. Eur J Biochem 1985; 146: 417-427.
62. Yother J, White JM. Novel surface attachment mechanism for the Streptococcus pneumoniae protein PspA. J Bacteriol 1994; 176: 2976-2985.
63. Rosenow C, Ryan P, Weiser JN et al. Contribution of novel choline-binding proteins to adherence, colonization and immunogenicity of Streptococcus pneumoniae. Mol Microbiol 1997; 25: 819-829.
64. Yother J, Leopold K, White J et al. Generation and properties of a Streptococcus pneumoniae mutant which does not require choline for growth. J Bacteriol 1998; 8: 2093-2101.
65. Yother J, Briles DE. Structural properties and evolutionary relationships of PspA, a surface protein of Streptococcus pneumoniae, as revealed by sequence analysis. J Bacteriol 1992; 174: 601-609.
66. McDaniel LS, McDaniel DO, Hollingshead SK et al. Comparison of the PspA sequence from Streptococcus pneumoniae EF5668 to the previously identified PspA sequence from strain Rx1 and ability of PspA from EF5668 to elicit protection against pneumococci of different capsular types. Infect Immun 1998; 66: 4748-4754.
67. Hollingshead SK, Becker RS, Briles DE. Diversity of PspA: mosaic genes and evidence for past recombination in Streptococcus pneumoniae. Infect Immun 2000; 68: 5889-5900.
68. Jedrzejas MJ, Hollingshead SK, Lebowitz J et al. Production and characterization of the functional fragment of pneumococcal surface protein A. Arch Biochem Biophys 2000; 373: 116-125.
69. Brooks-Walter A, Briles DE, Hollingshead SK. The pspC gene of Streptococcus pneumoniae encodes a polymorphic protein PspC, which elicits cross-reactive antibodies to PspA and provides immunity to pneumococcal bacteremia. Infect Immun 1999; 67: 6533-6542.
70. McDaniel LS, Ralph BA, McDaniel DO et al. Localization of protection-eliciting epitopes on PspA of Streptococcus pneumoniae between amino acid residues 192 and 260. Microb Pathogen 1994; 17: 323-337.
71. Nabors GS, Braun PA, Herrmann DJ et al. Immunization of healthy adults with a single recombinant pneumococcal surface protein A (PspA) variant stimulates broadly cross-reactive antibodies. Vaccine 2000; 18: 1743-1754.
72. Wu H-Y, Nahm M, Guo Y et al. Intranasal immunization of mice with PspA (pneumococcal surface protein A) can prevent intranasal carriage and infection with Streptococcus pneumoniae. J Infect Dis 1997; 175: 839-846.
73. Briles DE, Ades E, Paton JC et al. Intranasal immunization of mice with a mixture of the pneumococcal proteins PsaA and PspA is highly protective against nasopharyngeal carriage of Streptococcus pneumoniae. Infect Immun 2000; 68: 796-800.
74. Arulanandam BP, Lynch JM, Briles DE et al. Intranasal vaccination with pneumococcal surface protein A and IL-12 augments antibody-mediated opsonization and protective immunity against Streptococcus pneumoniae infection. Infect Immun 2001; 69: 6718-6724.

75. Yamamoto M, McDaniel LS, Kawabata K et al. Oral immunization with PspA elicits protective humoral immunity against Streptococcus pneumoniae infection. Infect Immun 1997; 65: 640-644.
76. Brooks-Walter A, Tart RC, Briles DE et al. The pspC gene encodes a second pneumococcal surface protein homologous to the gene encoding the protection-eliciting PspA protein of Streptococcus pneumoniae. ASM Annual Meeting 1997 (Abstract):35.
77. Hammerschmidt S, Talay S, Brandtzaeg P et al. SpsA, a novel pneumococcal surface protein with specific binding to secretory immunoglobulin A and secretory component. Mol Microbiol 1997; 25: 1113-1124.
78. Hammerschmidt S, Tillig MP, Wolff S et al. Species-specific binding of human secretory component to SpsA protein of Streptococcus pneumoniae via a hexapeptide motif. Mol Microbiol 2000; 36: 726-736.
79. Zhang J-R, Mostov KE, Lamm ME et al. The polymeric immunoglobulin receptor translocates pneumococci across human nasopharyngeal epithelial cells. Cell 2000; 102: 827-837.
80. Cheng Q, Finkel D, Hostetter MK. Novel purification scheme and functions for a C3-binding protein from Streptococcus pneumoniae. Biochemistry 2000; 39: 5450-5457.
81. Dave S, Brooks-Walter A, Pangburn MK et al. PspC, a pneumococcal surface protein, binds human factor H. Infect Immun 2001; 69: 3435-3437.
82. Janulczyk R, Iannelli F, Sjoholm AG et al. Hic, a novel surface protein of Streptococcus pneumoniae that interferes with complement function. J Biol Chem 2000; 275: 37257-37263.
83. Jarva H, Janulczyk R, Hellwage J et al. Streptococcus pneumoniae evades complement attack and opsonophagocytosis by expressing the pspC locus-encoded Hic protein that binds to short consensus repeats 8-11 of factor H. J Immunol 2002; 168: 1886-1894.
84. Weiser JN, Austrian R, Sreenivasan PK et al. Phase variation in pneumococcal opacity: relationship between colonial morphology and nasopharyngeal colonization. Infect Immun 1994; 62: 2582-2589.
85. Balachandran P, Brooks-Walter A, Virolainen-Julkunen A et al. The role of pneumococcal surface protein C (PspC) in nasopharyngeal carriage and pneumonia and its ability to elicit protection against carriage of Streptococcus pneumoniae. Infect Immun 2002; In Press.
86. Berry AM, Paton JC. Additive attenuation of virulence of Streptococcus pneumoniae by mutation of the genes encoding pneumolysin and other putative pneumococcal virulence proteins. Infect Immun 2000; 68:133-140.
87. Ogunniyi AD, Woodrow MC, Poolman JT et al. Protection against Streptococcus pneumoniae elicited by immunization with pneumolysin and CbpA. Infect Immun 2001; 69: 5997-6003.
88. Dintilhac A, Alloing G, Granadel C et al. Competence and virulence of S. pneuminiae: Adc and PsaA mutants exhibit a requirement for Zn and Mn resulting from inactivation of metal permeases. Mol Microbiol 1997; 25:727-739.
89. Berry AM, Paton JC. Sequence heterogeneity of PsaA, a 37-kDa putative adhesin essential for virulence of Streptococcus pneumoniae. Infect Immun 1996; 64 5255-5262.
90. Ogunniyi AD, Folland RL, Hollingshead S et al. Immunization of mice with combinations of pneumococcal virulence proteins elicits enhanced protection against challenge with Streptococcus pneumoniae. Infect Immun 2000; 68:3028-3033.
91. Lawrence MC, Pilling PA, Ogunniyi AD et al. The crystal structure of pneumococcal surface antigen PsaA reveals a metal-binding site and a novel structure for a putative ABC-type binding protein.. Structure 1998; 6:1553-1561.
92. Paton JC, Giammarinaro P. Genome-based analysis of pneumococcal virulence factors: the quest for novel vaccine antigens and drug targets. Trends Microbiol 2001; 9:515-518.
93. Gosink KK, Mann ER, Guglielmo C et al. Role of novel choline binding proteins in virulence of Streptococcus pneumoniae. Infect Immun 2000; 68:5690-5695.
94. Wizemann TM, Heinrichs JH, Adamou JE et al. Use of a whole genome approach to identify vaccine molecules affording protection against Streptococcus pneumoniae infection. Infect Immun 2001; 69:1593 1598.
95. Adamou JE, Heinrichs JH, Erwin AL et al. Identification and characterization of a novel family of pneumococcal proteins that are protective against sepsis. Infect Immun 2001; 69:949-958.
96. Brown JS, Ogunniyi AD, Woodrow MC et al. Immunization with components of two iron-uptake ABC transporters protects mice against systemic Streptococcus pneumoniae infection. Infect Immun 2001; 69:6702-6706.
97. Lee C-J, Lock RA, Mitchell TJ et al. Protection of infant mice from challenge with Streptococcus pneumoniae type 19F by immunization with a type 19F polysaccharide-pneumolysoid conjugate. Vaccine 1994; 12:875-878.

98. Michon F, Fusco PC, Minetti CA et al. Multivalent pneumococcal capsular polysaccharide conjugate vaccines employing genetically detoxified pneumolysin as a carrier protein. Vaccine 1998; 16:1732-1741.
99. Wortham C, L Grinberg, DC Kaslow, DE Briles, LS McDaniel, A Lees, M Flora, CM Snapper, JJ Mond. Enhanced protective antibody responses to PspA after intranasal or subcutaneous injections of PspA genetically fused to granulocyte-macrophage colony-stimulating factor or interleukin-2. Infect. Immun.;66:1513-1520.1998
100. Hvalbye BK, Aaberge IS, Lovik M et al. Intranasal immunization with heat-inactivated Streptococcus pneumoniae protects mice against systemic pneumococcal infection. Infect Immun 1999; 67:4320-4325.
101. Seong SY, Cho NH, Kwon IC et al. Protective immunity of microsphere-based mucosal vaccines against lethal intranasal challenge with Streptococcus pneumoniae. Infect Immun 1999; 67:3587-3592.
102. Jakobsen H, Schulz D, Pizza M et al. Intranasal immunization with pneumococcal polysaccharide conjugate vaccines with non-toxic mutants of Escherichia coli heat-labile enterotoxins as adjuvants protects mice against invasive pneumococcal infections. Infect Immun 1999; 67:5892-5897.
103. Malley R, Lipsitch M, Stack A et al. Intranasal immunization with killed unencapsulated whole cells prevents colonization and invasive disease by capsulated pneumococci. Infect Immun 2001; 69:4870-4873.
104. Paton JC, Morona JK, Harrer S et al. Immunization of mice with Salmonella typhimurium C5 aroA expressing a genetically toxoided derivative of the pneumococcal toxin pneumolysin. Microb Pathogen 1993; 14:95-102.
105. Nayak AR, Tinge SA, Tart RC et al. A live recombinant oral Salmonella vaccine expressing pneumococcal surface protein A induces protective responses against Streptococcus pneumoniae. Infect Immun 1998; 66:3744-3751.
106. Barry EM, Santiago AE, Sampson J et al. Multiple pneumococcal antigens expressed in attenuated S. typhi vaccine strains. Abstract. Third International Symposium on Pneumococci and Pneumococcal Diseases, Anchorage, Alaska, 2002.
107. Gilbert C, Robinson K, Le Page RW et al. Heterologous expression of an immunogenic pneumococcal type 3 capsular polysaccharide in Lactococcus lactis. Infect Immun 2000; 68:3251-3260.
108. Paton JC, Morona JK. Streptococcus pneumoniae capsular polysaccharide. In: Fischetti V, Novick R, Ferretti J, Portnoy D, Rood J, eds. Gram-Positive Pathogens. Washington DC: ASM Press, 2000:201-213.
109. Bosarge JR, Watt JM, McDaniel DO et al. Genetic immunization with the region encoding the alpha-helical domain of PspA elicits protective immunity against Streptococcus pneumoniae. Infect Immun 2001; 69:5456-5463.
110. Miyaji EN, Dias WO, Gamberini M et al. PsaA (pneumococcal surface adhesin A) and PspA (pneumococcal surface protein A) DNA vaccines induce humoral and cellular immune responses against Streptococcus pneumoniae. Vaccine 2001; 20:805-812.
111. Lesinski GB, Smithson SL, Srivastava N et al. A DNA vaccine encoding a peptide mimic of Streptococcus pneumoniae serotype 4 capsular polysaccharide induces specific anti-carbohydrate antibodies in Balb/c mice. Vaccine 2001; 19:1717-1726.

Chapter 20

New Generation Tuberculosis Vaccines for Targeted Populations

Uli Fruth and Michael J. Brennan

Every year, almost two million HIV-negative individuals die as a consequence of pulmonary tuberculosis (TB), and many hundreds of thousands more succumb to tuberculosis as a direct consequence of the breakdown of immunity caused by HIV.[1,2] These deaths occur despite the availability of effective drugs and a vaccine, BCG, which is the most widely used of all childhood vaccines.[3] The effectiveness of the BCG vaccine can be described, at best, as variable and drug treatment is long and burdensome, optimally requiring direct observation by a health worker. The fact that diagnosis of infection with *Mycobacterium (M.) tuberculosis,* at least in developing countries, is often made late, when bacteria already appear in the sputum; that reinfection or reactivation of *M. tuberculosis* occurs in drug-cured TB patients; and that multi-drug resistant *M. tuberculosis* strains commonly result from improper adherence to chemotherapy regimens, justifies the need for effective vaccines to help control the global epidemic of tuberculosis.

Mycobacterial Pathogenesis

An understanding of the pathogenic mechanisms of *M. tuberculosis* infection and colonization of susceptible hosts, as well as the role of the subsequent host immune response to the invading organism in the progression of TB, is crucial to the development of better vaccines and treatments for this widespread disease. A major advance in our ability to devise better approaches to investigating the immunopathogenesis of *M. tuberculosis* has been the unraveling of the genomic information found in *M. tuberculosis* and related mycobacterial organisms. Although complete genomic information is available on only two species, *M. tuberculosis*[4] and *M. leprae*,[5] partial information is available on a number of other species and the data suggests interesting differences among the various mycobacteria (see http://www.tigr.org and http://www.sanger.ac.uk). For instance, *M. leprae* the cause of leprosy, has less than one-half of the ~4000 genes found in *M. tuberculosis,* the causative agent of TB in humans. Cole et al[5] have remarked that lepromatous organisms have "just enough" genes left after reductive evolution compared with *M. tuberculosis* to survive within the human host. On the other hand, other mycobacteria like *M. smegmatis,* which prefer to live in the soil, far away from the ravages of an aggressive human immune system, have a much larger genome than *M. tuberculosis.*[6] At first glance, it would then appear to be helpful to have fewer genes if you intend to live within a more evolved organism and face the onslaught of the human immune system. Continued comparative analysis of mycobacterial genomes including those of *M. bovis*[7] and *M. avium* (http://www.tigr.org) will advance our understanding of mycobacterial pathogenesis. Some recent exciting outcomes resulting from genomic analysis of *M. tuberculosis* are discussed later in this chapter.

Another area of intense investigation in the field of TB is the study of how mycobacteria infect and persist within the host tissues. It has been observed that *Mycobacterium bovis*[7] (a

New Bacterial Vaccines, edited by Ronald W. Ellis and Bernard R. Brodeur.

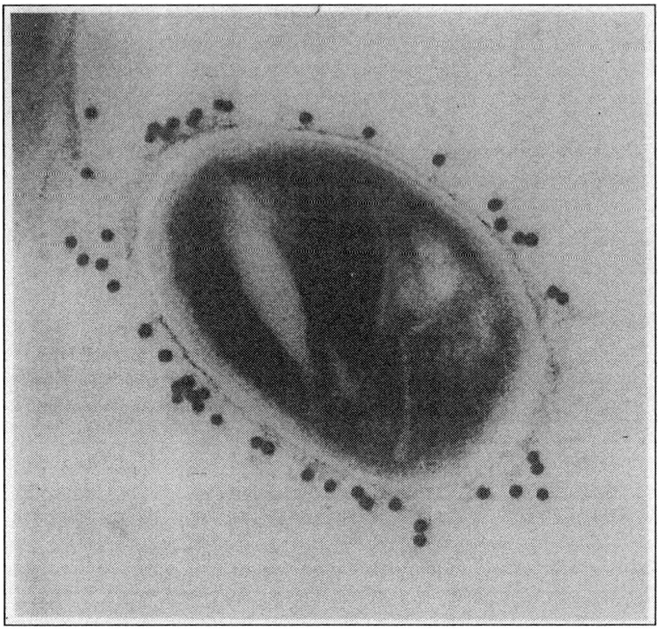

Figure 1. Immunoelectronmicroscopy of *M. tuberculosis* strain H37Ra showing localization of the HBHA adhesin protein on the surface of the *Mycobacterium*. The mycobacteria were incubated with the anti-HBHA monoclonal antibody E4 and anti-mouse IgG conjugated with colloidal gold as described in Menozzi et al.[50]

close cousin of *M. tuberculosis*) can occasionally infect humans, although it prefers to infect mammals such as cattle and even elephants resulting in a disease similar to that caused by *M. tuberculosis* in man. The reasons for this preference by quite similar bacteria for different hosts remain a mystery. One theory is that entry into the host occurs, but the organisms are efficiently eliminated by the immune system prior to colonization of host tissues. Alternatively, tropism for particular hosts may depend upon the bacterium, since there is evidence that certain mycobacterial surface components interact with complementary receptors that exist at the surface of specific host cells.[8,9,10] In the case of certain mycobacteria including *M. tuberculosis*, such receptors can be found on host immune defense cells like macrophages.[11] As observed for other pathogens, mycobacteria may have evolved surface "adhesins" that bind to "receptors" that exist only on certain host cells, thereby contributing to a preference for inhabiting only some host tissues (Fig. 1). Although there are candidates for mycobacterial adhesins (for example, the HBHA,[8] Erp[12] and Inv[13] proteins), the question of why certain mycobacterial species parasitize certain mammals like humans (*M. tuberculosis*), badgers (*M. bovis*), and birds (*M. avium*), while others seem to prefer the soil (*M. smegmatis, M. chelonae*) or perhaps muddy swamps (*M. ulcerans*), remains mostly unanswered. Nevertheless, understanding the mechanisms of mycobacterial infection, growth and persistence in host cells and tissues, especially the human lung, provides a foundation for investigating the cascade of events that follow in the complex immune response to *M. tuberculosis*.

Host Response to Infection with *Mycobacterium tuberculosis*

In studying TB, it is important to appreciate that the pathology of TB (particularly in the lung), although initiated by invading *M. tuberculosis*, is also a result of the complicated immune response to this intracellular organism. Our current understanding suggests that a cascade of host defense mechanisms is triggered when a relatively small number of inhaled *M.*

tuberculosis organisms reach the terminal airspaces of the lung and is ingested by alveolar macrophages. This initial event is followed by a phase of exponential growth of the bacilli at the site of infection, their spread to the proximal lymph nodes and eventual dissemination to other sites in the body. This process of replication and dissemination is commonly controlled by the onset of an effective immune response. The typical manifestation of cellular immunity against tuberculosis is the formation of immune-dependent granulomas (or tubercles), consisting of a core of *M. tuberculosis*-harboring macrophages surrounded by a layer largely composed of lymphocytes. However, it is important to understand that the bacteria walled off within the granuloma are almost never completely eliminated and infection may reactivate at a later date - the lifetime risk for this to happen in immunocompetent individuals is estimated at 5-10%. It is widely accepted that protective immunity against tuberculosis relies on the activation of T cells rather than B cells. $CD4^+$, $CD8^+$ as well as $\gamma\delta$ and double-negative $\alpha\beta$ T cells all are thought to participate in the immune response to infection. However, the relative importance of the different T-cell subsets during the progressive stages of the disease remains elusive. There can be no doubt as to the importance of $CD4^+$ T cells, since both the observed disease exacerbation in MHC class II knock-out mice[14] and the overwhelming susceptibility of HIV patients to TB support this assumption. Within the $CD4^+$ cell population, it is mainly the Th1 subset that appears to mediate protection in both animals and humans and indeed, exceptional susceptibility to tuberculosis has been described in individuals genetically deficient for the IFNγ receptor, the IL12 receptor or IL-12.[15] On the other hand, Th2 cytokines such as IL4 and IL13 can also be detected and are thought to be directly correlated with the extent of tuberculosis-related pathology.[16] It is known that TGFβ, a cytokine that contributes to the development of a Th2 immune response, is induced when macrophages contact lipoarabinomannan, a prominent constituent of the mycobacterial cell envelope.[17] This is one example of how *M. tuberculosis* can alter the host immune response by making it less effective and potentially harmful. It is assumed that such aberrant host responses contribute more to TB-associated pathology than inherent bacterial toxicities,[18] such as the ones mediated by cord factor, a *M. tuberculosis* glycolipid. This observation is of particular relevance for vaccine development. Every vaccine candidate, but in particular complex whole-cell or live vaccines as well as vaccines to be given against a background of previous exposure to mycobacteria, will have to be thoroughly screened for the possibility of exacerbating rather than enhancing the host immune system. This is meant to be only a brief overview of the host response to *M. tuberculosis*; much more thorough discussions of the immunopathogenesis of TB can be found in other excellent reviews.[19,20]

The Problem of Persistent Infection with *M. tuberculosis*

Reactivation of latent *M. tuberculosis* infection accounts for a significant proportion of tuberculosis cases and also necessitates a different approach toward vaccination. This study of the mechanisms of *M. tuberculosis* persistence is one actively being pursued by TB researchers with the objective of identifying important vaccine as well as drug targets specific for latent organisms. To date comparative genomics and molecular genetics have been most helpful for identifying mycobacterial antigens that are critical for maintaining latent infection of the host with *M. tuberculosis*. A good example is the finding that *M. tuberculosis* possesses genes that allow it to metabolize via the glyoxylate shunt pathway under anaerobic conditions that likely exist within the granuloma and other microenvironments inhabited by dormant *M. tuberculosis*.[21] These studies on the glyoxylate shunt enzyme, isocitrate lyase, show that it is critical for *M. tuberculosis* persistence within macrophages and mice. Other genes associated with lipid metabolism and in vivo persistence of *M. tuberculosis* have been identified by mutagenesis and genetic analysis.[22] An important discovery is the identification of mycolic acid cyclopropane synthetases, which synthesize cell wall lipids, as genes necessary for the persistence of *M. tuberculosis* in vivo.[23] Differential regulation of gene expression by *M. tuberculosis* living within host tissues is also an important topic of investigation, and *M. tuberculosis*-specific two-component signal-transduction systems have been implicated in persistent infection.[24,25] The expression of specific sigma factors have also been correlated with stress-like conditions of growth in *M. tuberculosis*.[26] In addition, there are some suggestions that *M. tuberculosis* can enter a dormant state similar to a spore-like life stage, but there is as of yet no strong evidence to support this view.[27] An unanswered question is where in the human does *M. tuberculosis* reside. Understanding the mechanisms of bacterial dissemination from initial sites of *M. tuberculosis* infection within the lung and the ability of *M. tuberculosis* to survive within nonphagocytic cells will help address this issue.

In addition to factors expressed by the bacterium that help it live within the host tissues, *M. tuberculosis* also produces factors that modify host-defense mechanisms and interfere with the ability of the host to eliminate the pathogen. *M. tuberculosis* shares with other microorganisms a number of tactics to combat host-killing mechanisms, including those initiated by reactive oxygen and nitrogen intermediates.[28] As an intracellular pathogen *M. tuberculosis* also has evolved specific methods for evading host-defense and killing mechanisms. For example, Ting et al[29] have provided evidence that infection of macrophages with *M. tuberculosis* inhibits transcription of IFNγ, subsequent activation of macrophages and the killing of *M. tuberculosis*. An important strategy used by *M. tuberculosis* for evading host recognition is its ability to "hide" in a cellular vacuole that does not fuse with the lysosome and thereby avoids lysosomal-killing mechanisms.[30] Defective transport and processing of class II molecules through the endosomal/lysosomal pathway may also be related to the down-regulation of class II antigen presentation by infected macrophages.[31] The discovery of the PE multi-gene family in *M. tuberculosis* has recently provided another exciting new possibility for immune evasion by *M. tuberculosis*. The PE family of *M. tuberculosis* is composed of ~100 highly homologous genes that are found only in mycobacteria.[4] PE_PGRS genes are a sub-group of the PE family that show significant homology with the EBNA1 protein of Epstein-Barr virus, a viral protein known to present antigens through the MHC I pathway.[32] This inhibition can be mediated by a small Gly-Ala peptide (GGAGAGAG) that interferes with the ubiquitin-proteasome pathway.[33] The PGRS domain of certain *M. tuberculosis* PE_PGRS proteins contains >30 –GGAGGX– repeats,[34] suggesting that this domain could inhibit *M. tuberculosis* antigen processing and the subsequent protective host immune response related to class I antigen presentation. Therefore, *M. tuberculosis* appears to have evolved a number of mechanisms including sequestration in endosomal compartments, inhibition of class I and II antigen presentation, and inhibition of macrophage activation to persist within an immunologically competent host.

In summary, with continued analysis of the mycobacterial genomes and advances in measuring molecular and systemic immune responses, our understanding of the nature of the infectious process continues to advance. In particular, our understanding of how mycobacteria infect and persist within host tissues and how the host responds to mycobacterial infection provides a foundation for a rationale approach to the development of an improved TB vaccine.

Lessons Learned from BCG Vaccine

What can we learn from the history of immunization with BCG vaccine? More than 300 million people a year are immunized with BCG,[3] and yet in 1997 there were ~1.8 billion people infected with *M. tuberculosis* and ~1.9 million deaths attributed to TB, which demonstrates that BCG is not a very effective vaccine.[1,2] The reasons for this are complex but in most cases may be due to the fact that the vaccine is given to neonates while most morbidity occurs in adults with pulmonary TB. BCG vaccine does appear to be effective against the complications of *M. tuberculosis* infection in infants and against pulmonary TB in some populations.[35] The origin of BCG, like many early vaccines, arose from the ideas of Pasteur and Koch for preventing serious disease by inoculating people with live but attenuated homogenous organisms. At first BCG was given orally and some protection (as well as some systemic reactivity) was noted in early studies.[36] Vaccination was also thought to correlate with a delayed-type hypersensitivity (DTH) response in humans measured by injecting a crude mixture of components secreted by *M. tuberculosis*, called tuberculin, subcutaneously. Other studies have suggested this correlation does not exist, but the tuberculin skin test is often used in countries where BCG is widely given to measure "vaccine take". In general, the true efficacy of BCG remains unclear. It seems to work in some populations but not others.[37] One recent study, suggests it protects against leprosy but not TB,[38] while another study performed in China suggests that the rates of TB meningitis in children are no different when you stop giving BCG at birth.[39]

BCG is a very good vaccine for protecting mice and guinea pigs against experimental TB. Yet we do not completely understand the immunological basis for why BCG halts bacterial growth and spread as well as prolongs survival in mice, guinea pigs, rabbits, monkeys and cattle. Neither the antigens present in BCG necessary for eliciting a protective immune response nor an immune response that correlates with protection have been clearly identified,[39] although much progress has been made in these areas [see discussion below]. Nevertheless, BCG remains the gold standard when comparing the efficacy of novel TB vaccines in preclinical studies, notwithstanding the obvious paradox that BCG does not work well in certain human populations.[34]

Improving the BCG Vaccine

So how can we improve on the BCG vaccine, and what kind of immunological responses should an effective TB vaccine elicit? An argument can be made that since BCG is widely used, has a good safety record and likely prevents complications caused by *M. tuberculosis* infection in infants, we should develop a better BCG. In fact, there is some evidence this can be accomplished. A recombinant BCG expressing the 85A antigen from a plasmid does offer more protection than BCG alone in the guinea pig model of TB.[41] However, there is no good immunological explanation for this improved efficacy. The potential effectiveness of new recombinant BCG vaccines in preventing adult pulmonary TB remains open to speculation, since BCG has shown 0% efficacy in certain geographical areas with high rates of pulmonary TB disease and a number of studies suggest that boosting with more immunizations of BCG does not enhance efficacy.[42] Also, BCG may cause BCGosis in immunocompromised populations, and safety parameters will need to be monitored carefully in human clinical studies. One solution may be the use of auxotrophic attenuated strains of BCG. Auxotrophic mutants of BCG have been identified that can be safely used in SCID mice as well as the highly susceptible guinea pig.[43,44,45] These strains could be used to construct attenuated recombinants that may reduce safety concerns associated with the use of live mycobacterial vaccines in immunocompromised human populations, although experience with other pathogens suggest that a fine-tuned balance between attenuation and immunity must be attained. A more efficacious BCG or attenuated *M. tuberculosis* strain has an advantage in that it may be accepted more readily into the existing global BCG immunization program than other, acellular TB vaccines. Also, BCG can be used to express antigens that protect against other endemic diseases and function as an expression vehicle for other vaccine genes such as malaria and HIV.[46]

The issue of heterologous immunity has been raised by a number of clinical studies of BCG vaccine, which have shown that it is less efficacious when used in certain regions closer to the equator.[47] For instance, the study by Fine et al[38] illustrates that the same BCG vaccine which shows significant efficacy in the UK shows no efficacy when used in Malawi (although it was effective against leprosy). Exposure of the Malawi population to environmental mycobacteria found in the soil such as *M. avium* and *M. chelonae* may be responsible for the diminished effects of BCG vaccine. Some particularly interesting animal studies supporting this interpretation have been performed by Brandt et al,[48] who found that introduction of soil mycobacteria into guinea pigs reduces the half-live of BCG in immunized animals as well as the protective efficacy compared to those animals given BCG only. Interestingly, pre-exposure to mycobacteria does not effect the colonization of guinea pigs by virulent *M. tuberculosis*. Moreover, when a novel adjuvanted subunit vaccine containing the mycobacterial antigens ESAT6 and 85A was used to immunize the animals, the vaccine gave the same efficacy whether the guinea pigs were pre-exposed to environmental mycobacteria or not. This kind of evidence provides additional justification for the further development of vaccines produced from individual components rather than live whole-cell vaccines and would suggest that subunit or DNA vaccines may be particularly useful in prime-boost strategies in geographical regions where exposure to environmental mycobacteria is common. These studies also provide a clue as to why boosting with live BCG following a primary immunization with BCG so far has proven to be ineffective.

There is no evidence that BCG immunization can prevent initial infection of the lung but BCG vaccine is effective against preventing the dissemination of *M. tuberculosis* to other tissues as noted in animal studies and in humans.[40,49] This may be why BCG vaccine effectively prevents TB meningitis and miliary TB in infants.[35] This inhibition of hematogenous colonization of mycobacteria also may be related to the efficacy of BCG that has been observed toward leprosy, which is caused by *M. leprae* that prefers to colonize peripheral tissues. Determining how *M. tuberculosis* disseminate from the initial foci in the lung may also be important for understanding persistent infection, since it is unclear where and how *M. tuberculosis* persist within infected humans. Certain vaccines may work better in preventing the spread of *M. tuberculosis* from the lungs and the resulting complications caused by disseminated *M. tuberculosis*. There is evidence that a mycobacterial surface protein, the heparin-binding hemagglutinin (HBHA), is involved in mediating *M. tuberculosis* infection of epithelial tissues[8,50] and a *M. tuberculosis* strain carrying a specific deletion in the *hbha* gene disseminates poorly from the lung.[51] This suggests that immunity targeted to this mycobacterial antigen could be useful for preventing the spread of *M. tuberculosis* to other tissues.

The investigation of HBHA and other mycobacterial proteins suggests that antibodies may play a role in the protective immune response to *M. tuberculosis*. The role of antibody response in tuberculosis is controversial since the primary immune response is considered to be mostly cellular,[19] but coordination of Th1-Th2 responses may be crucial to short- and long-term immunity against TB.[51,52] A major breakthrough would be the development of a vaccine that produced antibodies that could prevent initial infection of the host with *M. tuberculosis*. Although there is evidence suggesting that antibodies directed against the *M. tuberculosis* surface can enhance host survival and alter pathogenesis,[51,54] most experimental and epidemiological evidence suggests that this cannot be accomplished. Indeed, having active TB itself does not protect against reinfection or reactivation in all cases. Additional studies examining the entry of *M. tuberculosis* into the naso-bronchial network as well as mechanisms of invasion of individual cells are needed.

Novel Vaccine Approaches

Since relativly few of the immunocompetent individuals that are infected with *M. tuberculosis* become clinically ill, most people must be able to mount an immune response to *M. tuberculosis* sufficient to protect them for life. One could therefore claim that *M. tuberculosis* is more efficient as a vaccine than as a pathogen. Consequently, attempts to limit the replication of *M. tuberculosis* while preserving its capacity to induce a protective immune response represents a logical step in defining a new TB vaccine. Highly efficient tools to genetically manipulate microorganisms, such as transposon mutagenesis and allelic exchange technologies, have been adapted for use with mycobacteria over the last decade and have allowed the production of attenuated mutants of *M. tuberculosis*. The earliest of these mutants to become available were auxotrophs, lacking key genes for the synthesis of amino acids such as leucine or methionine.[44,45] These relatively crude constructs showed a tendency towards under- or over-attenuation, either killing the host or displaying poor protective efficacy, respectively. Newer more sophisticated technologies such as signature-tagged transposon mutagenesis[55] have allowed the creation of panels of mutants, graded by their degree of attenuation. Many of these mutants have been mapped to loci involved in membrane transport or lipid metabolism.[22] Stringent preclinical evaluation including ongoing measurement of safety parameters will show if any of these vaccine candidates perform better than BCG.

It is unknown which antigenic shortcomings render BCG sub-optimal as a vaccine. The fact that BCG's 'parent' organism, *M .bovis*, has primarily evolved within a bovine rather than a human host, is cited as one possible reason. This assumption has sparked numerous efforts to attenuate the human pathogen, *M. tuberculosis*. Moreover, the genome of the BCG strain has been deleted of several antigens, the equivalents of which are present in *M. tuberculosis*.[56] While these deletions may constitute the major attenuating mutations of BCG, the absence of certain known dominant antigens located in these genomic regions may also be an explanation of BCG's unreliable protective efficacy. This latter hypothesis has prompted a number of approaches aimed at either testing the protective capacity of the antigens located in these deletions[57] or reversing the supposed over-attenuation of BCG through various types of genetic manipulations. It is noteworthy that, in a reverse approach, deletion[57] of the RD1 region from the genome of *M. tuberculosis* is also being tested as a targeted means to attenuate the pathogen (WR Jacobs, personal communication).

While rational attenuation of mycobacteria certainly represents a scientifically exciting and challenging field of mycobacterial vaccine research, it is largely outweighed by attempts to define single protective antigens. Such approaches have been successful in the creation of many other vaccines and are often the first choice of the vaccine industry, due to their stability, ease of standardization and safety in the immunocompromised host. Proteins secreted by *M. tuberculosis* have received special attention as both subunit vaccines and 'add-ons' expressed in live vaccines because such antigens are among the first molecules of the pathogen to be encountered after infection. It has been argued that proteins secreted by live *M. tuberculosis* are good immunogens since killed *M. tuberculosis* are ineffective as TB vaccines.[58,59] Proteins that are differentially expressed under conditions mimicking the intracellular habitat of *M. tuberculosis* also have been considered for vaccine development.[60,61] However, most of the current approaches to define protective *M. tuberculosis* antigens are purely empirical. Antigens are selected from comprehensive 'collections' of *M. tuberculosis* proteins/peptides by virtue of either MHC[62] binding or their recognition by immune sera or primed T cells[63] and subsequent testing of protective qualities in appropriate animal models.

Antigens that are secreted from *M. tuberculosis*, having been isolated initially from the supernatants of mycobacterial cultures, are among the best characterized of the vaccine candidates under consideration. The 38 kD phosphate-binding protein,[64] the low molecular mass 'early secretory antigenic target' ESAT-6,[65] and in particular members of the family of fibronectin-binding secretory proteins, the antigen (Ag) 85 complex,[66] have been tested in a variety of delivery systems. These include adjuvanted protein subunits,[67] peptide epitope preparations,[68] DNA vaccines,[69] and live-vectored vaccines.[41] These vaccine preparations have shown good results in animal testing, often reaching levels of protection equivalent to BCG vaccine. Encouraging results have been obtained using antigens that were identified by screening *M. tuberculosis* expression libraries using patient sera or human T-cell clones.[63] After a first period of extreme analytical reductionism, down to the level of single proteins or even single epitopes, TB vaccine development has now entered into a second, synthetic phase, where different antigens and/or delivery systems are being combined to optimize their protective efficiency. Thus, fusion protein vaccines composed of either ESAT6 and Ag85B[70] or mtb72f (S. Reed, personal communication), composed of mtb32[71] and mtb39[63] have shown great promise in animal experimentation, and clinical evaluation will begin in the near future. Likewise, significant improvement of protective efficacy is observed in animals using multi-component as compared to single component DNA vaccines (Fig. 2).[72] In order to increase the immunogenicity and the protective efficacy of DNA vaccines, prime-boost strategies such as the use of DNA as a priming agent, following by a booster immunization using the same antigen in a protein-adjuvant formulation are being investigated. Finally, the first of the new TB vaccine candidates to go into a clinical phase I trial uses BCG as a priming agent and an Ag85A poxvirus construct as a boost to enhance protection against TB.[73]

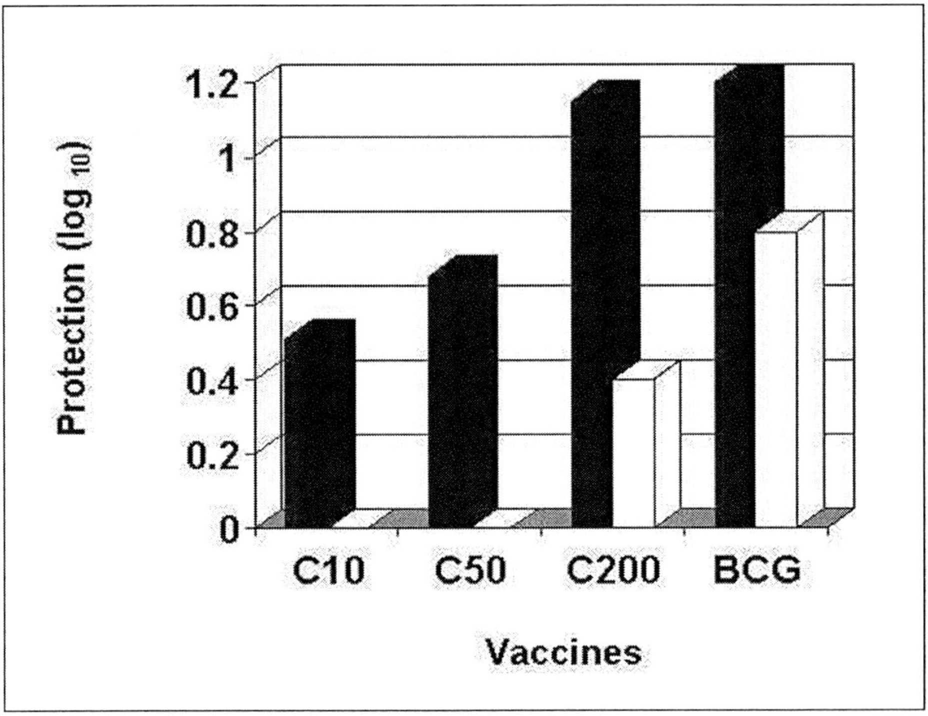

Figure 2. A combination of DNA-based vaccines protects mice in the mouse aerosol challenge model of tuberculosis. Three doses of 10 (C10), 50 (C50), and 200 (C200) μg each of a DNA vaccine composed of 10 candidate *M. tuberculosis* genes were given to mice prior to an aerosol challenge with virulent *M. tuberculosis* Erdman strain. Colony forming units (CFU) were determined for the lung (■) and spleen (□) thirty days following challenge and compared with mice receiving BCG vaccine. Protection is shown as the log differences based on CFU of the vaccinated animals compared with the unvaccinated group. (see Delogu et al [72] for details; we are grateful to Sheldon Morris, CBER, FDA for providing this data)

Due to the significant contribution of classically restricted, αβ receptor-carrying T cells in the protective immune response against *M. tuberculosis*, antigen selection is mostly geared towards identifying proteins/peptides. However, the findings that B cells,[54] γδ T cells and nonclassical restriction elements such as CD1 (reviewed in refs 74,75) participate in the immune response against *M. tuberculosis* also have prompted studies of nonpeptidic antigens such glycolipids[76] and lipoarabinomannan-conjugates[77] as TB vaccine candidates.

The "ideal" TB vaccine should elicit an immune response that is therapeutic as well as prophylactic in order to be effective in populations that are actively infected with *M. tuberculosis* or latently infected. Of interest here has been the proposed use of DNA vaccines as an immunotherapeutic vaccine to act synergistically with antibiotics in an integrated TB control program. One study has shown that a DNA vaccine expressing a mycobacterial heat-shock protein is an effective immunotherapeutic in an animal model of latent infection with *M. tuberculosis.*[78] Stewart et al[79] have recently constructed a regulatory mutant in *M. tuberculosis* that overexpresses Hsp70 and elicits an increased host response to the pathogen, which results in reduced survival of the *M. tuberculosis* strain in mice. These studies suggest that the host response to *M. tuberculosis* heat-shock proteins could be effective in eliminating persistent organisms. However, the use of heat-shock antigens that may promote autoimmune responses in humans is controversial, and the use of vaccines based on heat shock proteins in other model systems have not been successful and have produced untoward reactions. The safe use of these

Table 1. A summary of candidate tuberculosis vaccines tested in animal models of tuberculosis*

Vaccine Types	Examples	Results
Avirulent/ saprophytes	*M. vaccae*	Not active [m]
	M. microti	Marginal activity if given multiple times [m, gp]; more effective given orally? [m]
Auxotrophs	*M. tuberculosis*; BCG	Are gradually cleared but are immunogenic [m]
Mutants/gene knockouts	*M. tuberculosis*	Cleared but immunogenic [m]
Recombinants	rBCG-Ag85	Improved survival versus BCG [gp]
	rBCG-listeriolysin	May improve CD8-directed response [m]
Subunits	Culture filtrate pools	Good activity [m, gp]; benefiting from new improved adjuvants
	Ag85	Boosts BCG [m]
	Fusion proteins [72f]	Good results to date [m, gp, mon]
Viral delivery	Vaccinia-Ag85	Shows promise as BCG boost [m]
DNA vaccines	Multiple candidates	Promising results [m]
	Ag85	Good results [m, gp]; lung damage in post-exposure mode [m, gp]
	hsp60 [leprae]	Excellent results in iv model [m] Not active in aerosol model [m]; severe lung damage in post-exposure
	hsp60 [tuberculosis]	Not protective [m, gp]; severe lung damage
	Prime-boost strategies	Promising results [m]
BCG + vaccine	72f [protein or DNA]	Substantially increases survival compared to BCG alone [gp; mon]

Abbreviations: BCG= Bacillus Calmette-Guérin, hsp = heat shock protein, gp = guinea pig, mon = monkey, m = mouse

*We are grateful to Dr Ian Orme, CSU, Fort Collins, CO for providing the information in this table; see also reference 82

antigens in humans[80] will need to be carefully evaluated. It should also be noted that the heat-killed vaccine produced from the soil *Mycobacterium vaccae* also has shown some promise as an immunotherapeutic adjunct to antibiotic treatments.[81]

Preclinical Testing of New TB Vaccines

The role of preclinical investigations in the development of novel TB vaccines highlights the importance of having relevant animal models for TB to analyze immune responses and their relationship to efficacy. Table 1 shows a recent assessment of novel vaccine candidates that have been tested in standardized animal models for TB sponsored by the National Institutes of Health.[82] The comparison of various vaccine types has identified a number of promising vaccine candidates with good immunity and effectiveness ratings, while identifying others that are inactive or in some cases potentially harmful. The literature contains a number of examples where differences in animal models and in investigational protocols result in variable measures of vaccine effectiveness. For example, a DNA vaccine containing a heat-shock protein gene has been shown to be effective as an immunotherapeutic in one study[78] while showing no significant efficacy and evidence of tissue damage in another study.[83] It also has been known for some time that different strains of mice demonstrate inherent differences in susceptibility to *M. tuberculosis* infection and disease sequelae.[84] Recently, variable effectiveness of BCG vaccine also was demonstrated in two strains of nonhuman primates,[85] and a new TB vaccine shown to be effective in mice proved not to be effective in monkeys (S. Reed, personal communication). These findings provide a justification for performing preclinical studies in multiple animal models of disease. Animal models are also useful for determining meaningful endpoints of efficacy, which may be extrapolated to human clinical studies. For example, evidence from a number of investigators has shown that, although colonization of tissues (CFU) remains an important measure of protection after challenge in animal models, other parameters may be just as important. Vaccines which show no significant differences in CFU at certain time points, such as the commonly used timepoint of one month following challenge with virulent *M. tuberculosis*, can provide significant differences in survival rates.[86] Other measurements of vaccine effectiveness include histological examination of the inflammatory reaction in tissues, size of granulomas, mineralization, necrosis, and dissemination from the lung. In addition to advancing the identification of a new generation of TB vaccines, animal models also are required to establish important clinical parameters for measuring disease in human clinical studies and to enable investigators interested in the licensure of new TB vaccines to obtain safety and toxicology data prior to moving the vaccine into human clinical trials.[87]

TB Vaccines for Targeted Populations

A reasonable and compassionate case can be made for the development of improved TB vaccines to meet the needs of specific populations suffering most from tuberculosis.[88] This includes populations at high risk for developing TB such as persons living in close contact with others who have TB; immunocompromised individuals, including those who have AIDS or addiction problems; those who are latently infected with *M. tuberculosis*; those living in poverty and in poor living conditions; those who are unable to obtain routine antibiotic treatment; and infants or young children. In many countries where TB is prevalent, clinical studies and the ultimate introduction of improved vaccines into adult populations will be complicated by the fact that large percentages have been immunized with the BCG vaccine at birth. In certain countries, they may have also received booster doses of BCG vaccine. In the rationale design of an effective TB vaccine, the common vaccine questions relevant to an intracellular pathogen such as trying to prevent disease as well as transmission, and eliciting good memory response with proper boosting doses must be addressed. An effective TB vaccine also will need to elicit an effective immune response that works in those already infected with *M. tuberculosis* (one-third of the world's population) or infected with both *M. tuberculosis* and HIV. The fact that patients cured of TB can be reinfected suggests this is not going to be easy and that the vaccine will need to produce an immune response that is better than naturally occurring disease.

Progress Towards the Clinical Investigation of Novel TB Vaccines

It is likely that, as observed for AIDS vaccines,[89] we now will see the investigation of novel TB vaccine candidates in human clinical studies as the driving force for the development of better vaccines for tuberculosis. As shown in (Table 2), several promising candidate TB vaccines will soon be tested in human clinical trials. The candidates include *M. tuberculosis* antigens expressed in vaccinia or BCG, or antigens expressed as fusion proteins conjugated with adjuvant, as purified recombinant proteins plus adjuvant, as DNA-based vaccines, or as a string of peptides conjugated with adjuvant. In some cases, they will be tested in a prime – boost immunization strategy together with the licensed BCG vaccine. This testing of such a wide variety of vaccine types using different immunization strategies directed against a sole pathogen is unique in the history of vaccine development and will make the comparisons of clinical data interesting but also challenging. It will be important that this effort be coordinated by organizations such as the World Health Organization, the National Institutes of Health and other advocacy groups such as the Global Alliance for Vaccines and Immunization to foster communication among the investigators, to standardize clinical protocols and to include staff from endemic countries in the process.[88] This is vital for performing effective clinical efficacy

Table 2. Clinical studies of novel TB vaccines

TB Vaccine Candidates	Stage	Reference
Vaccinia-vectored Mtb Ag85	Phase I 2002 UK	McShane et al.[73]
Recombinant BCG-Ag 85	Phase I 2003 US	Horwitz et al.[41]
Subunit+ adjuvant-72f/AS2	Phase I 2003 US	S. Reed - personal communication
Mtb peptides (5) + adjuvant	*UD	Meister et al.[62]
HSP65 DNA vaccine	*UD	Tascon et al.[78]
Subunit + adjuvant-ESAT6/85A	*UD	Weinrich et al.[70]

* UD = undetermined at the time of publication

trials for the future introduction of effective vaccines into areas where the burden of disease is greatest.

Summary

Mycobacterium tuberculosis is a worthy opponent. More than one investigator, having attained success in elucidating the immunopathogenesis of another pathogen, has been humbled upon entering the field of mycobacteria research. The pursuit of effective vaccines has moved forward without a complete knowledge of the pathogenesis and immunology of *M. tuberculosis.* The need to find better ways to prevent and treat TB has been driven by the extent of morbidity and mortality associated with the diseases caused by *M. tuberculosis* and its close relatives. It is unlikely that one "ideal" vaccine to prevent *M. tuberculosis* infection and disease will be found, but the development of different vaccine types and innovative immunization strategies appears promising. However, the goal of clearing the host of this intracellular pathogen in those already infected with *M. tuberculosis* or coinfected with HIV will be a major challenge. It will likely require not only a coordinated effort but the combined implementation of new effective vaccines, diagnostics and drugs as well.

References

1. Dye C, Scheele S, Dolin P et al. Consensus statement: global burden of tuberculosis: estimated incidence, prevalence, and mortality by country. WHO Global Surveillance and Monitoring Project. J Am Med Assoc 1999; 282:677-686.
2. Murray CJ, Salomon JA. Modeling the impact of global tuberculosis control strategies. Proc Natl Acad Sci USA 1998 Nov 10; 95(23):13881-13886.
3. Fine PEM, Carneiro IAM, Milstein JB et al. Issues relating to the use of BCG in immunization programmes. [A discussion document]. Geneva: WHO/V&B/99.23, 1999.
4. Cole ST, Brosch R, Parkhill J et al. Deciphering the biology of Mycobacterium tuberculosis from the complete genome sequence. Nature 1998; 393(6685):537-544.
5. Cole ST, Eiglmeier K, Parkhill J et al. Massive gene decay in the leprosy bacillus. Nature 2001 Feb 22; 409(6823):1007-1011.
6. Merkel JS, Feldblyum T, Young B et al. Sequencing and assembly of the Mycobacterium smegmatis genome. Keystone Symposium: Molecular and Cellular Aspects of Tuberculosis Research in the Post Genomic Era 2001; Abst 131:62
7. Gordon SV, Eiglmeier K, Garnier T et al. Genomics of Mycobacterium bovis. Tuberculosis (Edinb) 2001; 81(1-2):157-163.
8. Delogu G, Brennan MJ. Functional domains present in the mycobacterial hemagglutinin, HBHA. J Bacteriol 1999; 181:7464-7469.
9. Ratliff TL, McCarthy R, Telle WB et al. Purification of a mycobacterial adhesin for fibronectin. Infect Immun 1993; 61:1889-1894.

10. Schlesinger LS, Horwitz MA. Phenolic glycolipid-1 of Mycobacterium leprae binds complement component C3 in serum and mediates phagocytosis by human monocytes. J Exp Med 1991; 174(5):1031-1038.
11. Schlesinger LS, Bellinger-Kawahara CG, Payne NR et al. Phagocytosis of Mycobacterium tuberculosis is mediated by human monocyte complement receptors and complement component C3. J Immunol 1990; 144:2771-2780.
12. Berthet FX, Lagranderie M, Gounon P et al. Attenuation of virulence by disruption of the Mycobacterium tuberculosis erp gene. Science 1998; 282(5389):759-762.
13. Arruda S, Bomfim G, Knights R et al. Cloning of an M. tuberculosis DNA fragment associated with entry and survival inside cells. Science 1993; 261:1454-1457.
14. Ladel CH, Daugelat S, Kaufmann SH. Immune response to Mycobacterium bovis Bacille Calmette Guerin infection in major histocompatibility complex class I and II-deficient knock-out mice: contribution of CD4 and CD8 t cells to acquired resistance. Eur J Immunol 1995; 25(2):377-384.
15. Ottenhoff TH, Kumararatne D, Casanova JL. Novel human immunodeficiencies reveal the essential role of type-I cytokines in immunity to intracellular bacteria. Immunol Today 1998; 19(11):491-494.
16. Seah GT, Scott GM, Rook GA. Type 2 cytokine gene activation and its relationship to extent of disease in patients with tuberculosis. J Infect Dis 2000; 181(1):385-389.
17. Dahl KE, Shiratsuchi H, Hamilton BD et al. Selective induction of transforming growth factor beta in human monocytes by lipoarabinomannan of Mycobacterium tuberculosis. Infect Immun 1996; 64(2):399-405.
18. Dannenberg AM Jr, Collins FM. Progressive pulmonary tuberculosis is not due to increasing numbers of viable bacilli in rabbits, mice and guinea pigs, but is due to a continuous host response to mycobacterial products. Tuberculosis 2001; 81(3):229-242.
19. Flynn JL, Chan J. Immunology of tuberculosis. Annu Rev Immunol 2001; 19:93-129.
20. Kaufmann SH, Anderson P. Immunity to mycobacteria with emphasis on tuberculosis: implications for rational design of an effective tuberculosis vaccine. Chem Immunol 1998;70:21-59.
21. McKinney JD, Honer ZB, Munoz-Elias EJ et al. Persistence of Mycobacterium tuberculosis in macrophages and mice requires the glyoxylate shunt enzyme isocitrate lyase. Nature 2000; 406(6797):735-738.
22. Cox JS, Chen B, McNeil M. Complex lipid determines tissue-specific replication of Mycobacterium tuberculosis in mice. Nature 1999; 402:79-83.
23. Glickman MS, Cox JS, Jacob Jr WR. A novel mycolic acid cyclopropane synthetase is required for coding, persistence, and virulence of Mycobacterium tuberculosis. Mol Cell 2000; 5:717-727.
24. Sherman DR, Voskuil M, Schnappinger D et al. Regulation of the Mycobacterium tuberculosis hypoxic response gene encoding alpha -crystallin. Proc Natl Acad Sci USA 2001 Jun 19; 98(13):7534-7539.
25. Zahrt TC, Deretic V. Mycobacterium tuberculosis signal transduction system required for persistent infections. Proc Natl Acad Sci USA 2001 Oct 23; 98(22):12706-12711.
26. Manganelli R, Dubnau E, Tyagi S et al. Differential expression of 10 sigma factor genes in Mycobacterium tuberculosis. Mol Microbiol 1999; 31(2):715-724.
27. Parrish NM, Dick JD, Bishai WR. Mechanisms of latency in Mycobacterium tuberculosis. Trends Microbiol 1998; 6(3):107-12.
28. Raupach B, Kaufmann SH. Immune responses to intracellular bacteria. Curr Opin Immunol 2001; 13(4):417-428.
29. Ting LM, Kim AC, Cattamanchi A et al. Mycobacterium tuberculosis inhibits IFN-gamma transcriptional responses without inhibiting activation of STAT1. J Immunol 1999; 163(7):3898-3906.
30. Clemens DL, Lee BY, Horwitz MA. Mycobacterium tuberculosis and Legionella pneumophila phagosomes exhibit arrested maturation despite acquisition of Rab7. Infect Immun 2000 Sep; 68(9):5154-5166.
31. Hmama Z, Gabathuler R, Jefferies WA et al. Attenuation of HLA-DR epression by mononuclear phagocytes infected with Mycobacterium tuberculosis is related to intracellular sequestration of immature class II heterodimers. J Immunol 1998; 161(9):4882-4893.
32. Levitskaya J et al. Inhibition of antigen processing by the internal repeat region of the Epstein-Barr virus nuclear antigen-1. Nature 1995; 375:685-688.
33. Levitskaya J et al. Inhibition of ubiquitin/proteasome-dependent protein degradation by the Gly-Ala repeat domain of the Epstein-Barr virus nuclear antigen 1. Proc Natl Acad Sci USA 1997; 94,12616-12621.

34. Brennan MJ, Delogu G. The PE multigene family: a 'molecular mantra' for mycobacteria. Trends Microbiol 2002; 10(5):246-249.
35. Fine PEM. Variation in protection by BCG: implications of and for heterologous immunity. Lancet 1995; 346:1339-1345.
36. Collins FM. Tuberculosis: the return of an old enemy. Crit Rev Microbiol 1993; 19:1-16.
37. Black GF, Fine PEM, Warndorff DK et al. Relationship between IFN-gamma and skin test responsiveness to Mycobacterium tuberculosis PPD in healthy, nonBCG-vaccinated young adults in Northern Malawi. Int J Tuberc Lung Dis 2001; 5(7):664-672.
38. Fine PEM, Floyd S, Stanford JL et al. Environmental mycobacteria in northern Malawi: implications for the epidemiology of tuberculosis and leprosy. Epidemiol Infect 2001; 126:379-387.
39. Zhang LX, Tu DH, He GX et al. Risk of tuberculosis infection and tuberculous meningitis after discontinuation of Bacillus Calmette-Guerin in Beijing. Am J Respir Crit Care Med 2000; 162(4 Pt 1):1314-1317.
40. McMurray DN, Collins FM, Dannenberg AM Jr et al. Pathogenesis of experimental tuberculosis in animal models. Curr Top Microbiol Immunol 1996; 215:157-179.
41. Horwitz MA, Harth G, Dillon BJ et al. Recombinant bacillus calmette-guerin (BCG) vaccines expressing the Mycobacterium tuberculosis 30-kDa major secretory protein induce greater protective immunity against tuberculosis than conventional BCG vaccines in a highly susceptible animal model. Proc Natl Acad Sci USA 2000; 97(25):13853-13858.
42. Comstock CW. Field trials of tuberculosis vaccines: how could we have done better? Contrl Clin Trials 1994; 15:247-276.
43. Chambers MA, Williams A, Gavier-Widen D et al. Identification of a Mycobacterium bovis BCG auxotrophic mutant that protects guinea pigs against M. bovis and hematogenous spread of Mycobacterium tuberculosis without sensitization to tuberculin. Infect Immun 2000; 68(12):7094-7099.
44. Jackson M, Phalen SW, Lagranderie M et al. Persistence and protective efficacy of a Mycobacterium tuberculosis auxotroph vaccine. Infect Immun 1999; 67(6):2867-2873.
45. McAdam RA, Weisbrod TR, Martin J et al. In vivo growth characteristics of leucine and methionine auxotrophic mutants of Mycobacterium bovis BCG generated by transposon mutagenesis. Infect Immun 1995; 63(3):1004-1012.
46. Ohara N, Yamada T. Recombinant BCG vaccines. [Review] [83 refs]. Vaccine 2001; 19(30):4089-4099.
47. Colditz GA, Brewer TF, Berkey CS et al. Efficacy of BCG vaccine in the prevention of tuberculosis. Meta-analysis of the published literature. JAMA 1994 Mar 2; 271(9):698-702.
48. Brandt L, Feino CJ, Weinreich OA et al. Failure of the Mycobacterium bovis BCG vaccine: some species of environmental mycobacteria block multiplication of BCG and induction of protective immunity to tuberculosis. Infect Immun 2002; 70(2):672-678.
49. Sutherland I, Lindgren I. The protective effect of BCG vaccination as indicated by autopsy studies. Tubercle 1979; 60(4):225-31.
50. Menozzi, FD, Rouse JH, Alavi M et al. Identification of a heparin-binding hemagglutinin present in mycobacteria. J Exp Med 1996; 184:993-1001.
51. Pethe K, Alonso S, Biet F et al. The heparin-binding haemagglutinin of M. tuberculosis is required for extrapulmonary dissemination. Nature 2001; 412(6843):190-194.
52. Bosio CM, Gardner D, Elkins KL. Infection of B cell-deficient mice with CDC 1551, a clinical isolate of Mycobacterium tuberculosis: delay in dissemination and development of lung pathology. J Immunol 2000; 164(12):6417-6425.
53. Glatman-Freedman A, Casadevall A. Serum therapy for tuberculosis revisited: reappraisal of the role of antibody-mediated immunity against Mycobacterium tuberculosis. Clin Microbiol Rev 1998; 11(3):514-532.
54. Teitelbaum R, Glatman-Freedman A, Chen B et al. A mAb recognizing a surface antigen of Mycobacterium tuberculosis enhances host survival. Proc Natl Acad Sci USA 1998; 95(26):15688-15693.
55. Camacho LR, Ensergueix D, Perez E et al. Identification of a virulence gene cluster of Mycobacterium tuberculosis by signature-tagged transposon mutagenesis. Mol Microbiol 1999; 34(2):257-267.
56. Mahairas GG, Sabo PJ, Hickey MJ et al. Molecular analysis of genetic differences between Mycobacterium bovis BCG and virulent M. bovis. J Bacteriol 1996 Mar; 178(5):1274-1282.
57. Brusasca PN, Colangeli R, Lyashchenko KP et al. Immunological characterization of antigens encoded by the RD1 region of the Mycobacterium tuberculosis genome. Scand J Immunol 2001; 54(5):448-452.

58. Andersen P, Askgaard D, Ljungqvist L et al. Proteins released from Mycobacterium tuberculosis during growth. Infect Immun 1991; 59(6):1905-1910.
59. Pal PG, Horwitz MA. Immunization with extracellular proteins of Mycobacterium tuberculosis induces cell-mediated immune responses and substantial protective immunity in a guinea pig model of pulmonary tuberculosis. Infect Immun 1992; 60(11):4781-4792.
60. Ramakrishnan L, Federspiel NA, Falkow S. Granuloma-specific expression of mycobacterium virulence proteins from the glycine-rich PE-PGRS family. Science 2000; 288:1436-1439.
61. Yuan Y, Crane DD, Barry CE 3rd. Stationary phase-associated protein expression in Mycobacterium tuberculosis: function of the mycobacterial alpha-crystallin homolog. J Bacteriol 1996 Aug; 178(15):4484-4492.
62. Meister GE, Roberts CG, Berzofsky JA et al. Two novel T cell epitope prediction algorithms based on MHC-binding motifs; comparison of predicted and published epitopes from Mycobacterium tuberculosis and HIV protein sequences. Vaccine 1995; 13(6):581-591.
63. Dillon DC, Alderson MR, Day CH et al. Molecular characterization and human T-cell responses to a member of a novel Mycobacterium tuberculosis mtb39 gene family. Infect Immun 1999; 67(6):2941-2950.
64. Young D, Kent L, Rees A et al. Immunological activity of a 38-kilodalton protein purified from Mycobacterium tuberculosis. Infect Immun 1986; 54(1):177-183.
65. Brandt L, Elhay M, Rosenkrands I et al. ESAT-6 subunit vaccination against Mycobacterium tuberculosis. Infect Immun 2000; 68(2):791-795.
66. Wiker HG, Harboe M. The antigen 85 complex: a major secretion product of Mycobacterium tuberculosis. Microbiol Rev 1992; 56(4):648-661.
67. Horwitz MA, Lee BW, Dillon BJ et al. Protective immunity against tuberculosis induced by vaccination with major extracellular proteins of Mycobacterium tuberculosis. Proc Natl Acad Sci USA 1995; 92(5):1530-1534.
68. Leao SC, Lopes JD, Patarroyo ME. Immunological and functional characterization of proteins of the Mycobacterium tuberculosis antigen 85 complex using synthetic peptides. J Gen Microbiol 1993; 139(pt7):1543-1549.
69. Montgomery DL, Huygen K, Yawman AM et al. Induction of humoral and cellular immune responses by vaccination with M. tuberculosis antigen 85 DNA. Cell Mol Biol 1997; 43(3):285-292.
70. Weinrich OA, van Pinxteren LA, Meng OL et al. Protection of mice with a tuberculosis subunit vaccine based on a fusion protein of antigen 85b and esat-6. Infect Immun 2001; 69(5):2773-2778.
71. Skeiky YA, Lodes MJ, Guderian JA et al. Cloning, expression, and immunological evaluation of two putative secreted serine protease antigens of Mycobacterium tuberculosis. Infect Immun 1999; 67(8):3998-4007.
72. Delogu G, Li A, Repique C et al. DNA vaccine combinations expressing either TPA-fusion proteins or ubiquitin-conjugated antigens induce sustained protective immunity in a mouse model of pulmonary tuberculosis. Infect Immun 2002; 70:292-302.
73. McShane H. Prime-boost immunization strategies for infectious diseases. Curr Opin Mol Ther 2002; 4(1):23-27.
74. Dieli F, Troye-Blomberg M, Farouk SE et al. Biology of gamma delta T cells in tuberculosis and malaria. Curr Mol Med 2001; 1(4):437-446.
75. Gumperz JE, Brenner MB. CD1-specific T cells in microbial immunity.Curr Opin Immunol 2001; 13(4):471-478.
76. Schaible UE, Kaufmann SH. CD1 and CD1-restricted T cells in infections with intracellular bacteria. Trends Microbiol 2000; 8(9):419-425.
77. Hamasur B, Kallenius G, Svenson SB. Synthesis and immunologic characterisation of Mycobacterium tuberculosis lipoarabinomannn specific oligosaccharide-protein conjugates. Vaccine 1999; 17(22):2853-2861.
78. Tascon RE, Colston MJ, Ragno S et al. Vaccination against tuberculosis by DNA injection. Nat Med 1996; 2:888-892.
79. Stewart GR, Snewin VA, Walzl G et al. Overexpression of heat-shock proteins reduces survival of Mycobacterium tuberculosis in the chronic phase of infection. Nat Med 2001; 7(6):732-737.
80. Battistini L, Salvetti M, Ristori G et al. Gamma delta T cell receptor analysis supports a role for HSP 70 selection of lymphocytes in multiple sclerosis lesions. Mol Med 1995; 1(5):554-562.

81. Mayo RE, Stanford JL. Double-blind placebo-controlled trial of Mycobacterium vaccae immunotherapy for tuberculosis in KwaZulu, South Africa, 1991-97. Trans R Soc Trop Med Hyg 2000; 94(5):563-568.
82. Orme IM, McMurray DN, Belisle JT. Tuberculosis vaccine development; recent progress. Trends Microbiol 2001; 9:115-118.
83. Turner OC, Roberts AD, Frank AA et al. Lack of protection in mice and necrotizing bronchointerstitial pneumonia with bronchiolitis in guinea pigs immunized with vaccines directed against the hsp60 molecule of Mycobacterium tuberculosis. Infect Immun 2000 Jun; 68(6):3674-3679.
84. Medina E, North RJ. Resistance ranking of some common inbred mouse strains to Mycobacterium tuberculosis and relationship to major histocompatibility complex haplotype and Nramp1 genotype. Immunology 1998 Feb; 93(2):270-274.
85. Langermans JA, Anderson P, van Soolingen D et al. Divergent effects of bacillius Calmette-Guerin (BCG) vaccination on Mycobacterium tuberculosis infection in highly related macaque species:implications for primate models in tuberculosis vaccine research. Proc Natl Acad Sci USA 2001; 98:11497-11502.
86. North RJ, Ryan L, LaCource R et al. Growth rate of mycobacteria in mice as an unreliable indicator of mycobacterial virulence. Infect Immun 1999 Oct; 67(10):5483-5485.
87. Brennan MJ, Collins FM, Morris SL. Propelling novel vaccines directed against tuberculosis through the regulatory process. Tuber Lung Dis 1999; 79(3):145-151.
88. Brennan MJ, Fruth U. Global Forum on TB Vaccine Research and Development. World Health Organization, June 7-8 2001, Geneva. Tuberculosis 2001; 81(5-6):365-368.
89. Esparza J, Osmanov S, Pattou-Markovic C et al. Past, present and future of HIV vaccine trials in developing countries. Vaccine 2002 May 6; 20(15):1897-1898.

Chapter 21

Typhoid Vaccines

Deborah House and Gordon Dougan

Introduction

Typhoid fever is a systemic illness caused by infection with the Gram negative bacterium *Salmonella enterica* sub-species 1 serovar Typhi (*S. typhi*). Patients with typhoid fever can be broadly divided into two groups, those with 'mild' disease (uncomplicated typhoid fever) and those with complications. The signs and symptoms of uncomplicated typhoid fever are relatively nonspecific, and their reported frequency is highly variable. The classic symptoms are pyrexia, headache and abdominal pain or discomfort. Fever rises in a step-wise manner during the first week of illness and can be as high as 40°C.[1,2] The disease is self-limiting in most patients and resolves within 4 – 5 weeks in the absence of chemotherapy.[1] Patients given a course of an appropriate antibiotic can recover within a week although weakness and debilitation may persist for several months.[3,4]

A minority of patients with typhoid fever develop complications, the most severe of which are gastro-intestinal (GI) haemorrhage and perforation of the gut wall.[5-7] Perforation is usually at a single site, occurring in the distal ileum in the centre of an ulcer.[8] The risk of mortality is substantially higher in patients with typhoid perforation than in those with uncomplicated disease (odds ratio 17.9 (6.27 – 51.18), with death normally associated with the subsequent development of peritonitis.[9,10]

A minority of typhoid patients who have apparently made a full recovery relapse several days, weeks or months after the initial infection, while another 1-4% of individuals become chronic carriers, i.e., healthy individuals who excrete *S. typhi* in their urine and faeces for ≥ 1 year.[11]

Epidemiology

There are ~16 million cases of typhoid fever per year worldwide.[12,13] The majority of these occur in developing countries, with an estimated mean incidence of $150/10^5$/year in South America and $900/10^5$/year in some parts of Asia.[13] The traditional view is that the incidence of typhoid fever is highest in school age children and young adults (5 – 19 years) and lowest in young children under three years of age and adults over the age of 35 years.[4,13] However, there are some data to suggest that the disease is common in young children aged between 1-5 years and that the disease goes undiagnosed in this group.[14,15]

Man is the only known host for *S. typhi*, and infected humans are believed to be the only significant source of the infection.[4] *S. typhi* is transmitted from person to person via the faecal-oral route, most commonly via fecally contaminated food or water. In endemic areas typhoid fever is most likely to originate from multiple sources and a general breakdown in sanitation. In nonendemic regions outbreaks of typhoid fever are usually associated with imported foods or typhoid carriers,[16,17] while isolated cases are generally associated with foreign travel or laboratory-acquired infections.

New Bacterial Vaccines, edited by Ronald W. Ellis and Bernard R. Brodeur.

Control of Typhoid Fever

The prompt diagnosis and administration of appropriate antibiotics to patients with acute typhoid fever, along with the identification and treatment of carriers minimizes the risk of transmission of *S. typhi*. However, the treatment of typhoid fever in many regions where the disease is endemic has become increasingly difficult following the emergence of multi-drug resistant (MDR) *S. typhi*, i.e., strains resistant to Chloramphenicol, Ampicillin and Trimethoprim. More recently nalidixic acid (quinolone)-resistant *S. typhi* have been reported.[18] Thus typhoid fever may become untreatable in certain areas where alternative antibiotics, such as third-generation cephalosporins, are expensive. In developed countries, improvements in the quality of the water and sewage disposal resulted in a dramatic reduction in the incidence of typhoid fever.[11] Unfortunately the costs of such interventions is prohibitive in many regions where typhoid fever is endemic.[13] An alternative approach for the control of the disease in these regions is the introduction of mass immunisation schedules,[19] or targeted programmes aimed at those most at risk.

Licensed Typhoid Vaccines

There are currently three typhoid vaccines licensed for use in humans: parenteral whole-cell killed vaccines, purified Vi capsular polysaccharide (Vi-CPS), and the live-attenuated oral vaccine Ty21a.[20,21]

Killed-Parenteral Vaccines

S. typhi was first isolated in the 1880's and the first vaccine, consisting of heat killed *S. typhi*, was developed shortly afterwards in 1896. Over the following years a variety of vaccine preparations using different methods of inactivation and preservation were developed but the efficacy of these was not properly evaluated until the 1960's when the WHO initiated a series of controlled field trials lasting over 12 years. The vaccines tested were the acetone-inactivated and dried K vaccine and the heat-killed, phenol-preserved L vaccine. The vaccines were prepared at the Walter Reed Army Institute of Research from the standard *S. typhi* strain Ty2V, and both vaccines had been shown to be effective against an oral challenge with *S. typhi* (Quailles strain) in volunteer studies.[22] The WHO trials were undertaken in Yugoslavia, Guyana, Poland and the USSR.[23] Both vaccines generated a significant degree of protection against typhoid fever, although the K vaccine had a higher rate of efficacy than that of the L vaccine (Table 1). Unfortunately, systemic and local reactions were common with both preparations, most likely due to the high lipopolysaccharide (LPS) content. The most common systemic reaction was pyrexia, resulting in absenteeism with many vaccinees, while local reactions included pain and redness at site of injection. The heat-inactivated phenol-preserved vaccine is licensed for use in civilians, but due to the high frequency of adverse reactions it is not recommended for general use by the WHO.[28]

Vi Capsular Polysaccharide (Vi-CPS)

A number of parenteral subunit typhoid vaccines have been developed, but the only ones to have been licensed are based on purified Vi-CPS. This antigen was first described by Felix and Pitt in 1934, who coined the term Vi, or virulence, antigen following the observation that Vi-expressing *S. typhi* were more virulent in a mouse potency test than strains which lacked the antigen.[29] Vi-CPS is a linear homopolymer of a(1→4) galacturonic acid that is N-acetylated at C2 and O-acetylated at C3.[30] The antigen forms a capsule over the surface of the bacterium and can mask other surface antigens such as the LPS, or O, antigen.[29] The expression of Vi-CPS is dependent upon the presence of the ViaB genetic locus, which is located on a 118-kbp loop of DNA at 98 minutes on the *S. typhi* chromosome.[31] Nine of the eleven genes within the locus are responsible for the synthesis and polymerization of the antigen (*tviaB* to *tviE*), and transport of the polymer to the cell surface (*vexA* to *vexE*). The first gene in the locus (*tvi*A) is a regulator of Vi-CPS expression, while the last gene of the operon (*orf11*) is of unknown

Table 1. Summary of WHO whole-cell parenteral K and L vaccine trials: 2-dose regime 4 weeks apart (adapted from ref. 23).

Study and Period of Study	Age (Years)	Vaccine Type	Number Vaccinated	Number of Typhoid Cases	Duration of Follow-Up (Years)	Efficacy (vs Control Group)
Yugoslavia 1960-1963[a]	< 15	Acetone dried (K)	2 423	11	3	76.6
		Heat-phenol (L)	2 467	17		63.8
		Control (TT)	2 446	47		
	≥ 15	Acetone dried (K)	2 605	5		82.1
		Heat-phenol (L)	2 601	20		28.6
		Control (TT)	2 593	28		
Guyana 1960-1964[b]	5 – 15	Acetone dried (K)	24 046	5	3.5	94.4
		Heat-phenol (L)	23 431	20		77.4
		Control (TT)	24 241	90		
Poland 1961-63[c]	5 – 15	Acetone dried (K)	81 534	4	2.0	87.1
		Control (TT)	83 734	31		
USSR 1962-63[d]	School children	Heat-phenol (L)	36 112	13	1.5	73.0
	and young adults	Control (TT)	36 999	50		

TT = tetanus toxoid.
a. Ref. 24
b. Ref. 25
c. Ref. 26
d. Ref. 27

function. The expression of Vi-CPS is under the control of the two-component sensor-regulators *RcsB-RcsC* and *OmpR*-EnvZ.[32,33] The *rcsB* and *rcsC* genes are located within the ViaA locus, which is also present in *E. coli* where it is involved in the regulation of colonic acid capsule synthesis.

Early vaccine studies with purified Vi-CPS were disappointing, with the antigen proving to be poorly immunogenic.[34] However, these antigen preparations were treated with acid, which removes all of the *O*-acetyl and part of the *N*-acetyl moieties, and partially de-polymerises the polysaccharide.[30] The utilisation of a milder extraction technique originally developed for the purification of meningococcal polysaccharide antigens resulted in the purification of nondenatured Vi-CPS which retained the antigenic acetyl moieties and was immunogenic and nonreactogenic in vivo.[35-37] The efficacy of the purified Vi-CPS vaccine was evaluated in two large field trials in Nepal and South Africa and was found to be *ca* 60-75% over 17-21 months and 55% over three years.[38-40] Furthermore, no serious adverse reactions were reported.

Live-Attenuated Oral Vaccine Ty21a

The first oral typhoid vaccines tested were whole-cell killed vaccines. No adverse reactions were observed but they did not give protection against typhoid fever in experimental challenge studies or in controlled field trials in endemic areas. A major breakthrough in the development of live-oral typhoid vaccines came with the development of Ty21a by Germanier and Furer.[41] Ty21a is a *galE* mutant which was derived from *S. typhi* Ty2 by chemical mutagenesis

(N-methyl-N'-nitro-N-nitrosoguanidine). *gal*E mutants lack the enzyme uridine diphosphate (UDP)-galactose-4-epimerase and as a result are rough-type strains (although when galactose is supplied exogenously galE mutants can synthesis smooth LPS). Ty21a does not express the Vi antigen, suggesting that the strain harbors a further mutation(s) in one or more of the genes required for Vi expression. There are also reports of differences in the outer membrane protein (OMP) profile of Ty2 and Ty21a, although this is not a consistent finding.[42,43]

There have been several different formulations of Ty21a evaluated including liquid preparations, which are administered with sodium bicarbonate, and gelatin and enteric-coated capsules. Large-scale vaccine trials in endemic areas using the two formulations have shown Ty21a to be a safe vaccine for use in humans.[44,45] The avirulence of Ty21a was thought to be due, in part, to the strong bacterial lysis that follows the uptake of galactose and the accumulation of galactose-1-phosphate and UDP-galactose within the bacterial cell. However, EX462 (a defined *gal*E mutant of Ty2) causes bacteremia and fever in humans when given orally, indicating that other unknown mutations contribute to the avirulence of Ty21a.[46]

The efficacy of Ty21a was evaluated in a series of large-scale controlled field trials in Alexandria, Egypt, Santiago, Chile and Indonesia.[44,45,47-50] The results of these studies showed that both the number of doses and dosing schedule was important, with a minimum of three doses given on alternate days being required to induce significant long-lasting protection (Table 2). Furthermore, the formulation of the vaccine was critical, with liquid formulations having a higher efficacy than enteric capsules, although this was only significant in one of the two studies in which the two formulations were tested in the same trial.[49,50] A recent follow-up study in Chile showed that the protection afforded by Ty21a was long-lasting, with enteric capsules giving 62% protection over seven years and the liquid formulation 78% protection over five years.[51]

Immunological Basis of Protection

The pathogenic process of typhoid fever is highly complex. Following ingestion, the bacteria pass through the stomach into the small intestine where they are thought to adhere and penetrate M cells or epithelial cells in the distal ileum. After breaching the mucosal barrier, the bacteria enter the bloodstream and are disseminated throughout the body. There then follows a period of bacterial replication, probably in the organs of the reticulo-endothelial system, before the bacteria are shed back into the bloodstream in large numbers. This results in the onset of clinical symptoms and marks the end of the incubation period, which is typically 10-14 days. Thus, the protective immune mechanisms elicited by immunization could act at any one of several stages in the infective process.

Despite the large number of typhoid vaccine studies, there are very little data on correlates of protection. Three of the major surface antigens of *S. typhi* are the O (somatic, LPS), H (flagella), and Vi (virulence) antigens and most field and laboratory studies that investigated the immune response to the licensed vaccines have looked at the antibody response to these three antigens. The role of these antigens in vivo is unclear, although the flagella antigen may have a role in attachment to gut epithelial cells, given that hair- and flagella-like appendages have been observed at the point of interaction between *S. typhi* and epithelial cells in vitro.[52,53] The Vi capsule is believed to be expressed when *S. typhi* is in the blood.[30] This antigen, along with the long carbohydrate side-chains of the LPS molecule, is believed to be anti-opsonic and anti-phagocytic, thus protecting the bacteria from complement(C')-mediated lysis and uptake by professional phagocytes.[54-56] Thus anti-flagella antibodies at mucosal surface may interfere with attachment and inhibit invasion of the gut epithelium, while anti-LPS and anti-Vi antibodies, when bound to the bacterium, may facilitate the activation of the classical C' pathway, and promote phagocytosis of extracellular bacteria via C' and Fc receptors on the surface of professional phagocytes. In addition, anti-LPS antibodies may bind to free LPS, preventing its interaction with LPS receptors on the surface of host cells and the subsequent activation of inflammatory mediator release, such as TNFa, by these cells.[57]

Table 2. Summary of Ty21a field trials using liquid and enteric-coated capsule formulations: 36 months surveillance, children received 3 doses of vaccine or placebo within 1 week

	Alexandria, Egypt(1978-81)[a]		Santiago, Chile (1982)[b]		Santiago, Chile (1986-89)[c]		
	Liquid	Placebo	Enteric Capsules	Placebo	Liquid	Enteric Capsules	Placebo
Age 5 – 9 years							
Number of children	16 486	15 902	7034	7193	22 586	21 128	5989
Cases	1	22	10	25	10	44	15
Incidence/10^5	6.1	138	142	348	44.3	208	251
Efficacy	95.6	-	59.1	-	82.3	16.9	-
(95% CI)	(77-99)%	-	(16-80)%	-	(61-92)%	(0-53)%	-
Age ≥ 10 years							
Number of children	-	-	15 134	14 711	14 037	13 568	4313
Cases	-	-	13	45	13	19	13
Incidence/10^5	-	-	85.9	306	92.6	140	301
Efficacy	-	-	71.9	-	69.3	53.5	-
(95% CI)	-	-	(48-55)%	-	(35-86)%	(7-77)%	-

a. Ref. 44
b Ref. 45
c Ref. 49

The anti-O antibody response following immunization with the heat-killed, phenol-preserved L vaccine peaks seven days after immunization and remains elevated for six months.[58] In the first WHO vaccine trial using freshly prepared L vaccine, serum anti-H agglutinating antibodies were found to be the most reliable indicator of vaccine efficacy.[23] It is of interest that an acetone-inactivated whole-cell parenteral vaccine made from a nonmotile mutant of Ty2 lacking the H antigen did not provide any protection against typhoid fever in a large controlled field trial in Egypt.[59] However, human volunteer studies with the parenteral whole-cell killed K and L vaccines found no association between vaccine-induced protection and either serum O and H agglutinating antibody titers or serum bactericidal activity.[22]

Vi-CPS behaves like a type-2 T-cell-independent antigen, in that it elicits a serum antibody response that is not amenable to boosting and which is impaired in HIV-infected persons with a low $CD4^+$ cell count.[60-62] The serum antibody response to Vi-CPS is predominantly of the IgG isotype. These antibodies persist for at least 3 years after vaccination, even in individuals living in nonendemic regions where there is minimal reexposure to the antigen.[40,63] It has been estimated that a serum anti-Vi IgG level of 1 mg/mL is protective.[40]

Human volunteer studies have shown that, when grown in the presence of galactose, the live-oral vaccine Ty21a is immunogenic, eliciting both antibody and cell-mediated immune responses.[64] The O-9,12 specific antibody-secreting cell (ASC) response peaks within one week of immunisation, is predominantly of the IgA isotype, and is directed against the carbohydrate side-chains of the LPS molecule.[65-67] In vitro studies have shown that serum and $CD4^+$ cells from these vaccinees can mediate antibody-dependent cell-mediated cytotoxicity (ADCC) that is bactericidal for *S. typhi* and *S. paratyphi* A and B.[68,69] The ASCs response elicited by the vaccine appears to be directed to the mucosa, since the majority of antigen-specific ASCs isolated from the peripheral blood of vaccinees express a4 and b7 (the gut homing receptor LPAM-1), while the proportion of cells expressing L-selectin (the peripheral lymph node homing receptor) is reduced.[67] Furthermore, there is a significant increase in anti-LPS IgA in intestinal secretions following oral Ty21a, although the dose used in the study was substantially higher than that in commercial vaccine preparations.[65] Field studies have shown that the anti-LPS IgG seroconversion rate increases with the number of doses of Ty21a and roughly correlates with the level of protection, although it does not necessarily follow that these antibodies are mediating protection.[70] As Ty21a does not express Vi-CPS and does not elicit a Vi antibody response its mode of protection differs from that of Vi-CPS based vaccines.

New Typhoid Vaccines

The World Health Organisations' Global Programme on Vaccines recommends the use of typhoid vaccines in school-based immunization programs as a means of controlling typhoid fever.[28] As pointed out in these recommendations, the major limitation of whole-cell killed parenteral vaccines is the high frequency of adverse side-effects, and these are not recommended for routine use. Although Vi-CPS and Ty21a have been shown to be safe and effective in older children and adults, and the practicality of administering Ty21a as part of a school-based immunisation programme has been demonstrated, neither of these vaccines are widely used in areas where typhoid is endemic. One reason for this underutilization is that health authorities in these regions maintain they have insufficient resources to administer typhoid vaccines to school-age children and have expressed a preference to administer the vaccines to infants (0-12 months of age) through the Expanded Programme of Immunisation (EPI).[71] Unfortunately, infants and young children do not respond well to bacterial capsular polysaccharides, such as Vi-CPS, and Ty21a has not consistently been shown to be immunogenic in young children.[21,72,73] Consequently there has been a desire to develop new typhoid vaccines that are safe, immunogenic and protective in children under five years of age.

One approach that has been taken in the development of new typhoid vaccines has been to improve the immunogenicity of Vi-CPS by conjugation to a carrier protein, the rationale being that the protein carrier will elicit a T-cell memory response, resulting in a higher serum IgG response that can be boosted. One vaccine that is looking particularly promising is a Vi-*Pseudomonas aeruginosa* recombinant exoprotein A (Vi-rEPA) conjugate. Volunteer studies have shown that Vi-rEPA is safe and that it elicits a significantly greater serum anti-Vi IgG response than Vi-CPS alone.[61] Subsequent studies in laboratory animals and humans showed that conjugates prepared using the linker ADH (Vi-rEPA$_2$) were more immunogenic than those prepared using SPDP (Vi-rEPA$_1$).[74,75] The Vi-rEPA$_2$ conjugate elicited a significant increase in serum anti-Vi IgG, IgA and IgM levels in both children aged 5-14 years and, more importantly, 2-4 years. Fever was not observed in any of the vaccinees, although some reported discomfort at the site of injection. A recent study conducted in southern Vietnam reported an efficacy of 91% for the Vi-rEPA conjugate in children aged 2-5 years over a 2-year period.[76] This is extremely high, and it will be interesting to see if the vaccine is as effective in other typhoid endemic regions.

A second approach has been to develop genetically-defined live-attenuated vaccines that can be administered orally, ideally as a single dose. The rationale behind this approach is based largely on the results from studies of *S. typhimurium* in the mouse, which is often used as an animal model of typhoid fever. These studies have shown that live vaccines can protect both innately susceptible (*Nramp-/-*) and resistant (*Nramp+/+*) mice against a lethal challenge with virulent *S. typhimurium*, while whole-cell killed or parenteral vaccines can only protect innately resistant mice.[77-79] Live vaccines elicit T-cell responses, and the expression of immunity induced by live vaccines in innately susceptible mice is impaired in animals functionally defective in cellular immune functions such as CD4$^+$ and/or CD8$^+$ T cells, NK cells, IL-12, TNFa and IFNg.[80-86] Thus the superior efficacy of live vaccines appears to be due to their ability to elicit T-cell responses.

Several potential live *S. typhi*-based vaccine candidates for use in humans have been developed, including strains harboring mutations in genes encoding biosynthetic, e.g., *aroC aroD*,

Table 3. New live-attenuated oral typhoid vaccines

Vaccine	Attenuation/Characteristics	Parent Strain	References
541 Ty	Δ*aroA* Δ*purA*	CDC10-80	87
543 Ty	Δ*aroA* Δ*purA*, Vi-	541 Ty	
CVD 908	Δ*aroC* Δ*aroD*	Ty2	46, 88, 89
CVD906	Δ*aroC* Δ*aroD*	ISP 1820, phage-type 46	
χ3927	Δ*cya* Δ*crp*	Ty2	89
χ4073	Δ*cya* Δ*crp* Δ*cdt*	Ty2	
CVD 908-*htrA*	Δ*aroC* Δ*aroD* Δ*htrA*	Ty2	90
CVD 906-*htrA*	Δ*aroC* Δ*aroD* Δ*htrA*	Ty2	
Ty800	Δ*phoP* Δ*phoQ*	Ty2	91, 92
Ty445	Δ*phoP* Δ*phoQ* Δ*htrA*	Ty2	
PBCC211	Δ*aroA* Δ*aroD* Δ*htrA*	CDC10-80	93
BRD691	Δ*aroA* Δ*aroC*	Ty2	94
BRD1116	Δ*aroA* Δ*aroC* Δ*htrA*	Ty2	
CVD 909	Δ*aroC* Δ*aroD* Δ*htrA*, constitutive Vi	Ty2	95
ZH9	Δ*aroC* Δ*ssaV*		96

and regulatory proteins, e.g., *phoP phoQ* (Table 3). These vaccines are, for the most part, immunogenic in nonimmune adult volunteers, yielding systemic (serum anti-LPS IgG) and mucosal (anti-LPS IgA ASCs) immune responses which are as high as, if not better than, those observed with a single dose of Ty21a. Adverse reactions and 'silent-bacteraemia' can occur at high dosage levels with some vaccine strains; thus, strains with additional attenuating lesions have been developed. Two vaccine candidates that look particularly promising are *S. typhi* derivatives harbouring two aro mutations (*aroC aroD*) with an additional attenuating lesion in *htrA* (CVD906-*htrA* and CVD908-*htrA*), a stress response gene that encodes a periplasmic protease.[90] Both candidate vaccines are as immunogenic as the double aro (*aroC aroD*) parent strains CVD 906 and CVD 908, but fewer adverse reactions are reported, and 'silent bacteraemia' is uncommon. They also elicit both humoral, secretory and cell-mediated responses.[90,97] More recently Hindle et al reported on the safety and immunogenicity of *S. typhi* Ty2 *ΔaroCΔssaV* vaccine strain (ZH9).[96] *SsaV* forms part of the type-three secretion system apparatus of Salmonella pathogenicity island 2.

The serological response to the Vi antigen is generally low with live-attenuated oral vaccines.[89] The efficacy of these vaccines theoretically could be increased if they elicited an anti-Vi antibody response. A strain of Ty21a that expresses the Vi-CPS antigen has been constructed but did not elicit a detectable anti-Vi antibody response in naïve human adults.[98,99] This is perhaps not surprising, since serum anti-Vi antibodies are not always detectable in persons with naturally acquired *S. typhi* infections until late in the disease (after the second week of fever) [House, unpublished data], possibly because the antigen is poorly immunogenic or because it is not expressed in sufficient quantities until late in the infection. Wang et al reported on the vaccine candidate CVD 909, in which the Vi promoter P_{tvia} was replaced with the constitutive promoter P*tac*, resulting in a strain which expressed Vi antigen constitutively.[95] In vivo studies in mice immunized intranasally showed a higher level of seroconversion to the Vi antigen and higher serum anti-Vi IgG titers in mice receiving CVD909 than in animals receiving the parental strain CVD 908-*htrA*. The presence of the Vi-CPS did not appear to interfere with the antibody response to other antigens, since the anti-LPS IgG response was similar with the two vaccines. Furthermore, CVD 909 had an efficacy of 62% against an intra-peritoneal challenge with virulent *S. typhi*, compared to 10% with CVD 908-*htrA*.

The Future

Although typhoid fever is not a major killer, the burden of disease is substantial in some developing countries with limited health care systems and public health resources. With the emergence of MDR and quinolone-resistant *S. typhi*, this situation is likely to worsen. As there is no known animal reservoir for *S. typhi*, typhoid fever is amenable to eradication, either by a combination of treatment of carriers and improvements in sanitation and water purity (as has occurred in the Western world) or by the introduction of targeted vaccine campaigns in conjunction with the provision of safe drinking water (as was demonstrated in Thailand).[19] Since there are limited resources in many typhoid-endemic regions, targeted vaccine campaigns would appear to be the most cost-effective option for the control of typhoid fever in the short term. We now have a better understanding of the pathogenic process of typhoid fever, and the whole-genome sequence of *S. typhi* is now available (http://www.sanger.ac.uk/Projects/S_typhi). This means that we can take a more rationale approach to the development of new typhoid vaccines that are effective in both young children and adults.

Unfortunately one important question remains unanswered, and that is why the current licensed typhoid vaccines do not give greater protection against typhoid fever. It may simply be a matter of inoculating dose, and that no matter how immunogenic a vaccine, the immune system is overwhelmed when the inoculating dose is high. Alternatively the type or magnitude of the immune response elicited by the different vaccines may be inappropriate or inadequate in certain individuals.

The Vi-CPS based vaccines can confer a high degree of protection against typhoid fever, particularly when the polysaccharide is conjugated to the protein carrier rEPA. However, there are still a minority of persons who are not protected with these vaccines. It is possible that vaccine fails to 'take' in certain individuals with a particular genetic background, as has been documented with pneumococcal polysaccharide antigens.[100] Alternatively, the vaccine may fail to give protection in persons infected with Vi$^-$ *S. typhi*.[101,102] *S. typhi* that do not express the Vi-CPS antigen can cause disease in humans, but data as to the clinical importance of such strains are not available.[2,46] Clinical isolates of *S. typhi* can fail to agglutinate with anti-Vi antisera, but whether these strains are truly Vi$^-$ (i.e., lack one or more of the genes required for the expression of Vi-CPS) has not been demonstrated.[103,104] The expression of Vi-CPS is tightly regulated in response to different environmental conditions, and strains which fail to agglutinate may simply have 'switched off' the expression of Vi-CPS, as can occur when *S. typhi* is passaged on laboratory media.

There is some debate as to which type of immune response (humoral or cellular), and thus which type of vaccine (killed or live), is required to protect against typhoid fever. Data from murine studies clearly demonstrate that the relative importance of cellular and humoral responses is dependent upon the genetic background of the host. Mice with fully functional macrophages (Nramp1$^{+/+}$) can be protected by immunization with subunit or killed vaccines, which elicit humoral immune responses, while innately susceptible mice (Nramp1$^{-/-}$) with defective macrophage function require immunization with live vaccines, which elicit both cellular and humoral responses.[78] Which of the two models better represents the situation in typhoid fever in humans is unclear; however, live-attenuated oral vaccines, which elicit both humoral and cellular response theoretically should protect both 'susceptible' and 'resistant' individuals.

Although the currently licensed vaccines do not confer complete protection against typhoid fever, they may be effective in inducing herd-immunity within vaccinated populations and general vaccination programs in endemic areas warrant further consideration.[28,105] Safety and immunogenicity are clearly important issues in the development of any vaccine; however, these are irrelevant if the vaccine cannot be introduced because of logistic or financial reasons. Other factors that need to be taken into consideration are, e.g., the route of immunisation, the number of doses, in addition to ease of production, quality control, and storage and transportation of the vaccine. One advantage of live-oral vaccines such as Ty21a is that they do not require medically trained personnel to administer them. However, these vaccines ideally should be effective as a single dose, since one of the main criticisms of Ty21a is the multiple-dose regime, which although practical in school-based immunization schedules would not be useful as part of the EPI scheme.

Future studies of typhoid vaccines should determine the immunological status of vaccinees, both before and after immunization, if we are to find reliable correlates of vaccine-induced protection and determine why vaccines fail to protect certain individuals.

References

1. Huckstep RL. Typhoid fever and other salmonella infections. London: E & S Livingstone Ltd, 1962.
2. Hornick RB, Greisman SE, Woodward TF et al. Typhoid fever: pathogenesis and immunologic control (first of two parts). New Eng J Med 1970; 283:686-691
3. Smith MD, Duong NM, Hoa NT et al. Comparison of ofloxacin and ceftriaxone for short-course treatment of enteric fever. Antimicrob Agents Chemother 1994; 38:1716-1720.
4. Forsyth JRL. Typhoid and paratyphoid. In: Topley, Wilson, eds. 9th ed. Vol 3, Chp 24. 1998: 459-478.
5. Bitar R, Tarpley J. Intestinal perforation in typhoid fever: a historical state-of-the-art review. Rev Infect Dis 1985; 7:257-271.
6. Butler T, Knight J, Nath SK et al. Typhoid fever complicated by intestinal perforation: a persisting fatal disease requiring surgical management. Rev Infect Dis 1985; 7:244-256
7. van Basten JP, Stockenbrugger R. Typhoid perforation. A review of the literature since 1960. Trop Geog Med 1994; 46:336-339.
8. Azad AK, Islam R, Salam MA et al. Comparison of clinical features and pathological findings in fatal cases of typhoid fever during the initial and later stages of the disease. Am J Trop Med Hyg 1997; 56:490-493.
9. Butler T, Islam A, Kabir I et al. Patterns of morbidity and mortality in typhoid fever dependent on age and gender: review of 552 hospitalised patients with diarrhoea. Rev Infect Dis 1991; 13:85-90.
10. Stuart BM, Pullen RL. Typhoid. Clinical analyses of three hundred and sixty cases. Arch Internal Med. 1946; 78:629-661.
11. Miller SI, Hohmann EL, Pegues DA. Salmonella (including Salmonella typhi). In: Mandell GL, Bennettt JR, Dolin R, eds. Principles and Practice of Infectious Diseases. Chpt 200. 1994:2013-2033. Churchill Livingstone, New York.
12. Edelman R, Levine MM. Summary of the international workshop on typhoid fever. Rev Inf Dis 1986; 4:329-349.
13. Ivanhoff B. Typhoid fever: global situation and WHO recommendations. Southeast Asian J Trop Med Pub Health.1995; 26(2):1-6.
14. Sinha A, Sazawal S, Kumar R et al. Typhoid fever in children aged less than 5 years. Lancet 1999; 354:734-737.
15. Ferreccio C, Levine MM, Manterola A. Benign bacteremia caused by Salmonella typhi and paratyphi in children younger than 2 years. J Pediatrics 1984; 104:899-901.
16. Galloway H, Clark NS, Blackhall M. Paediatric aspects of the Aberdeen typhoid outbreak. Arch Dis Child 1966; 41:63-68.
17. Birkhead GS, Morse DL, Levine WC. Typhoid fever at a resort hotel in New York: a large outbreak with an unusual vehicle. J Infect Dis 1993; 167:1228-1232.
18. Wain J, Hoa NT, Chinh NT et al. Quinolone-resistant Salmonella typhi in Viet Nam: molecular basis of resistance and clinical response to treatment. Clin Infect Dis 1997; 25:1404-1410.
19. Bodhidatta L, Taylor DN, Thisyakorn U. Control of typhoid fever in Bangkok, Thailand, by annual immunization of schoolchildren with parenteral typhoid vaccine. Rev Inf Dis 1987; 9:841-845.

20. Tacket CO, Levine MM. Human typhoid vaccines – old and new. In: DAA Ala'Aldeen, CE Hormaeche, eds. Molecular and Clinical Aspects of Bacterial Vaccine Development. England: John Wiley and Sons, 1995:119-178.
21. Lindberg AA. Vaccination against enteric pathogens: from science to vaccine trials. Curr Opin Microbiol 1998; 1:116-24.
22. Hornick RB, Greisman SE, Woodward TF et al. Typhoid fever: pathogenesis and immunologic control (second of two parts). New Eng J Med 1970; 283:739-746.
23. Cvjetanovic B, Uemura K. The present status of field and laboratory studies of typhoid fever and paratyphoid vaccines. Bull WHO 1965; 32:29-36.
24. Yugoslav Typhoid Commission. A controlled field trial of the effectiveness of acetone-dried and inactivated and heat-phenol-inactivated typhoid vaccines in Yugoslavia. Bull WHO 1964; 30:623-630.
25. Ashcroft MT, Singh B, Nicholson CC et al. A seven-year field trial of two typhoid vaccines in Guyana. Lancet 1967; 2:1056-1059.
26. Polish Typhoid Committee. Controlled field trials and laboratory studies on the effectiveness of typhoid vaccines in Poland 1961-1964. Bull WHO 1966; 34:211-222.
27. Hejfec LB, Salmin LV, Lejtman MZ et al. A controlled field trial and laboratory study of five typhoid vaccines in the USSR. Bull WHO 1966; 34:321-339.
28. Ivanhoff B, Levine MM Lambert PH. Vaccination against typhoid fever: present status. Bull WHO 1994; 72:957-971.
29. Felix A, Pitt RM. A new antigen of B. typhosus. Lancet 1934; July:186-191.
30. Robbins, JD, Robbins JB. Reexamination of the protective role of the capsular polysaccharide (Vi antigen) of Salmonella typhi. J Infect Dis 1984; 150:436-49.
31. Liu SH, Sanderson KE. Rearrangement in the genome of the bacterium Salmonella typhi. Proc Natl Acad Sci USA 1995; 92:1018-22.
32. Arricau N, Hermant D, Waxin H et al. The RcsB-RcsC regulatory system of Salmonella typhi differentially modulates the expression of invasion proteins, flagellin and Vi antigen in response to osmolarity. Mol Microbiol 1998; 29:835-850.
33. Pickard D, Li J, Roberts M et al. Characterisation of defined ompR mutants of Salmonella typhi: ompR is involved in the regulation of Vi polysaccharide expression. Infect Immun 1994; 62:3984-3993.
34. Landy M. Studies on Vi antigens: immunization of human beings with purified Vi antigen. Am J Hyg 1954; 60:52-62.
35. Wong KH, Feeley JC. Isolation of Vi antigen and a simple method for its measurement. App Microbiol 1972; 24:628-633.
36. Szewczyk B, Taylor A. Immunochemical properties of Vi antigen from Salmonella typhi Ty2: presence of two antigenic determinants. Infect Immun 1980; 29:539-544.
37. Tacket CO, Ferreccio C, Robbins JB et al. Safety and immunogenicity of two Salmonella typhi Vi capsular polysaccharide vaccines. J Infect Dis 1986; 154:342-345.
38. Acharya IL, Lowe CU, Thapa R et al. Prevention of typhoid fever in Nepal with the Vi capsular polysaccharide of Salmonella typhi. A preliminary report. N Eng J Med 1987; 29:1101-1104.
39. Klugman KP, Gilbertson IT, Koornhof HJ et al. Protective activity of Vi capsular polysaccharide vaccine against typhoid fever. Lancet 1987; 2:1165-1169.
40. Klugman, KP, Koornhof HJ, Robbins JB et al. Immunogenicity, efficacy and serological correlate of protection of Salmonella typhi Vi capsular polysaccharide vaccine three years after immunisation. Vaccine 1996; 14:435-438.
41. Germanier R, Furer E. Isolation and characterisation of a galE mutant Ty21a of Salmonella typhi: a candidate strain for a live oral vaccine. J Infect Dis 1975; 131:553-558.
42. Silva BA, Gonzalez C, Mora GC et al. Genetic characteristics of the Salmonella typhi strain Ty21a vaccine. J Infect Dis 1987; 155:1077.
43. Cryz SJ, Furer E. Further characterisation of the Salmonella typhi Ty21a vaccine strain. J Infect Dis 1988; 157:1276-1277.
44. Wahdan MH, Cerisier SY, Sallam S et al. A controlled field trial of live Salmonella typhi strain Ty21a oral vaccine against typhoid: three-year results. J Infect Dis 1982; 145: 292-295.
45. Levine MM, Ferrecio C, Black RE et al. Large-scale field trial of Ty21a live oral typhoid vaccine in enteric-coated capsule formulation. Lancet 1987; 1049-1052.
46. Hone DM., Attridge SR, Forrest B et al. A galE via (Vi antigen-negative) mutant of Salmonella typhi Ty2 retained virulence in humans. Infect Immun 1988; 56:1326-1333.
47. The Chilean Typhoid Committee, Black RE, Levine MM et al. Efficacy of one or two doses of Ty21a Salmonella typhi vaccine in enteric-coated capsules in a controlled field trial. Vaccine 1990; 8:81-84.

48. Ferreccio C, Levine MM, Rodriguez H et al. Comparative efficacy of two, three, or four dooses of Ty21a live oral typhoid vaccine in enteric-coated capsules: a field trial in an endemic area. J Infect Dis 1989; 159:766-769.
49. Levine MM, Ferreccio C, Cryz S et al. Comparison of enteric-coated capsules and liquid formulation of Ty21a typhoid vaccine in randomised controlled field trial. Lancet 1990; 336:891-894.
50. Simanjuntak CH, Paleologo FP, Punjabi NH et al. Oral immunisation against typhoid fever in Indonesia with Ty21a vaccine. Lancet 1991; 338:1055-1059.
51. Levine MM, Ferreccio C, Abrego P et al. Duration of efficacy of Ty21a, attenuated Salmonella typhi live oral vaccine. Vaccine 1999; 17:S22-S27.
52. Yokoyama H, Ikedo M, Kohbata S et al. An ultrastructural study of HeLa cell invasion with Salmonella typhi GIFU 10007. Microbiol Immunol. 1986; 31:1-11.
53. Huang XZ, Tall B, Schwan WR et al. Physical limitations on Salmonella typhi entry into cultured human intestinal epithelial cells. Infect Immun 1998; 66:2928-2937.
54. Esposito M. Agar plaque formation by mouse spleen cells in response to vaccination with Vi antigen in typhoid vaccines. J Bacteriol 1969; 99:356-357.
55. Looney RJ, Steigbigel RT. Role of the Vi antigen of Salmonella typhi in resistance to host defence in vitro. J Lab Clin Med 1986; 108:506-16.
56. Jiminez-Lucho V, Leive LL, Joiner KA. Role of the O-antigen of lipopolysaccharide in Salmonella in protection against complement action. In: BH Inglewski, Clark VL, eds. Molecular Basis of Bacterial Pathogenesis: The Bacteria. Volume XI. Academic Press, 1990.
57. Casadevall A. Antibody-mediated protection against intracellular pathogens. Trend Microbiol. 1998; 6:102-107.
58. Chaicumpa W, Wechsathanarak Y, Tantivanich S et al. Antibody responses to heat-killed, phenol preserved parenteral typhoid vaccines. Southeast Asian J Trop Med Public Health 1985; 16:371-376.
59. Wahdan MH, Sippel JE, Mikhail IA et al. Controlled field trial of a thoid vaccine prepared with a nonmotile mutant of Salmonella typhi Ty2. Bull WHO 1975; 52:69-72.
60. Mond JJ, Lees A, Snapper CM. T-cell independent antigens type 2. Annul Rev Immunol 1995; 13:655-692.
61. Szu SC, Taylor DN, Trofa AC et al. Laboratory and preliminary clinical characterisation of Vi capsular polysaccharide-protein conjugate vaccines. Infect Immun 1994; 62:4440-4444.
62. Kroon FP, van Dissel JT, Ravensbergen E et al. Impaired antibody response after immunisation of HIV-infected individuals with the polysaccharide vaccine against Salmonella typhi (Typhim-Vi"). Vaccine 1999; 17:2941-2945.
63. Tackett CO, Levine MM, Robbins JB. Persistence of antibody titres three years after vaccination with Vi polysaccharide vaccine against typhoid fever. Vaccine 1988; 6:307-308.
64. Viret JF, Favre D, Wegmuller B et al. Mucosal and systemic immune responses in humans after primary and booster immunizations with orally administered invasive and noninvasive live attenuated bacteria. Infect Immun 1999; 67:3680-3685.
65. Forrest BD. Identification of intestinal immune response using peripheral blood lymphocytes. Lancet 1988; 81-83.
66. Kantele A, Arvilommi H, Kantele JM et al. Comparison of the human immune response to live oral, killed oral or killed parenteral Salmonella typhi Ty21a vaccine. Microb Pathogen 1991; 10:117-126.
67. Kantele A, Kantele JM, Savilahti E et al. Homing potentials of circulating lymphocytes in humans depends on the site of activation. Oral but not parenteral, typhoid vaccination induces circulating antibody-secreting cells that all bear homing receptors directing them to the gut. J Immunol 1997; 158:574-579.
68. D'Amelio R, Tagliabue A, Nencioni L et al. Comparative analysis of immunological responses to oral (Ty21a) and parenteral (TAB) typhoid vaccines. Infect Immun 1988; 56:2731-2735.
69. Tagliabue A, Villa L, de Magistris MT et al. IgA-driven T cell mediated anti-bacterial immunity in man after live oral Ty21a vaccine. J Immunol 1986; 137:1504-1510.
70 Levine MM, Taylor DN, Ferrecio C. Typhoid vaccines come of age. Pediatr Infect Dis J 1989; 8:374-381.
71. Levine MM. Presented at the Third Asia-Pacific Symposium on Typhoid Fever and Other Salmonellosis, Denpasar, Bali, Indonesia. 1997; December 8-10.
72. Murphy JR, Grez L, Schlesinger L et al. Immunogenicity of Salmonella typhi Ty21a vaccine for young children. Infect Immun 1991; 59:4291-4293.
73. Cryz SJ, Vanprapar N, Thisyakorn U et al. Safety and immunogenicity of Salmonella typhi Ty21a vaccine in young Thai children. Infect Immun 1993; 61:1149-1151.

74. Kossacza Z, Bystricky S, Bryla DA et al. Synthesis and immunological properties of Vi and Di-O-acetyl pectin protein conjugates with adipic acid dihydrazide as the linker. Infect Immun 1997; 65:2088-2093.
75. Kossaczka Z, Lin FYC, Ho VA et al. Safety and immunogenicity of Vi conjugate vaccines for typhoid fever in adults, teenagers, and 2- to 4-year old children in Vietnam. Infect Immun 1999; 67:5806-5810.
76. Lin FYC, Ho VA, Khiem HB et al. The efficacy of a Salmonella typhi Vi conjugate vaccine in two-to-five-year-old children. New Eng J Med 2001; 344:1263-1269.
77. Hormaeche CE, Khan CMA, Mastroeni P et al. Salmonella vaccines: mechanisms of immunity and their use as carriers of recombinant antigens. In: DAA Ala'Aldeen, Hormaeche CE, eds. Molecular and Clinical Aspects of Bacterial Vaccine Development. Chp 4. John Wiley and Sons Ltd, 1995:119-153.
78. Eisenstein TK, Huang D, Schwacha MG. Immunity to Salmonella infections. In: Paradise LJ, Bendinelli M, Friedman H, eds. Enteric Infections and Immunity. Chp 4. New York and London: Plenum Press, 1996:57-78.
79. Makela PH, Hormaeche CE. Immunity to Salmonella. In: S. Kaufmann, ed. Host Response to Intracellular Pathogens. Chapter 10. USA: RG Landers Co., 1996:143-166.
80. Harrison JA, Villarreal-Ramos B, Mastroeni P et al. Correlates of protection induced by live Aro- Salmonella typhimurium vaccines in the murine typhoid model. Immunology 1997; 90:618-625.
81. Nauciel C. Role of CD4+ T cells and T-independent mechanisms in acquired resistance to Salmonella typhimurium infection. J Immunol 1990; 145:1265-1269.
82. Tite JP, Dougan G, Chatfield SN. The involvement of tumour necrosis factor in immunity to Salmonella infection. J Immunol 1991; 147:3161-316.
83. Mastroeni P, Villarreal-Ramos B, Hormaeche CE. Role of T cells, TNFa and IFNg in recall of immunity to oral challenge with virulent salmonellae in mice vaccinated with live attenuated aro- salmonella vaccines. Microbial Pathogen 1992; 13:477-491. 84. Nauciel C, Espinasse-Maes F. Role of gamma interferon and tumor necrosis factoalpha in resistance to Salmonella typhimurium infection. Infect Immun 1992; 60:450-454.
85. Schafer R, Eisenstein TK. Natural killer cells mediate protection induced by a Salmonella aroA mutant. Infect Immun 1992; 60:791-797.
86. Mastroeni P, Harrison JA, Chabalgoity JA ET AL. Effect of interleukin 12 neutralisation on host resistance and gamma interferon production in mouse typhoid. Infect Immun 1996; 64:189-196.
87. Levine MM, Herrington D, Murphy JR et al. Safety, infectivity, immunogenicity, and in vivo stability of two attenuated auxotrophic mutant variant strains of Salmonella typhi, 541Ty and 543Ty, as live oral vaccines in man. J Clin Invest 1987; 79:888-902.
88. Tacket CO, Hone DM, Losonsky GA et al. Clinical acceptability and immunogenicity of CVD908 Salmonella typhi vaccine strain. Vaccine 1992; 10:443-446.
89. Tacket CO, Hone DM, Curtis R III et al. Comparison of the safety and immunogenicity of DaroC DaroD and Dcya Dcrp Salmonella typhi strains in adult volunteers. Infect Immun 1992; 60:536-541.
90. Tacket CO, Sztein MB, Losonsky GA et al. Safety of oral Salmonella typhi vaccine strains with deletions in htrA and aroC aroD and immune response in humans. Infect Immun 1997; 65:452-456.
91. Hohmann EL, Oletta CA, Killeen KP et al. phoP/phoQ-deleted Salmonella typhi (Ty800) is a safe and immunogenic single-dose typhoid fever vaccine in volunteers. J Infect Dis 1996; 173:1408-1414.
92. Hohmann EL, Oletta CA, Miller SI. Evaluation of a phoP/phoQ-deleted, aroA-deleted live oral Salmonella typhi vaccine strain in human volunteers. Vaccine 1996; 14:19-24.
93. Dilts DA, Riesenfeld-Orn I, Fulginiti JP et al. Phase I clinical trials of aroA aroD and aroA aroD htrA attenuated S. typhi vaccines; effect of formulation of safety and immunogenicity. Vaccine 2000; 18:1473-1484.
94. Lowe DC, Savidge TC, Pickard D et al. Characterisation of candidate live oral Salmonella typhi vaccine strains harbouring defined mutations in aroA, aroC, and htrA. Infect Immun 1999; 67:700-707.
95. Wang JY, Noriega FR, Galen JE et al. Constitutive expression of the Vi polysaccharide capsular antigen in attenuated Salmonella enterica serovar Typhi oral vaccine strain CDV 909. Infect Immun 2000; 68:4647-4652.
96. Hindle Z, Chatfield SN, Phillimore J et al. Characterisation in volunteers of Salmonella enterica derivatives harbouring defined aroA and SPI2 type III secretion system (ssaV) mutations. Infect Immun Submitted 2001.
97. Sztein MB, Wasserman SS, Tacket CO et al. Cytokine production patterns and lymphoproliferative responses in volunteers orally immunised with attenuated vaccine strains of Salmonella typhi. J Infect Dis. 1994; 170:1508-1517.

98. Cryz SJ, Furer E, Baron LS et al. Construction and characterisation of a Vi-positive variant of the Salmonella typhi live oral vaccine strain Ty21a. Infect Immun 1989; 57:3863-3868.
99. Tacket CO, Losonsky G, Taylor DN et al. Lack of immune response to the Vi component of a Vi-positive variant of the Salmonella typhi live oral vaccine strain Ty21a in human studies. J Infect Dis 1991; 163:901-904.
100. Musher DM, Groover JE, Watson DA et al. Genetic regulation of the capacity to make immunoglobulin G to pneumococcal capsular polysaccharides. J Invest Med. 1997; 45:57-68.
101. Arya SC. Efficient vaccination strategy against typhoid fever. Vaccine 1997;18:2321.
102. Arya SC. Efficacy of Vi polysaccharide vaccine against Salmonella typhi. Vaccine 1999;17:1015.
103. Keddy KH, Klugman KP, Robbins JB. Efficacy of Vi polysaccharide vaccine against strains of Salmonella typhi: reply. Vaccine 1998; 16:871-872.
104. Hormaeche CE. Letter to the editor. Vaccine 1999; 17:1016.
105. Levine MM, Ferreccio C, Black RE et al. Progress in vaccines against typhoid fever. Rev Infect Dis 1989; 11:S552-S5667.

Chapter 22

Vaccines against *Vibrio cholerae*

James D. Campbell and James B. Kaper

Overview

Cholera, the acute diarrheal disease caused by *Vibrio cholerae* serogroups O1 and O139, continues to cause endemic disease and epidemic outbreaks in many parts of the world. The highest incidence of disease is found in poor countries with inadequate waste disposal and contaminated water supplies. Over nearly two centuries, it has caused seven pandemics, the last of which began in 1961 and continues today. The impact that cholera has had on the health of the world's population, even in the last decade, remains substantial. In 1991, cholera returned to Latin America causing hundreds of thousands of cases;[1] in 1994, epidemic cholera rapidly swept through the Rwandan refugee camps in Zaire leading to an estimated 70,000 cases and 12,000 deaths.[2] In the year 2000, it was reported in 56 countries and in every region of the world. In 2000 and 2001, large numbers of cases were reported in many countries including the Niger, Guinea, Burkina Faso, Ivory Coast, Mali, Chad, and Afghanistan. India suffered tens of thousands of cases after severe flooding, and over 86,000 cases were reported in Kwazulu-Natal in South Africa. Cholera has also found its way to the islands of Micronesia, the Marshalls, and Madagascar.[3] The worldwide case-fatality rate, as reported by the World Health Organization, was 3.6% in 2000. Although much progress has been made, it is clear that current efforts to curb the devastation of cholera remain inadequate.

Clinically, cholera causes a spectrum of disease states ranging from asymptomatic shedding of bacteria to cholera gravis. In fact, two-thirds to three-quarters of cholera infections are inapparent, and among persons with symptoms, only a minority will have severe purging. Classical biotype strains lead to a higher proportion of patients with moderate and severe diarrhea.[4] Some patients will become extremely ill from dehydration very quickly; others will slowly worsen. Patients with cholera gravis may purge enough fluid (1000 mL/hour) to cause death from dehydration within hours of onset of illness. The classic signs and symptoms of dehydration are seen in patients with cholera gravis: weak or absent peripheral pulses, hypotension, sunken eyes, poor skin turgor, and decreased urine output. Patients also may have a flat affect and muscle cramps, as well. Stools may have a peculiar fishy odor and are referred to as "rice-water" due to the clear watery stool mixed with mucus.

The primary treatments for cholera are rapid, large-volume fluid replacement and antibiotics. Fluids may be given enterally using oral rehydration solutions for mild and moderate cases; intravenous rehydration should be used in severe cases. Antibiotics are an adjunct to fluid therapy and have been shown to decrease the duration of both diarrhea and shedding of the organism.[5,6] Antibiotics should be chosen based on the susceptibility pattern of *V. cholerae* in the particular setting. Tetracyclines or fluoroquinolones have proven efficacy.

Cholera is acquired from contaminated water or food. The bacterium is orally ingested and, after an incubation period of a few hours to several days, colonizes the small intestine without invading cells or tissues and produces a potent secretogenic toxin. Factors important in cholera pathogenesis include those affecting colonization and those leading to toxin production. Toxin coregulated pili (TCP) are required for colonization, and expression of these filamentous

New Bacterial Vaccines, edited by Ronald W. Ellis and Bernard R. Brodeur.

surface structures is correlated with expression of cholera toxin (CT).[7] In volunteer studies, strains of *V. cholerae* unable to produce TCP did not colonize humans. Subjects who ingested these strains did not shed the organism, had no diarrhea, and failed to mount an immune response.[8] Nevertheless, antibodies against TCP are not generated by volunteers who ingest wild-type *V. cholerae*, even though anti-CT and vibriocidal antibodies are seen.[9]

The organism also elaborates CT, which causes a secretory diarrhea due to the enzymatic activity of the toxin A subunit (CTA). The toxin alone is sufficient to cause voluminous watery diarrhea,[10] but removal from the organism of *ctx* genes encoding CT does not completely prevent diarrhea.[11] Cholera toxin is a dimeric molecule, with a B subunit (CTB) responsible for binding to the host cell surface and CTA with the specific enzymatic activity. Host cell adenylate cyclase is activated to transform ATP to cAMP when CTA binds to a cellular G protein, G_s. Through the elevation of intracellular cAMP in intestinal epithelial cells, CT leads to severe watery diarrhea.[4] Additional toxins, such as the accessory cholera toxin (ACE)[12] and the zonula occludens toxin (ZOT),[13] have been shown to have enterotoxic effects in vitro and in animal studies, but their role in cholera pathogenesis is unknown.

V. cholerae organisms are subgrouped into biotype, serogroup, serotype, and by the ability to make CT. The most important distinction is serogroup (also called serovar), which is based on the lipopolysaccharide (LPS) O antigen. There are nearly 200 different serogroups but only two serogroups (O1 and O139) routinely express CT and cause epidemic cholera. Within strains of the O1 serogroup there are two distinct serotypes, Inaba and Ogawa. Serogroup O1 strains are also typed into one of two biotypes, classical or El Tor. All recent outbreaks, with the exception of some O139 outbreaks in Bangladesh and in eastern India in the 1990s, have been caused by O1 El Tor strains. Immune responses are made against LPS and other surface proteins as well as against CTB. There is apparently no appreciable protective cross-immunity between O1 and O139 strains, but there is substantial cross-protection between biotypes and serotypes within strains of the O1 serogroup.[4] Knowledge of the immunobiology of the organism has directed efforts in vaccine development.

Immunobiology

Evidence for immunologic protection against cholera following infection comes from two sources: epidemiologic studies of natural infection and volunteer challenge studies.

Protection After Infection

There is evidence to support that natural cholera infection will protect subjects from future cholera illness in most circumstances. Bangladeshi household contacts with elevated vibriocidal antibody titers, indicating previous *V. cholerae* infection, had a significant reduction in risk of cholera when compared to household contacts with low vibriocidal titers.[14] However, this infection-induced protection may be biotype-specific, since in one study lasting for 42 months investigators found that only classical and not El Tor O1 strains led to significant prevention against future cholera.[15] There have been reports of reinfection with cholera,[16] but the reported rates have not been compared with rates of infection in subjects at similar risk but without prior natural infection. Taken together, these studies suggest that infection is protective, at least for classical O1 strains, but that protection is incomplete.

Protection In Volunteer Challenge Studies

Previous cholera infection of healthy volunteers in an experimental setting protects the volunteer from subsequent cholera illness.[17;18] University of Maryland investigators have used this model to test the efficacy of several cholera vaccines[18-20] and have accumulated data on the protection afforded by infection with wild-type *V. cholerae* as well. Previous infection with classical *V. cholerae* O1 prevents illness in 100% of subjects later challenged with the same biotype, whereas El Tor cholera provides ~90% protection against subsequent El Tor challenge. The protection afforded by experimental infection with the classical strain continues for at least three years, the longest duration tested.[21] Protection is seen against challenge using both the homologous and heterologous serotypes. Rechallenge studies in volunteers have also established the immunizing capacity of an initial clinical episode of O139 cholera against homologous challenge three months later.[22]

Another important finding emerging from these studies is the effect of previous cholera infection on future colonization with *V. cholerae*. Individuals with a history of classical biotype infection do not become colonized by the classical strain upon rechallenge, whereas one-third of individuals ingesting El Tor biotype, following an original El Tor challenge, shed the organism in their stool. Complete protection from cholera resulting from previous infection is most likely due to an immune response that prevents colonization of the gut upon subsequent ingestion of cholera organisms.

Immunogenic Antigens

The immune response to infection with *V. cholerae* can be separated into responses against bacterial surface structures and responses against the toxin. Although strong responses are found against both, the antibacterial response has proven more crucial for protection. When a strain of *V. cholerae* lacking both CTA and CTB (JBK70) was used to vaccinate volunteers, it led to protection equivalent to that of the toxin-producing parent strain.[11] Oral vaccines containing only killed *V. cholerae* organisms lead to protection, whereas CT toxoids do not.[10] Still, the addition of CT toxoid to a vaccine that induces anti-bacterial immune responses may provide synergistic protection.[23]

The best assay for determining protection following exposure to *V. cholerae* or a cholera vaccine is serum vibriocidal antibody response. In this assay, subject serum is added with complement to a standard culture of *V. cholerae*, and the amount of bacterial killing is measured. The antibodies measured in this functional assay are directed against the LPS and other cell-surface structures. The majority of vibriocidal activity is due to antibodies directed against LPS, but a smaller portion of the vibriocidal response consists of antibodies directed against a protein component that has not been definitively identified.[4] Unfortunately, antibodies against any single surface molecule have not been shown to be adequate surrogates for the vibriocidal assay in determining protection. Although serum vibriocidal antibody titers are the best correlates for immune protection, they may be markers for another immune response, intestinal sIgA, which is actually performing the protective mucosal function. Also, some proteins against which infected subjects make antibody are only expressed in vivo.[24;25]

Although not protective by themselves in human disease, antibodies against CT are made following infection. CT is a heterodimer consisting of a pentamer of CTB subunits that bind to the host cell surface and a single CTA subunit that is the active enzymatic portion. Antibodies are directed against CTB and can be measured by enzyme-linked immunosorbant assay (ELISA).

Strategies for a Cholera Vaccine Based on Epidemiology and Immunobiology

Rational strategies for cholera vaccine development should take into account the realities of the populations who will most need the vaccine and the current knowledge of the immune responses that are most important for protection.

The recipients of a cholera vaccine would fall into three primary groups: citizens of countries in the areas of the developing world where cholera is endemic or epidemic; refugees who relocate to cholera-prone regions, or individuals living in such areas following natural disasters; and travelers to cholera-prone areas. Developers should therefore aim to manufacture a cholera vaccine that is inexpensive and simple to produce and that is formulated for the tropics (withstands heat, is easy to administer, etc.). It should elicit a protective response quickly, given its potential use in emergencies and in travelers. It should be amenable to use in children, since they are the least likely to have encountered natural disease. The vaccine also should provide durable protection with minimal side effects.

The vaccine should impart antibacterial immunity in order to preclude adherence of cholera organisms to the intestinal mucosal surface during future episodes of exposure to *V. cholerae*. This immunity is conferred by intestinal sIgA antibodies against the O antigen and other surface antigens, but is best measured by the vibriocidal assay. Mucosal presentation of the antigen is expected to induce the optimal mucosal effector response. Although not necessary for protection, inclusion of some portion of CT may adjuvant the immune response.

Efforts to Date (Table 1)

Parenteral Vaccines

The first parenteral cholera vaccine was tested in 1884, within a year of the discovery by Robert Koch of the bacterium responsible for cholera. Since those early efforts, numerous injectable cholera vaccines have been tested, which can be grouped into one of two broad classes: whole-cell and subunit vaccines. These earlier vaccine efforts have been reviewed elsewhere.[26]

Parenteral Killed Whole-Cell Vaccine (WCV)

The currently licensed vaccine in the U.S. is a whole cell *V. cholerae* killed by phenol. It is not widely used given its poor efficacy, its short-term protection, and its side-effect profile. It protects against cholera for 3-6 months in ~50% of subjects but causes injection site pain, erythema, and induration as well as fever and other constitutional symptoms.[27]

Parenteral Subunit Vaccines

Various antigens such as LPS and CT have been tested in injectable subunit vaccines. The newest parenteral vaccine, which is in early stages of development, consists of *V. cholerae* O1 LPS conjugated to one of two CT variants. The reactogenicity profile of this vaccine in volunteers does not mimic that seen following killed WCV, and the new O polysaccharide (Ps) protein conjugate vaccine elicits anti-LPS antibody, vibriocidal titers, and IgG against CT.[28]

Oral Vaccines

In the past three decades there has been a steadily increasing understanding of the importance of the mucosal immune system in protecting against intestinal pathogens. With this increased understanding, most investigators have turned their focus to orally administered cholera vaccines. Two oral cholera vaccines have been licensed by regulatory authorities in a number of countries: CTB-WCV[29] and CVD103-HgR.[30;31]

BS-WC

This inactivated oral vaccine contains three different strains of heat-inactivated and formalin-inactivated *V. cholerae* O1 bacteria, representing a mixture of classical and El Tor biotypes and Inaba and Ogawa serotypes. A single dose consists of 10^{11} bacteria and 1.0 mg CTB, suspended in buffer. Three doses of the vaccine conferred ~85% protection over six months and ~50% protection over three years in a field trial in Bangladesh.[32] The current commercial formulation utilizes a recombinant CTB (rCTB) to help diminish production costs and is well tolerated by adults and children.[33] Two doses of the rCTB-WCV given two weeks apart conferred ~86% protective efficacy upon a group of Peruvian soldiers.[34] In contrast, in a subsequent large placebo-controlled field trial of efficacy in Lima, Peru that included children as well as adults, the same regimen had 0% efficacy during a 12-month period of follow-up.[35] However, following the administration of a third dose of vaccine one year later, significant (61%) protection was conferred over the next year of observation, including against both hospitalized cases (82% efficacy) and against field cases (49% efficacy).[35]

The rCTB-WCV vaccine, manufactured by SBL Vaccin AB (Stockholm, Sweden) and marketed under the names Dukoral® or Colorvac®, is licensed in six Latin American countries

Table 1. *Vaccines against* Vibrio cholerae *currently licensed and under development*

Type	Vaccine	Route	Schedule	Stage of Development
Parenteral	Killed WCV	IM	Single dose	Licensed (but not widely used)
	O conjugate	IM	Not determined	Phase I/II
Oral Killed	rCTB-WCV (O1)	Oral	0, 2 weeks (boost at 1 year)	Licensed in some countries
	rCTB-WCV (O1/O139)	Oral	0, 2 weeks (boost at 1 year)	Phase II
Oral Live	CVD 103-HgR (classical O1 Inaba)	Oral	1 dose	Licensed in some countries
	CVD 111 (El Tor O1 Ogawa)	Oral	1 dose	Phase II
	CVD 103-HgR plus CVD 111	Oral	1 dose	Phase II
	Peru 15 (El Tor O1 Ogawa)	Oral	1 dose	Phase II
	CVD 112 (O139)	Oral	1 dose	Phase II
	Bengal 15 (O139)	Oral	1 dose	Phase II
	638 (El Tor O1 Ogawa)	Oral	1 dose	Phase II

and in Sweden and Norway. The vaccine is given in a glass of water together with an alkaline buffer in two doses, two weeks apart; a booster dose is recommended after 1 or 2 years.

Bivalent O1-O139 rBS-WC

An oral bivalent rCTB-O1/O139 WCV has been prepared by adding formalin-inactivated *V. cholerae* O139 to the oral recombinant O1 rCTB-WCV.[36] When tested in a Phase 1 trial in Swedish adults, a two-dose regimen of this vaccine was well tolerated and immunogenic. Significant vibriocidal responses were observed against O1 organisms in 10 of 12 (83%) subjects and against O139 organisms in 8 of 12 (67%). The vaccine induced both antitoxic and antibacterial mucosal antibody responses. The proportion of bivalent vaccine recipients with side effects was found to be very similar to the proportion of monovalent recipients with side effects.[36]

CVD 103-HgR

Recombinant live oral cholera vaccine CVD 103-HgR was engineered by deleting from a wild-type *V. cholerae* O1 classical Inaba strain 94% of the gene encoding the CTA_1 subunit and by inserting into the hemolysin A (*hlyA*) locus a gene encoding resistance to mercury.[30;37] CVD 103-HgR is a licensed vaccine in many countries and available under the trade names Orochol® and Mutacol®. CVD 103-HgR is expected to soon be considered for licensure in the USA by the Food and Drug Administration.

The safety and immunogenicity of a single oral dose of this vaccine in subjects as young as 3 months and as old as 65 years of age, including subjects infected with the human immunodeficiency virus (HIV), has been established in a number of randomized, placebo-controlled, double-blind clinical trials with active surveillance (involving more than 7,000 subjects) in countries in Asia, Latin America, Africa, Europe and North America.[38-46] A single dose of CVD 103-HgR confers on adult volunteers significant protection against experimental challenge with pathogenic *V. cholerae* O1 of either biotype or serotype.[30;31;47] Protection is evident as early as eight days after vaccination and lasts for at least six months (the shortest and longest intervals tested).[31] The single-dose efficacy and rapid onset of protection are attractive characteristics of CVD 103-HgR.

In a randomized, placebo-controlled, double-blind field trial in Indonesia, 67,508 pediatric and adult subjects received a single dose of CVD 103-HgR vaccine or placebo.[48] Vaccine did not confer significant long-term protection over the 4 year follow-up (13.5% vaccine efficacy overall), but in an "intent to vaccinate" analysis assessing vaccine efficacy in relation to blood group, persons of blood group O were modestly protected by vaccine (p=0.06, vaccine efficacy = 45%). Unfortunately, too few cases (5 in controls, 2 in vaccinees) occurred in the first four months of follow-up after vaccination to allow a valid comparison with the previous studies using adult volunteers. The most likely reason for decreased efficacy in field-trial subjects in the developing world is their lower post-vaccination vibriocidal titers when compared to volunteers in challenge studies.[41;42;44;46;49-51]

The phenomenon of decreased immunogenicity of live oral vaccines when given to young children living in poorer countries compared to children in industrialized countries has been found with both oral polio vaccine and rotavirus vaccine.[52;53] In order to achieve high seroconversion rates of vibriocidal antibody in Indonesian children and Peruvian adults living in underprivileged conditions, it was necessary to give a 10-fold higher dose (5×10^9 cfu) of CVD 103-HgR[41;46] than the dose (5×10^8 cfu) that is consistently immunogenic in North Americans and Europeans.[38;40] Factors that may partially explain this barrier to successful intestinal immunization are small bowel bacterial overgrowth[54-58] and heavy infection with intestinal helminths.[59] In addition, the ability of malnourished children to mount immune responses may be altered, with certain cell-mediated responses being particularly affected.[60]

Among the licensed oral vaccines, CVD 103-HgR is unique in having a single-dose immunization schedule. In safety/immunogenicity studies in Chilean infants and toddlers[45] and in preschoolers in Indonesia and Peru,[42;61] the formulation of CVD 103-HgR used was a suspension. In the toddler and infant age groups, the taste of the vaccine and the recommended volume were problematic,[45] but the vaccine was well-tolerated and vibriocidal antibody seroconversion was similar (66% vs. 63%) in subjects receiving the full volume of vaccine and those who drank a smaller fraction of the vaccine volume.

Other Attenuated *V. Cholerae* O1 and O139 Live Oral Vaccine Strains

Three other attenuated *V. cholerae* O1 vaccine strains have been reported to have well tolerated, immunogenic, and protective in small clinical trials in volunteers: Peru 15,[62] CVD 111,[63] and 638.[64] Peru 15 is a nonfilamentous, nonmotile strain of an El Tor *V. cholerae* O1 in which the genes encoding CT, ACE, and ZOT have been deleted, along with some flanking sequences, and the gene encoding CTB has been reinserted into the chromosome so as to inactivate *recA*, the gene responsible for homologous recombination. None of the 44 subjects receiving doses of 10^6-10^9 bacteria had diarrhea following vaccination, although other minor gastrointestinal side effects were occasionally noted. Four-fold rises in vibriocidal titers were seen in 38 of 44 vaccinees.[65] Three of five volunteers challenged following vaccination had no diarrhea, and the volumes of diarrhea in the two volunteers not completely protected were low (<1L).[62]

CVD 111 is a *V. cholerae* O1 El Tor Ogawa strain that has had the *ctx, zot, cep,* and *ace* genes deleted, while the genes for CTB and a mercury-resistance marker have been inserted into the hemolysin A gene (*hlyA*). Three of 25 volunteers receiving this vaccine had mild diarrhea, but 23 of 25 developed high-titer vibriocidal antibodies. Vaccine efficacy was 81% following challenge with the parent strain.[66]

A combined CVD 111/CVD 103-HgR bivalent vaccine was evaluated in phase 2 trials in adult community volunteers in the U.S., in Peruvian military personnel,[63] and in several hundred

U.S. military personnel in Panama.[67] The vaccine was safe and immunogenic. The addition of CVD 111 led to an increase in the vibriocidal seroconversion rate and in Ogawa vibriocidal titers when compared to CVD 103-HgR alone. All dosages were well tolerated in Peruvian subjects,[63] but some mild diarrhea was seen in a minority of U.S. volunteers (8 of 103 receiving the bivalent vaccine compared to 0 of 67 receiving CVD 103-HgR alone or placebo in the Panama study).[67] An attenuated O1 El Tor Ogawa strain, 638, has been developed by investigators in Cuba.[64] This strain is deleted of the *ctx, zot, cep,* and *ace* genes and is also deleted of a gene encoding a hemagglutinin/protease (Hap) that has been implicated in reactogenicity of CT-negative *V. cholerae* vaccine strains. In an initial phase 1 study, four of 42 subjects who ingested strain 638 and one of 14 who received placebo experienced loose stools. The vaccine elicited significant vibriocidal antibody titers, but protective efficacy data in a challenge study have not been reported.

Two attenuated O139 strains, Bengal 15[68] and CVD 112,[69] have also been shown to be reasonably well tolerated, immunogenic, and protective in experimental challenge studies. Bengal 15 is a nonmotile derivative of an O139 strain with deletion of the *ctxA*, *ace*, zot, and cep genes along with flanking sequences and insertion of cloned *ctxB* into the *recA* gene. The vaccine was found to have an efficacy rate of 83% in a challenge study of human volunteers. None of the 20 recipients of Bengal 15 given at a dose of either 10^6 or 10^8 cfu suffered from diarrhea, although 1 of 4 given 10^6 cfu of an earlier motile strain (Bengal 3) did have diarrhea.[68] CVD 112 was constructed by deleting from another O139 strain the core region (*ctxAB, zot, and ace*) and reinserting into *hlyA* the CTB gene and a mercury-resistance gene.[69] This vaccine was 84% effective against challenge with the parent O139 strain in a study of healthy adult volunteers. At the lower dose (10^6 cfu), no adverse events were noted; but at the higher dose (10^8 cfu), 3 of 6 volunteers had diarrhea.

If protection against O1 and O139 is desirable in the same vaccine, one may test a vaccine that contains an attenuated strain of both serogroups. An alternative strategy is to use a vaccine that is derived from an O1 wild-type strain, such as CVD 103-HgR, as a carrier for immunogenic O139 antigens. A strain called CH25 is a derivative of CVD 103-HgR into which genes that encode a portion of the O polysaccharide and the O139 capsular Ps were transferred into the parent strain and genes required for O1 LPS expression were deleted.[70] Parenteral administra tion in rabbits led to antibody responses, but no human trials have been reported to date.

Combined Cholera and Typhoid Vaccine

Coadministration of CVD 103-HgR with the first dose of the live attenuated oral typhoid vaccine Ty21a has been tested for safety and immunogenicity.[71;72] In one study,[72] four-fold rises in vibriocidal antibody responses against the homologous serotype (Inaba) were seen in 94% of recipients and against the heterologous serotype (Ogawa) in 80%. Serum IgG anti-*S. typhi* O antibody responses were equivalent to the responses after separate administration, and the adverse reactions were not enhanced by simultaneous administration. In the other study,[71] peak and geometric mean vibriocidal titers were increased in those receiving the combined vaccine regimen when compared to CVD 103-HgR followed by placebo.

The Future

The next several years of research into cholera vaccines will deal with a number of topics including basic science, formulation, testing, and regulatory issues. Most of these issues concern live attenuated cholera vaccines rather than the killed rCTB-WCV, for which the great majority of development has been accomplished. One of the biggest issues concerns the use of volunteer studies versus field studies. The attenuated *V. cholerae* strain CVD 103-HgR proved highly efficacious in protecting adult North Americans against challenge with wild-type *V. cholerae*, yet provided meager protection in a field trial in Indonesia. Was the Indonesian experience truly reflective of the actual vaccine efficacy, or would another field trial demonstrate significant efficacy? A precedent can be seen in trials of rCTB-WCV discussed above, where a two-dose regimen in one field trial in Peru gave 86% protection yet another two-dose trial in Peru gave 0% protection. Based on this experience, CVD 103-HgR should be studied in another field trial to examine the reasons for the discrepancy between the high rate of protection seen in North Americans and the low level seen in Indonesians. If such volunteer trials cannot be used to predict field efficacy, another set of questions arises as to the best way to evaluate cholera vaccines. Discordant field trial and volunteer results have important implications for licensure of cholera vaccines. An argument can be made that for licensure of a cholera vaccine for travelers and military personnel from the U.S. or other industrialized countries, the results of volunteer studies using U.S. subjects are more relevant than results of field trials using subjects in developing countries. These testing and regulatory issues are relevant to other attenuated cholera vaccines such as Peru-15 and 638 as they move through development.

There are several formulation issues that are unresolved, ranging from issues affecting individuals to issues affecting an entire country. The taste and volume of the fluid used to resuspend the organisms can affect acceptance, particularly in small children. A major issue is the need for a combined O1 and O139 vaccine versus O1 vaccine alone. When the O139 serogroup first emerged in the early 1990s, it was believed that it would rapidly spread throughout the world and that any useful cholera vaccine would need to incorporate both O1 and O139 strains. However, O139 did not spread widely and is currently present only in Bangladesh and eastern India in a minority of cholera patients. Vaccines intended for the rest of the world containing both O1 and O139 strains would increase production expenses of an already marginally profitable class of vaccines. Other formulation issues include the combination of cholera vaccines with other enteric vaccines such as typhoid vaccines.

Finally, other basic science and epidemiological questions remain; e.g., what is the mechanism by which *ctx*- negative *V. cholerae* strains can still cause mild diarrhea in some individuals? How did the O139 serogroup emerge in the early 1990s, having never been seen prior to this time, and could another novel and lethal serogroup of *V. cholerae* emerge in the future? The recent determination of the genome sequence of *V. cholerae*[73] will greatly enhance our ability to answer such basic questions about *V. cholerae*. Although significant progress has been made in the development of new cholera vaccines, these and other questions still remain unanswered in the search for a safe and widely effective cholera vaccine despite more than 115 years of vaccine development efforts.

References

1. Ries AA, Vugia DJ, Beingolea L et al. Cholera in Piura, Peru: a modern urban epidemic. J Infect Dis 1992; 166:1429-1433.
2. Public health impact of Rwandan refugee crisis: what happened in Goma, Zaire, in July, 1994? Goma Epidemiology Group. Lancet 1995; 345:339-344.
3. WHO Report on Global Surveillance of Epidemic-prone Infectious Diseases. Internet http://www.who.int/emc-documents/surveillance/docs/whocdscsrisr2001.html/cholera/cholera.htm. 2001.
4. Kaper JB, Morris JG Jr, Levine MM. Cholera. Clin Microbiol Rev 1995; 8:48-86.
5. Lindenbaum J, Greenough WB, Islam MR. Antibiotic therapy of cholera. Bull World Health Organ 1967; 36:871-883.
6. Wallace CK, Anderson PN, Brown TC et al. Optimal antibiotic therapy in cholera. Bull World Health Organ 1968; 39:239-245.
7. Taylor RK, Miller VL, Furlong DB et al. Use of phoA gene fusions to identify a pilus colonization factor coordinately regulated with cholera toxin. Proc Natl Acad Sci USA 1987; 84:2833-2837.
8. Herrington DA, Hall RH, Losonsky G et al. Toxin, toxin-coregulated pili, and the toxR regulon are essential for Vibrio cholerae pathogenesis in humans. J Exp Med 1988; 168:1487-1492.
9. Hall RH, Losonsky G, Silveira AP et al. Immunogenicity of Vibrio cholerae O1 toxin-coregulated pili in experimental and clinical cholera. Infect Immun 1991; 59:2508-2512.
10. Levine MM, Kaper JB, Black RE, Clements ML. New knowledge on pathogenesis of bacterial enteric infections as applied to vaccine development. Microbiol Rev 1983; 47:510-550.
11. Levine MM, Kaper JB, Herrington D et al. Volunteer studies of deletion mutants of Vibrio cholerae O1 prepared by recombinant techniques. Infect Immun 1988; 56:161-167.

12. Trucksis M, Galen JE, Michalski J et al. Accessory cholera enterotoxin (Ace), the third toxin of a Vibrio cholerae virulence cassette. Proc Natl Acad Sci USA 1993; 90:5267-5271.
13. Fasano A, Baudry B, Pumplin DW et al. Vibrio cholerae produces a second enterotoxin, which affects intestinal tight junctions. Proc Natl Acad Sci USA 1991; 88:5242-5246.
14. Glass RI, Svennerholm AM, Khan MR et al. Seroepidemiological studies of El Tor cholera in Bangladesh: association of serum antibody levels with protection. J Infect Dis 1985; 151:236-242.
15. Clemens JD, van Loon F, Sack DA et al. Biotype as determinant of natural immunising effect of cholera. Lancet 1991; 337:883-884.
16. Woodward WE. Cholera reinfection in man. J Infect Dis 1971; 123:61-66.
17. Cash RA, Music SI, Libonati JP et al. Response of man to infection with Vibrio cholerae. I. Clinical, serologic, and bacteriologic responses to a known inoculum. J Infect Dis 1974; 129:45-52.
18. Levine MM, Nalin DR, Craig JP et al. Immunity of cholera in man: relative role of antibacterial versus antitoxic immunity. Trans R Soc Trop Med Hyg 1979; 73:3-9.
19. Levine MM. Immunity to cholera as evaluated in volunteers. In: Ouchterlony O, Holmgren J, editors. Cholera and related diarrheas. Basel: Karger, 1980:195-203.
20. Levine MM, Black RE, Clements ML et al. Volunteer studies in development of vaccines against cholera and enterotoxic E. coli: a review. Acute enteric infections in children. New prospects for treatment and prevention. Elsevier: North Holland Biomedical Press, 1981:443-459.
21. Levine MM, Black RE, Clements ML et al. Duration of infection-derived immunity to cholera. J Infect Dis 1981; 143:818-820.
22. Morris JG, Jr., Losonsky GE, Johnson JA et al. Clinical and immunologic characteristics of Vibrio cholerae O139 Bengal infection in North American volunteers. J Infect Dis 1995; 171:903-908.
23. Peterson JW. Synergistic protection against experimental cholera by immunization with cholera toxoid and vaccine. Infect Immun 1979; 26:528-533.
24. Jonson G, Svennerholm AM, Holmgren J. Vibrio cholerae expresses cell surface antigens during intestinal infection which are not expressed during in vitro culture. Infect Immun 1989; 57:1809-1815.
25. Richardson K, Kaper JB, Levine MM. Human immune response to Vibrio cholerae O1 whole cells and isolated outer membrane antigens. Infect Immun 1989; 57:495-501.
26. Levine MM, Pierce NF. Immunity and Vaccine Development. In: Barua D, Greenough WB, eds. Cholera. New York: Plenum Medical Book Company, 1992: 285-327.
27. Graves P, Deeks J, Demicheli V, Pratt M, Jefferson T. Vaccines for preventing cholera. Cochrane Database Syst Rev 2000;CD000974.
28. Gupta RK, Taylor DN, Bryla DA, Robbins JB, Szu SC. Phase 1 evaluation of Vibrio cholerae O1, serotype Inaba, polysaccharide-cholera toxin conjugates in adult volunteers. Infect Immun 1998; 66:3095-3099.
29. Holmgren J, Svennerholm AM, Jertborn M et al. An oral B subunit: whole cell vaccine against cholera. Vaccine 1992; 10:911-914.
30. Levine MM, Kaper JB, Herrington D et al. Safety, immunogenicity, and efficacy of recombinant live oral cholera vaccines, CVD 103 and CVD 103-HgR. Lancet 1988; 2:467-470.
31. Tacket CO, Losonsky G, Nataro JP et al. Onset and duration of protective immunity in challenged volunteers after vaccination with live oral cholera vaccine CVD 103-HgR. J Infect Dis 1992; 166:837-841.
32. Clemens JD, Sack DA, Harris JR et al. Field trial of oral cholera vaccines in Bangladesh: results from three- year follow-up. Lancet 1990; 335:270-273.
33. Sanchez J, Holmgren J. Recombinant system for overexpression of cholera toxin B subunit in Vibrio cholerae as a basis for vaccine development. Proc Natl Acad Sci USA 1989; 86:481-485.
34. Sanchez JL, Vasquez B, Begue RE et al. Protective efficacy of oral whole-cell/recombinant-B-subunit cholera vaccine in Peruvian military recruits. Lancet 1994; 344:1273-1276.
35. Taylor DN, Cardenas V, Sanchez JL et al. Two-year study of the protective efficacy of the oral whole cell plus recombinant B subunit cholera vaccine in Peru. J Infect Dis 2000; 181:1667-1673.
36. Jertborn M, Svennerholm AM, Holmgren J. Intestinal and systemic immune responses in humans after oral immunization with a bivalent B subunit-O1/O139 whole cell cholera vaccine. Vaccine 1996; 14:1459-1465.
37. Ketley JM, Michalski J, Galen J et al. Construction of genetically marked Vibrio cholerae O1 vaccine strains. FEMS Microbiol Lett 1993; 111:15-21.
38. Kotloff KL, Wasserman SS, O'Donnell S et al. Safety and immunogenicity in North Americans of a single dose of live oral cholera vaccine CVD 103-HgR: results of a randomized, placebo- controlled, double-blind crossover trial. Infect Immun 1992; 60:4430-4432.

39. Perry RT, Plowe CV, Koumare B et al. A single dose of live oral cholera vaccine CVD 103-HgR is safe and immunogenic in HIV-infected and HIV-noninfected adults in Mali. Bull World Health Organ 1998; 76:63-71.
40. Cryz SJ Jr, Levine MM, Kaper JB et al. Randomized double-blind placebo controlled trial to evaluate the safety and immunogenicity of the live oral cholera vaccine strain CVD 103-HgR in Swiss adults. Vaccine 1990; 8:577-580.
41. Suharyono, Simanjuntak C, Witham N et al. Safety and immunogenicity of single-dose live oral cholera vaccine CVD 103-HgR in 5-9-year-old Indonesian children. Lancet 1992; 340:689-694.
42. Simanjuntak CH, O'Hanley P, Punjabi NH et al. Safety, immunogenicity, and transmissibility of single-dose live oral cholera vaccine strain CVD 103-HgR in 24- to 59-month-old Indonesian children. J Infect Dis 1993; 168:1169-1176.
43. Migasena S, Pitisuttitham P, Prayurahong B et al. Preliminary assessment of the safety and immunogenicity of live oral cholera vaccine strain CVD 103-HgR in healthy Thai adults. Infect Immun 1989; 57:3261-3264.
44. Lagos R, Avendano A, Prado V et al. Attenuated live cholera vaccine strain CVD 103-HgR elicits significantly higher serum vibriocidal antibody titers in persons of blood group O. Infect Immun 1995; 63:707-709.
45. Lagos R, San Martin O, Wasserman SS et al. Palatability, reactogenicity and immunogenicity of engineered live oral cholera vaccine CVD 103-HgR in Chilean infants and toddlers. Pediatr Infect Dis J 1999; 18:624-630.
46. Gotuzzo E, Butron B, Seas C et al. Safety, immunogenicity, and excretion pattern of single-dose live oral cholera vaccine CVD 103-HgR in Peruvian adults of high and low socioeconomic levels. Infect Immun 1993; 61:3994-3997.
47. Tacket CO, Cohen MB, Wasserman SS et al. Randomized, double-blind, placebo-controlled, multicentered trial of the efficacy of a single dose of live oral cholera vaccine CVD 103-HgR in preventing cholera following challenge with Vibrio cholerae O1 El tor inaba three months after vaccination. Infect Immun 1999; 67:6341-6345.
48. Richie EE, Punjabi NH, Sidharta YY et al. Efficacy trial of single-dose live oral cholera vaccine CVD 103-HgR in North Jakarta, Indonesia, a cholera-endemic area. Vaccine 2000; 18:2399-2410.
49. Su-Arehawaratana P, Singharaj P, Taylor DN et al. Safety and immunogenicity of different immunization regimens of CVD 103- HgR live oral cholera vaccine in soldiers and civilians in Thailand. J Infect Dis 1992; 165:1042-1048.
50. Glass RI, Holmgren J, Haley CE et al. Predisposition for cholera of individuals with O blood group. Possible evolutionary significance. Am J Epidemiol 1985; 121:791-796.
51. Tacket CO, Losonsky G, Nataro JP et al. Extension of the volunteer challenge model to study South American cholera in a population of volunteers predominantly with blood group antigen O. Trans R Soc Trop Med Hyg 1995; 89:75-77.
52. Patriarca PA, Wright PF, John TJ. Factors affecting the immunogenicity of oral poliovirus vaccine in developing countries: review. Rev Infect Dis 1991; 13:926-939.
53. Hanlon P, Hanlon L, Marsh V et al. Trial of an attenuated bovine rotavirus vaccine (RIT 4237) in Gambian infants. Lancet 1987; 1:1342-1345.
54. Fagundes-Neto U, Viaro T, Wehba J et al. Tropical enteropathy (environmental enteropathy) in early childhood: a syndrome caused by contaminated environment. J Trop Pediatr 1984; 30:204-209.
55. Fagundes NU, Martins MC, Lima FL et al. Asymptomatic environmental enteropathy among slum-dwelling infants. J Am Coll Nutr 1994; 13:51-56.
56. Khin MU, Bolin TD, Duncombe VM et al. Epidemiology of small bowel bacterial overgrowth and rice carbohydrate malabsorption in Burmese (Myanmar) village children. Am J Trop Med Hyg 1992; 47:298-304.
57. Lagos R, Fasano A, Wasserman SS et al. Effect of small bowel bacterial overgrowth on the immunogenicity of single-dose live oral cholera vaccine CVD 103-HgR. J Infect Dis 1999; 180:1709-1712.
58. Shedlofsky S, Freter R. Synergism between ecologic and immunologic control mechanisms of intestinal flora. J Infect Dis 1974; 129:296-303.
59. Cooper PJ, Chico ME, Losonsky G et al. Albendazole treatment of children with ascariasis enhances the vibriocidal antibody response to the live attenuated oral cholera vaccine CVD 103-HgR. J Infect Dis 2000; 182:1199-1206.
60. Glass RI, Svennerholm AM, Stoll BJ et al. Effects of undernutrition on infection with Vibrio cholerae O1 and on response to oral cholera vaccine. Pediatr Infect Dis J 1989; 8:105-109.
61. Lagos R, Losonsky G, Abrego P et al. Tolerancia, immunogenicidad, excresion y transmision de la vacuna anti0colera oral viva-attenuada, CVD 103 HgR, estudio pareado de doble ciego en ninos Chilenos de 24 a 59 mesas. Bol Hosp Infant Mex 1996; 53:214-220.

62. Kenner JR, Coster TS, Taylor DN et al. Peru-15, an improved live attenuated oral vaccine candidate for Vibrio cholerae O1. J Infect Dis 1995; 172:1126-1129.
63. Taylor DN, Tacket CO, Losonsky G et al. Evaluation of a bivalent (CVD 103-HgR/CVD 111) live oral cholera vaccine in adult volunteers from the United States and Peru. Infect Immun 1997; 65:3852-3856.
64. Benitez JA, Garcia L, Silva A et al. Preliminary assessment of the safety and immunogenicity of a new CTXPhi- negative, hemagglutinin/protease-defective El Tor strain as a cholera vaccine candidate. Infect Immun 1999; 67:539-545.
65. Sack DA, Sack RB, Shimko J et al. Evaluation of Peru-15, a new live oral vaccine for cholera, in volunteers. J Infect Dis 1997; 176:201-205.
66. Tacket CO, Kotloff KL, Losonsky G et al. Volunteer studies investigating the safety and efficacy of live oral El Tor Vibrio cholerae O1 vaccine strain CVD 111. Am J Trop Med Hyg 1997; 56:533-537.
67. Taylor DN, Sanchez JL, Castro JM et al. Expanded safety and immunogenicity of a bivalent, oral, attenuated cholera vaccine, CVD 103-HgR plus CVD 111, in United States military personnel stationed in Panama. Infect Immun 1999; 67:2030-2034.
68. Coster TS, Killeen KP, Waldor MK et al. Safety, immunogenicity, and efficacy of live attenuated Vibrio cholerae O139 vaccine prototype. Lancet 1995; 345:949-952.
69. Tacket CO, Losonsky G, Nataro JP et al. Initial clinical studies of CVD 112 Vibrio cholerae O139 live oral vaccine: safety and efficacy against experimental challenge. J Infect Dis 1995; 172:883-886.
70. Favre D, Cryz SJ Jr, Viret JF. Construction and characterization of a potential live oral carrier-based vaccine against Vibrio cholerae O139. Infect Immun 1996; 64:3565-3570.
71. Cryz SJ Jr, Que JU, Levine MM et al. Safety and immunogenicity of a live oral bivalent typhoid fever (Salmonella typhi Ty21a)-cholera (Vibrio cholerae CVD 103-HgR) vaccine in healthy adults. Infect Immun 1995; 63:1336-1339.
72. Kollaritsch H, Furer E, Herzog C et al. Randomized, double-blind placebo-controlled trial to evaluate the safety and immunogenicity of combined Salmonella typhi Ty21a and Vibrio cholerae CVD 103-HgR live oral vaccines. Infect Immun 1996; 64:1454-1457.
73. Heidelberg JF, Eisen JA, Nelson WC et al. DNA sequence of both chromosomes of the cholera pathogen Vibrio cholerae. Nature 2000; 406:477-483.

Index

A

A-hemolysin 53
Acute rheumatic fever (ARF) 155, 156, 162-164, 167
Adenoids 69
Adhesin 112, 115, 133, 135, 136, 139, 161, 185, 222, 246, 247, 283, 284, 288-290, 292, 302, 303, 312, 313
Adjuvant 10, 22, 24, 26, 27, 30, 33-35, 67, 69-71, 73, 74, 84, 86, 88-90, 104, 118, 134, 144, 159, 162, 178, 182, 183, 194-197, 207, 222, 224, 237, 286, 289-291, 301, 304, 317, 319, 320, 342
Aeromonas hydrophila 272
Ag85A 32, 317
Ag85B 317
Alpha C protein 177, 185
Alpha toxin 284, 290-292
AltaStaph 287
Aluminum salt 89, 90
Animal model 8, 9, 13-15, 28, 33, 34, 46, 48, 50, 56, 69, 72, 80, 85, 88, 104, 111, 112, 116, 118, 119, 142, 167, 178, 184, 186, 192, 195, 205, 207, 219-221, 244, 249, 250, 251, 260, 264, 268, 273, 283, 284, 300, 303, 304, 317-320, 331
Anthrax toxin 31
Antigen 1, 2, 4-8, 10, 12-15, 17, 19, 22, 25, 27, 28, 30-37, 45-56, 61, 63-74, 80, 82, 84-90, 98, 99, 101-105, 110, 112, 114-121, 128-130, 132, 136-145, 160-165, 167, 176-180, 185, 187, 193, 194, 196, 197, 204-207, 211, 212, 219-224, 232, 237-239, 244, 246-253, 260, 262-265, 267-274, 284, 290, 294, 296-298, 300, 302-306, 313-320, 327-330, 332, 333, 340-342, 345
Antigen secretion 53
Antigen-presenting cell (APC) 31, 34-36, 54, 55, 69, 71, 103, 105
Antigenic variation 13, 129, 132, 133, 135, 139, 204
Antitoxin 120
AroC 47, 331, 332
AroD 47, 331, 332
Attenuated bacteria 45, 54, 57, 69, 83
Attenuation 47, 50, 57, 67, 71, 83, 143, 193, 315-317, 333
Autoimmune 70, 158, 163, 318

B

B cells 34, 65, 66, 68, 69, 134, 192, 195, 231, 233, 250, 264, 265, 272, 297, 313, 318
B-cell lymphomas 33
Bacille Calmette-Guérin (see BCG)
Bacillus anthracis 1, 32, 33, 52, 53, 55
Bacteria 1-10, 12, 13, 28, 30-33, 36, 37, 45, 46, 52, 65, 67, 69, 71, 73, 80, 81, 83-85, 87, 88, 90, 93, 98, 111, 113, 115, 117, 120, 134, 136, 140, 141, 165, 174, 176, 203-205, 217-222, 246-252, 262, 266, 284, 289, 290, 301-305, 311-313, 329, 339, 342, 344
Bacterioferritin 32
BCG 8, 32, 67, 81, 83, 311, 314-317, 319, 320
BCG vaccine 83, 311, 314-317, 319, 320
Beta C protein 22, 177
Bioterrorism 46, 53, 55, 84
Biovar 93, 94
Biowarfare 55
Bordetella pertussis 1, 81, 85, 86, 270
Borrelia burgdorferi 31, 63, 81, 86, 202-208, 210-212
Broncho-Vaxom® 249, 250, 253
Bubonic 55
Burkholderia cepacia 13, 262
BVH-11 27, 28
BVH-3 27, 28

C

C. diphtheriae 86
C. pneumoniae 8, 32, 93, 94, 96, 98-100, 103, 105
C. psittaci 32, 93, 96-99, 104, 105
C5a peptidase 160, 161, 164, 165, 178, 185
Campylobacter jejuni 13
Cancer 30, 35, 46, 57, 58, 83, 175, 193, 264
Capsular polysaccharide (CPS) 4, 31, 73, 112, 175, 176, 178, 185, 187, 221, 222, 229, 230, 283, 284, 287, 327, 328, 330, 331, 333

Carbohydrate 25, 130, 160, 161, 174, 176, 178, 180, 238, 247, 270, 329, 330
Carcinoembryonic antigen 132, 247
CD1c 68
CD3+ 33
CD4+ 32, 34, 36, 101, 103, 105, 141, 163, 192, 195, 196, 250, 269-272, 296, 313, 330, 331
CD8+ 32, 34, 36, 37, 46,-48, 53, 54, 68, 101, 103, 195, 196, 250, 265, 269, 271, 272, 313, 331
CD11a 195
CD11b 192
CD11b/CD18 192
CD18 192
CD40 272
CD40 ligand 272
CD46 135, 136
CD54 192
CD66 132, 133, 138, 139, 142
CD80 34, 192
CD86 192
CD103 195
CD154 34
CEA 132
CEACAM 132, 133, 138
Cell-mediated immunity (CMI) 32, 35, 37, 48, 54, 70, 72, 84, 269, 270, 272, 273
CFA/I fimbria protein 31
CFC-101 266, 267
CGH 3
Chemotherapy 83, 283, 311, 326
Chlamydia spp 13
Chlamydia trachomatis 93-96, 98-101, 103-105, 128
Cholera 45, 63, 69, 75, 81-85, 113, 114, 117, 120, 144, 159, 194, 196, 301, 304, 339-346
Cholera toxin 69, 83, 117, 144, 159, 194, 196, 301, 304, 340
Choline binding protein A (CbpA) 302
Chronic inflammation 196
Chronic obstructive pulmonary disease 218, 244, 245
Ciprofloxacin 129
Clinical trial 30, 33, 52, 57, 82, 83, 86, 87, 93, 103, 110, 112, 115-118, 129, 158, 159, 177, 178, 180-184, 187, 192, 197, 208, 233, 234, 249, 250, 264, 266, 273, 274, 283, 286, 287, 296, 297, 320, 343, 344
Clostridium tetani 33, 81, 82, 86
Clumping factor 283, 290, 292
Cna 289, 290
Cochleate 67, 71
Collagen 164, 247, 283, 284, 288-290, 292
Collagen-binding protein 283, 289, 292
Colonization 51, 52, 57, 73, 74, 83, 104, 111, 114-119, 142, 159, 160, 162, 175, 185, 186, 192, 193, 206, 217, 219, 220-222, 230, 245, 246, 248, 249, 264, 271, 296, 299, 303, 304, 311, 312, 315, 316, 320, 339, 341
Colonization factor antigen (CFA) 31, 114, 116-119
Common polysaccharide antigen (CPA) 264
Community-acquired infection 283
Complement 2, 6, 19, 73, 130, 157, 160, 161, 164, 167, 185, 207, 220, 221, 230, 234, 295, 301, 329, 341
Complete genome hybridization 3
Conjugate 4, 12, 18, 19, 22, 24, 26, 67, 70, 73, 82, 86, 87, 98, 115, 116, 119, 120, 159, 177-187, 223, 229-236, 238, 239, 251, 252, 258, 259, 262, 264, 266, 268, 269, 285, 286, 294, 297-300, 304-306, 313, 318, 320, 331, 333, 342
Conjugate vaccine 12, 19, 26, 86, 87, 119, 177, 178, 180-187, 229-236, 239, 264, 269, 285, 286, 294, 297, 298-300, 304, 305, 342
COPD 218, 220, 245, 247, 248
Corynebacterium diphtheriae 1, 81, 86
CovR 164-166
CP5/CP8/rEPA vaccine 286
CPAF 98, 103
CPMV-D 289
CPS (see Capsular polysaccharide)
Cross-protection 4, 6, 7, 207, 208, 211, 272, 297, 340
Crp 48, 51, 52
CT 67, 69, 70, 74, 83, 85, 86, 89, 114, 194, 196, 304, 340-342, 344, 345
CTLA-4 34
Cystic fibrosis (CF) 244, 245, 260, 262, 264-269, 271-274
Cystic fibrosis transmembrane (CFTR) 269, 271
Cytotoxic T lymphocyte (CTL) 32-36, 47, 48, 54, 67, 83, 84, 101, 265, 269, 271

D

DAEC 110, 113, 115, 120
DAP 88
DC 35, 36, 103, 105, 269, 272
Delayed-type hypersensitivity (DTH) 314
Delivery 10, 23, 25, 30, 34-36, 45-47, 54, 55, 63, 71, 82, 84, 88-90, 144, 159, 160, 175, 184, 224, 244, 251, 260, 273, 274, 292, 305, 306, 317, 319
Delivery vehicle 34, 35, 55, 273
Dendritic cell 35, 55, 65, 103, 105, 144, 269, 272
Diaminopimelic acid 49, 71, 88
Diarrhea 45, 48, 51, 69, 89, 110, 113-116, 118-120, 197, 339, 340, 344-346
Diarrheal disease 110, 113, 114, 120, 339
Diphtheria 1, 13, 45, 81, 86, 183, 233, 260, 298
DIVAS 185
DNA microarray 3, 9, 58, 165
DNA vaccine 30-37, 55, 72, 88-90, 103, 105, 144, 266, 305, 316-320
Domains 20, 31, 54, 68, 89, 93, 94, 98, 101, 102, 132, 135, 137, 142, 143, 162, 204, 289-302, 314

E

EAggEC 110, 113, 114, 120, 121
Edema Factor (EF) 31
Edible plant vaccine 72
EHEC 110, 113, 114, 119, 120
EIEC 110, 113, 114, 120
Elementary body (EB) 8, 93, 96, 98, 99, 104
Enterotoxigenic *Escherichia coli* 13, 31, 81, 85, 110
Enterotoxin 63, 67, 69, 70-74, 113, 114, 121, 284, 291, 304
Enterotoxin adjuvants 69, 70
Env 36
EPEC 110, 113-115, 119
Epidemic 113, 229, 232, 236, 237, 311, 339-341
Epidemiology 80, 157, 174, 202, 217, 219, 326, 341
ESAT6 315, 317, 320
Escherichia coli 4, 5, 7, 8, 10, 13, 16, 19, 27, 30, 31, 36, 52-54, 69-82, 85, 86, 96, 98, 104, 110-118, 134, 142, 143, 196, 207, 237, 268, 272, 273, 300, 303, 304, 328
ETEC 31, 85, 110, 113-119
Exoproteins 284, 290-292, 331
Exotoxin 116, 119, 157, 160, 161, 260, 264, 269, 284
Exotoxin A 116, 157, 160, 161, 260, 264, 269
Expression library immunization (ELI) 31
Extracellular matrix 206, 247, 288
Extracellular protein 162-165

F

Fet 136
Fibrinogen-binding protein 283, 290, 292
Fibronectin 89, 132, 160-162, 165, 204, 206, 247, 284, 317
Fibronectin-binding protein 89, 160-162, 165, 204, 283, 289, 292
Fimbria 31, 246, 251
Fimbriae 74, 111, 112, 114-119, 246, 251
Flagella 51, 203, 267, 268, 274, 329
Flagellar 110, 196, 204
Follicle-associated epithelium (FAE) 65, 68, 69
Formulated DNA 88
Formulation 12, 19, 30, 35, 36, 69, 71, 84, 86, 88-90, 145, 158, 159, 185, 249-251, 253, 294, 296-299, 304, 305, 317, 329, 331, 342, 344-346
Francisella tularensis 55-57

G

GAS carbohydrate 160
Gastritis 74, 192, 193, 195, 196
Genome 2-4, 7-9, 13, 15, 45, 57, 58, 83, 85, 94, 96-99, 103, 105, 162-167, 185, 203, 238, 249, 303, 305, 311, 314, 317, 333, 346
Genomic 1-3, 9, 10, 12, 14, 15, 20, 27, 31, 85, 93, 103, 105, 129, 143, 163, 165, 167, 196, 197, 238, 239, 245, 249, 292, 311, 313, 317
Genomic Neisseria Antigen (GNA) 143
Glucose 176, 264
GM-CSF 34, 304
Gonorrhea 73, 128, 129, 133, 134, 139-144
GRA 160, 161, 163
GroEL 98-100, 104, 137
Group A Streptococcus 155-167, 195
Group B Streptococcus 9, 12, 15, 19-27, 174-187
Gut-associated lymphoid tissue (GALT) 46, 51, 56

H

H. felis 193, 195, 196
Haemin (X factor) 244
Haemophilus influenzae type b 86, 144, 178, 184, 221, 222, 230, 247, 250, 294
Haemorrhage 326
Hap 246-248, 345
Hb 136, 137
HBHA 312, 313, 316
Heat shock protein (HSP) 32, 99, 204, 212, 269, 318, 319
Heat-labile enterotoxin 69, 70, 113, 304
Heat-stable enterotoxin 114
Helicobacter pylori 8, 13, 50, 51, 74, 80, 192-197, 270
Hemoglobin 136
Hemorrhagic 110, 113, 114, 120
Heparan sulfate proteoglycan (HSPG) 132, 133, 139, 140
Heparin-binding hemagglutinin 316
Hepatitis B 33, 49, 50, 53, 72, 82, 87
Heterologous antigen 46-49, 51-53, 56
Hia 246-248, 252
Hib 82, 86, 87, 184, 185, 294, 297, 298
HIV gp160 33
HlyAs 53
HMW1 246-248, 252
HMW2 246-248, 252
Hop 197
Host 3, 4, 9, 36, 37, 46, 48-54, 58, 72, 80, 83, 84, 93, 96, 98, 99, 103, 105, 110-113, 116, 118, 128-133, 136, 139, 140, 142, 157, 159-161, 163-165, 167, 185, 192-196, 202-208, 230, 247, 248, 262, 265, 268, 272, 284, 288, 295, 300, 303, 305, 306, 311-314, 316-318, 321, 326, 329, 333, 340, 341

I

Ice nucleation protein (INP) 52, 53
IEL 68
IFN-γ 32, 36, 68, 270, 313, 314, 331
IgA 47, 48, 50, 63, 65, 66, 68-70, 72-75, 104, 116, 117, 135, 138-141, 143, 159, 160, 162, 182, 186, 195-197, 220, 237, 250, 251, 289, 302, 330-332
IgG 47, 48, 50, 63, 65, 69, 73-75, 87, 104, 112, 115, 134, 135, 139-141, 158-160, 175, 176, 178, 180-187, 196, 197, 207, 220, 231, 235, 250, 251, 264, 268, 270, 273, 285-287, 289, 295, 300, 313, 330-333, 342, 345
IgM 65, 74, 101, 140, 144, 182, 250, 264, 265, 267, 285, 286, 331
IL-1 68, 139, 140, 192
IL-2 34, 250, 271
IL-4 34, 68, 193, 196, 272, 313
IL-6 68, 139, 140, 192, 248
IL-7 68
IL-8 68, 139, 140, 192, 248
IL-10 68, 270, 271
IL-12 32, 34, 192, 193, 272, 304, 313, 331
IL-18 34
IMMUNO vaccine 267
Immuno-stimulating complex 71
Immunoassay 219, 220
In silico 7, 8, 103
Intercellular adhesion molecule-1 (ICAM-1) 68, 248
Intra-epithelial lymphocyte 68, 195
Intratracheal (IT) immunization 250
Invasive disease 87, 156, 162, 230, 294, 296-299, 302, 305
Iron-regulated protein 136, 237
ISCOM 67, 71, 105
Ixodes pacificus 202
Ixodes persulcatus 202
Ixodes ricinus 202
Ixodes scapularis 202

K

K1 capsular antigen 112
KDO 130, 264
Killed 6, 12, 16, 56, 69, 105, 115, 117, 129, 158, 230, 244, 249-251, 253, 270, 271, 295, 304, 317, 319, 327, 328, 330, 331, 333, 341, 342, 345
Klebsiella ozaenae 250
Klebsiella pneumoniae 250
Klebsiella spp 13

L

L-glyero-D-manno-heptose and 3-deoxy-D-mann 264
L-selectin 34, 68, 330
LACK 32
Lactobacilli 67, 72
Lactococcus lactis 304
Lactoferrin 136, 137, 222, 301
Laminin 163, 247
Langerhans cell (LC) 35
Leishmania manor 33
Lethal Factor (LF) 31, 32, 136-139
Lipoprotein 5, 27, 52, 56, 86, 96, 136, 137, 204, 206, 208, 251, 252, 302, 303
Lipoprotein D 251, 252
Liposome 19, 67, 71, 134
Live attenuated vaccine 104, 143
Live vector vaccine 118, 120
Live-attenuated oral typhoid vaccine 333, 345
LmSTI1 32
Lipooligosaccharide (LOS) 129-131, 133-135, 137-140, 143, 221, 223, 237, 238, 247, 248, 251, 252
Lipopolysaccharide (LPS) 15, 47-52, 55-57, 74, 87, 93, 96, 98, 99, 110, 119, 229, 236, 260, 262-264, 266, 267, 269, 270, 272, 274, 327, 329-333, 340-342, 345
LT 67, 69, 70, 85, 86, 89, 113, 114, 116-119, 196, 197, 304
LT adjuvant 197
Lyme disease 13, 31, 81, 86, 202, 203, 205-208, 210, 212, 222
LYMErixtm 208, 210

M

M (membranous or microfold) cells 46, 65, 89, 329
M protein 72, 157-165, 167
M. chelonae 312
M. smegmatis 311, 312
M. ulcerans 32, 312
MAb (see Monoclonal antibody)
Macrophage-derived chemokine 272
MAdCAM 1 66
Major outer membrane protein 93
Malaria 33, 34, 45, 63, 82, 84, 86, 87, 315
Maternal antibod 23, 24, 175
Maternal immunity 25
MCP-I 192
MDC 272
Meningitec 234
Meningitidis 4, 6, 12, 13, 15, 73, 81, 85, 86, 112, 229, 230, 238, 298
Meningococcal conjugate vaccine 229, 230, 232, 234, 239
Meningococci 17, 131, 133, 137, 143, 230, 232
Meningococcus 4, 6, 7, 9, 85, 87, 129, 137, 229, 230, 234
Menjugate 234
MEP 260, 262, 265, 266, 274
Mga 164, 166
Microbial cell surface components 288
Microparticle 35, 36, 67
MIP-1a 192
MOMP 32, 93, 94, 96, 98-105
Monoclonal antibody (MAb) 14-22, 96, 99-102, 104, 116, 120, 131, 133-135, 143, 163, 207, 264, 267, 271, 273, 290, 305, 313
Moraxella catarrhalis 13, 73, 217-224, 250, 253
Mortality 1, 25, 55, 56, 112, 155, 156, 157, 162, 246, 248, 250, 260, 267, 273, 283, 288, 289, 290, 294-297, 305, 321, 326
MSCRAMMS 288
MTb 32
Mtb32 317
Mtb39 317
Mtb72f 317
Mucin 50, 222, 246, 247, 268
Mucoid exopolysaccharide 262, 265
Mucosa-associated lymphoid tissue (MALT) 51, 65, 66, 68, 69, 71, 74
Mucosal addressin 66
Mucosal immunity 46, 63, 65, 68, 73, 84, 88-90, 158, 159, 186, 250
Mutagenesis 4, 8, 83, 161, 185, 300, 303, 313, 316, 328
Mutant 4, 8, 10, 17, 36, 45-56, 69, 86, 88, 89, 117-119, 136, 138, 160-162, 164, 183, 193, 195-197, 233, 273, 283, 290-292, 300, 302, 303, 315, 316, 318, 319, 328-330
Mutation 9, 10, 36, 47-51, 56, 57, 86, 89, 118, 130, 133, 138, 143, 207, 208, 272, 295, 300, 302, 317, 329, 331, 332
Mycobacterium bovis 8, 32, 83, 311, 312
Mycobacterium leprae 13, 32, 311, 316
Mycobacterium tuberculosis 8, 33, 88, 269, 311-321
Mycobacterium vaccae 319
Mycoplasma pulmonis 31

N

N. lactamica 15
N. polysaccharea 15
NAD (V factor) 118, 244
Naked DNA 35, 55, 88
NALT 68
Nasal carriage 73, 284, 301, 302
Nasal lymphoid tissue 68
Native conformation 37, 237
Native outer membrane vesicle 237
Neisseria gonorrhoeae 6, 13, 15, 128
Neisseria meningitidis 4, 6, 12, 13, 73, 81, 85, 86, 112, 229, 230, 238, 298
NeisVac-C 234
Neonatal meningitis 112
Newborn 24, 25, 94, 110, 174, 175, 179, 183, 184, 274
NF-kB 192, 248
NIPH OMV vaccine 237
Non typable *Haemophilus influenzae* 13, 298
Nosocomial 218, 260, 264, 273, 283, 291
Neisserial surface protein A (NspA) 15-19, 143, 238
NTHI 244-253

O

O antigen 110, 120, 130, 260, 262-264, 269, 274, 340, 342
OapA 246, 247
OMP26 251, 252
OMV vaccine 236, 237-239
Opacity (Opa) Proteins 15, 130, 132, 133, 135, 137-142
Oral immunization 53, 56, 84, 117, 120, 193, 195-197, 249-251, 253
Oral vaccine 84, 117, 118, 249-251, 253, 327, 328, 330, 332-334, 341, 342, 344
OspA 31, 86, 204-208, 210-212, 222
OspC 31, 204-206, 212
Otitis 73, 87, 217, 219-222, 224, 244, 245, 248, 252, 294
Otitis media 73, 87, 217, 219-222, 224, 244, 245, 252, 294
Outer membrane protein (OMP) 15, 52, 56, 87, 132, 135-137, 143, 221, 222, 229, 230, 236, 237, 239, 246-248, 252, 262, 263, 266, 267, 291, 298, 329
Outer membrane protein (OMP) F vaccine 262, 263, 266
Outer membrane vesicle (OMV) 15, 85, 236-239

P

P. falciparum 33, 34, 47
P2 16, 24, 246, 248, 251, 252
P39 32
P5 246, 247, 251, 252
P6 248, 251, 252
PA 31, 32, 55
Passive therapy 274, 284
Pathogenic 9, 10, 13, 46, 55, 83, 85, 111, 118, 139, 165, 205, 230, 244, 248, 249, 251, 283, 284, 303, 311, 329, 333, 344
Peptidase 160, 161, 164, 165, 178, 185
Peptide 2, 4, 5, 7, 10, 19, 21, 31, 33, 35, 51, 52, 67, 70, 82, 84, 86, 87, 89, 103, 105, 114, 116, 119, 132, 134, 135, 142, 158-160, 197, 237, 249, 251, 252, 262, 266, 268, 269, 289, 290, 292, 297, 305, 314, 317, 318, 320
Peptide-based 85, 135
Peptide-based vaccine 135
Pertussis 1, 13, 81, 85, 86
Pertussis toxoid 85
Peyer's patch 36, 51, 52, 65, 66, 89, 249, 270
Pharyngitis 155-159, 162-164, 167
PhtA 303
PhtB 303
PhtD 303
PIgR 66, 68, 74, 302
PilE 133, 135, 136
Pili 113, 119, 133, 135, 136, 138-140, 221, 246, 248, 268, 339
PilQ 133, 136, 142
Plasma cell 65, 66, 68, 73, 74
Plasmid 2, 30-37, 46-51, 54, 55, 71-73, 83, 88, 105, 113, 114, 117, 119, 120, 203, 204, 273, 305, 315
Plasmodium falciparum 33, 47
Plasmodium yoelii 33
PLG 35, 36, 71
Pmi 51
Pmp genes 96-99
Pmr 51, 52
Pneumococcal Surface Antigen A (PsaA) 302-305
Pneumococcal Surface Protein A (PspA) 31, 73, 301-305
Pneumococcal Surface Protein C (PspC) 301-303
Pneumococci 28, 295-305

Pneumococcus 6, 85, 87, 294, 296, 303
Pneumolysin 300-304
Pneumonia 8, 27, 28, 93, 94, 103, 175, 218, 245, 260, 265-273, 283, 294, 296, 300, 304
Pneumonic plague 55, 56
Poly (N-vinyl pyrrolidone) 35
Poly-lactide-coglycolide 35, 71
Polymeric Ig receptor 68
Polypeptides 15, 20, 27, 31, 81, 82, 84-86, 160, 162
Polysaccharide 1, 4, 12, 15, 31, 47, 70, 73, 74, 80, 82, 84, 86, 87, 93, 110, 112, 116, 163, 175-178, 180, 221, 222, 229-232, 234, 244, 260, 262, 264, 265, 270, 283, 284, 287, 288, 294, 295, 297, 327, 328, 331, 333, 340, 342, 345
Polysaccharide intercellular adhesin 284, 288
Polysaccharide-based 82, 86, 87
Polysaccharide-protein conjugate vaccine 229, 297
Polysaccharides 221, 283, 284, 287, 295
Pomp genes 97
Por 129, 130, 133, 135, 140
PorA 133, 142, 237-239
Porin 16, 31, 96, 129, 133, 136, 142, 197, 222, 238, 251, 252
PoxA 51, 52
Pregnant women 23, 112, 174, 175, 178, 180-182, 184, 187, 210
Protective antigen 4- 7, 31, 45, 52, 53, 55, 71, 104, 120, 160-162, 165, 250, 264, 273, 302, 305, 306, 317
Protein antigen 6, 30, 31, 34, 36, 37, 69, 70, 72, 73, 85, 90, 117, 177, 185, 269, 294, 296, 300, 304, 306
Protein D 251
Proteomics 2, 4, 7, 9, 12, 15, 196, 239
Proteus spp 13
PRP-D 231
Ps 4, 6, 12, 19, 26, 84, 86, 87, 112, 115, 116, 119, 120, 244, 288, 294, 295-300, 304, 305, 342, 345
Pseudogen 263
Pseudomonas aeruginosa 13, 31, 82, 86, 87, 116, 119, 260, 262-274, 285, 331
Pseudomonas aeruginosa exotoxoid A 285
Pseudomonas syringae 52
PT 85, 86
PVP 35

R

R28 protein 160-162
RANTES 192
Recombinant bacteria 81, 83
Recombinant polypeptide 81, 84-86
Recombinant protein 6, 7, 13, 14, 27, 28, 32-34, 88, 96, 104, 105, 143, 144, 207, 249, 289, 291
Recombinant vector 84
REPA 285, 286, 331, 333
Resistance 49, 51, 52, 104, 128, 129, 132, 133, 139, 148, 149, 151, 153, 167, 174, 222, 260, 264, 270, 271, 283, 295, 299, 305, 343-345
Respiratory tract infection 94, 155, 217-219, 224, 250
Reticulate bodies (RB) 8, 93, 96
Reverse vaccinology 4, 6-8, 238
Rgg 165
Rhamnose 176, 264
Rheumatic heart disease (RHD) 155, 157, 163, 167
Rheumatic fever (RF) 155-157, 163, 164
Rib 22, 162, 177
Rmp 130, 134, 137, 138, 140, 142

S

S. typhi 541Ty 47
S. typhi chi 48, 49
S. typhi chi4073 48
S. typhi chi4632 49
S. typhi CVD 908 47, 48
S. typhi CVD 908-htrA 48
S. typhi Ty445 49, 50
S. typhi Ty800 50, 51
S. typhimurium LH1160 51
S. typhimurium VNP20009 57
S. typhimurium VNP20029 57
Safety 12, 33, 47, 48, 50, 52, 57, 70, 71, 80, 112, 116, 117, 134, 138, 159, 178, 183-185, 197, 208, 210, 224, 234, 238, 273, 274, 285-287, 315-317, 320, 332, 334, 343-345
Salmonella enterica 45, 197, 270, 273, 326
Salmonella typhi 45-51, 53, 57, 58, 81, 83, 84, 326-333, 345
Salmonella typhimurium 36, 46-58, 82, 159, 196, 331
SBA 234, 235, 237

SCPA 160, 161
SEA 291
SEB 291
Secretion 7, 53, 54, 65, 66, 68-70, 73, 75, 86, 98, 111, 114, 116, 119, 128, 140, 141, 164, 248, 250, 268, 270, 331, 332
Sepsis 27, 110, 112, 113, 116, 162, 184, 237, 271, 273, 289-291, 300, 302, 303
Sequence 2, 4, 6-9, 15, 19-21, 27, 30, 31, 34, 52, 72, 85, 86, 94, 96-99, 101-103, 114, 118, 132, 135, 142, 160, 162-166, 185, 204, 238, 247, 251, 289, 292, 300-305, 333, 344-346
Serogroup 4, 6, 7, 9, 13, 15-19, 27, 28, 82, 87, 104, 110, 113, 229, 230, 232, 234, 262-264, 266, 267, 269, 272, 273, 339, 340, 345, 346
Serogroup B *Neisseria meningitidis* 13
Serotype 4, 6, 9, 12, 13, 15, 19-22, 24-26, 31, 87, 99, 101, 102, 110, 113, 114, 116-119, 126, 157-162, 164, 165, 173, 175, 176, 178-183, 185, 187, 244-246, 264, 277-279, 285, 287, 294-300, 304, 305, 340-342, 344, 345
Serum bactericidal assay 222, 234
Sexually transmitted disease (STD) 73, 74, 103, 133, 175
Shigella spp 13, 30, 36, 47, 54, 56, 71, 73, 81, 83, 114, 118-120
SIgA 47, 49, 56, 116, 118, 119, 159, 341, 342
Signature-tagged mutagenesis (STM) 4, 8-10, 185
Sinusitis 218, 245, 250, 294
Sip 19-22, 24-27, 178
SLC 34
SOD 53
ST 114, 116-119
StaphGAM 287
StaphVAX 285-287
Staphylococcal enterotoxin A 291
Staphylococcal enterotoxin B 291
Staphylococcus aureus 13, 89, 250, 271, 283-292
Streptococcal heme-associated protein (Shp) 161-163
Streptococcal protective antigen 160-162, 165
Streptococcal pyrogenic exotoxin A (SpeA) 157, 160, 161, 166
Streptococcal pyrogenic exotoxin B (SpeB) 157, 160-162
Streptococcal pyrogenic exotoxin C (SpeC) 160, 161, 167
Streptococcus agalactiae 9, 13, 174
Streptococcus mutans 13
Streptococcus pneumoniae 6, 7, 9, 12, 13, 15, 20, 26, 27, 31, 33, 73, 81, 85, 185, 217, 221, 250, 253, 294, 295, 298-303, 305, 308-310
Streptococcus pyogene 13, 89, 155, 161, 250
Streptococcus pyogenes (group A) 13, 20
Streptococcus viridans 250
Subunit 1, 8, 10, 12, 31, 50, 67, 69, 70, 72, 74, 80, 81, 84-86, 89, 90, 104, 110, 115, 117-120, 129, 135, 136, 144, 159, 239, 246, 301, 304, 315-317, 319, 320, 327, 333, 340-343
Superantigen 157, 161, 291
Superoxide dismutase 53
Surface antigen 7, 15, 33, 53, 72, 82, 87, 110, 116, 129, 137, 140, 176, 205, 220, 237, 248, 302, 327, 329, 342
Surface immunogenic protein 19, 178

T

T cell 1, 32, 33, 36, 37, 47, 66, 68, 70, 103, 159, 163, 192, 193, 195, 196, 206, 231, 250, 269-272, 313, 318, 331
T-cell 13, 32, 34, 36, 53, 70, 87, 101, 103-105, 163, 192, 195, 196, 231, 233, 251, 270, 271, 285, 291, 297, 313, 317, 330, 331
T-cell–independent (TI) immunogens 87
T-helper cells 65, 103
TAPET 57
TB 311-321
TbpA 137, 141, 143, 222, 237
TCRab 68
TCRgd 68
Tetanus 13, 31, 48, 81, 86, 87, 177, 180, 184, 187, 230, 234, 260, 268, 298, 329
Tf 136-140
TGF-β 68, 313
TH1 response 32, 67, 141, 144, 193, 250, 271
TH2 response 67, 141, 196, 250, 253, 270, 271, 305, 316
TI immunogens 87
Ticks 202, 203, 205-208, 210, 212
TNF-α 68, 139, 140, 192, 248, 329, 331
Toll-like receptor (TLR) 10, 34, 206, 248

Tonsils 68, 69, 163
Toxic shock syndrome toxin-1 291
Toxin 1, 10, 31, 32, 48, 63, 64, 69, 70, 83, 85, 86, 89, 114-117, 119, 120, 144, 158, 159, 194, 196, 233, 268, 283, 284, 290-292, 298, 300, 301, 304, 339-341
Toxin coregulated pili (TCP) 339, 340
Toxoid 13, 31, 48, 82, 85, 86, 87, 89, 119, 120, 180, 187, 230, 234, 260, 290, 291, 298, 329, 341
Tpb 237
Transfection 35, 36, 271, 272
Transferrin 136, 143, 222, 252
Transferring binding protein 237
TSA 32
Tuberculosis 8, 32, 33, 81-83, 88, 269, 311-321
Tularemia 55, 56
Tumor 30, 33, 35, 55, 57, 196
Tumor-amplified protein expression therapy 57
Ty21a 47, 53, 57, 83, 327-332, 334, 345
Typhoid 45, 47, 49, 51, 75, 81, 83, 119, 326-331, 333-346

U

Ulcer 32, 192, 193, 195, 326
Ulcerative keratitis 260
UPEC 110-112, 115
Urinary tract 13, 110, 111
Urinary tract infection 13, 110, 111
Uropathogenic *E. coli* 110, 111
UTI 111, 112, 115

V

V factor 244
Vaccinology 4, 6-8, 12, 238
VCAM-1 68
Vector 2, 5, 12, 16, 30, 32, 33, 36, 45-58, 67, 71, 81, 84, 88, 90, 103, 118-120, 144, 159, 160, 202, 208, 210, 212, 272, 305
Vi antigen 329, 332, 333
Vi capsular polysaccharide (Vi-CPS) 327, 328, 330-333
Vi-Pseudomonas aeruginosa recombinant 331
Vi-rEPA 331
Vibrio cholerae 69, 81-85, 120, 339-346
Vibriocidal 340-345
Virulence 3-5, 8, 9, 47-51, 58, 67, 83, 84, 110-114, 116, 119, 158, 162-167, 178, 179, 186, 196, 230, 245, 246, 252, 260, 268, 273, 284, 289, 290, 292, 295, 299-303, 327, 329

W

Waldeyer's ring 69
Whole Bacteria 84
Whole bacteria 81, 84, 220, 273

X

X factor 244

Y

Yersinia outer protein E 54
Yersinia pestis 55, 56
YopE 54